WOMEN'S WISDOM

3,577 TIPS, FACTS & ADVICE Every Woman Must Know about Her HEALTH *and* LIFESTYLE

Edited by Sharon Faelten

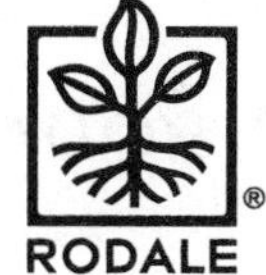

RODALE

Printed in the United States of America on acid-free ♾, recycled paper ♻

Cover Photographers: Hilmar, PhotoDisc
Interior Illustrators: Karen Kuchar (how-to illustrations), Susan Ishige (part opener cartoons)

Library of Congress Cataloging-in-Publication Data

Women's wisdom : 3,577 tips, facts & advice every woman must know about her health and lifestyle / edited by Sharon Faelten.
p. cm.
Includes index.
ISBN 1-57954-201-8 hardcover
1. Women—Health and hygiene—Popular works. I. Faelten, Sharon.
RA778 .W785 2000
613'.04244—dc21 00-033311

Distributed to the book trade by St. Martin's Press

2 4 6 8 10 9 7 5 3 1 hardcover

Visit us on the Web at www.rodalebooks.com, or call us toll-free at (800) 848-4735.

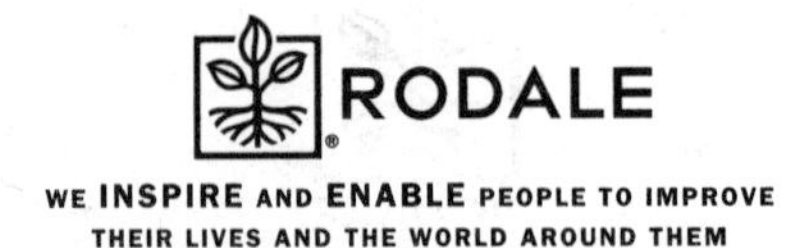

About *Prevention* Health Books

The editors of *Prevention* Health Books are dedicated to providing you with authoritative, trustworthy, and innovative advice for a healthy, active lifestyle. In all of our books, our goal is to keep you thoroughly informed about the latest breakthroughs in natural healing, medical research, alternative health, herbs, nutrition, fitness, and weight loss. We cut through the confusion of today's conflicting health reports to deliver clear, concise, and definitive health information that you can trust. And we explain in practical terms what each new breakthrough means to you, so you can take immediate, practical steps to improve your health and well-being.

Every recommendation in *Prevention* Health Books is based upon reliable sources, including interviews with highly qualified health authorities. In addition, we retain top-level health practitioners who serve on the Rodale Books Board of Advisors to ensure that all of the health information is safe, practical, and up-to-date. *Prevention* Health Books are thoroughly factchecked for accuracy, and we make every effort to verify recommendations, dosages, and cautions.

The advice in this book will help keep you well-informed about your personal choices in health care—to help you lead a happier, healthier, and longer life.

Notice

This book is intended as a reference volume only, not as a medical manual. The information given here is designed to help you make informed decisions about your health. It is not intended as a substitute for any treatment that may have been prescribed by your doctor. If you suspect that you have a medical problem, we urge you to seek competent medical help. If you take vitamins, herbs, or other alternative remedies, let your health care practitioner know.

Women's Wisdom Staff

Editor: Sharon Faelten

Writers: Judith Springer Riddle, Arden Moore, Nanci Kulig, Alison Rice, Eric Metcalf, Rick Ansorge, JoAnne Czarnecki, Jennifer Bright Kaas, Joan Price, Kelly Garrett, Brett Bara, Lisa Bennett, Sarah Robertson, Karen Cheney

Art Director: Darlene Schneck

Cover and Interior Designer: Richard Kershner

Assistant Manager, Editorial Research: Shea Zukowski, Sandra Salera Lloyd

Primary Research Editor: Anita C. Small

Lead Researcher: Molly Donaldson Brown

Editorial Researchers: Barb Fexa, Jennifer Bright Kaas, Rebecca Kleinwaks, Jennifer S. Kushnier, Janice McLeod, Mary S. Mesaros, Karen Jacobs, Elizabeth B. Price, Valerie Rowe, Staci Sander, Elizabeth Shimer, Holly Ann Swanson, Lucille Uhlman, Teresa A. Yeykal, Nancy Zelko

Senior Copy Editor: Kathy D. Everleth

Editorial Production Manager: Marilyn Hauptly

Layout Designer: Daniel MacBride

Associate Studio Manager: Thomas P. Aczel

Manufacturing Coordinators: Brenda Miller, Jodi Schaffer, Patrick T. Smith

Rodale Healthy Living Books

Vice President and Publisher: Brian Carnahan

Vice President and Editorial Director, *Prevention* Group: Anne Alexander

Director of New Title Development: Tammerly Booth

Director of Series Development: Gary Krebs

Editorial Director: Michael Ward

Vice President and Marketing Director: Karen Arbegast

Product Marketing Manager: Tania Attanasio

Book Manufacturing Director: Helen Clogston

Manufacturing Managers: Eileen Bauder, Mark Krahforst

Research Manager: Ann Gossy Yermish

Copy Manager: Lisa D. Andruscavage

Production Manager: Robert V. Anderson Jr.

Digital Processing Group Managers: Leslie M. Keefe, Thomas P. Aczel

Office Manager: Jacqueline Dornblaser

Office Staff: Susan B. Dorschutz, Julie Kehs Minnix, Tara Schrantz, Catherine E. Strouse

Rodale Books Board of Advisors

cation for otolaryngology at Manhattan Eye, Ear and Throat Hospital, both in New York City

Jeffrey R. Lisse, M.D., professor of medicine and director of the division of rheumatology at the University of Texas Medical Branch at Galveston

JoAnn E. Manson, M.D., Dr.P.H., professor of medicine at Harvard Medical School and chief of preventive medicine at Brigham and Women's Hospital in Boston

David Molony, L.Ac., Dipl.C.H., executive director of the American Association of Oriental Medicine, a diplomate in Chinese herbology of the National Certification Commission for Acupuncture and Oriental Medicine, and a licensed acupuncturist in Catasauqua, Pennsylvania

David J. Nickel, O.M.D., L.Ac., Dipl.C.H., a doctor of Oriental medicine, licensed acupuncturist, diplomate in Chinese herbology of the National Certification Commission for Acupuncture and Oriental Medicine, chairman and CEO of PrimeZyme, and a nutritionist in Santa Monica, California

Susan C. Olson, Ph.D., clinical psychologist, life transition/psychospiritual therapist, and weight-management consultant in Seattle

Mary Lake Polan, M.D., Ph.D., professor and chair of the department of gynecology and obstetrics at Stanford University School of Medicine

David P. Rose, M.D., Ph.D., D.Sc., chief of the division of nutrition and endocrinology at Naylor Dana Institute, part of the American Health Foundation in Valhalla, New York, and an expert on nutrition and cancer for the National Cancer Institute and the American Cancer Society

Mark Stengler, N.D., a naturopathic and homeopathic doctor, director of natural medicine at Personal Physicians clinic in La Jolla, California, and associate clinical professor at the National College of Naturopathic Medicine in Portland, Oregon

Shawn M. Talbott, Ph.D., executive editor for SupplementWatch in Provo, Utah

Lila Amdurska Wallis, M.D., M.A.C.P., clinical professor of medicine at Weill Medical College of Cornell University in New York City, past president of the American Medical Women's Association (AMWA), founding president of the National Council on Women's Health, director of continuing medical education programs for physicians, and master and laureate of the American College of Physicians

Andrew T. Weil, M.D., director of the program in integrative medicine and clinical professor of medicine at the University of Arizona College of Medicine in Tucson

E. Douglas Whitehead, M.D., associate attending physician in urology at Beth Israel Medical Center and New York University Downtown Hospital and cofounder and director of the Association for Male Sexual Dysfunction, all in New York City, and associate clinical professor of urology at Albert Einstein College of Medicine in the Bronx

Robert E. C. Wildman, R.D., Ph.D., assistant professor of nutrition at the University of Louisiana at Lafayette

David Winston, an herbalist; founding and professional member of the American Herbalists Guild; and president of Herbalist and Alchemist and dean of the Herbal Therapeutics School of Botanical Medicine, both in Washington, New Jersey

Carla Wolper, R.D., nutritionist and clinical coordinator at the obesity research center at St. Luke's–Roosevelt Hospital Center and nutritionist at the center for women's health at Columbia-Presbyterian/Eastside, both in New York City

Contents

D

E-F

J-K-L

P-Q

Introduction

Uncommon Knowledge from Inside Experts

Like most women, I've had my share of kitchen burns. One night, I was cooking dinner and accidentally burned my foot. I was in the kitchen barefoot, and I dropped a steaming hot ravioli. It really hurt. Another time, I was pulling a tray of hot hors d'oeuvres out of the oven and burned my wrist on the oven door.

Having edited a number of home remedies books, I knew in both cases exactly what to do for the burn: run cold water over it immediately. What I really needed to know was how to prevent future kitchen burns.

Shortly after these incidents, I edited the chapter on burns for this manuscript. Aha! There's the answer—from a woman chef in one of the busiest kitchens in New York City.

You don't have to be a klutz to need the info in this book. With 332 health and lifestyle topics, conveniently arranged from A to Z, you'll find practical advice for dozens of concerns, from Accident Proneness to Zinc.

I think you'll like what you see. Women who were shown a sneak preview of the book commented that they were impressed and amazed that each chapter, however brief, seemed to tell them everything they needed to know in so little space. They appreciated that they didn't have to slog through a lot of verbiage to get to the point. This format is perfect for busy women. You can find out what you need to know in just a minute or two.

Even if you consider yourself well-schooled in health, I think you'll like what you read.

For example, did you know that washing your hair too often can make it oily? That the benefits of fruits and vegetables outweigh the risks of pesticide residues? That eating the wrong kind of yogurt can cause, not cure, abdominal distress? That you can get all the calcium you need without drinking milk? That there are 14 ways to get more soy in your diet without eating tofu? That two of the best foods you can eat for a healthy heart are wine and chocolate?

Page after page is packed with new information—information I never before encountered in the many previous books I've written and edited, including a few maverick ideas from unusual sources.

You'll find advice on jet lag from a female astronaut with NASA. Tactics on better concentration from a female billiards champion. Strategies for staying alert from a female pilot for UPS. (The last catalog item you ordered probably traveled on her plane!).

This is much more than a health reference book, though. It's jam-packed with "Gee, I didn't know that!" advice for your lifestyle. Read about Alimony (will payments cover the so-called divorce tax?); Road

Rage (aromatherapy can keep you calm behind the wheel), and its indoor counterpart, Cubicle Rage (remedies for the hemmed-in feeling); and Hot Tubs (suits or no suits?).

With so many topics, you may wonder, *Where do I start?* Well, it's easy.

If you have a health problem, check the contents or the index. If, on the other hand, you're generally in good health but yearn to learn more, feel free to browse. When you light on what interests you the most, flag those pages with colored sticky notes.

Mark up the book and keep it handy. Share what you learn with your sister, mother, coworkers, and girlfriends. I can personally guarantee that not a day will go by when you don't have need for the wisdom in this book.

Sharon Faelten

Sharon Faelten
Editor
Prevention Health Books
for Women

A

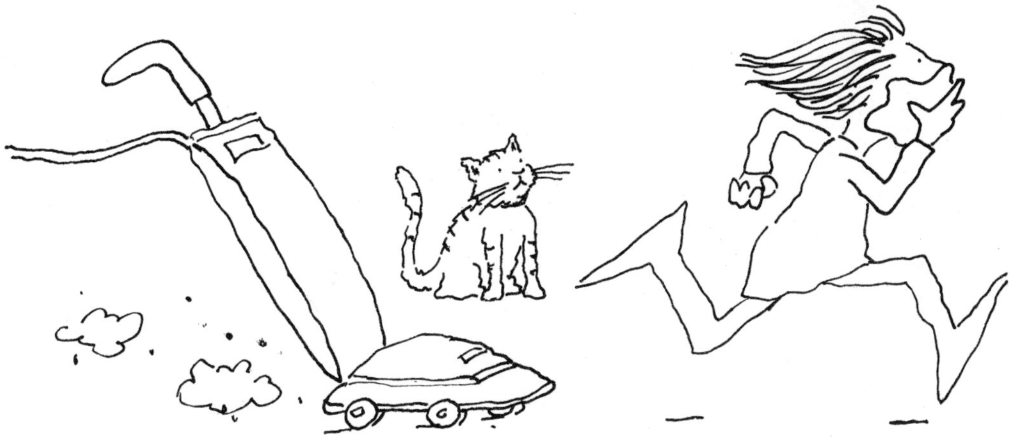

How do women who are allergic to dust
clean without kicking up a snootful of allergens?
To find out, turn to page 14.

Accident Proneness

How to Stay Out of the Hospital

Are you learning the medical names for every bone in your body the hard way—by repeated trips to the emergency room?

Have you had more than your share of cuts, scrapes, twists, and overturns that landed you in the hospital for stitches or x-rays?

Then you're among the people J. Crit Harley, M.D., calls accident prone. And he could spot you in a heartbeat.

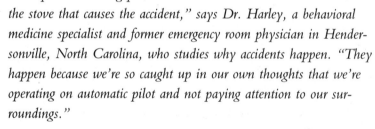

"It's not the child's toy on the step or the boiling pot on the stove that causes the accident," says Dr. Harley, a behavioral medicine specialist and former emergency room physician in Hendersonville, North Carolina, who studies why accidents happen. "They happen because we're so caught up in our own thoughts that we're operating on automatic pilot and not paying attention to our surroundings."

Dr. Harley can't promise to make everyone accident-free, but he can help improve your chances of staying out of the hospital if you follow this advice.

Be in the here and now. On any typical day, between 40,000 to 60,000 thoughts—big and small—fill our heads. Most of these fall in the "should have" and "what if" categories as we lament the past and ponder the future. Devote more time to thinking about what's happening here and now.

Take a deep breath before moving. Each time you're about to do something like climb the stairs, use a sharp knife, or reach for a boiling ››

BEWARE OF THE SINGLE EXTROVERT WHO SMOKES

Dr. Harley is especially savvy at spotting people prone to accidents. Topping the list:

People with outgoing personalities. Extroverts are either too busy anticipating praise or letting their minds move on to the next thing so that they aren't focused on the task at hand.

People preoccupied with kicking a bad habit like smoking. In fact, a 10-year study in the United Kingdom reported that the rate of workplace accidents goes up as much as 10 percent more during No Smoking Day (the British version of the Great American Smokeout) than the week before or after. Dr. Harley suggests that withdrawal may affect clear thinking.

People going through romantic breakups. People going through personal problems are withdrawn and less focused, setting themselves up for falls or spills. If they're wondering why "Everything seems to happen to me," this could be one of the reasons.

pot, stop for a full second. Breathe in deeply and then slowly exhale. Think, even say out loud, "I'm about to climb the stairs or cut this carrot or reach for this pot." This one-second action will help make you conscious of the task at hand.

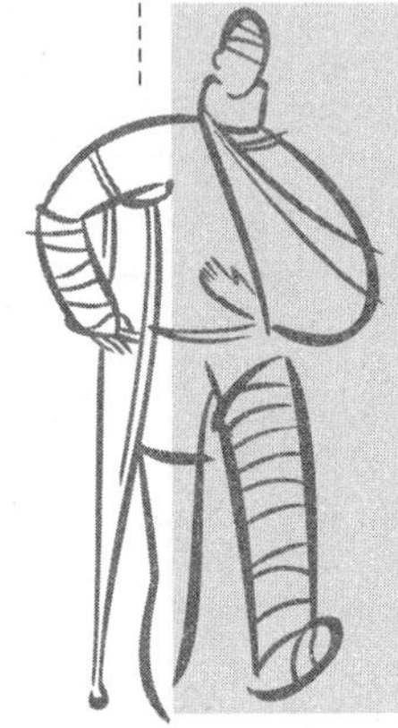

DON'T MAKE THIS MISTAKE

Don't label yourself as a klutz. It can be a self-fulfilling prophecy.

"As we look back on our childhoods, we are selective with our memories," says Dr. Harley. "If we view ourselves as klutzes, we tend to remember only all the accidents we had. If we think of ourselves as coordinated, we tend not to remember the accidents."

Give stress a rest. Clear your mind of the tiff you had with your husband this morning or the extra workload your boss dumped in your lap before you pick up the knife to slice onions or head up the stairs with an armful of groceries. "Those problems won't get resolved while you're climbing the stairs, so tell yourself that this is not the time or place to think, worry, or argue in your head," says Dr. Harley.

Book fretting time. Devote 5 to 10 minutes each day to thinking about issues that make you feel worried or anxious. And do it sitting down in a familiar and safe place so it becomes a healthy, problem-resolving habit. ■

Acne

The Right Way to Pop a Pimple

Ask your doctor if it's okay to squeeze a pimple, and chances are you'll get a stern warning against do-it-yourself extraction. Unless you know what you're doing, trying to squeeze a pimple can make matters worse.

"There's a right way and a wrong way to pop pimples," says Leslie S. Baumann, M.D., director of cosmetic dermatology at the University of Miami. "It can mean the difference between blemish-free skin or permanent scars."

The fastest and safest way to get rid of a pimple is for a dermatologist to inject it with a mild steroid solution, which will make the pimple disappear within a day or two, says Dr. Baumann. If you're nowhere near your dermatologist when a pimple breaks the surface of your skin, you may be able to safely pop the blemish on your own—provided the pimple has a whitehead filled with pus over its top. If it doesn't, leave the pimple alone.

Dr. Baumann offers this four-step strategy to pop pimples safely, provided you proceed carefully.

Aerobic Exercise

10 Ways to Burn 100 Calories in Just 15 Minutes

Think you're way too busy to exercise—and reap its benefits? Think again.

Burning just 100 extra calories a day will help you trim 10 pounds in a year, and it will also help you cut your risk for heart disease, diabetes, and high blood pressure, says Holli Spicer, a personal trainer and spokeswoman for the American Council on Exercise in San Diego. And best of all, you can do it in 15 minutes a day.

Here are 10 ways to set that flab on fire—whether at work, at play, or in the gym. (These figures are based on a 150-pound woman. If you weigh less, it will take you longer; if you weigh more, it will take you even less time to burn the same number of calories.)

1. Walk one mile. Get on your treadmill or hit the pavement, walking as if you're in a hurry. You'll know you're going too fast if you can't talk without huffing and puffing, says Spicer.

2. Cycle at 10 mph. The trick to a fast calorie burn on two wheels is to pedal at a steady 10-mph pace and add some variety to your workout. For instance, ride up and down hills, increase or decrease resistance, or pedal quickly on the easiest gear—while keeping the speedometer on target, suggests John Emmett, Ph.D., professor of physical education at Eastern Illinois University in Charleston. ››

1. Wash your face with antibacterial soap and warm water to open up your pores and kill bacteria.

2. Sterilize a straight pin by holding it over the flame of a match until the point turns black.

3. Very gently **pierce the surface of the whitehead** on the pimple.

4. Wrap your pointer fingers in tissue, then **apply equal pressure to all sides and squeeze** the sides of the pimple until all of the pus comes out. (Don't try this if you have long nails—you'll leave scars.) If no pus emerges, try piercing the whitehead again and squeezing the sides.

DON'T MAKE THIS MISTAKE

Never pierce a pimple with a straight pin that isn't sterilized. You can develop an infection. And don't squeeze the pimple too hard. That will force pus and bacteria deeper into your skin, creating a cyst and possibly a permanent scar.

5. Apply a topical antibiotic ointment or benzoyl peroxide and do no touch the area again unless a large amount of pus reaccumulates, then repeat the procedure, advises Dr. Baumann. If nothing happens, leave it alone and wait for the pimple to disappear on it's own. ■

3. Do a quick round of weight training. To get the most burn for your effort at the gym, target your major muscle groups with: leg presses, leg extensions, hamstring curls, leg presses, bench presses, seated rows, and lat pulldowns. Shoot for two sets of 8 to 10 reps, moving from one exercise to another without resting.

4. Jump around. Unless you're in great shape, jump rope for 1 to 2 minutes. Then take a break. March in place, do jumping jacks, sit-ups, or push-ups, says Dr. Emmett. When you catch your breath, jump rope for another minute or two, and repeat these exercises.

5. Start a game of tennis. If you love competition, find a buddy who's good at playing tennis. Not only will you have fun racing around the court, but that 15 minutes will turn into 30, and before you know it, you'll have burned 200 or more calories.

6. Swim 20 laps. Or however many you can finish in 15 minutes, doing the breaststroke or front crawl, says Dr. Emmett.

7. Play your favorite CD and dance in place. The faster the tempo, the more calories you'll burn, says Dr. Emmett.

8. Toss a Frisbee. You won't see it on one of those morning fitness shows, but playing outside in the yard with your kids, spouse, or even the dog is a surefire way to torch calories.

9. Plant some shrubs. Digging holes and planting shrubs or small trees is one of the best gardening workouts, says Dr. Emmett. Ditto for shoveling mulch onto flowerbeds.

10. Mow the lawn (or part of it). For a truly aerobic workout, trade your power mower for a manual model and cut your grass using your own fuel, says Dr. Emmett. ■

Afternoon Slump

Three Easy Moves to De-Fog and Energize

At 3:00 P.M., when a fog drifts across her mind and fatigue creeps over her body, Judith Lasater, Ph.D., doesn't douse herself with a mega-mug of coffee. Instead, this San Francisco physical therapist and author of Relax and Renew: Yoga for Stressful Times *assumes a few yoga poses.*

"If you're sitting at a desk all day, your blood tends to pool in your abdomen away from your head, and your muscles become static. The end result, unfortunately, is mental and physical fatigue," says Dr. Lasater. "But this is where yoga can help. Yoga will clear your mind by getting your blood circulating throughout your body again. It will warm your muscles and wake up your sleepy nervous system."

To snap out of your next afternoon slump, try these three easy yoga moves, courtesy of Dr. Lasater.

1. Wall stretch (stretches shoulders, upper back, and hamstring muscles). Stand straight, facing a wall, with your feet shoulder-width apart and about arm's length from the wall. Take one step back-

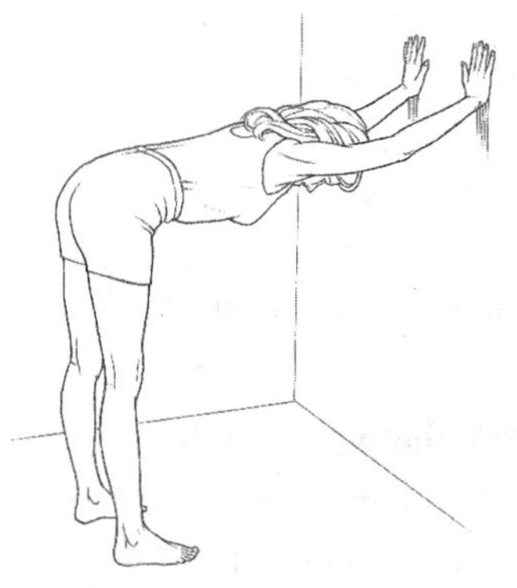

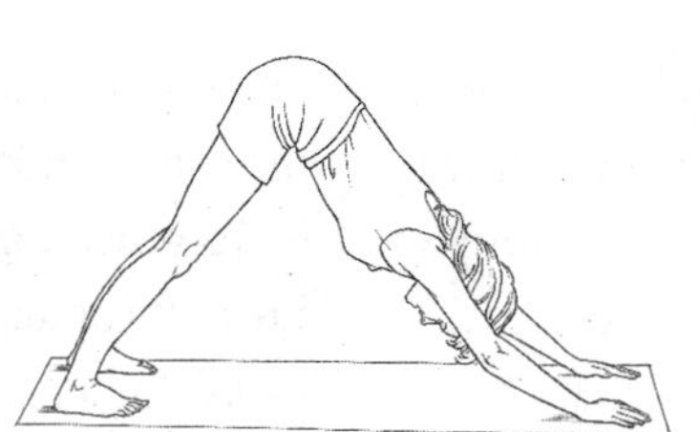

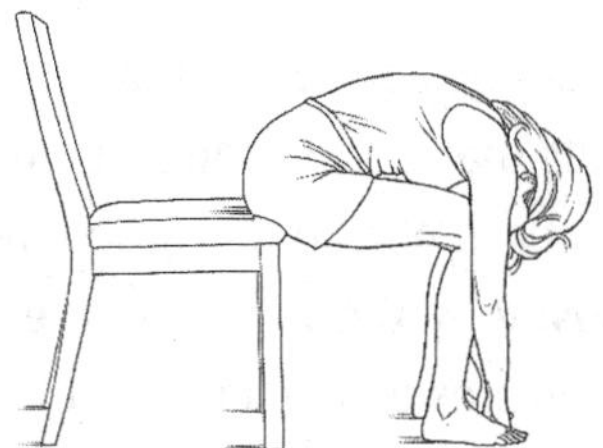

ward. Bending from the hips, raise your arms and place your palms on the wall (shoulder-width apart as shown above), keeping your back and arms straight. (Bend your hips until your spine is parallel to the floor.) Back up your feet until your back is flat and your feet are directly under your hips. Keep your knees straight, your legs firm, and your head and neck in line with your arms.

Breathe gently while holding this position for up to 30 seconds. To come out of the stretch, inhale as you walk your feet forward and stand up.

2. Downfacing dog pose (above center; stretches lower back, shoulders, and hamstring muscles). Kneel down and place your hands on the floor in front of you. (An exercise mat will help avoid slipping and cushion your hands and knees when you're kneeling.) With your knees bent, place your feet flat on the floor or mat. Walk your feet backward and your hands far forward, keeping your arms straight and your feet flat on the floor or mat, until your body is in the shape of an inverted V. Keep your head and neck in line with your arms. Your hands and feet should be slightly wider than shoulder-width apart and flat on the floor or mat.

Remain in position for 2 minutes, inhaling and exhaling slowly. To come out of the pose, bend your knees, walk your hands toward your feet, and slowly stand up.

3. Chair forward bend (above right; stretches lower back). Sit near the edge of a chair with your feet firmly on the floor, slightly wider than hip-width apart. Slowly bend forward until your chest rests on your thighs. Let your head hang down naturally. Allow your arms to dangle by your sides. Close your eyes. Breathe quietly for 2 minutes. To come up, place your hands on the sides of the chair seat and press down as you inhale and lift your torso. ■

DON'T MAKE THIS MISTAKE

Don't practice the chair forward bend if you're more than 3 months pregnant or if you have a hiatal hernia, retinal problems, eye pressure, or a sinus infection.

Age Spots

See Spot Fade—With Lemon Juice

Ironically, age spots—those nagging little brown spots that start to show up on our skin when we approach 40—aren't caused by age at all. **They're caused by the sun.** Exposure to ultraviolet rays stimulates production of melanin, a natural coloring pigment in the skin that also causes a tan. Over time, permanent clusters of melanin appear on areas repeatedly exposed to the sun—like your face and hands.

To erase age spots, dab on some lemon juice. It contains citric acid, an alpha hydroxy acid (AHA) found in many antiaging creams. AHAs loosen dead skin and accelerate your skin's ability to replace them with new ones. Over time, any

Aging

20 Foods That Keep You Young

You don't have to spend thousands of dollars on cosmetic surgery or hundreds of dollars on expensive wrinkle creams to look younger. The real key to rejuvenation is what you put in your mouth.

"A diet rich in nutrients, full of fiber, and low in calories will dramatically slow down the rate at which you age," says Michael F. Roizen, M.D, a preventive gerontologist and professor of medicine, anaesthesia, and critical care at the University of Chicago and author of RealAge: Are You as Young as You Can Be? *"A bad diet can make you look and feel 12 years older than you really are."*

Case in point: Eating foods high in saturated fats and calories will increase your risk for clogged arteries (atherosclerosis), cancer, diabetes, heart attack, and strokes—debilitating diseases that spell "old age" to baby boomers, he says.

After poring over 25,000 medical studies, Dr. Roizen and the RealAge scientific team concluded that the solution is simple: Eat a wide variety of fruits, vegetables, whole grains, and fish. These foods are packed with a host of antiaging nutrients, from antioxidants such as carotenoids and flavonoids to isoflavones and omega-3 fatty acids. Unlike cosmetic surgery and wrinkle creams, they don't cover up the signs of aging. They fight aging from the inside out.

For instance, antioxidants neutralize free radicals, renegade molecules that attack and damage cells and lead to cancer and other degenerative diseases that accelerate aging. Carotenoids, which are natural antioxidants found in yellow, orange, red, and dark leafy green fruits and vegetables, help prevent LDL ("bad") cholesterol from sticking to your artery walls. Flavonoids, antioxidants found in plants, work a slightly different way. Some think they act like a Teflon coating to stop your blood from sticking to ar-

superficial pigmentation—like age spots—fades. Lemon juice is a natural bleaching agent.

Here's what to do.

1. After you've washed and dried your face, **saturate a cotton ball with pure lemon juice and pat it over the age spots.** Don't get any closer to your eyes than the length of your lashes, or your eyes will sting something fierce. You may notice some tingling as the citric acid starts to work, but it should subside in a few minutes.

2. If there's no sign of irritation after 2 to 3 weeks, **dab lemon juice on the spots twice a day, once in the morning and once at night.** Some women notice improvement in 8 weeks; in others, it takes a year.

Helpful Hints

Citric acid increases sensitivity to sunlight. So before going outdoors, allow the lemon juice to dry, then apply sunscreen. Also, you can prevent additional age spots by always wearing sunscreen with an SPF of at least 15 whenever you go outdoors. ■

teries. You can find flavonoids in red wine, green tea, citrus and other fruits, oregano, and many vegetables. Isoflavones, found in soy beans, tofu, tempeh, soy milk, and many beans, aid in cutting your risk for breast, ovarian, and uterine cancer. Salmon and tuna are rich in omega-3 fatty acids, good fat that in some women dramatically lowers cholesterol levels and blood pressure. In fact, eating fish at least once a week can cut your risk of heart attack in half and make your "Real Age" more than a year younger.

Dr. Roizen's antiaging formula? Try to eat five to six servings of vegetables and legumes and two to three pieces of fruit each day. (A serving size is equal to ½ cup or will roughly fit in the palm of your hand.) His top picks:

1. Spinach
2. Broccoli, steamed
3. Tomatoes, cooked
4. Onions
5. Strawberries
6. Papaya
7. Canned pink salmon (bones included)
8. Canned tuna in water
9. Black or green tea
10. Black-eyed peas
11. Kidney beans
12. Acorn squash
13. Sweet potatoes
14. Whole wheat bread
15. Soy foods
16. Fat-free milk
17. Fat-free plain yogurt
18. Calcium-fortified orange juice
19. Chile peppers (2 to 3)
20. Red or white grapes (or wine made from them)

DON'T MAKE THIS MISTAKE

Don't overcook your vegetables. Overcooking boils away all the antiaging nutrients. You should cook green vegetables just until they turn bright green.

Helpful Hint

Make vegetables your new snack food. Buy a bag of precut baby carrots and other vegetables, such as celery, broccoli, cauliflower, peppers, radishes, and even mushrooms and keep them in the refrigerator. Eaten raw, these veggies retain rejuvenating nutrients that cooking can deplete. ■

Air Bags

Survive a Crash and Inflation

Q: What's the difference between a windbag and an air bag?

A: One will bore you to death, the other will save your life.

Tucked out of sight in the steering wheel or dashboard as you drive, air bags were designed to provide an instant cushion between your head, neck, and chest and the steering wheel and dashboard during a collision. In order to inflate quickly on impact, these balloon-like apparatuses burst from their compartments at speeds up to 200 miles per hour. So women who need to sit closer to where an air bag is deployed to reach the brake and accelerator or who don't wear seat belts have occasionally suffered minor cuts, bruises, and abrasions from the force of its inflation. A few have died.

Adults under 5 feet 2 inches, most of whom are women, are at greatest risk. But anyone—male or female, short or tall—can avoid air-bag injuries.

"Air bags have saved a lot of lives," says Mitch Fuqua, a spokesperson for AAA (American Automobile Association) in Heathrow, Florida. "Women are much safer with air bags than without them," he says.

To avoid an air-bag injury, follow these guidelines set by the National Highway Traffic Safety Administration and AAA.

Buckle up. Secured across your hips, chest, and shoulders, seat belts keep you a safe distance from the air bag and prevent you from flying forward into a deployed air bag when you brake. (Most serious injuries from air bags occurred when occupants were driving unbelted or seated too close to the wheel.)

If your steering wheel tilts, direct it toward your chest, not your head. This directs the air bag, if deployed, toward your chest instead of the more vulnerable head and neck areas.

Sit at least 10 inches from the wheel. The farther away from the steering wheel you sit, the less force you'll experience when the air bag deploys. Air bags can cause the most injury within the first 2 to 3 inches of inflation, so placing yourself 10 inches away should provide ample protection. Measure the 10 inches from the center of your breastbone to the center of the air-bag cover.

Recline your seat. To help achieve that safety margin, recline your seat. If that makes it tough to see the road, raise your car seat or sit on a firm, nonslippery cushion.

Forget about driving with your hands in the 10 o'clock and 2 o'clock position, which you learned in driver education. Instead, hold the steering wheel in the 9 and 3 position. That keeps your arms apart and leaves space for the air bag to inflate, says Fuqua. And don't slump forward toward the steering wheel as you drive. ■

DON'T MAKE THIS MISTAKE

Holding the wheel at the 12 o'clock position can result in a broken arm if the air bag deploys while you're driving, says Fuqua.

Airline Food

In-Flight Meal Tips from a Frequent Flyer

Debi Tracy-Hirsch eats right, even when she's at 30,000 feet. As operations manager of a New Jersey–based event management company who logs up to 100,000 miles a year in the air, Tracy-Hirsch does what a lot of frequent flyers do: She orders a "special meal" when she books a flight. So Tracy-Hirsch dines on a fruit plate, seafood, or a vegetarian meal instead of a gravy-soaked chicken breast or sauce-smothered fettuccine.

Most major airlines offer one, if not several, different choices to accommodate passengers with certain diet requirements—meat-free, low-fat, or low-sodium meals, for example. Dietitians applaud the strategy because special meals tend to usually feature lighter fare that will be easier to digest than whatever the standard meal is.

"Flying puts stress on all body systems, especially the digestive system," says Kristin Larney, R.D., a registered, licensed dietitian at Mercy Medical Center in Baltimore. "The lighter and healthier the meal, the less passengers will be prone to indigestion, upset stomachs, and heartburn."

You can order a special meal when you book your flight or anytime up to 24 hours before flight time. Larney also offers other flight-friendly food strategies.

Good: Slip a sports nutrition bar into your carry-on. These bars can fill you up for a long time, and they're designed to cause minimal stomach upset.

Better: Scout the airport food courts and snack shops. Skip the pepperoni pizza, though. Better choices, says Larney, are unsalted soft pretzels, fresh fruit smoothies (with fat-free milk), garden salads (keep the salad dressing packet sealed until ready to eat), hard rolls (less fatty and sugary than croissants and muffins), and a bag of dried apricots.

Best: Pack some food in a waterproof lunch bag with a chilled ice pack. Larney suggests grapes, melon chunks, or orange slices sealed in plastic bags; low-fat pudding in individual serving packs; a veggie pita (hold the mayonnaise); or a peanut butter-and-apple butter sandwich on whole wheat bread.

Helpful Hint

If you want to pack a sandwich to take with you, make it with a firm low-fat or fat-free cheese such as mild Cheddar, provolone or mozzarella. ■

DON'T MAKE THIS MISTAKE

If you're bored between flights, don't distract yourself by noshing constantly on snacks. This smorgasbord-in-the-sky approach can lead to bloating, stomachaches, heartburn, or nausea by the time you land, cautions Larney. You'll pack on some weight, too: Together, high-fat snacking and meals can supply you with 3,500 calories, which works out to a pound of gained weight for just 1 day of travel, she says. Concentrate on nonedible activities such as reading a bestseller, solving crossword puzzles, or writing notes to friends.

Airline Travel

Survival Tactics against Airborne Germs

Airlines may be the safest way to travel, but they're not always the healthiest. Seating is tight on most planes, so a sniffle from someone in business class could leave you with a first-class cold. The confines of a pressurized cabin expose you to other maladies, too, from ear and head pain to dry skin and swollen feet.

"The inside of a plane has a great potential for spreading illness," says Lauri Kane, Sc.D., a health program administrator in Baltimore. By the time you reach your destination, you could land with the makings of a cold, the flu, or other respiratory infection, says Dr. Kane, who flies frequently.

Here's what experts recommend to germproof airline travel.

Fortify yourself with echinacea. A day or so before your flight, start shoring up your resistance to germs with echinacea. Take a dropperful of echinacea tincture in a glass of water or a 500-milligram capsule four times a day until takeoff, says Mark Stengler, N.D., a naturopathic physician in San Diego and author of *Natural Physician: Your Guide for Common Ailments*. Do not use echinacea if you have tuberculosis or an autoimmune condition such as lupus or multiple sclerosis because it stimulates the immune system. Also avoid it if you're allergic to closely related plants such as ragweed, asters, and chrysanthemums.

Bolster your immunity with vitamin C. Three days before an upcoming flight, start taking 1,000 milligrams of vitamin C a day to help bolster your body's resistance to infection, says Dr. Stengler. (If you get diarrhea from this much vitamin C, cut back the dosage.)

Adjust the overhead air jet. As soon as you reach your seat, redirect your air vent so that it is not pointing directly at you, says Gary N. Gross, M.D., clinical professor of medicine at the University of Texas Southwestern Medical School in Dallas. This will limit your exposure to possible pollutants in the air and minimize the dryness of your nasal passages. A wet nose helps shed viruses and helps to warm, humidify, and filter the air we breathe, says Dr. Gross.

Dab antibiotic ointment in your nostrils. A tiny amount of a topical antibiotic ointment such as Bacitracin dabbed around the bottom of your nostrils before you get on the plane may act as a germ barrier, says Dr. Gross. Or, you could just use a nasal moisturizing gel such as Ayr Saline Nasal Gel to keep the nasal membranes moist.

Carry disposable antiseptic wipes. Available at pharmacies and supermarkets, use these germ-killing wipes to wash your hands and face before and after the in-flight meals, before using the tray table as a desk, after using the in-flight lavatory, and when you retrieve your checked-in

PASS UP THE PILLOW

Don't cozy up to the square, paper-coated pillows provided by the airlines, especially if they look as though they've seen a lot of mileage. Otherwise, you're setting yourself up for a face-to-face encounter with any germs left by a previous passenger.

luggage (wipe down the handle).

Drink to your health. Dr. Kane urges airline passengers to drink a lot of water before and during a flight. Airplane interiors are notoriously dry. And fluid will help flush germs from your system.

Helpful Hint

Take a decongestant before boarding to prevent pressure from building in your ears during takeoff and landing. The decongestant is especially helpful if you have a slight cold, says Dr. Gross. He suggests using a decongestant nose spray (like Afrin) before the flight and a saline nose spray during the flight to keep the tissues moist. (Skip decongestants if you have high blood pressure, though.) ■

Alimony

Never Pay "Divorce Tax"

Like severance pay from work, alimony is income. The IRS wants its share. So when negotiating alimony with her ex, a woman needs to consider the effect on her taxes, says Mary Frances Lyle, a partner with the law firm Bruce, Weathers, Corley, Dughman, and Lyle in Nashville and cochairperson of the Alimony and Spousal Support Committee of the American Bar Association.

Here's what Lyle recommends.

• When deciding how much you'll need to live on, **consider how much more you'll owe in income tax** and increase the amount of alimony you request accordingly. (If you're paying alimony, it's tax-deductible.)

• When you change your marital status on your W-4 form, also **adjust your tax withholding** to account for your new financial status.

DON'T MAKE THIS MISTAKE

The lawyer who drew up your will or handled the sale of your house may not be the best lawyer to handle your divorce. Hire an attorney who specializes in divorce law, who knows the legal and financial ins and outs of divorce. To find someone in your area, contact your county's chapter of the American Bar Association.

Keep alimony and child support payments separate. If you pay child support as part of one big alimony payment, you can claim both amounts as a tax deduction. But if you receive the combined alimony/child support payment, you have to claim the entire amount as income and pay tax on all of it. To keep the whole thing fair, Lyle recommends that child support payments, which are neither deductible nor required to be claimed as income, be separate from alimony. ■

Allergies

Are You Allergic to Housework?

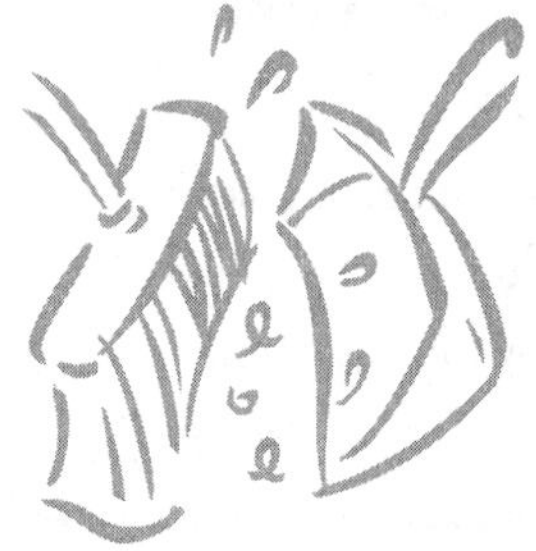

How can a woman with allergies rid her house of dust mites and molds—notorious for triggering symptoms—while stirring up the very allergens responsible for her symptoms?

"Most allergens in the house are dust mite particles, which tend to lie in the carpet or upholstery until they're disturbed," says Carol Wiggins, M.D., an allergy specialist in Atlanta. Yet you have to disturb the area in order to clean.

You could give up cleaning entirely, and delegate all the dusting, scrubbing, mopping, and vacuuming to your kids. But let's face it: Unless you're lucky enough to have a very cooperative family—or you can afford a regular cleaning service—you're going to end up doing at least some of the cleaning.

By taking these simple steps, you can keep the allergen population down without aggravating your symptoms:

Try the ER look. You can buy the same kind of light-

Anger

Control Your Temper in Any Situation

Have you ever watched a pyrotechnics-loving friend light a long string of firecrackers on the Fourth of July? The match passes the flame to the fuse, which quietly crackles for a moment as bystanders grow tense, waiting for the . . . BANG POW BANG BANG BANG that becomes an extended battery of noise.

A burst of temper can grow like that firecracker display. If you want to avoid it, learn to keep hot situations from lighting your fuse instead of trying to stop your anger after it has started, suggests Marcia J. Slattery, M.D., a psychiatrist with the Mayo Clinic in Rochester, Minnesota.

Pay attention to your warning lights. Whether you're the type who readily vents or quietly turns anger inward, many women don't notice when they're becoming angry. The next time you're in a temper-provoking scenario, take a quick inventory of your feelings. Do you get a knot in your stomach? Or ask a trusted friend to give you her impression of how you act when you're angry. Do you start to twitch? Tap your foot? Does your voice get tense? Then listen to your warning signs sooner.

Think before you act. Before you say exactly what's on your miffed mind, take a few moments to consider ways to deal with the situation without making it worse. Walk away if you have to, then come back and continue.

Chase the little aggravations away. If you allow petty annoyances to accumulate, you push your temper to its limits. Let annoyances pass, and forget about them.

weight paper surgical masks you see on *ER* at pharmacies. "They're inexpensive, and really do protect you," says Dr. Wiggins.

Switch to a HEPA vacuum bag. Vacuum cleaners with special seals and HEPA (high-efficiency particulate air) filters keep the dust mites out of the air while you're sucking them out of the carpet. But they cost a lot more than regular vacuum cleaners. So Dr. Wiggins suggests trying individual HEPA filter bags on the vacuum cleaner you already have. "They're only a little more expensive than regular bags, and they'll trap the dust mites so they won't bother you," she says.

Seal off bed mites. If you have allergies, chances are you've already considered covering your mattresses, boxsprings and pillows with zip-on plastic casing to trap the allergens inside. This will help as much when you're cleaning the bedroom or changing the bedding as it will when you're sleeping. Be sure to wipe down the plastic with a damp cloth periodically.

Pay attention to pillows. Sure, you wash the pillowcases, but what about the actual pillows? It doesn't matter if they're feathered or synthetic—pillows are havens for dust mites. So wash your pillow in hot water once a week or more.

Dry out high-moisture spaces. Allergens thrive in damp air. Run a dehumidifier regularly in damp, poorly ››

Compartmentalize your life. Find a proper balance between all the aspects of your life, such as your friends, family, work, exercise, and hobbies, Dr. Slattery suggests. When your life becomes focused on one narrow pursuit—for example, work—you tend to lose perspective on all the things that are important and react too quickly to problems that shouldn't be such a big deal.

Write a list of all the things that make your life complete or draw them out on a pie chart. Hang it up on your office wall or put it in your purse. The next time you're in a huff, look at the piece of paper and weigh this minor aggravation against all the good things in your life, Dr. Slattery suggests.

End problems before they begin. If your child keeps doing something that always triggers a battle, write out a contract when you're both calm that specifies what the consequences will be the next time he does it. If he breaks the agreement, don't get mad—just pull out the contract and follow the plan you've established.

Don't assume others are out to get you. If you encounter a slow clerk in the supermarket checkout line, remember that the cashier didn't wake up that morning determined to make your life miserable. She's doing the best she can, just like you are. Instead of losing your temper—and escalating the situation—treat her with a positive attitude.

Put your problems in perspective. Keep in mind that at any given time, disasters are changing people's lives all around the globe. Though you may be exasperated when your computer freezes up, this inconvenience isn't worth getting upset over when you compare it with a real tragedy. ■

ventilated spaces like bathrooms or the basement. Running an air conditioner, if you have one, helps, too. That will keep the mold and dust mite population down so you can clean the area more comfortably.

Clean the bathroom regularly. The surest way to avoid mold allergies is to keep mold in check, says Dr. Wiggins. Don't keep any carpets or mats in there, and wash the shower curtain frequently along with the towels and washcloths. Once a week is fine, she adds.

Helpful Hint

While you'll need a very dilute solution of bleach to effectively kill mold, try to avoid strong-scented cleaners. "Some women with allergies are sensitive to the cleaning products themselves," says Dr. Wiggins. "You may need to use trial and error to find products that agree with you. But generally, the less fragrant the better." ■

Angina

Cut Your Heart Attack Risk by a Third

When it comes to controlling angina pectoris—those heavy, pressurelike chest pains from restricted blood flow to the heart—women have a key advantage: An angina attack is very often her first indication that she has heart disease. Some "advantage," you might be thinking. But compare it to men: Their *first hint of a troubled ticker is more often a heart attack—or sudden death.*

"The fact that women are more likely than men to have angina before getting a heart attack provides a window of opportunity to prevent that heart attack," says Nanette Wenger, M.D., professor of medicine and cardiology at Emory University School of Medicine and chief of cardiology at Grady Memorial Hospital in Atlanta.

Modern medical treatment can usually keep angina from causing you more pain, Dr. Wenger says. But much, if not most, of your strategy to prevent progression of the disease is in your own hands.

Take aspirin every day. The anticlotting power of simple aspirin (50 to 325 milligrams a day, depending on what your doctor recommends) can cut your risk of heart attack by a third or more.

Add vitamin E to the mix. There's evidence that women with angina can reduce their chances of a heart attack by as much as 77 percent if they take 400 to 800 international units of vitamin E supplements daily. If you are considering taking amounts above 400 IU, discuss this with your doctor first. One study using low-dose supplements showed increased risk of hemorrhagic stroke.

Get mellow. Avoiding emotional stress now has a double benefit. For one thing, feelings of anger or hostility seem to be connected with heart attack risk. For another, strong emotions are (along with overexertion

CHELATION DOESN'T WORK

No matter what you've heard, forget chelation therapy, injections of compounds promoted as an alternative treatment for chest pains and heart disease There's absolutely no credible evidence that it works. And despite claims to the contrary, it may not be safe.

and heavy meals) a trigger of angina attacks.

Ask your doctor for an exercise prescription. Shedding extra pounds and getting more exercise can improve heart health considerably. But if you have angina, both should be customized for you based on an exercise test, not guesswork.

Ask about nonsurgical treatment. A procedure called Enhanced External Counterpulsation (EECP) may be just as effective as balloon angioplasty or bypass surgery for chronic angina. EECP provides more blood (and therefore more oxygen) to the heart by periodically compressing a series of cuffs around your legs and backside. And it costs less than surgery. ■

Antioxidants

Why Do We Get Old? The Answer Is Radical

When our bodies are exposed to factors like pollution, sunlight, and even everyday wear and tear, cells produce unstable molecules, damaging our cells, putting dings in our DNA, and contributing to a variety of diseases from heart disease to cancer.

Day by day, bit by bit, free radicals may also cause changes in the body that we normally associate with aging, from forgetfulness to poor immunity.

Vitamins A, C, and E along with selenium, beta-carotene, and other substances collectively known as antioxidants are the heroes in this drama. They step in between free radicals and your body's healthy molecules, preventing damage associated with disease and aging.

Foods rich in antioxidants provide protective compounds that enter your bloodstream and assist your healthy molecules against the pillaging free radicals—and perhaps early aging.

"Antioxidant supplements are fine, but I prefer eating foods rich in antioxidants instead," says James A. Joseph, Ph.D., chief of the neuroscience laboratory in the human nutrition center at ››

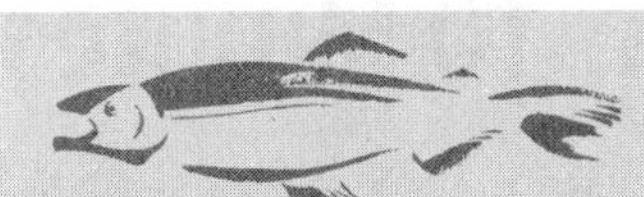

THE PERFECT ANTIAGING MEAL

If you're looking for a meal loaded with antioxidants, Dr. Joseph shares one of his healthy and tasty favorites.

Grilled salmon topped with plum tomatoes, scallions, oregano, garlic, basil, and parsley
Steamed broccoli
Steamed spinach
Fresh blueberries

Tufts University in Boston.

He should know. Dr. Joseph and his colleagues conducted a series of studies identifying certain fruits, vegetables, and other foods that do an exceptionally good job of slowing the aging process in your body and your brain. Eating them can sharpen your memory, improve learning, and improve overall health.

Dr. Joseph and his Tufts colleagues recommend eating at least five servings per day of these foods, which score high in anti-aging antioxidants:

- Vegetables: carrots, cooked tomatoes or tomato sauce, kale, spinach, broccoli
- Fruits: blueberries, oranges, strawberries, raisins
- Other: vegetable oils (in moderate amounts), fish, whole grain cereals, garlic

Anxiety

Calm Nervous Tension in 10 Minutes Flat

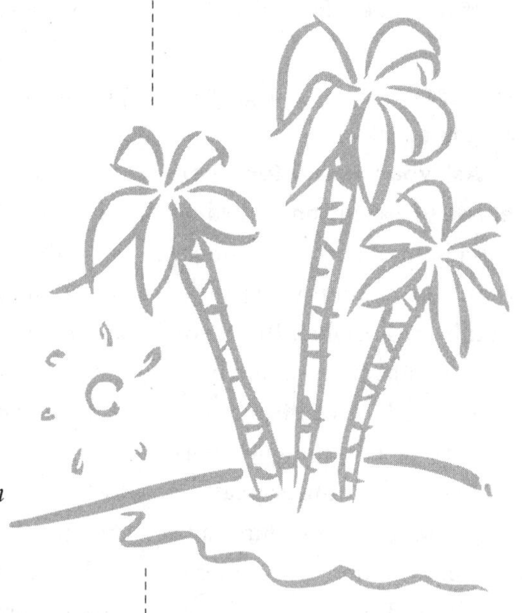

Anxiety is like bad television reception: Disorienting. Out of control. And not always easy to fix.

"When we're confronted with problems and don't have solutions, the emotional response is anxiety," says Susan Heitler, Ph.D., a clinical psychologist in Denver and author of the audiotape Anxiety: Friend or Foe? *"Women are especially likely to experience anxiety when they're vaguely disturbed about a problem, like having too much to do and too little time in which to do it."*

If your nerves are on edge, try Dr. Heitler's anti-anxiety tips, designed to help ease your emotional state and regain control in 10 minutes flat.

Devise an action plan. "The very best antidote to anxiety is to gather information," says Dr. Heitler. Pull out a sheet of paper and write down exactly what is bugging you. Then review your list and write down what you need to handle the problems. "For example, if you're losing your job, write down your fears of not having enough money to pay bills or whether you'll find another job quickly. Perhaps you can get information from your family about loan possibilities

Dr. Joseph practices what he researches. "My wife and I have been vegetarians for 15 years, and we go through 9 pounds of plum tomatoes a week," he says. "Tomatoes contain lycopenes, excellent antioxidant compounds."

Helpful Hint

While it's best to eat the freshest fruits and vegetables possible, you can still get antioxidants from out-of-season foods. For example, blueberries are just about as high in antioxidants out of season as when they're picked fresh. Dr. Joseph says that the antioxidant properties remain intact in blueberries washed, put in sealed plastic bags, and stored in your freezer for up to a year. ■

or talk to human resources about other positions within your company," she says.

Take the fantasy route. Sit down in a comfortable chair, close your eyes, and picture yourself lying on a beautiful beach on a tropical island. Inhale and exhale deeply as you visualize yourself basking in the sunshine, listening to the ocean waves, and seeing the palm trees rustling in the wind. "Soon enough, your breathing and heart rate will slow down, your stress level will drop, your anxiety will disappear, and your thoughts will clear," says Dr. Heitler.

Avoid the superwoman trap. If you usually have 20 errands to run and household chores to do, decide which are the most important and postpone the rest. "You may have to cut back the number of hours you spend on work, split the chores and errands with your husband, or hire some help," says Dr. Heitler.

Find time to have fun. Make personal time a priority. Schedule fun things on your calendar and don't let other matters interfere—even if it means leaving your job on time (for a change) or saying no to another obligation.

"At the end of the work day, make it a point to leave your job emotionally as well as physically. When you get home, order out for dinner and relax by lying down and listening to music, reading, and playing with the kids, the dog, or the cat," says Dr. Heitler. "Making time to relax and unwind a priority is essential to good health."

The good thing about feeling anxious: It's a barometer, giving you feedback on what's going on in your life. "So listen to your anxious feelings and begin shortening your to-do list to a manageable size," she says. ■

DON'T MAKE THIS MISTAKE

Don't rely on anti-anxiety drugs like Xanax to help you cope with the normal stresses of everyday life, says Dr. Heitler. Prescription sedatives are potentially addictive and should only be taken for short-term crises, if recommended by your doctor.

Aromatherapy

Tired, Blue, or Stressed Out? Boost Your Spirit with Scents

If you've ever come home to the aroma of chicken noodle soup, you know how scents can soothe your soul. But they may do more than simply lift your spirits by reminding you of your favorite childhood meal. When inhaled or applied to the skin, aromatic plant extracts known as essential oils can chase away headaches, relieve stress, fight infections and alleviate PMS, according to aromatherapists, who believe that the scents and chemicals of essential oils affect the mind and body.

"When you inhale an aroma, it goes to your brain and affects chemicals there," explains Mindy Green, educational director of the Herb Research Foundation in Boulder, Colorado, and author of Aromatherapy: A Complete Guide to the Healing Art.

Green practices what she preaches. While the rest of us reach for another cup of coffee to deal with the day's stress or fatigue, Green pulls out a mist bottle of essential oils diluted in water and sprays her office with scent, as needed.

Here, Green shares her favorite combinations. Simply fill a 4-ounce spray bottle with water, add the essential oils suggested and spray as needed. (You can find essential oils at many health food stores as well as aromatherapy shops.)

If you're stressed: Five drops of lavender, 2 drops of

SNIFF AWAY THE POUNDS

Peppermint can calm an upset stomach, freshen your breath, and as an essential oil, energize a tired mind. It may also help you lose weight.

Your body's olfactory nerves (located in in your brain) use aromas to regulate your satiety center. Simply put, aromas help tell your brain when you've eaten enough, explains Alan R. Hirsch, M.D., neurological director of the Smell and Taste Treatment and Research Foundation in Chicago and author of *Dr. Hirsch's Guide to Scentsational Weight Loss*. That's why diet experts recommend that people chew their food thoroughly. It slows down their eating, but it also allows the aromas to reach the olfactory bulb and tell you that you're full before you overeat.

Dr. Hirsch wanted to explore whether scent alone could help people lose weight. So he gathered more than 3,000 people and gave them inhalers containing the aromas of peppermint, banana, or green apple. For 6 months, these men and women sniffed the inhalers any time they were hungry or tempted by food. At the end of the study, the group with the inhalers had lost an average of 5 pounds per month, while those without inhalers did not.

You can try this technique yourself by filling a small vial with peppermint or apple shampoo, peppermint leaves, or essential oils to sniff when the need arises. "Just choose something with a strong scent," Dr. Hirsch says. Perfumed lotions or candles may be too weak to stimulate your satiety center.

DON'T MAKE THIS MISTAKE

If you're pregnant or have heart disease, high blood pressure, asthma, epilepsy, or cancer, talk to your health care practitioner before using any essential oil. While aromatherapy is generally safe, the chemicals in certain oils could aggravate some health problems by stimulating the nervous system, irritating sensitive airways, or affecting your condition in other ways.

Roman chamomile, and 3 drops of bergamot. Lavender and Roman chamomile are both relaxing scents; bergamot enhances your mood without making you edgy.

If you're feeling down: One drop of ylang-ylang, 3 drops of clary sage, and 5 drops of bergamot. This soothing combination will lift your spirits without making you excitable.

If you need an afternoon pick-me-up: Five drops of rosemary, 1 of peppermint, and 3 of lemon. "They're all mental energizers," Green says. ■

Arthritis

Do Joint Pain Supplements Really Work?

Walk into any health food store, and you'll find an array of nutritional supplements with tongue-twisting names such as chondroitin sulfate and glucosamine promising to ease your joint pain. Do they really help? Or are they just useless additions to a long list of alleged arthritis remedies, like copper bracelets and snake venom?

Evidence suggests they're worth a try.

In normal joints, cartilage cushions and protects the ends of your bones. Composed of cells known as chondrocytes and connective tissue such as chondroitin, glucosamine sulfate, collagen, and proteoglycans, cartilage is a tough substance, perfect for helping your joints absorb the impact of aerobics or running. "But it's harder to replenish than something like skin, which has a good blood supply," explains Sol Grazi, M.D., assistant professor of family medicine at University of Colorado School of Medicine in Denver. "Normally, things in the body that wear out get rejuvenated and replaced. In osteoarthritis, the joint gets worn out and beaten up to a greater extent than the cartilage can be made to replace it. The joint doesn't have enough material to make the cartilage it needs."

Without that essential cushioning, a joint becomes inflamed, swollen, and painful to use.

Here's a primer on the most commonly used joint pain supplements available in drug stores and health food stores.

Glucosamine. Supplements of glucosamine work by providing your body with the raw materials to heal cartilage. Sometimes, they also reduce inflammation. "This is the most documented and effective natural remedy for repairing joint cartilage," says Woodson Merrell, M.D., executive director of the Center for Health and Healing at Beth Israel Medical Center in New York City. Made from ❯❯

crustacean shells, glucosamine seems to stimulate the creation of new cartilage. Though it takes longer to work, it can be as effective as ibuprofen for arthritis pain and inflammation—and with fewer side effects. Dr. Merrell suggests taking 500 milligrams three times daily until your pain subsides.

Chondroitin sulfate. Often sold in combination with glucosamine, chondroitin sulfate is reputed to slow cartilage breakdown and reduce joint pain. Researchers are still studying whether people with arthritis benefit most by taking chondroitin alone, glucosamine alone, or a combination of the two. "If you're going to use one, you might as well use both, because they could work in different ways," says Roland W. Moskowitz, M.D., professor of medicine at Case Western Reserve University in Ohio. The generally recommended dose is 1,200 milligrams daily.

Helpful Hint: If you're using glucosamine or chondroitin, consider taking up to 5 milligrams of manganese supplements per day also, says Chris Leffler, M.D., medical director of NeuroMetrix in Cambridge, Massachusetts. In one study, Dr. Leffler found that a combination of the three helped Navy divers with osteoarthritis of the knee. If you don't have enough manganese in your diet, your body will have trouble taking advantage of these arthritis supplements because it needs this trace element for the chemical reactions that make cartilage.

SAMe (S-adenosylmethionine). Used as a treatment for depression in Europe, SAMe boosts mood in those who are depressed by keeping serotonin circulating in the brain, just as some antidepressants do. But SAMe, a molecule that moves throughout the body, also helps arthritis, Dr. Grazi says. "SAMe gets into the joint and serves as a building block to make more of the substances a joint needs." In addition to regenerating cartilage, SAMe also reduces inflammation, which allows the cartilage cells known as chondrocytes to repair the injured joint. To take advantage of SAMe's benefits, take 200 to 800 milligrams daily until your joint pain lessens, Dr. Grazi recommends.

NETTLE HELPS REDUCE NEED FOR ARTHRITIS DRUG

Taking nettle leaf—a widely available herb—along with diclofenac (an anti-inflammatory drug prescribed for sudden flare-ups of arthritis) may enable women with arthritis to take less of the drug for pain relief. A study conducted in Germany showed that men and women who took nettle leaf and a low dose of diclofenac experienced just as much pain relief as others who took a full dose of the prescription drug.

The less diclofenac you need for pain relief, the lower the risk of serious side effects. The nettle may enhance the drug's antirheumatic effectiveness, say the study authors.

Use of nettles for arthritis is new but experimental. Talk with your doctor before trying nettles or changing your dosage of any prescription medication. Also, if you have allergies, be aware that nettles may worsen your symptoms.

MSM (methylsulfonylmethane). A sulfur-containing compound found in trace amounts in food, MSM is not as well-researched as other joint remedy supplements. It seems to relieve arthritis pain and inflammation by increasing the effectiveness of cortisol, the body's own natural inflammation fighter. MSM may dampen chronic joint pain, says Stanley Jacob, M.D., professor of surgery at the Oregon Health Sciences University in Portland. Take 1,000 milligrams twice a day with food for the first 2 to 3 days, he says. Then, each week, add another 1,000 milligrams to your daily intake until the pain subsides. A typical dose of MSM ranges from 2,000 to 8,000 milligrams a day. If you develop gastrointestinal problems such as cramping, cut back to a lower dose. (Don't combine MSM with blood thinning drugs such as aspirin or warfarin.)

Helpful Hint: Arthritis relief supplements work more slowly than arthritis drugs, so "if you want to try an arthritis relief supplement, give them at least 4 to 6 weeks," Dr. Merrell says. ■

Artificial Nails

Is Your Manicure Hazardous?

Thanks to the miracles of acrylic, plastic, glue, powder, and gel, you don't have to have naturally strong nails to have long, perfectly uniform manicured nails. Many women also find that artificial nails are a convenient answer to easily broken or badly chewed nails.

Artificial nails can look like the real thing—maybe even better. If applied for a special occasion, they're safe. Worn regularly, however, they can cause problems. Your fingernails are living tissue. Choked off from oxygen by the artificial coverings, your nails can become thin or brittle and break easily. Or they can develop nail fungus, not a pretty sight.

If you must have perfect nails for a special occasion and want to keep your nails healthy, follow these "rules of thumb," recommended by Ida Orengo, M.D., associate professor of dermatology at Baylor College of Medicine in Houston.

Wear press-on nails only for the special occasion, but no longer. You can wear acrylic and gel nails longer because they allow your natural nails to breathe a bit more. But even so, they should be removed after 1 month.

Have artificial nails applied and removed by a professional manicurist. Ripping or peeling acrylic or gel nails when trying to remove them yourself may damage the nail plate. A manicurist will use a solvent that will gently and safely separate artificial nails from your own nails.

Watch your natural nails closely for any changes. If they seem brittle or separate from the covering, or if they become thinner and more fragile, have the artificial nails removed. Wait several weeks before reapplying.

Helpful Hint

Whether or not you wear artificial nails, dry your hands thoroughly after you wash them. Nail fungus thrives in moisture under nail tips. ■

Artificial Sweeteners

Scout Out Hidden Calories in Sugar-Free Sweets

If you've switched to sugar-free desserts, pastries, and snacks to save calories but don't seem to be losing weight, take a closer look at what you're eating. Just because a food is "sugar-free" doesn't necessarily mean that it contains fewer calories than regular goodies. You could end up consuming nearly as many calories from sugar-free foods as you would if you stuck to the real thing.

Take a look at the Nutrition Facts labels for two packages of chocolate sandwich cookies, for example. One contains 13 grams of sugar and 140 calories for 3 cookies. The second supplies no sugar, but weighs in at 120 calories—nearly the same as the 3 regular cookies. The fat content is the same.

Where do the calories come from? Very often, artificial sweeteners, which are—surprise!—carbohydrates.

Although the sugar content looks lower in the "diet" cookies, the number of carbohydrates (19 grams) is practically the same. "So buying products marketed as 'sugar-free' and 'no sugar added' isn't necessarily saving you a significant number of calories," says Karen Chalmers, R.D., director of nutrition services at the Joslin Diabetes Clinic in Boston.

Not all artifical sweeteners contain calories. Saccharin (Sweet 'N Low), aspartame (Equal, Nutrasweet), acesulfame-K (Sweet One), and sucralose (Splenda) are truly calorie-free. Others, including maltodextrin, polydextrose, sorbitol, mannitol, xylitol, isomalt, and hydrogenated starch hydrolysate (or HSH) contain almost as many calories per teaspoon as sugar.

"Artificial sweeteners—especially those with calories—offer no great benefit," says Chalmers. "They were originally created to help people with diabetes avoid sugar, thought to be the culprit behind high blood sugar. Now we know that carbohydrates in any form, be it table sugar or a sweet-tasting synthetic, are okay for people with diabetes, as long as they limit their portion sizes."

Her advice: If you're watching your waistline or blood sugar levels, don't automatically assume that a sugar-free product is lower in calories than a non-sugar-free version. Instead, read labels.

Helpful Hints

Large amounts of sweeteners like mannitol or sorbitol (called sugar alcohols) have a laxative effect and can cause digestive problems. Non-caloric sweeteners such as aspartame do not. So if you experience digestive problems after eating sugar-free food, read ingredient labels and avoid sweeteners that are suspect.

"Remember, one packet of regular sugar has 16 calories," says Chalmers. "Even people with diabetes can use sugar. I wouldn't use five or six packets of it, but one won't hurt." ■

Take a Close Look at Those "Sugar-Free" Cookies

Here are the Nutrition Facts labels for two kinds of chocolate cookies. The label on the right, for sugar-free cookies, has just 20 fewer calories, the same amount of fat, and nearly as many carbohydrates as regular cookies (*left*). You might as well eat the real thing.

To size up your favorite cookies, compare total calories, fat, and carbohydrates, not sugar content. The sugar-free version may not save you calories, fat, or sugars.

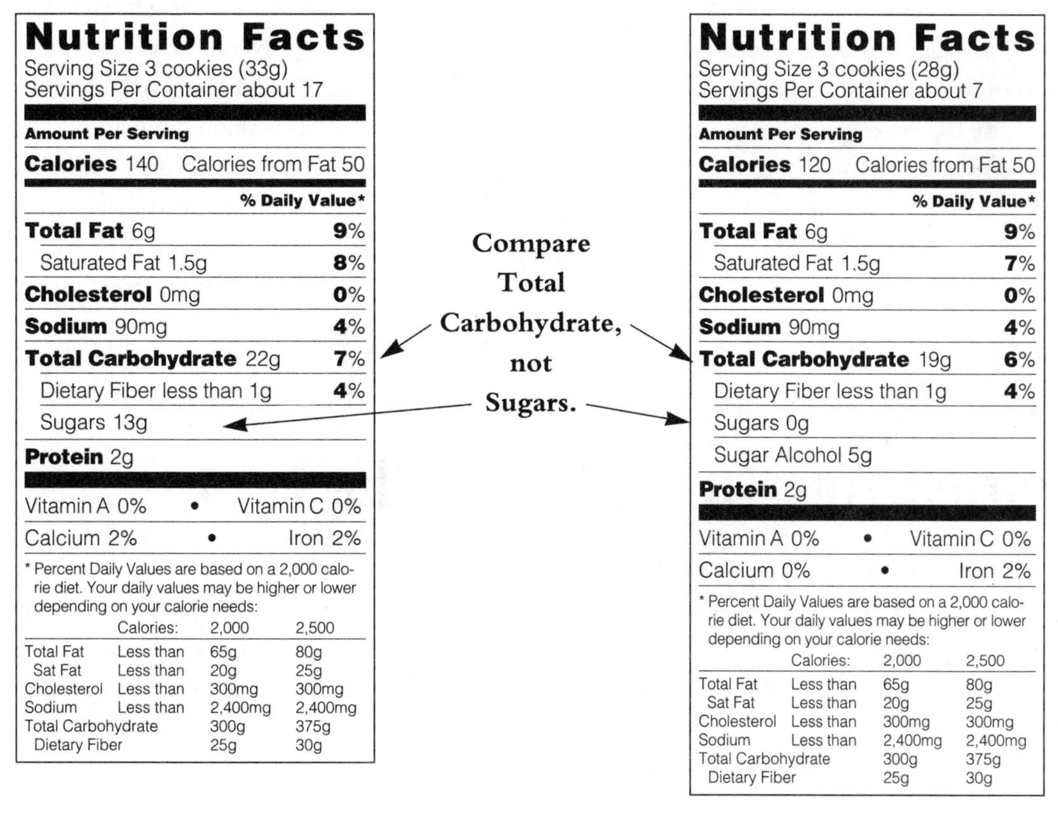
Compare
Total
Carbohydrate,
not
Sugars.

Nutrition Facts

Serving Size 3 cookies (33g)
Servings Per Container about 17

Amount Per Serving	
Calories 140	Calories from Fat 50
	% Daily Value*
Total Fat 6g	**9%**
Saturated Fat 1.5g	**8%**
Cholesterol 0mg	**0%**
Sodium 90mg	**4%**
Total Carbohydrate 22g	**7%**
Dietary Fiber less than 1g	**4%**
Sugars 13g	
Protein 2g	
Vitamin A 0% •	Vitamin C 0%
Calcium 2% •	Iron 2%

* Percent Daily Values are based on a 2,000 calorie diet. Your daily values may be higher or lower depending on your calorie needs:

	Calories:	2,000	2,500
Total Fat	Less than	65g	80g
Sat Fat	Less than	20g	25g
Cholesterol	Less than	300mg	300mg
Sodium	Less than	2,400mg	2,400mg
Total Carbohydrate		300g	375g
Dietary Fiber		25g	30g

Nutrition Facts

Serving Size 3 cookies (28g)
Servings Per Container about 7

Amount Per Serving	
Calories 120	Calories from Fat 50
	% Daily Value*
Total Fat 6g	**9%**
Saturated Fat 1.5g	**7%**
Cholesterol 0mg	**0%**
Sodium 90mg	**4%**
Total Carbohydrate 19g	**6%**
Dietary Fiber less than 1g	**4%**
Sugars 0g	
Sugar Alcohol 5g	
Protein 2g	
Vitamin A 0% •	Vitamin C 0%
Calcium 0% •	Iron 2%

* Percent Daily Values are based on a 2,000 calorie diet. Your daily values may be higher or lower depending on your calorie needs:

	Calories:	2,000	2,500
Total Fat	Less than	65g	80g
Sat Fat	Less than	20g	25g
Cholesterol	Less than	300mg	300mg
Sodium	Less than	2,400mg	2,400mg
Total Carbohydrate		300g	375g
Dietary Fiber		25g	30g

Assertiveness

Say Goodbye to the Invisible Woman

Contrary to the dictionary definition, assertiveness is not a form of aggression.

"Assertiveness means refusing to be invisible," says Bonnie Jacobson, Ph.D., director of the New York Institute for Psychological Change and author of If Only You Would Listen. *"For women, it means putting yourself out there to be recognized."*

Sounds pretty reasonable. With the exception of jewel thieves, we tend to want to be recognized. Unfortunately, many women end up being taken advantage of because they're too timid, especially when it comes to asking for what they need or want.

If that's you, Dr. Jacobson offers some basic building blocks for getting your way.

Concentrate on one thing at a time. Think of something specific you want to ask for. "The first step in assertiveness making clear what it is that you want," Dr. Jacobson says. Do you need help getting something done around the house? Do you need help at work on a particular project? Do you have a problem with a product or service? "You

Asthma

Retrain Your Lungs to Breathe Easy

If you have asthma, your doctor has probably explained that the bronchial tubes in your lungs are narrower than they should be. During an asthmatic episode, the lining of the tubes swells and muscles surrounding the tubes constrict, making breathing difficult or labored.

Almost instinctively, many people who get asthma attacks start to take shallow, gasping breaths. Bad move. What you should do instead is take slow, deep breaths—even more slowly than you normally breathe. In fact, deep, slow breathing can prevent asthma attacks in the first place.

"Slow breathing exercises control reflexes that govern our blood pressure and other involuntary functions," says Paul M. Lehrer, Ph.D., professor in the department of psychiatry at the University of Medicine and Dentistry of New Jersey Robert Wood Johnson Medical School in Piscataway. "These involuntary functions become more efficient and may help prevent an asthma attack."

If you have asthma, try practicing the following technique for 20 minutes two times every day, which may help alleviate symptoms. (For best results, use a watch with a second hand to time your breaths).

• Breathe in and exhale slowly and regularly, once

might even want to write it down," says Dr. Jacobson.

Brainstorm. Not sure what you want? Talking it out with a friend can help clarify your thoughts and even give you ideas on what to say when the time comes.

Put your request in concrete terms. "I'd like it if you made dinner the 2 days a week that I have to work late" is concrete. "I wish you'd help out around here" isn't. Wishy-washy requests are counterproductive, according to Dr. Jacobson. "Vagueness induces in the other person a feeling that they have to take care of you," she says. "Then they start to resent you."

DON'T MAKE THIS MISTAKE

Screaming and shouting won't work. Instead, be clear and centered when making a request.

Collaborate. Being assertive doesn't mean creating an adversarial situation. Your goal is cooperation. "You want to help the other person give you what you want," Dr. Jacobson says. "Make it as friendly as possible and be very willing to assist."

Listen. It takes two to have a conversation, and being assertive doesn't change that. Listening to what the other person has to say isn't just polite—it's strategically sound. "If they're resisting giving you whatever it is you're asking for, hearing the other person's side lets you see where the resistance is coming from," says Dr. Jacobson. ■

every 10 seconds (about six long, slow breaths a minute).

• Don't inhale too deeply—you'll hyperventilate.

• Exhale through pursed lips, to control the release of air.

• Breathe from your abdomen, not your upper lungs. (Pull in your abdomen as you inhale and release your abdominal muscles as you exhale.)

• If you start feeling lightheaded, take shallower breaths.

Helpful Hint

To make it a habit, practice this breathing exercise at the same times every day. ■

Athlete's Foot

Treats for Sweeter Feet

Gym shoes and moist socks. Pumps and nylons. Tennis shoes on hot macadam. All are welcome mats to the fungal infections called athlete's foot.

"A closed-in, sweaty foot is the perfect environment for the tiny organisms that cause athlete's foot," says Cheryl Burgess, M.D., a dermatologist at the Center for Dermatology and Dermatologic Surgery in Washington, D.C. The result isn't pretty: Your feet or the spaces between your toes may burn and itch. The sides and bottoms of your feet may become dry and scaley. You may experience peeling and a white, cottony appearance between your toes. Uggh!

Athlete's foot fungi love the moist combination of bare feet and gym showers, swimming areas, and bathroom floors, says Karen Deasey, M.D., chief of dermatology at Bryn Mawr Hospital in Pennsylvania. She recommends the following strategies to prevent athlete's foot. ››

• Wash and dry your feet carefully, especially between your toes.

• Put on clean socks or clean hose every day.

• Don't wear the same shoes 2 days in a row. Alternate shoes instead.

• Dust the insides of your shoes with cornstarch or baby powder when going without stockings.

• Don't go barefoot. Wear sandals outside and flip-flops in the gym locker-room and shower.

THE TEA TREE OIL CURE

Over-the-counter antifungal creams generally clear up athlete's foot.

For a nondrug approach, try tea tree oil.

"It's cheap and safe, and it works as well or better than over-the-counter medications," says Dr. Weil.

You can pick up a bottle of 100 percent tea tree oil at health food stores and herb stores. Apply a light coating to the affected area three or four times a day and continue to apply it for 2 weeks after symptoms are gone, says Dr. Weil.

Helpful Hints

If you're prone to frequent fungal infections, add one or two cloves of raw garlic a day to your diet. It's a natural fungus fighter, says Andrew T. Weil, M.D., director of the program in integrative medicine and clinical professor of internal medicine at the University of Arizona College of Medicine in Tucson.

Use an antifungal cream or powder once a week when you know you'll be in sweaty shoes.

If you get itchy toes every time you wear a certain pair of shoes, get rid of them. They're probably contaminated with fungus, says Dr. Deasey. ■

DON'T MAKE THIS MISTAKE

If you're using an antifungal cream to treat athlete's foot, don't stop too soon. Your symptoms may be relieved in a week, but you should continue to use the cream for at least 30 days, says Dr. Burgess. "You want to kill the fungus, not just slow it down. Otherwise, it starts growing again when you stop using the cream."

B

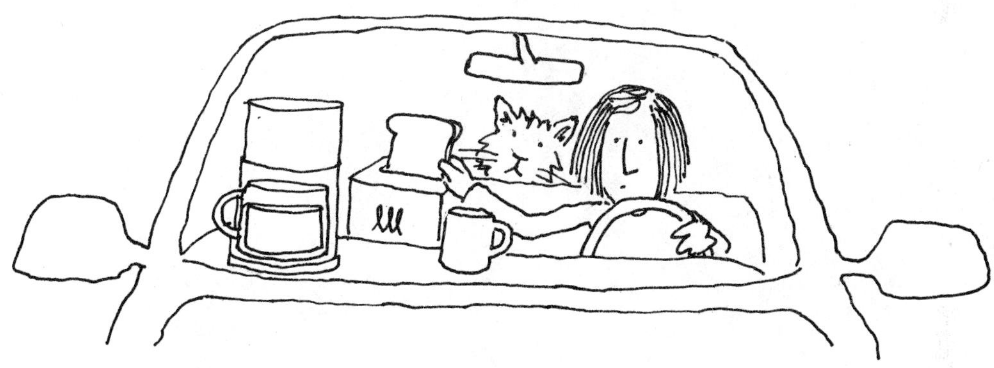

If you leave the house in a rush every morning, you can still eat a "real" breakfast—without creating a driving hazard. See page 54.

Back Pain

37 Cures for an Out-of-Whack Back

Walking around bent over in pain like Quasimodo will get you plenty of sympathy. Or maybe just strange looks from the office staff. Either way, if your lower back is out of whack, you need relief quickly. But you also need long-term solutions for protecting your back from pain and injury.

Here are 37 back-saving tips from the best "back engineers" in the country: Rowland Hazard, M.D., of the Spine Institute of New England in Williston, Vermont, and the Vermont Back Research Center in Burlington; Mary Lynn Mayfield, patient educator at the Texas Back Institute in Plano, Texas; and Lynne Nicolson, M.D., chief of physical medicine and rehabilitation at the Sunnyview Rehabilitation Center in Schenectady, New York.

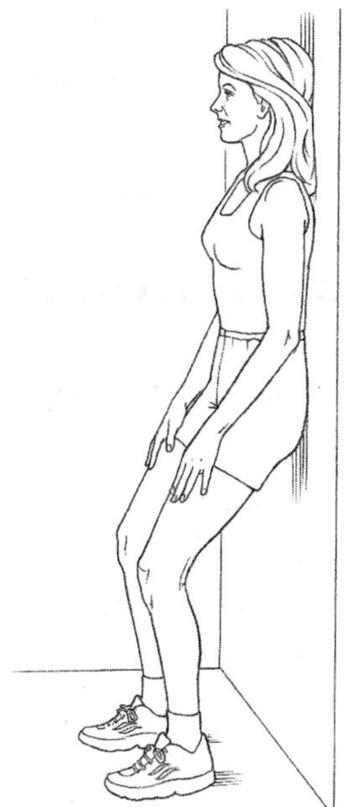

On-the-Spot Relief

1. Keep a freezable gel pack on hand. When back pain first strikes, put a towel between the pack and your skin and leave it in place once an hour, for up to 20 minutes an hour. Don't fall asleep with it in place.

2. Take a warm shower. Or once the pain starts to subside, take a hot soak in the tub.

3. Lean with your back pressed against a wall (as shown) if you're on the go and your back starts to hurt. Stand with your feet 12 to 18 inches away from the wall and your knees slightly bent. You might also use this position for putting on socks or underwear when your back is aching.

Massage and Support Devices

4. Lumbar support pillow. A well-designed pillow is the Original McKenzie Lumbar Roll, a cylindrical, foam support that works well on almost any type of seat, including car seats, regardless of your size and weight. Available through your physical therapist or from Orthopedic Physical Therapy Products, P.O. Box 47009, Minneapolis, MN 55447-0009.

5. Vibrating back pads. While these back massagers won't cure you, they feel great when you're in pain. Available in variety stores and department stores.

6. BackCycler. This air pillow slowly inflates and deflates, keeping your spine in motion as you sit, while you control the pressure. Even better than a back massager, this moves the spine and shifts the pattern of stress. Available from Ergomedics, Inc., 15 Tigan St., Winooski, VT 05404. ››

Stretch Away the Pain

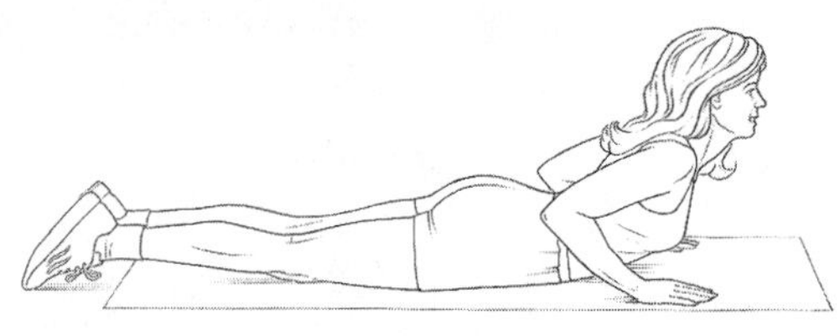

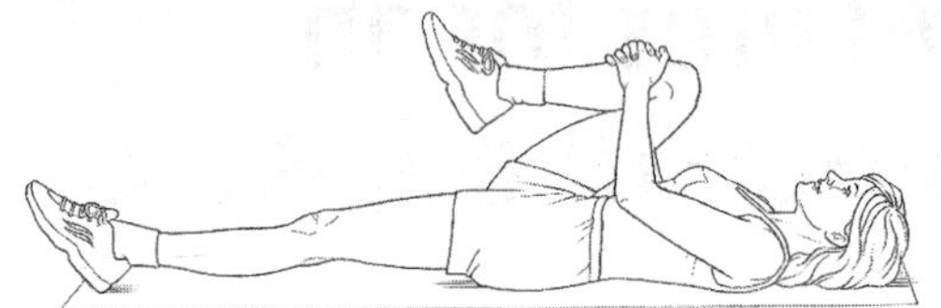

7. Knee to chest stretch (*above*): Lie on your back and bring one knee to your chest. Alternate knees, then do both knees together.

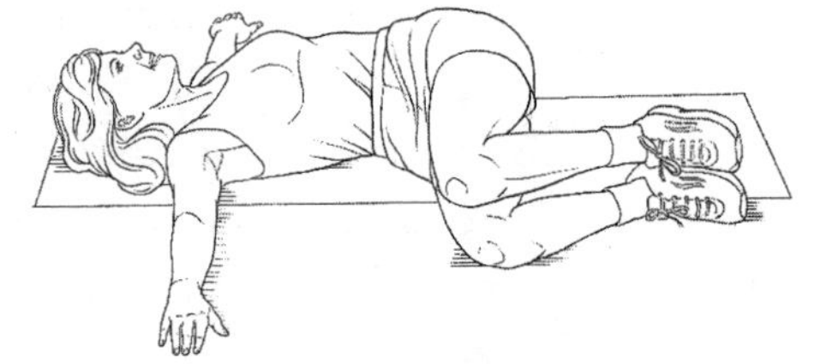

8. Modified cobra stretch (*above left*): Lie on your stomach and press with your arms, pushing your chest up from the floor.

9. Rotation stretch (*center left*): Lie on your back, knees pulled up, arms outstretched. Lower your knees to one side, keeping your head and neck in line with your body. Relax. Change sides.

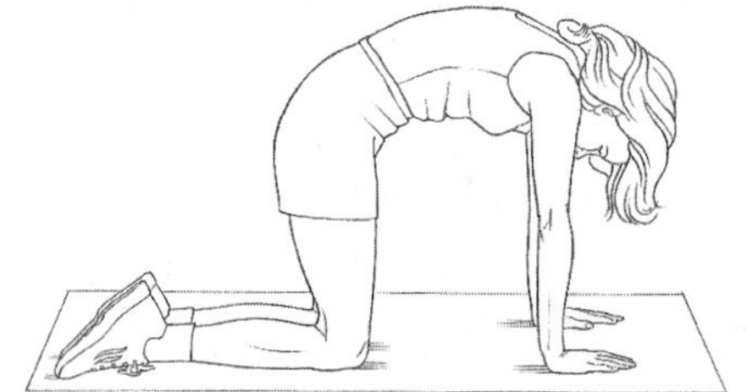

10. Cat stretch (*lower left*): On your hands and knees, slowly round and then arch your back, alternating between the two movements.

Heal Yourself with Motion

11. Keep active. Doctors used to advise rest for back pain, but now they know that moving around works better. Staying in good physical condition—with regular aerobic exercise like walking, resistance training, and stretching—also protects against future back pain. Be sure to warm up and cool down with some stretching exercises.

12. Walk in water. Walking in a pool or lake may be more comfortable than walking on dry land because your spine doesn't have to bear your weight.

13. Do the side stroke. If swimming, the breaststroke and crawl make your pain worse because they arch the back. You may be more comfortable doing the side stroke.

14. Buy, rent, or borrow an exercise bike. Bicycling is ideal for women with back trouble because it's non-weight-bearing. An exercise bike is easier than cycling outdoors because you avoid bumps and bad weather.

Helpful Hint

Make sure your seat and handlebars are adjusted for comfort.

Around the House

15. Storing kitchen goods: Make a circle with your arms overhead. Store cookware and canned goods on shelves within reach of your fingertips. Store only things that you don't need very often in the highest and lowest cabinets.

16. When you're standing at the kitchen sink: Open a lower cabinet and prop one foot on the base.

17. To vacuum: Long strokes strain your back. Instead of bending over and stretching forward, trying to cover a large area in one pass, vacuum a foot or two at a time, then move to another spot. (Better yet, milk the situation and beg someone else to do the vacuuming.)

18. To make a bed: Don't bend from the waist or reach as you pull the sheet and blankets into place. Instead, put your knee on the bed so your spine is straight and stabilized.

19. Garden plot. Don't bend from the waist to yank weeds or plant seeds. Get down to the dirt by using foam kneepads sold in garden centers or by sitting on a stool. Pace yourself and avoid staying in one position for too long.

Sleep Etiquette for Your Back

20. Lie on your back and put pillows under your knees. Or, if you sleep on your side, put a pillow between your knees. Sleeping on your stomach may be tough on your back. But if that's the only way you can sleep, put a small pillow under your hips.

21. Sleep on your side with a 4-foot-long body pillow. Hold the pillow against your chest, between your knees, and under one foot (great for pregnant women). And it doesn't snore!

22. To get out of bed, don't sit up at first. Instead, roll to the side, then push your upper body up and drop your feet off the side with your knees bent.

At Your Desk

23. Make sure your computer screen is at eye level. Ask your eye care practitioner for eyewear or contact lenses designed for computer users, which correct your vision for the distance from your eye to the monitor.

24. Ask for an ergonomically designed chair. Or support your lower back by placing a rolled-up towel or pillow between your back and the chair.

25. When working at a desk or computer, sit all the way back in the chair. Keep your chair close enough to your desk so that you don't have to lean forward. Don't cross your legs.

In the Bathroom

26. Brush your teeth in the shower so that you can stand up straight instead of bending over the sink.(Don't confuse the shampoo with the toothpaste.)

27. Rest one foot on a shower chair (available in medical supply stores) while shaving your legs in the shower. ❯❯

Smarter Ways to Stand, Bend, Lift and Carry Stuff

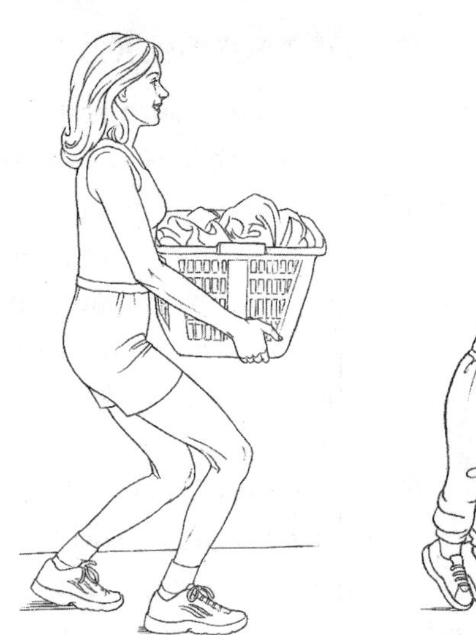

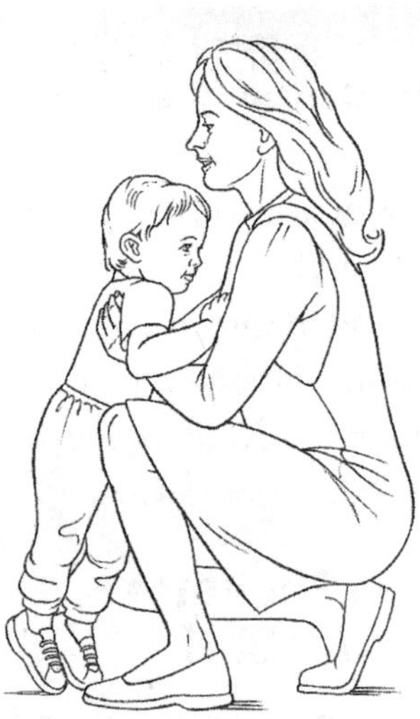

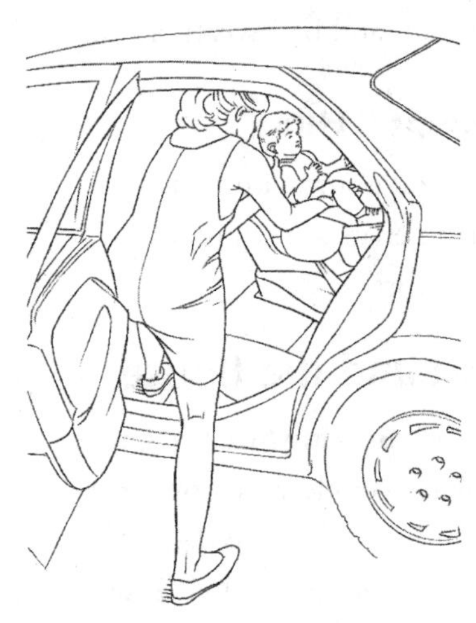

28. Stand up straight. Good posture puts less wear and tear on the spine. Check yourself in mirrors, windows, shiny car doors, or any reflective surface. Keep your head right above your shoulders.

29. Pivot, don't twist. Injuries occur when people lift objects and twist to put them down at their side. Instead, face the object, then pivot your body before you put it down.

30. To lift something (*above left*): Use correct form for bending (bend at the knees, not at the waist), stretching (don't twist), and lifting (pull the object in close to you, and pull straight up).

31. To lift a child (*above center*): Place the child in front of you, close against your body, between your knees. Pick him straight up without twisting. Then carry him close to your body.

32. To lift a toddler into a car seat (*above right*): Put your foot on the floor of the car so that you have a more balanced support. Go slow and avoid jerky movements.

33. To exit a car: Push the seat all the way back before you get out of the car. Then swing both legs out together and place your feet on the ground before you start to stand.

34. To push a grocery cart loaded down with heavy items like cat litter and a case of soda: Stay close enough so that your elbows are bent as you push the cart. Walk with it, rather than pushing and then catching up.

35. To lift groceries out of the car trunk: Pull them toward you, getting the weight closer to your body. Put your knee on the bumper for stability before you lift.

Back-Friendly Fashion Tips

36. Switch from a heavy handbag to a little organizer bag. Buy one with a built-in billfold and room for only a comb, lipstick, and keys, or use a fanny pack.

You don't really need to take all your earthly possessions with you when you go out to lunch.

37. Switch to low-heeled pumps or flats. High-heel shoes throw your posture off—aggravating a bad back—and give you a greater risk of tripping. ■

Bad Breath

Fresh Out of Mouthwash? Try This

Even the most dedicated nonsmoking brushers and flossers sometimes find themselves with unexpected elbow room at social gatherings. The fact is, bad breath often just isn't your fault. Certain foods—including very healthy foods—can turn the breath of life into the kiss of death.

One solution is to stop eating. A better one is to fight nature with nature by taking advantage of a smorgasbord of natural breath fresheners that let you overcome odor without wearing out a path to your medicine cabinet.

Breath-Saving Foods

If garlic or onion flavored your meal, try these antidotes at the end of it.

Eat your greens. The chlorophyll molecules in just about any fresh, green, leafy vegetable render the molecules responsible for bad odors inert. "I haven't found anything that masks bad breath better than chlorophyll," says John Heinerman, Ph.D., director of the Anthropological Research Center in Salt Lake City. So fresher breath relief can be as simple as chewing on lettuce or parsley. About 10 or 15 sprigs should do it.

Helpful Hint

Wrapping parsley sprigs around a celery stalk and chewing it all helps your breath stay fresh longer than eating parsley alone.

Chomp a carrot. Chlorophyll isn't the only breath help from the garden. "Chewing a raw carrot is another good way to get rid of bad breath," Dr. Heinerman says.

Have an apple for dessert. The natural sugars in apples help to overcome halitosis.

Get Fresh with Spices

Your spice rack offers aromatic alternatives that sweeten your breath in different ways. Here's what works.

Allspice. Stir ½ teaspoon of powdered allspice into ½ cup of warm water and swish it in your mouth for a minute, then spit it out. Better than the powder, though, are dried allspice berries. (They look like big brown peppercorns.) Simply steep a handful of berries in boiling water, strain, let it cool, then rinse or gargle. ››

Clove. This sweet-smelling spice works well with cinnamon. Put four whole cloves and 2 tablespoons of shredded cinnamon sticks in a quart of water and bring it to a boil. Cover and simmer for 5 minutes and then let the tea sit for about 20 minutes more. Strain it and enjoy a cup while it is still warm for long-lasting fresh breath.

Cardamom. Borrow from Middle Eastern cuisine: Just chew on a few seeds (don't swallow) and let cardamom's natural antiseptic action kill bad-breath bacteria.

Peppermint. As a mealtime tea, this famously refreshing herb takes care of breath problems that come from your digestive tract. Tea bags are fine, or try steeping your own using a tablespoon of dried leaves (2 tablespoons if they're fresh) per cup of water. If you are using fresh leaves, steep for at least 10 minutes for maximum potency. ■

MAKE YOUR OWN NATURAL MOUTHWASH

Natural mouthwashes can work better than the brand-name varieties. Here's one that Dr. Heinerman recommends.

Apple Cider Mouthwash

- In a small saucepan, combine four or five cinnamon sticks with 2 cups of apple cider.
- Bring the mixture to a boil, lower the heat, and let it simmer for 5 minutes.
- Cover and steep for another 30 minutes.

Use this intense but sweet-flavored mouthwash warm or cold as needed. Store it in a tightly covered jar in the fridge, Dr. Heinerman suggests. It will keep for up to a week.

Bad News

Smart Ways to Happily Stay Informed

A serial killer is on the loose. Terrorists have struck again. The stock market is about to crash. There was a shootout in a high school and a high-speed chase on the interstate. Somewhere a war is raging. Stay tuned for film at 11.

With a ready supply of bad news and an abundance of outlets to carry it around the world—TV, radio, newspapers, and the Internet—you don't have to go long without learning some depressing information.

But, you can stay well-informed without becoming overwhelmed by a downpour of bad news, says Stuart Fischoff, Ph.D., professor of media psychology at California State University, Los Angeles, and senior editor of the *Journal of Media Psychology.*

Except for urgent breaking news—like an impending hurricane—Dr. Fischoff suggests that you try to get your news from a newspaper rather than television. Newspapers tend to be less upsetting: They generally deliver more detail and less sensationalism than television. Plus, newspapers usually stack the important news at the beginning of stories, so you can stop reading when you've had enough. (Do take time to read any boxes that accompany the main story—they often contain "how to" information, so you feel less helpless in response to the danger reported.)

When you do choose to watch televised news, keep the following tips in mind.

• When you've heard what you really need to know about a news story, stop watching. Often, we get addicted to a story, following it second by second, and the more it upsets us the more we watch, says Dr. Fischoff.

• Don't assume a string of similar events is an irreversible trend. "Take shootings at high schools, for example," says Dr. Fischoff. "Bear in mind that these events tend to occur in cycles—an event occurs, it produces copycat behavior patterns, it peaks, and it drops off rather dramatically, then it waits for the next violent scenario du jour, then that goes through its cycle as well."

• Remember that just because a bad thing happens to someone else—a school shooting, a robbery at the cash machine—it won't necessarily happen to you or your loved ones. "Yes, the incidents are profoundly disturbing, especially if you're a teacher or have kids of your own. But even with copycat incidents, the likelihood of a shooting taking place at your particular school is low." This is especially true today, with heightened security and zero-tolerance policies now in force.

• Monitor your emotions as you watch the day's events instead of letting them build up. Take note of what makes you feel bad and what makes you feel optimistic, and how that affects your view of the outside world.

• Get out and live a balanced life so that news reports aren't your only source of information.

"People who don't get outside to test reality enough and who use the news as the window to the world, find the world a far more negative, dark place," Dr. Fischoff says. "For the most part, people don't live in as crime-ridden a world as the news would have us believe."

Helpful Hint

If watching the 11 o'clock news interferes with sound sleep, skip it, or watch an earlier broadcast. ■

Beans

20 No-Fuss Ways to Eat Less Beef and Reap the Nutritional Benefits of Beans

You've probably heard that beans are a great source of fiber, but this "musical fruit" has a lot more to toot about. Loaded with vitamins, minerals, and protein, "beans are an excellent food," says David Lineback, Ph.D., food scientist, chemist, and director of the Joint Institute for Food Safety and Applied Nutrition at the University of Maryland in College Park. But unlike a bottle of supplements, a bag of beans won't bust your budget.

Here are a few of the natural health defenders you'll find inside every little bean.

Fiber. This dietary wonder not only helps shrink your appetite and lower cholesterol but it also reduces your risk of digestive disorders and breast and colorectal cancer. In fact, preliminary studies suggest that the fiber in fava (broad) beans may prevent or slow the progression of colon cancer. Experts recommend 20 to 35 grams of fiber a day. At 7.5 grams of fiber per ½ cup, a handful of black beans mixed into rice or ½ cup of chickpeas tossed on top of a salad goes a long way to meet your fiber quota for a meal. In contrast, meat has no fiber.

Calcium. While beans may not contain as much of this bone-hardening mineral as milk (150 milligrams per ½ cup), they still make quite a dent in your Daily Value. Just ½ cup of white beans has about 95 milligrams of calcium; black-eyed peas (cowpeas) contain a whopping 106 milligrams. In contrast, meat has no calcium.

Folate. All beans contain this B vitamin that helps prevent birth defects and lower risk of cardiovascular disease. A mere ½ cup of Roman and Great Northern beans holds more than 100 micrograms—25 percent of the recommended daily intake. Getting 400 micrograms each day from food may reduce the risk of colon cancer in women by as much as 31 percent, according to a 14-year study including nearly 90,000 nurses. Meat has no folate.

Iron. Eat beans before donating blood. According to the Stanford Medical School Blood Center, eating foods rich in iron and vitamin C 6 hours before donating blood helps replenish your blood supply more quickly. Another reason to grab a can—verve! Subtle iron deficiencies can steal your energy to work, learn, or play. Just ½ cup of Roman, lima, or navy beans provides at least 2 milligrams of iron, nearly 20 percent of the RDA for premenopausal women.

Phytoestrogens. Beans are loaded with mild, estrogen-like plant hormones that appear to lower your risk of breast and endometrial cancers. Estrogens found in soybeans appear most beneficial. Meat has none.

Protein. Beans are an ideal protein source for vegetarians because they contain a full set of amino acids, the basic units of proteins. "That makes them an excellent source of pro-

THE SECRET OF FLATULENCE-FREE BEANS

For all their nutritional superiority, beans have one humbling attribute: If you're not used to eating them, your body creates gas when digesting oligosaccharides, the carbohydrates in beans.

Start with ½ cup of lower-fiber beans, like pink or red, at dinner. If you experience digestive upset, wait a couple of days, then try again. If your colon remains calm, replace the pink beans with ½ cup of high-fiber beans, like Roman or Great Northern. If all goes well, switch to a full cup or add other fiber foods to your diet in a few days.

Try Beano. If even small amounts of meticulously presoaked beans give you gas, reach for a gas suppressor, like Beano. It prevents fermentation of oligosaccharides and their embarrassing by-product.

tein," says Dr. Lineback. Always try to mix beans with other, more cooperative foods, like pasta, rice, potatoes, tomatoes, carrots, or chicken.

Here are 20 ways to add beans to your meal at home, in restaurants, and at salad bars.

At Home

You don't have to spend hours soaking, rinsing, and cooking huge vats of dried beans to reap their benefits. Canned beans are just as nutritious and flavorful, since they retain their original moisture and texture. So keep plenty on hand. If sodium is a concern for you, soak and rinse the beans before use.

1. Mix red or black beans with rice (add beans to rice about 10 minutes before it's finished cooking).

2. Add a can of Great Northern, kidney, or cannellini beans to soups or stews.

3. For lunch, open a can of lentil or split pea soup.

4. Add tofu (bean curd) to stir-fries or breakfast smoothies.

5. Serve baked beans whenever your family asks for burgers at home.

6. Mix canned beans with vegetables in an omelet.

7. Top homemade pizza with vegetables, kidney beans, and chickpeas.

8. For a quick dip, puree beans with chili powder and serve with pita wedges or baked chips.

9. Snack on roasted soy nuts (available at health foods stores and some supermarkets).

On the Menu

Ordering chili instead of a burger or a bean burrito instead of a cheese enchilada are obvious ways to help yourself to beans when dining out. Here are other dishes to look for.

10. Pasta e fagioli (Italian bean and meat soup)

11. Tuscan soup (sometimes made with two or three types of white beans)

12. Cassoulet (white bean and meat casserole)

13. Hoppin' John (Cajun stew usually made with black-eyed peas or kidney beans)

14. Falafels (made from pureed chickpeas)

15. Vegetarian burgers (frequently made from black beans)

16. Miso (bean paste)

17. Frijoles (Mexican beans)

Under the Sneeze Guard

Next time you belly up to the salad bar, pass on the potato salad and try these salad toppers.

18. Three bean salad

19. Hummus

20. Chickpeas ■

Beef

If You Want It, You Can Have It

You don't have to say goodbye to beef to stay healthy. While eating too much beef—or any other food containing saturated fat—seems to contribute to heart disease and an increased risk of certain kinds of cancer, small amounts of lean meat are actually good for you.

Just one 3-ounce slice of sirloin—the size of a deck of cards—supplies you with almost 50 percent of your daily need for zinc and 17 percent of needed iron and nutrients vital for immunity, energy, and learning. You'd have to eat five chicken breasts to get that much zinc and 3½ cups of raw broccoli for the iron. Beef is also an efficient way to get protein.

The key to making beef part of a health-building diet is to choose wisely. Fattier cuts, like prime rib and regular ground beef, are major sources of saturated fat, which can raise your cholesterol levels, clog your arteries, and expand your waistline. And studies have found that improperly grilling and pan-frying beef increases your risk for cancer. When dry heat, like open flames and hot grills, touches meat, cancer-causing compounds form on its surface. The hotter the temperature and the longer meat is exposed to dry heat, the greater the number of carcinogens. Another cancer-begetter: fat drippings. When beef juices drop down on hot charcoal or flames, cancer causers are conceived. The resulting waft of smoke carries them back up to the beef. Sounds scary, but "as long as you don't eat grilled or pan-fried meat every day and you cook smart, you may decrease the risk of cancer associated with these compounds," says Rashmi Sinha, Ph.D., an epidemiologist specializing in beef and cancer at the National Cancer Institute.

Here are some simple techniques for cutting out the cancer creators and saturated fat.

Order child-size portions. Experts recommend eating no more than 6 ounces of cooked beef a day. That's about the size of two decks of cards.

Look for lean. Choose lower-fat grades, such as "select" or "choice," and pick lean cuts—anything with "loin" or "round" in its name. These meats have just a little more saturated fat than a chicken leg—less than 4.5 grams per 3-ounce serving.

Make it moist. Roast, braise, or stew beef more often than you grill it. These techniques cook meat with hot liquids rather than fiery dry heat, so they don't pose as great a cancer threat.

Take it slow. Turn your gas grill dial down to low or raise your hibachi rack up a slot to slow cook your steak.

Avoid direct heat. To prevent smoky carcinogen-creating flame-ups when gas grilling, light one burner and place your meat over the other unlit burner, recommends Steven Raichlen, author of *Barbeque Bible* and *Steven Raichlen's Healthy Latin Cooking.* With charcoal grills, stack two piles of charcoal with a drip pan in between. Cook the meat over the drip pan.

Request medium-well. Order your burger medium-well. This way, the cancer threat will be reduced, but it's still hot enough to kill bacteria. (To destroy harmful bacteria such as *E. coli*, ground beef must be cooked to an internal temperature of 160°F).

Helpful Hint

If you order beef when dining out, consider Cajun-style blackened beef. The flour-and-herb coating is charred rather than the meat, so this spicy dish is not a major source of carcinogens. ■

MIGHTY MARINADES THAT FIGHT CANCER

Besides adding flavor and tenderizing leaner (usually tougher) cuts of beef, marinades form a protective coating between the grill and the meat, slashing cancer-causing compounds normally formed during grilling by as much as 94 percent. Yet dripping oil can also create cancer-causing smoke and charring. To solve this problem, choose an acidic ingredient like orange juice or lemon juice, add a few herbs, and make a marinade without using oil. Or use a dry-rub to season beef before grilling.

Try these two coatings suggested by Steven Raichlen, author of *Barbeque Bible* and *Steven Raichlen's Healthy Latin Cooking*.

Dry Rub: Combine 1 teaspoon each of dried rosemary leaves and cracked black pepper and add salt to taste. Rub about ½ teaspoon of this blend on each side of your steak.

Marinade: Combine 1 cup of orange juice, ½ onion, 2 garlic cloves, 1 chipotle chile (canned), ½ teaspoon each oregano and cinnamon, and salt and pepper to taste. Puree all the ingredients in blender.

Beer

The Next "Health Drink" and All-Purpose Antiseptic?

While high-priced athletes and high-concept commercials publicly pitch beer's taste appeal, high-minded scientists have been scrutinizing the beverage for its unadvertised—but far more invaluable—properties. Their findings: Beer not only tastes great but also shows promise as a weapon against cancer and other health problems.

"Research on the benefits of beer is long overdue," says Donald Buhler, Ph.D., a leading beer scientist and professor of environmental and molecular toxicology at Oregon State University in Corvallis. "An occasional brew may be very healthy for you."

Scientists like Dr. Buhler are discovering how beer plays a protective role in blocking cancer-causing cells from entering the body, as well as slowing or even halting tumor growth. ››

So far, the research has been done on lab mice, but Dr. Buhler is optimistic that flavonoids in hops—the bitter-tasting chemicals that give beer its distinctive taste—will be part of a new generation of anticancer drugs for womankind.

Beer appears to behave much like a bodyguard, albeit at the cellular level. Tests by Japanese researchers show that beer—especially dark beer like stout—protects against cancer-causing carcinogens found in cooked hamburger.

And that's not all. Among the most surprising benefits of beer are that it:

Acts as an antioxidant. The flavonoids in hops help

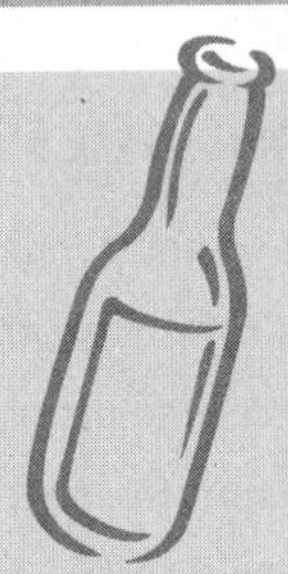

DON'T MAKE THIS MISTAKE

Rejoice in beer's newly found medicinal role, but don't celebrate by drinking a six-pack. For women, limiting yourself to one to two beers a day is still the best advice for your overall health. Consuming higher amounts has been linked to breast cancer. And of course, if you currently avoid alcohol for health or religious reasons, there's no reason to start to drink.

Beta-Carotene

Top Picks in the Produce Bin

Pumpkin pie supplies so much beta-carotene that it's practically a nutritional supplement.

In fact, almost any dark green, orange, or yellow fruit or vegetable contains protective amounts of beta-carotene, plus generous amounts of related substances called carotenoids that are converted into vitamin A in the body.

But beta-carotene's role goes beyond being vitamin A's backup. A single serving of a food rich in beta-carotene every day could help you avoid breast cancer. In one study, women age 40 and older who ate more of beta-carotene a day from food were much less likely to develop breast cancer than women who ate foods containing little or no beta-carotene. As a bonus, foods rich in beta-carotene may help you avoid heart disease.

Unlike some other nutrients, nutrition experts have not set a Daily Value for beta-carotene. Instead, they recommend eating one food rich in

10 TASTY WAYS TO GET BETA-CAROTENE

Baked sweet potato (½ cup)	9.5 mg
Pumpkin pie (1 slice)	8.5 mg
Baby carrots (⅔ cup)	6.2 mg
Canned apricot halves (4)	5.9 mg
Steamed spinach (½ cup)	4.7 mg
Raw spinach salad (1 cup)	3.1 mg
Cantaloupe chunks (1 cup)	2.4 mg
Sweet red pepper (½ cup chopped)	1.6 mg
Romaine lettuce (1 cup)	1.1 mg
Steamed broccoli (½ cup)	0.8 mg

keep blood pressure and cholesterol at safe levels by taking on free radicals, the wayward oxygen molecules that damage tissue in the body.

Serves as a tasty source of vitamin B_{12}. All varieties of beer contain a small amount of this essential vitamin otherwise found primarily in animal products. A healthy supply of vitamin B_{12} helps against anemia. That's good news, especially for vegans who do not eat meat or dairy foods. Of course, the average beer contains only 0.07 microgram of B_{12}, so vegetarians might still need to take supplements to get their Daily Value of 6 micrograms even if they do have an occasional cold one.

Doubles as an antiseptic. The next time you scrape a knee at a family picnic and find yourself short a first aid kit, open a cold beer. Pour some beer directly on the wound to help kill germs on the spot. The alcohol and flavonoids in beer possess antibacterial properties.

Helpful Hint

Certain beers pack more hops than others. It all depends on how they're brewed. Microbrews, stouts, and ales have the highest amounts of hops. ■

beta-carotene a day. "With so many foods rich in beta-carotene, there's no need to take supplements," says Georges Halpern, M.D., Ph.D., D.Sc., professor emeritus at the University of California School of Medicine at Davis and visiting professor at the University of Hong Kong School of Traditional Medicine. "What's more, many of the dark green, yellow, and orange foods also contain other carotenoids, such as alpha-carotene, lycopene, zeaxanthin and lutein, that also help fight disease."

To select produce with the most carotenoids, food experts offer a couple of pointers.

• Buy at least one dark green vegetable. Although yellow and orange foods contain high amounts of beta-carotene, the dark green, leafy foods like spinach, kale, and chard rate as the best sources.

• Look for squashes like butternut or acorn without soft spots in the skin, says Carla Wolper, R.D., nutritionist and clinical coordinator at the Obesity Research Center at St. Luke's/Roosevelt Hospital Center in New York City. The outside should be hard, and the inside should be bright orange. Since beta-carotene is a pigment, the darker the flesh the more beta-carotene it contains. ■

DON'T MAKE THIS MISTAKE

Don't confuse beta-carotene with vitamin A, which can be toxic at high levels. The Daily Value for vitamin A is 5,000 IU. People who take much more—that is, more than 50,000 IU of vitamin A daily for weeks or even months—can develop headaches, blurred vision, hair loss, dry skin, diarrhea, and enlargement of the liver and spleen. Doses above 10,000 IU must be taken under medical supervision only.

Bickering

Don't Take the Bait

In the Woody Allen movie Radio Days, *a husband and wife argue over which ocean is bigger, the Atlantic or the Pacific.*

That's the essence of bickering. Unlike full-blown arguing, bickering consists of little snipes over seemingly trivial issues. In the end, it usually makes no difference who's right and who's wrong. Still, persistent bickering can be corrosive to a relationship.

"Hostile language is as toxic as chemical waste," says Suzette Haden Elgin, Ph.D., applied psycholinguist in Huntsville, Arkansas and author of The Gentle Art of Verbal Self-Defense series. *"It's as toxic for the people dishing it out as it is for the people receiving it."*

So for the sake of everybody's health, it's best to either avoid bickering or short-circuit it before it escalates into a big fight. Here's how.

Remember, it takes two to bicker. "A large percentage of our bickering consists of verbal attack patterns and taking the bait," Dr. Elgin says. "If you refuse to take the bait, the other person can't continue to bicker alone."

Recognize bicker bait. Some husbandly examples: "Why do you always hide my socks?" "If you really loved me, you wouldn't spend so much money." "If you really cared about your health, you'd stay on your diet."

Agree with him. In a neutral voice, say, "It's really annoying to not be able to find your socks." Dr. Elgin says, "That'll stop him in his tracks. He can try a new attack, but the first one is over."

Refuse to feed him his next line. "If you say, 'I do stick to my diet,' that gives him an opportunity to say, 'But what about yesterday when you ate that doughnut?'" Dr. Elgin says. "Women who refuse to be a partner in bickering are going to get far less of it."

Neutralize hurtful comments. "Hostile language almost always has lots of personal language," says Dr. Elgin. "Instead, respond with a bland platitude, such as 'Money is a problem in every marriage'—it doesn't have any I's or you's in it," Dr. Elgin says.

Helpful Hint

When you can't think of a platitude, use this all-purpose emergency sentence: "You can't tell which way the train went by looking at the tracks."

"You can find meaning in it, and it is, in fact, true," Dr. Elgin says. "People will say, 'I never thought about it that way' or 'Wow, that's deep.'"

"If someone's interested in the platitude and wants to dis-

DON'T MAKE THIS MISTAKE

Unlike a lawyer's closing argument, bickering doesn't have to have a beginning, a middle, and an end. "A lot of people tell me they can't quit in the middle," Dr. Elgin says. "Sure you can. All you have to do is stop and say, 'This is all wrong. Let's start over again.'"

cuss it, fine. It's a conversation," Dr. Elgin says. "If not, they'll wander off." Either way, you've accomplished your goal, which is to not bicker.

You can use the sentence only once with the same person, though. If you said it to your husband more than once it wouldn't work. ■

Bicycling

Why You Need a "Girl's Bike"

Sure, bicycling is great exercise. It's also a romantic way to tour France and a cost-effective way to commute. But spend an afternoon on a unisex bike, and your neck, shoulders, and back feel as though you've been stretched on a torture rack.

Enter Georgena Terry, the heroine of women cyclists. No matter how hard she tried, she, too, couldn't find a bicycle to fit her correctly. An avid cyclist and a mechanical engineer, Terry set up shop in her basement making her own frames. Her female friends started coming to her for frames that fit. So she founded Terry Precision Cycling for Women in Macedon, New York, which now distributes female-friendly bicycles to bike shops across the country.

There's more to men's versus women's bikes than the absence of the top tube (connecting the handlebars and the seat tube), explains Terry.

"What makes a real difference is the length of the top tube," she says. "On most bikes, the distance between the handlebars and the seat is too long for most women." Consequently, female cyclists feel too stretched out. Besides, she adds, it's not safe. "You're not in control of the bike if it doesn't fit your body."

Here are Terry's expert tips for finding the perfect bike for your body.

- Stand over the bike. If you can't straddle the top tube with at least ¾ inch clearance on a road bike and 2 inches on a mountain bike, the bike is too big.
- Take the bike out for a test ride. You should comfortably reach the handlebars and handle the brakes easily without locking your elbows.
- Ask the dealer to adjust the saddle height, handlebar height, and the distance between the handlebars and the seat. The width of the handlebars should match the width ››

DON'T MAKE THIS MISTAKE

Don't wear underwear or panty liners with cycling shorts—you lose the non-chafing advantages of the anatomically designed padding.

What Makes a Woman's Bike Female-Friendly?

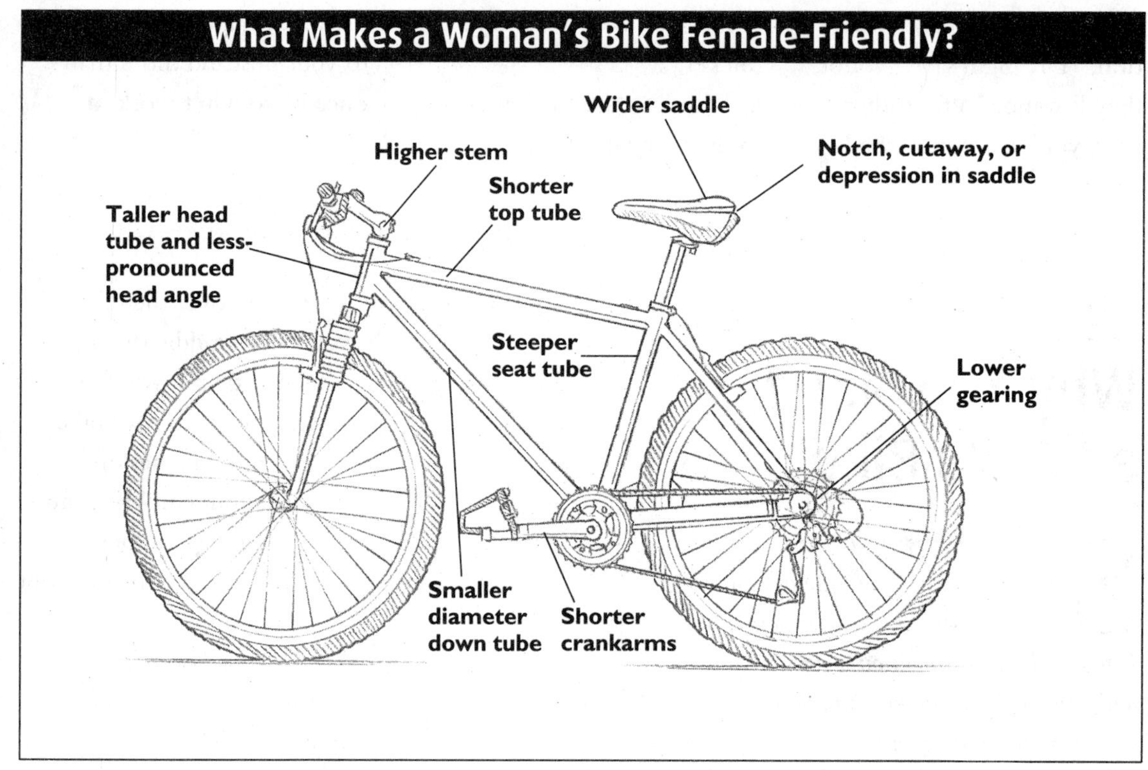

of your shoulders. Your leg should be able to extend fully (without locking your knee) at the lowest point in the revolution, and you should be able to pedal smooth circles without your hips moving from left to right.

• Choose a woman's saddle, which is wider in the back to accommodate a woman's pelvis. Anatomically correct saddles (sometimes gel-cushioned) keep pressure off soft tissues. If you are prone to chafing, bruising, or yeast infections, get a saddle with a notch, depression, or cutaway under the crotch for air circulation and zero pressure on sensitive areas. (If you're on a romantic bicycle trip with your honey, this is especially important. Otherwise, making love for the next few days will be painful.)

• Accessorize for comfort. "Any part of your body that is in contact with the bike is a candidate for specialized clothing," says Terry. That includes cycling shorts with inside padding and no seams in the crotch, padded gloves (or lightweight gloves and foam-padded handlebar tape) and stiff-soled biking shoes.

Helpful Hints

If you have a woman's saddle and you're still uncomfortable, your bike frame may be forcing you to lean too far forward. "If you can sit more upright, that puts your weight toward the back of the saddle," says Terry. ■

Bikini Line Bumps and Rashes

Take the "Ouch" Out of Hair Removal

In Manhattan, women know where to go to have bikini line hair removed: J. Sisters International. There, seven Brazilian sisters (whose names all begin with "J") introduced a bikini wax that enables women to wear the teeniest of itsy-bitsy polka-dot bikinis without revealing upper leg hair.

Even if skimpy swimwear isn't your style, you probably want a smooth bikini line for swimsuit season.

Removing hair at the bikini line isn't as simple as, say, shaving your legs or underarms. Without proper precautions, shaving can leave unsightly red bumps along the bikini line. Waxing can leave you hairless for weeks, but unless it's done right, it may result in ingrown hairs. "The ingrown hair just burrows under the skin and gets infected, which may require surgery to remove," explains J. Michael Maloney, M.D., a Denver dermatologist who does such operations monthly. So waxing is best left to experienced salon professionals who know how to minimize the pain, irritation and risk of ingrown hairs.

Other than wearing a swimsuit with a skirt, here's what Dr. Maloney says you can do to avoid bikini line bumps, rashes, and ingrown hairs.

Smooth on AHAs. "There's some evidence that using alpha-hydroxy lotion, which exfoliates the skin surface, can also reduce ingrown hairs," Dr. Maloney says. Whether you shave or have your bikini line professionally waxed, smooth AHA lotion daily on your bikini line.

If you shave, trade soap for shaving cream. "Shaving cream helps soften the hair shaft itself so that it's easier to cut," Dr. Maloney says. "It also reduces the friction of the razor, so the blade glides over your skin, decreasing the chances for razor burn."

Shave in the direction of hair growth. Bikini line hair grows in at all angles, so this may be challenging, but shaving in the direction hair generally grows reduces ingrown hairs.

Choose vitamin C cream. Apply this antioxidant cream after you shave or wax for its anti-inflammatory effects. Use this in addition to using the AHA lotion, Dr. Maloney says. The vitamin C cream will soothe irritated skin, while the AHA prevents razor burn and ingrown hairs, he explains.

In an emergency, use hydrocortisone cream. If you develop bikini line bumps despite careful shaving, try 1 percent hydrocortisone cream (such as Cortaid Intensive Therapy). "You can't use it repeatedly in thin-skinned areas such as the bikini line, though," cautions Dr. Maloney. "It will cause the skin to thin out even more and shrivel up."

Helpful Hint

If you find waxing too painful and shaving leaves your skin irritated, try a chemical depilatory formulated especially for the bikini area. Just follow the directions exactly. ■

Birthday Blues

Midlife Is Not a Crisis

Early in life, we look forward to upcoming birthdays. At 16 we can drive, at 18 we can vote, at 21 we can legally enjoy drinks with friends if we want to. But how do women feel about getting older when they reach midlife?

Studies of women between the ages of 35 and 60 indicate that 80 to 90 percent feel positive about midlife. More than 80 percent felt positive about their physical appearance and their futures. Others were bothered by signs of aging, such as wrinkles and weight gain. Some felt panicky and worried about loss of memory and other mental power; others did not.

"Birthdays needn't be a negative experience," says Carol Goldberg, Ph.D., clinical psychologist and president of Getting Ahead Programs, a New York–based corporation that conducts workshops on stress management, health, and wellness. Dr. Goldberg offers the following suggestions for transforming birthdays into a day for celebration.

Use your birthday as an opportunity to take stock of what you've achieved, and see the glass half full rather than half empty. "Think of each birthday as a graduation. Feel a sense of accomplishment over what you've achieved," says Dr. Goldberg, "and know that you have more knowledge than ever to move forward."

One 39-year-old office manager in the Seattle Midlife Women's Health study said that getting older reflected maturation—"a transition from young and immature to old and mature."

Set new goals for the upcoming year or decade. Reassess your priorities and give yourself something to work toward that is important to you. Take a class, learn a new hobby, or become involved with a charity that has always interested you. The 39-year-old officer manager, for example, decided to go back to school and get her teaching certificate. "This gave me a sense of direction," she says.

Make a list of all the positive things associated with growing older. Chances are, you have more wisdom, more money, and less responsibility. Relish all the opportunities available to you that you didn't have when you were younger. In the Seattle study, one woman described midlife as "a time when your family is raised and you start to think more about what you would like to do without the heavy responsibility of children." Another

DON'T MAKE THIS MISTAKE

Viewing birthdays as a reminder that you have fewer years left to live may be a self-fulfilling prophecy, Dr. Goldberg says. Studies show that men and women who are depressed don't live as long as happier people. "Depressed people feel helpless and hopeless, and those are not emotions conducive to living a long, healthy life," says Dr. Goldberg. If your birthday causes more than a mild case of the blues or makes you aware that you are depressed, see a professional to help work through your depression.

woman, age 47, described her daughter going to college as giving her a sense of freedom.

Don't allow a negative body image to keep you down. If growing older has led you to feel unhappy about your body, do something to change that—you'll feel years younger, says Dr.Goldberg. Start an exercise regime, stop smoking, and eat healthfully. Buy some new clothes to update your wardrobe, get a new hairstyle, change your makeup, or update the frames of your glasses. All of these things will show that you have control over your body, says Dr. Goldberg, and will make you feel younger.

WHAT OTHER WOMEN SAY ABOUT BIRTHDAYS

In one study of 131 women conducted at the University of Washington in Seattle, women between the ages of 35 and 55 described midlife in their own words.

"A time when you make a shift in your priorities and attitudes about life."

"A dividing line between knowing what you want and what you don't want."

"A transitional period after raising children . . . figuring out life for yourself and your husband."

"Little more than a halfway point where one might reflect back on life to make sure there isn't something you might miss; reprioritizing time."

If you're approaching a midlife birthday of your own, take a cue from the women interviewed. Overall, they spoke of midlife as "a time of taking stock, looking back to see what's happened, where life has brought you so far, and the direction you're going in, and if you like it or don't like it."

Focus on your physiological age, not your chronological age. Your chronological age is based on the years and months that have passed since you were born, but your physiological age is based on your level of health and fitness, compared to the norm for your age group and sex, says Susan Johnson, Ed.D., director of continuing education at the Cooper Institute in Dallas. "Men and women who exercise regularly, don't smoke, have low stress, and follow a healthy diet can have a physiological age up to 20 years younger than an unfit person of the same chronological age," says Dr. Johnson. Adopting these healthy habits at any time will help lower your physiological age, so it's never too late to start. You'll feel like a kid again!

Start your own business, change careers, learn a language, or take a trip. In other words, do something big that you've always wanted to do but couldn't. Now you have more freedom, personally and financially, and you have more wisdom—so go for it! "A meaningful life change will give you something exciting to anticipate in the future," says Dr. Goldberg. In the Seattle study, women mentioned that having the time and money to travel and pursue leisure activities like gardening were among the most satisfying aspects of reaching midlife.

Celebrate in a way that makes you happy. That may mean treating yourself to a day at the spa, or taking the phone off the hook and spending all day reading a novel you haven't had time for, or throwing a huge bash with all your friends. ■

Blisters

Rescue Tactics for Walkers (and Everyone Else)

If you spent all day, every day, padding around the house in fuzzy slippers, you'd never get a blister. But real life occasionally demands something a little dressier—or serviceable. Walking around in tight-fitting dress shoes can leave you with a painful hot spot on your heel or big toe. So can wearing a new pair of sandals, walking shoes, inline skates, or ski boots.

"Blisters are caused by the force of rubbing against skin," explains Thomas M. Novella, D.P.M., associate professor of orthopedic science at the New York College of Podiatric medicine, who's treated thousands of recreational athletes. "Rubbing separates the layers of the skin, similar to what happens when you try to open a thin plastic bag in the produce aisle."

To prevent blisters in the first place:

• Always wear shoes that fit properly—not too snug, not too loose—to minimize rubbing as you walk or run.

• Smear a layer of petroleum jelly on your foot under your sock (or under hose, when you're wearing dress shoes).

• Switch from cotton socks to synthetics when you take a walk, hike, or work out. Socks made with synthetic fibers and blends are softer than cotton, even when wet, reducing friction.

• Wear a nylon sock liner under an athletic sock. (You can find sock liners, along with synthetic socks, at any sporting goods store.)

If despite these precautions you start to feel a blister-in-the-making, wrap it with an over-the-counter blister product like Second Skin, available at sports shops. (In a pinch, you can use an adhesive bandage.)

If it's too late and you already have a blister, don't pop it unless it's very painful. By opening up the area, you risk infection, says Dr. Novella.

Bloating

Periodic Puffiness? Skip These Foods

Many women crave chocolate—any kind of chocolate—during their periods. Paradoxically, this melt-in-your-mouth treat can actually contribute to bloating, says Meena Rao, M.D., assistant professor of obstetrics and gynecology at Emory University School of Medicine in Atlanta.

Right before you get your period, levels of the female hormone progesterone drop sharply, infusing your body tissue with fluid. That's why it's so hard to zip up your favorite blue jeans during this time of the month. Eat the wrong foods, and you can really puff up.

Here's what to avoid if you're bloated.

Salty snacks. Chips, pretzels, crackers, and other high-sodium foods make you retain water, says Dr. Rao.

And never pull off the thin "roof" of the blister, exposing tender skin underneath and further risking infection.

If you must pop a blister, do it carefully. Here's how, says Dr. Novella.

- Wash the area thoroughly with soap and water.
- Wipe the blister with skin disinfectant like Betadine solution, and let it dry.
- Sterilize a needle in a flame. Or use a sterile lancet from a pharmacy.
- Gently prick the side of the blister with the needle. Do not jab the skin underneath.
- Press the fluid out with a sterile gauze pad.
- Apply an adhesive bandage over blister. ■

Boredom

Effortless Ways to Escape Tedium

The next time you're idly flipping through the TV channels, staring dully at the walls of your office cubicle, or stranded at an airport for hours, remember Vickie Kloeris.

For 91 days, the NASA scientist lived in a small, airtight capsule in Houston's Johnson Space Center with three other researchers to simulate living conditions on a lengthy space flight.

Despite the cramped surroundings and limited social circle that surrounded her for 3 months, Kloeris says she rarely grew bored.

Here are some of the ways she enlivened her days, along with related hints from Norman Sundberg, Ph.D., professor emeritus of psychology from the University of Oregon in Eugene, who has studied boredom.

Get up and about. We often grow bored when we feel powerless to change our surroundings, Dr. Sundberg says. If you've been stuck in the same corner of the world for too long, shake up your point of view by moving ❯❯

Sweets. Candy, cookies, cakes, pastries, ice cream, and other yummy goodies are a big no-no. Fat and sugar encourage your body to store water. "Your body retains and uses water to process sugar, so in the interim, you'll feel bloated," says Dr. Rao.

Gas-producing foods. Broccoli, Brussels sprouts, cabbage, corn, eggplant, garlic, onions, and radishes are perfectly healthy foods. But for some, they produce intestinal gas, contributing to bloatedness, especially around your period.

Helpful Hint

You should drink more water when you're bloated, not less. In fact, the more water you drink, the less your body will retain. Why? Because you'll keep your kidneys busy flushing out salt and sugar that contribute to the problem. As long as you're increasing fluids, have a cup or two of peppermint or chamomile tea. Both herbs are carminatives—they help dissipate or expel gas. ■

around, ideally to see something or someone different.

Kloeris had only about 600 square feet to bounce around in, so to "move in place," she logged a multitude of miles on a treadmill and stationary bike. When you have a break at work, walk around the building or down an unfamiliar hallway.

Entertain yourself. Each Wednesday night, Kloeris and her comrades watched silly movies to see who could come up with the funniest comments about them. "It was a big morale booster," she says.

As you sit on the bus or at the airport, look at passersby and imagine where they've been or where they're going. Does that woman really think those shoes look nice with those slacks? Does that young man's mother know he got his eyebrow pierced?

Look at the little things. Dr. Sundberg, whose hobby is photography, has learned that there are always details in our surroundings that might not appear interesting until we focus in on them. You may live in a neighborhood that has become boringly familiar, but you can make it seem fresh when you take an observant look at people, places, and objects around you as if you've never seen them before.

Helpful Hint

Start your day well-rested, Dr. Sundberg suggests. When you're tired, you have less energy to beat boredom. ■

Bossiness

Why You Need a Take-Charge Attitude

As a nurse, Susan Bramson of Greeley Hill, California learned how to get along smoothly with doctors who had big egos and little patience.

Later, when she spent 27 years as part of a management consulting business, collaborating with her husband, the late Robert Bramson, Ph.D., on *Coping with Difficult Bosses,* she saw how her experience in difficult workplace situations could apply to others.

Bramson says that the answer to dealing with difficult bosses—authoritarians, nit-pickers, or people who hang over your shoulder—is rooted in the so-called Serenity Prayer, which encourages you to change the things you can and learn to accept the things you can't. You can use this philosophy at work by changing your end of the relationship, which is easier and less frustrating than trying to change your supervisor. Shifting your own attitude can help you feel less like a victim.

To turn the relationship around, try these tips.

Learn to make decisions like your boss does. If she won't make up her mind until she reads a 10-page report detailing all the facts and potential outcomes, don't burst into her office with a great idea until you've done your homework on it, Bramson says. Conversely, if she likes to make snap decisions with quick outcomes, don't test her patience with too much information. Instead, boil your research down into a quick paragraph.

Bottled Water

Drink Your Fill—For Free

Traditional health advice concerning water is simple: Drink eight 8-ounce glasses a day. If you drink your quota in bottled water, 5 years' worth can easily cost more than $1,000. The same amount of tap water costs about $1.66.

Bottled water has certain advantages. It's convenient—you can carry it everywhere. If your tap water has an off flavor or smells bad, bottled water tastes better. If your local water supply has problems, bottled water might be your best bet. But don't be misled; bottled water is not 100 percent pure.

"All water—bottled or tap—contains traces of other ingredients," says James Symons, Sc.D., a University of Houston professor emeritus of civil engineering and a water-quality expert. "That's because water dissolves at least a little of everything it touches. And it's virtually impossible for suppliers to rid water of all traces of impurities." The government sets safety limits for nearly 100 impurities. (If you have your own well, though, the »

DON'T MAKE THIS MISTAKE

If you're displeased with the way your supervisor treats you, take it up only with her. Don't complain to other co-workers who can't change the situation—you'll only spread bad feelings without accomplishing anything, says Jim Miller, of Arlington, Texas, and author of *Best Boss, Worst Boss* and *The Corporate Coach*.

Change tactics. If your supervisor still shoots down an idea, don't continue to persist with the same line of reasoning. If you feel the idea is still worth pursuing, come up with a fresh angle with new data to support your view.

Meet her more than halfway. If your boss is managing your every move, offer to meet with her daily at a set time to discuss your plans. If you show her you've nailed down every detail, she may not feel the need to watch you so closely.

Realize your boss is under pressure, too. Maybe she's watching you so closely because she's trying to catch any mistake that would reflect badly on her. By going out of your way to work with her, she'll feel more assured in your skills, and she'll give you more freedom.

Remember that trying extra hard to please your boss is different from letting her walk all over you. "You need to keep your own sense of integrity and strength of position within yourself. No one has the right to make a doormat out of you," Bramson says. ■

water quality is your responsibility.)

If safety is a concern, bottled water may be your only option. If it's convenience you're after, you can simply refill empty water bottles with tap water and carry them with you to the gym or wherever. Either way, here's how to keep your store-bought water fresh, or give your tap water a from-the-bottle feel, says Dr. Symons.

Buy it from a popular location. As bottled water sits on the shelf, any bacteria inside have a chance to grow and multiply. So be sure to purchase it from a store that has plenty of turnover. If the cap is dusty, buy it elsewhere.

Keep it cool. Once you open a bottle of water, you

Breakfast

Grab-and-Go Starters

Even if you hate to eat breakfast—or simply don't have time—you owe it to yourself to eat something in the morning. When you wake up, your body has been without fuel for at least 10 to 15 hours. Your brain needs energy—immediately. Some combination of carbohydrates and protein is the best way to juice it up.

Carbohydrates give your system an almost immediate zing. Protein, on the other hand, breaks down a little slower—providing late-A.M. oomph. Plus, it increases your levels of dopamine, a neurotransmitter that wakes up your noggin, helping you think more clearly.

Traditional breakfast foods like cereal, whole grain bread, oatmeal, pancakes, and fruit supply carbohydrates. Fat-free milk, fat-free yogurt, egg whites or egg substitute, omelets, and lean ham provide protein. (Egg whites are an excellent source of low-fat protein; yolks hold all the cholesterol and fat).

Still, some women can't bring themselves to eat breakfast—or they're too rushed to make anything elaborate before heading off to work. No problem. Just try these quick and easy excuse busters.

"Skipping breakfast saves me a lot of calories."

This is counterproductive. "Women who skip meals usually make up the calories and then some at lunch," warns Susan Bowerman, R.D., former nutrition consultant for the Oakland Raiderettes (cheering squad) and Raiders and executive assistant to the director of the UCLA Center for Human Nutrition in Los Angeles. Instead, make a low-fat breakfast smoothie with 1 cup of fat-free plain yogurt and fruit, like berries, melon, or a banana. You'll pack plenty of brain fuel and nutrients into less than 300 calories.

"I hate breakfast foods."

A turkey sandwich—or microwaved chicken breast and rice—are perfectly good foods. It makes no difference what time you eat them.

"I don't like a big meal in the morning."

So grab a snack. Reach for a piece of fruit or a snack bag full of dry high-fiber cereal on the must treat it like a food, he says. Pop it back into the refrigerator when you're not drinking it.

If the H_2O from your well or municipal water company has a funny taste or smell, try filling a clean, empty water jug from the faucet and chill it in the fridge. It's more likely to have no or very little flavor and smell when it's cold.

Make it zesty. You can improve the flavor of tap water by adding just a few drops of lemon juice to it.

Just beat it. Another way to remove some of the odd taste from your tap water is to pour it into a blender and process it for a few minutes. Blending vaporizes the compounds responsible for the funny taste, improving the flavor. ■

way out the door. An hour or two later, have a cup of yogurt or a glass of milk or snack on leftover turkey to get your protein. You don't need to eat everything at once. Scattering a few light snacks supplies your morning fuel and may also prevent overeating at lunch.

"I can't eat anything before noon."

Have a drink. "Blend a cup of soy or skim milk with ½ cup of orange juice and frozen fruit, like bananas and strawberries," recommends Bowerman. This sweet and creamy shake provides plenty of carbohydrates and protein to rouse your brain and energize your muscles.

"All I need in the morning is a cup of coffee" (or cola).

Although caffeine in coffee and soda can jolt your neurons awake, the effect is short-lived. And while you will get that much needed morning zing from sugar in regular colas or naturally sweetened coffee, there's one problem: Since you haven't eaten a late-morning energizer, like protein, your pep will die in an hour or two. So you'll start craving sources of instant energy—typically in sweet starches, like doughnuts, sweet rolls, or more coffee. "That's why many women need to keep drinking coffee and colas throughout the morning—to stay alert," says Bowerman.

Instead, eat complex carbohydrates and protein, like fat-free cottage cheese on toast or a fruit smoothie. They'll supply what you need to get through the morning roller-coaster effect on blood sugar levels.

Helpful Hint

Want to pack 8 to 10 grams of fiber, as well as a whole lot of calcium, fat-free protein, and carbohydrates into your breakfast for less than 300 calories? Combine a high-fiber cereal (at least 5grams of fiber per serving) with fat-free milk and some fruit, like apples, grapes or berries. ■

WATCH THOSE MEGA-BAGELS

Though bagels are low in fat, they can be high in calories. "A typical bagel from a bagel shop can weigh as much as 4 ounces—the equivalent of 4 slices of bread," says Bowerman. "That's a lot of calories, even without cream cheese or jelly." Instead, scoop out the inner breading and use fat-free cream cheese—or eat only half a bagel, plus a banana or apple.

Breast Cancer

A Shopping Cart Full of Prevention

Among cancer diagnoses, breast cancer scares women most. Yet despite the frightening aspects of the disease, "there are several things you can do to cut your risk of breast cancer," says Suzanne Dixon, R.D., research epidemiologist at Josephine Ford Cancer Center of Henry Ford Health System in Detroit. "There's no way to guarantee that you'll never get it. But if you eat a low-fat, high-fiber, nutrient-dense diet, exercise regularly, and limit how much alcohol you drink, you'll greatly reduce your risk."

Here's Dixon's easy five-step plan for increasing your chances of staying breast cancer–free.

Step 1: Think produce and plant foods. Every time you go to the grocery store, put lots of fruits and vegetables in your cart. (The brighter and more colorful, the better.) Reach for blueberries, strawberries, raspberries, mangoes, papaya, cantaloupe, carrots, eggplant, broccoli, bell peppers, sweet potatoes, spinach, kale, and Brussels sprouts. They contain powerful nutrients that act as antioxidants such as beta-carotene, vitamin C, and vitamin E, preventing the cell damage that leads to cancer, says Dixon. And if produce is out of season, try frozen fruits and vegetables—they can be just as good as fresh.

Step 2. Go for whole grains. Look for whole grain breads and cereals, oats, and barley, as well as legumes like lentils, black-eyed peas, and navy and kidney beans. All of these plant foods, whole grains, and legumes contain large amounts of phytochemicals and flavonoids—vitamin-like substances that can help ward off cancer.

One study found that women with a family history of breast cancer who munched on more vegetables and less beef and pork had less damage to their DNA, the genetic material that controls cell function. Damaged DNA leads to cancer. Another study reported that women who ate carrots and spinach more than twice a week had only half the risk of breast cancer of women who ate none.

Step 3: Work that body. Aerobic exercise keeps your weight down and reduces the estrogen levels in your body, which may decrease your risk of breast cancer. Some research suggests that excess estrogen in the body can cause genetic cell damage that leads to cancer. "Women who don't exercise and are overweight have a higher risk than leaner women who do exercise," says Dixon.

Case in point: Women who exercised at least 4 hours a week had a 37 percent lower breast cancer risk compared with women who didn't exercise at all, according to a Norwegian study. In other research, postmenopausal

DON'T MAKE THIS MISTAKE

If friends send you e-mail messages warning about products or ingredients (like sodium lauryl sulfate in shampoo) that are said to cause breast cancer, don't believe what you read. On the Internet, false rumors spread like urban legends. For updates on causes and treatments, go to Web sites for reputable sources, such as www.aicr.org or www.cancer.org. If you can't find an answer to a question you have, ask your doctor.

women who were moderately active (walking, gardening, or doing housework several times a week) had a 50 percent reduced risk of breast cancer compared with sedentary women.

Step 4: Curb the cocktails. "Alcohol boosts circulating estrogen and other hormones, linked to breast cancer, and some research suggests that alcohol itself is carcinogenic," says Dixon. "So I would suggest that women have three drinks or less per week," says Dixon.

In one particular study, consuming an average of one drink a day raised the risk of breast cancer 11 percent. The risk doubled for each additional daily drink (one drink equals a 5-ounce glass of wine, a 12-ounce can of beer, or a mixed drink made with 1.5 ounces of 80-proof distilled spirits).

Step 5: Enjoy soy. Japanese women have been eating foods made from soybeans for centuries. And as a result, they have one-quarter as much breast cancer as American women. A few studies, however, have questioned whether soybeans really lower breast cancer risk. But the evidence of their positive health benefits is still strong.

Soy is brimming with isoflavones—compounds that act like weak estrogens in your body and block the body's own stronger, cancer-promoting estrogens from inhabiting breast cells, says Dixon. Additionally, research suggests that the estrogen-like effects of isoflavones are not the only way that soy can help minimize the risk of cancer. Soy isoflavones may decrease the chances that cells will become cancerous in the first place. One serving of soy milk, soy cheese, tempeh, soy nuts, and tofu packs 30 to 50 milligrams of these compounds, which is all you need each day.

What's a serving? One cup of soy milk, ½ cup of tofu, 3 tablespoons of roasted soy beans, 1 soy protein shake or bar. You can try soy milk in puddings or on cereal, blend tofu in fruit smoothies, or make a soy-butter-and-jelly sandwich for lunch. (Soy sauce and soybean oil have very little of the isoflavones.)

Helpful Hint

Brew some tea. In a Japanese study, women recovering from breast cancer who drank 5 to 8 cups of green tea a day had the lowest rate of metastasis and recurrence compared with women who drank less or none at all. In other words, their cancer didn't tend to spread or recur. Green tea contains EGCG (epigallocatechin gallate), a potent antioxidant that can stop cancer growth. ■

Breast Pain and Swelling

Soothe Tender Breasts with an Herbal Wrap

Right before your period, something as simple as a hug can be unbearable. When your estrogen levels are at their highest, your breasts become achy. Discomfort ranges from mild tenderness in some women to excruciating pain in others.

Sometimes, tender fluid-filled cysts can appear in your breasts' milk glands. Doctors refer to this as fibrocystic breast disease (although it's not really a disease). It's caused by accumulated fluid and strands of fibrous tissue, and it's very common.

If you've seen your doctor and she has assured you that you have nothing serious to worry about, here are two herbal compresses you can apply to your breasts to relieve the pain and inflammation, courtesy of Mindy Green, a founder and professional member of the American Herbalists Guild and director of education services for the Herb Research Foundation in Boulder, Colorado.

Wrap them in ginger. This pungent herb is a powerful anti-inflammatory that will relieve the soreness and reduce swelling, says Green. Grate ¼ cup of the fresh herb. Sprinkle the shavings evenly on a thin cloth. Fold it in half. Then, wet it with hot water. Apply it to each breast for 10 to 20 minutes. Repeat two or three times a day, if possible.

If using powdered ginger—the kind found in your spice rack—is more convenient, add 1 teaspoon of powdered ginger

FOUR WAYS TO DISSOLVE HARMLESS BREAST LUMPS

If you have been diagnosed with fibrocystic breasts, these doctor-recommended strategies may help reduce lumps—or at least get rid of the pain.

Strike oil. Evening primrose oil is an anti-inflammatory that can relieve tenderness and help shrink breast cysts. Take one or two 500-milligram capsules three times a day.

Cut the caffeine. Coffee, tea, cola, and chocolate all contain methylxanthines, naturally occurring substances that may contribute to the problem.

Pop extra E. Some studies have shown that, taken in significant doses, vitamin E can prevent breast lumps from returning. Vitamin E encourages your body to get rid of excess estrogen, which seems to aggravate the condition. Take 400 to 600 IU a day. (Get your doctor's go-ahead first.)

Feast on fiber. Build your diet around plant foods, such as fruits, vegetables, and legumes, and whole grain bread, pasta, and cereals. A low-fat, high-fiber diet lowers estrogen levels, which means less lumpiness and discomfort.

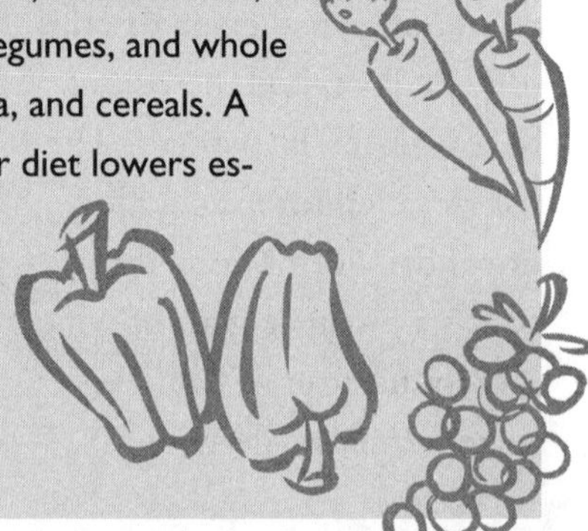

NEWS FLASH

If you ever need breast cancer surgery, check your calendar. A study found that women who undergo breast cancer surgery after day 12 and before day 3 of their menstrual cycles have a better long-term prognosis than those who have the surgery at other times.

to 2 cups of hot water. Dip a wash cloth in the solution and apply it to your skin.

Soothe with castor oil. Castor oil is great for relieving tenderness and breaking up fibrous tissue, says Green. Dip a dry washcloth in some castor oil and apply it to your breasts. Place a hot-water bottle on top of the washcloth for 20 to 30 minutes. Or, rub the castor oil directly onto your breasts. Cover them with plastic wrap and a thin towel. Place a hot-water bottle on top for the same amount of time.

Helpful Hint

If you have sensitive skin, rub some vegetable oil on your breasts before applying the ginger compress. The oil may help prevent your skin from turning red and overheating. ■

Breast Reconstruction Surgery

Stretches to Speed Recovery

One out of three women who has a mastectomy for breast cancer elects to have breast reconstruction immediately after surgery. Using either an implant or skin and fat "borrowed" from the abdomen, surgeons can recreate a fairly natural looking new breast, with a reasonable facsimile of a nipple.

You can—and should—do everything you can do to speed healing from postmastectomy reconstruction, says G. Patrick Maxwell, M.D., director of the Institute for Reconstructive Surgery at Baptist Hospital in Nashville.

"The whole purpose of breast reconstruction is emotional and physical healing," says Dr. Maxwell. The faster you heal physically, the more fully you'll heal emotionally.

Specifically, it's critical that you perform certain stretches to prevent excessive scarring, stiffness, and a "frozen shoulder," says Dr. Maxwell. "The body tries to curl up as it forms scars, making you hunch down and your arm flex inward," he explains.

As soon as any swelling and tenderness from your reconstruction has subsided, Dr. Maxwell suggests stretching your arms and back with the following exercises. (Check with your surgeon to be sure these are appropriate for you and report any pain you may feel during or after doing these stretches.)

Arm stretch: Stand with your side to the wall. Lift ››

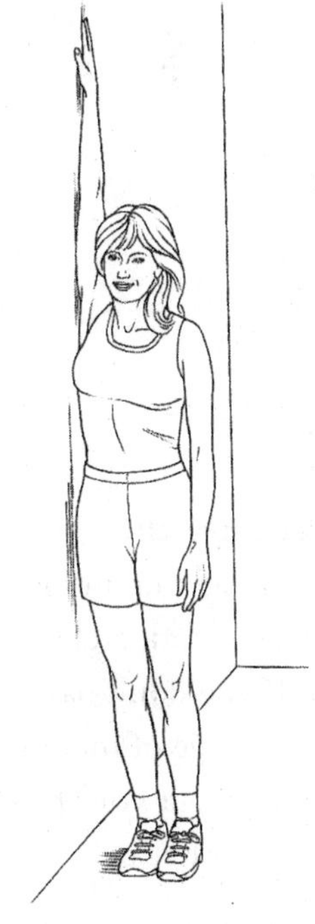

your arm and touch the wall with your arm at a right angle to the wall. Keep stepping closer to the wall, moving your arm up until it is extended over your head and your armpit is pushing into the wall. (It may take a few weeks before you can get your arm all the way up.) Change sides and do the other arm.

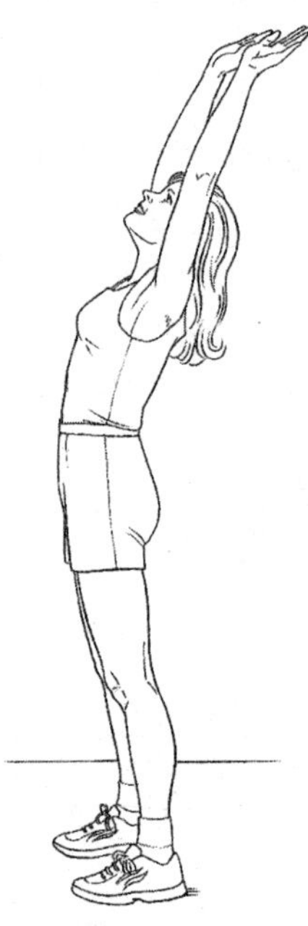

Back stretch: Extend your hands straight up in the air and bend backward, arching your back. If you don't have enough range of motion in your arms, put your hands on your upper buttocks instead. ■

Brittle Nails

Out with Quick-Drying Polish

What woman hasn't found herself flailing her arms wildly, trying to speed-dry her nails while her husband waits so that they can leave for a party? Or putting on a pair of pantyhose with half-dry nails, only to botch the polish and the stockings?

Quick-dry nail polishes are incredibly convenient. Your nails dry in 60 seconds or less. But they have a couple of drawbacks.

"Quick-drying nail polishes chip faster than regular polish, and they can also make your nails more brittle," says Diane Hengstler, a supervisor and manicurist at Gordon Phillips beauty school in Philadelphia. The quick-drying varieties contain more formaldehyde and alcohol than regular polish, so they dry faster. But those same ingredients dry out your nails and make them prone to splitting, peeling, and breaking.

So if you're nails are brittle, use regular polish instead, says Hengstler. **To speed-dry your nails naturally,** dump a tray of ice cubes into your bathroom sink and fill it with cold water. Then, after each coat, dip your newly painted nails into the cold water for a minute or two. When you take your hands out of the water, your nail polish will be miraculously dry.

"The cold water acts as a curing agent to set the polish," explains Hengstler. (Drying your nails with your blow dryer on the cool setting also works, though not as quickly as cold water.)

Helpful Hint

Stash a few tubes of petroleum jelly that's marketed for chapped lips in convenient places: your purse, desk drawer, and car. A few times a day, rub it on your nails and cuticles. **It's an easy, inexpensive remedy for dry, brittle nails.** ■

Broken Condoms

Next-Day Contraception

In 1220 B.C.*, tribesmen in Egypt fashioned the first condoms: sheaths of animal skin to protect their private parts from infection, injury, and insect bites. In the 1500s, an Italian invented a glans-shaped linen sheath that he claimed protected men from syphilis. By the 1700s, condoms made of animal gut were used as contraceptives. Yet despite thousands of years of evolving technology, science has yet to guarantee perfection. Condoms still break.*

It if happens to you, pick up the phone and dial your doctor immediately. If used within 72 hours after unprotected sex, emergency contraception—a special combination of birth control pills—will reduce the chance of pregnancy by 75 percent, says Robert Hatcher, M.D., professor of gynecology and obstetrics at Emory University in Atlanta and co-author of Contraceptive Technology *and* Emergency Contraception.

A fertilized egg takes 5 to 7 days to travel from the fallopian tubes to the uterus to become implanted. Emergency contraception prevents pregnancy by keeping the fertilized egg from becoming implanted. If the regimen is started too late after the egg is implanted, it doesn't work—the pregnancy continues with little or no risk to the fetus. But emergency contraception is not an abortion.

Also, don't call it the "morning-after pill," urges Dr. Hatcher. Depending on the formulation, it's a series of one, two, four, or five pills taken over 12 hours and effective up to 72 hours after unprotected intercourse. It's not taken only on the morning following intercourse (although it's best if you start the series immediately). "Emergency contraception is available, effective, and safe," says Dr. Hatcher. "And the sooner it's initiated, the better."

If you don't have a regular doctor or nearby women's health/family planning center, you can call a toll-free hotline (1-888-NOT-2-LATE) for a directory of health care providers in your area who can prescribe emergency contraceptives.

Helpful Hints

A condom is most likely to break before ejaculation, ››

DON'T MAKE THIS MISTAKE

Emergency contraception is not as effective as regular, consistent contraception, so use it only as a back-up on an emergency basis.

DON'T USE A CONDOM AS A WATER BALLOON

A condom is more likely to break because the people using it, not the people who made it, goofed. Experts who studied how often condoms break and why offers these inside tips.

- Don't open the wrapper with your teeth. For that matter, don't use *any* sharp object (scissors, knife, pencil) to open the condom. It should tear open easily using only your fingers.
- Don't unroll the condom before putting it on. Place it on the head of the erect penis and unroll it down the shaft.
- Don't use the condom inside out.
- Don't test the condom by filling it with water before sex.

not after, when the risk of pregnancy is very small—provided you notice it in time and he withdraws. If the condom slips off after ejaculation, however, pregnancy is more likely. "To avoid slippage, the man must grasp the base of the penis and the condom after ejaculation and withdraw the condom and penis together soon after.

Worried about future breaks? Try a female condom. Made of plastic, they're 40 times as strong as male condoms, which are made of latex. Their breakage rate is only 0.2 percent, says Mary Ann Leeper, president of the Female Health Company, which makes the Reality Female Condom. ■

Bronchitis

Antibiotics May Be the Last Thing You Need

Call it "broncho-sore-is": Congestion, coughing, wheezing, and fever leave you sicker than an ailing prehistoric reptile. When the bronchial tree becomes inflamed with bronchitis, airways narrow and the surfaces of the airways become damaged, generally wreaking havoc on your lungs. It's often caused by the same viruses that are responsible for upper respiratory tract infections—in fact, bronchitis sometimes goes hand in hand with the common cold. It can also be brought on by smoking or air pollution.

Meanwhile, with every coughing episode, you feel as though your lungs are being ripped out of your chest.

Don't rush for the antibiotics. Bronchitis is usually caused by a viral infection, and antibiotics are effective only against bacterial infections. Still, many women (and men) coax their physicians into prescribing antibiotics because they think it will help them beat the infection. But taking antibiotics when they're not completely necessary can actually do more harm than good, says Irwin Ziment, M.D., professor and chief of medicine at Olive View–UCLA Medical

Broken Nails

Good As New in No Time

So there you were, making a snow globe out of a baby food jar from directions in *Martha Stewart Living*. Suddenly, just as you were gluing a tiny pine tree to the lid of the jar, you broke a nail clear off. There's blood everywhere, your finger is throbbing in pain, and the snow globe project is history.

Okay, breaking a nail isn't the drama of a good soap opera, but it can be traumatic to you. Depending on how far down it breaks—and whether it breaks off cleanly or is still partially attached—a broken nail can leave you feeling like you're all thumbs for weeks. Everyday tasks like shampooing your hair or typing at a computer are impossible or hurt like the dickens.

Center in Sylmar, California, and an expert in respiratory pharmacology. It creates a void by eliminating harmless bacteria, and then other, more harmful, bacteria can come in. Antibiotics should be reserved for use only when other treatments have failed and symptoms persist or worsen over a few days, he says.

If you've been diagnosed with bronchitis, the following strategies can speed recovery and help prevent future episodes.

Drink lung-friendly herbal tea. Herbs such as mullein, horehound, coltsfoot and seneca have all been used successfully as expectorants, says Dr. Ziment. To make a tea out of any of these herbs (which are available at health food stores), steep 1 to 2 teaspoonfuls of the dried leaves in 8 ounces of hot water. Steep for 10 minutes, strain, and drink while still warm. If you want, add a teaspoon of honey as a sweetener. The steam from the hot tea will help to thin the mucus, and the expectorant properties of the herbs will help you cough it up. Do not use coltsfoot for more than a week. Seneca isn't intended for long-term use either, and it shouldn't be used at all if you have gastritis or gastric ulcers.

Swig chicken soup. And be sure to add lots of hot, pungent spices like pepper, garlic, and curry powder, says Dr. Ziment. The warm fluid and the pungent spices will help break up stagnant mucus in your beleaguered lungs, and these natural expectorants will aid in getting rid of the mucus.

DON'T MAKE THIS MISTAKE

If you have bronchitis, don't take a cough suppressant, says Anne Davis, M.D., associate professor of clinical medicine at New York University Medical Center. Coughing is one of your body's methods of fighting the disease, by helping to expel phlegm and mucus. If you take a drug to stop coughing, you'll undermine your body's natural defense. If you have a persistent, unproductive cough (lasts more than 3 days), you should see your doctor to rule out more serious conditions.

Gargle. Dr. Ziment suggests this home remedy: Add 1 teaspoon each of horseradish, honey, and Tabasco sauce to a glass of water. Gargle and ››

No need to suffer. Just go to the nearest nail salon and have one artificial nail, tip, or silk wrap applied to the broken nail. If your finger is bleeding, you need to wait until it stops to have the new nail applied. The artificial nail or wrap will help protect sensitive exposed skin that hurts when you bump it.

And don't worry: Whether you like to wear your nails long or short, you won't have to touch the rest of your nails. "A professional manicurist can make the artificial nail look just like the other nails," says Diane Hengstler, a supervisor and manicurist at Gordon Phillips beauty school in Philadelphia.

You can keep the artificial nail in place for up to a month, or until your own nail grows back completely. ■

then swallow the mixture several times a day. It may have an unpleasant effect, but that's partly why it works: the pungent spices will stick to your throat and stimulate the secretion of water in your airways, which results in a thinning of the sticky mucus.

Once you've had bronchitis, you're more susceptible to getting it again. To help prevent future episodes and the development of chronic bronchitis, Dr. Ziment suggests the following:

• Eat garlic and hot spices every day. If you're concerned about smelly side effects, garlic pills usually work just as well.

• Exercise your lungs and chest muscles to keep them strong. Swimming, walking, and jogging are all good choices because they strengthen the respiratory muscles and help keep mucus flowing.

• Deep breathing or exercises like tai chi (a series of fluid movements based on martial arts) or yoga help the lungs open up and prevent them from getting sticky.

• Don't smoke. It's one of the surest ways to develop chronic bronchitis.

CHEST CONGESTION? TRY THIS HERBAL RUB

Mix ½ teaspoon of the essential oil myrrh (available at most health food stores) with 1 tablespoon of sweet almond or sunflower oil. Apply to your chest as needed. When used as a chest rub, myrrh helps get rid of thick phlegm caused by severe colds and bronchitis. The essential oil may be toxic at high concentrations—that's why you must dilute it in a carrier oil such as sunflower or sweet almond.

Helpful Hint

The antioxidants found in fruits and vegetables (vitamins A, C, and E) appear to have a protective effect on the lungs and seem to help prevent lung problems like bronchitis. Eating five servings of fruits and vegetables (including garlic and onions) every day is the best way to get this protective effect, says Dr. Ziment. ■

Bruises

Wipe Out Black-and-Blue Marks with Blueberries

When shin and table—or knee and sidewalk or forehead and trunk lid—collide, they leave behind a nasty reminder of your, uh, lack of attention: a brilliant black-and-blue bruise.

Unlike cuts, which bleed on the skin's surface, bruises are caused by blood collecting in the tissue right under the skin. And they aren't easy to hide. In the days that follow, they take an autumnal path from usually red at first to purplish black to blue to brown and finally yellow, visual signs that the spilled blood under the tissue is slowly being reabsorbed by your body.

You can't do much to cover up bruises, but you can help speed up their disappearing act by eating blueberries. Blueberries are a rich source of flavonoids and a good source of vitamin C, which together improve blood circulation (which reduces swelling) and help form collagen, the tissue that holds skin cells together, says Mark Stengler, N.D., a naturopathic physician in San Diego. Blueberries contain a type of flavonoid called proanthocyanidins, which are known for strengthening the walls of capillaries weakened by bruising.

Or try pineapple. This tropical fruit contains bromelain, a protein-digesting enzyme that works to stop inflammation of the bruised area.

So next time you need a cure for what nailed you, try one or any combination of the following, all rich in bruise-banishing healing agents (stick to fresh if possible).

Blueberries: one handful twice a day

Pineapple: ½ cup twice a day

Mango: one peeled fruit once a day

Cantaloupe: ½ once a day

Strawberries: 1 cup once a day

To speed up healing even faster, take these vitamins with your fruit cure.

Vitamin C: 1,000 milligrams once a day

Vitamin E: 400 IU once a day

Vitamin A: 10,000 IU once a day

These necessary antioxidants will repair damaged cells, strengthen blood vessel walls, form collagen, and reduce inflammation. ■

Bunions

When Pain Is Afoot, Try These Soothing Steps

Even if you never leave your hometown, you'll still probably walk the equivalent of four laps around the earth in your lifetime. That's 8,000 to 10,000 strides per day for a lifetime total of 115,000 miles. It's easy to overlook the workhorse role of feet—until they ache.

Women can often blame unrelenting foot pain on bunions, those unflattering bony protrusions that lead to tenderness, inflammation, and a crippled big toe. Although bunions can be an inherited trait, tight-fitting, pointed-toe shoes make the problem worse because of the constant pressure and friction placed on the big toe every time you squeeze it into a shoe, says Kathleen Stone, D.P.M., a podiatrist in Glendale, Arizona. But you can take steps toward a pain-free stride. Here's a day-long plan from Dr. Stone.

Wake up with a foot massage. Before you get out of bed, spend 5 to 10 minutes rubbing and kneading your entire foot—not just where the bunion is. Move each toe gently back and forth. This do-it-yourself massage will loosen the muscles, improve joint mobility, and get blood flowing before your feet hit the ground.

Park a pair of shoes by your bedside. Make a habit of stepping into a pair of moccasins or sneakers when you get out of bed. Either shoe provides adequate cushion and toe-wiggle room until you're ready to put on your work shoes.

Rise up against the pain. During your lunch hour and late afternoon, prop your feet on a box or upturned trash basket for 10 minutes. The longer you stay on your feet during the day, the more they are apt to swell and hurt from the pressure of your own body weight. Elevating your feet, even slightly, relieves the pressure and the pain, says Dr. Stone. ››

IS YOUR FOOTWEAR *TOO* COMFY?

Avoid walking around in flip-flops or household slippers. Sure, they're comfortable, but they offer no support or cushioning. "These types of footwear do not control the forces that lead to the deformity. In fact, they contribute to problems," says Glenn Gastwirth, D.P.M., a podiatrist and executive director of the American Podiatric Medical Association in Bethesda, Maryland.

Take a cool plunge. After dinner, reduce swelling by treating your feet to a 10-minute soak in a tub of cool water. Warm water might feel soothing at first, but it can actually make pain and swelling worse. Cool water, on the other hand, permeates

Burnout

Put Yourself First for a Change

As director of the Career Development Office at Smith College in North Hampton, Massachusetts, Barbara Reinhold, Ed.D., sees plenty of women who start out their adult lives with energy and enthusiasm, only to end up feeling exhausted, cynical, and ineffective at midlife.

The women Dr. Reinhold counsels say they feel squeezed from all sides. At work, their bosses pile on projects. At home, their husbands won't help with the housework and their children expect them to be cook, chauffeur, laundress, nurse, and financier. "On top of that, many find themselves taking care of aging parents," says Dr. Reinhold, author of Toxic Work: How to Overcome Stress, Overload, and Burnout and Revitalize Your Career. *Burnout can affect anyone, but women in jobs that combine heavy workloads with minimal control—like waitressing—are more susceptible than executives.*

"Burnout happens when the stresses are too strong and the rewards too few," says Dr. Reinhold. You might be contributing to burnout without even realizing it, she adds, if you believe that you must work like a slave to be loved, be a good person, or prove that you're as good as others.

Burnout can manifest itself as any one of a multitude of problems, including frequent colds or bouts of the flu or bronchitis, neck or joint pain, headache, upset stomach, moodiness, troubled sleep, tension with family and friends, even heart disease. If you're burned out, don't expect the problem to go away by itself. Take steps to change the situation. Here's how.

Ask for help. If your job consists of a never-ending series of crises, meet with your supervisor to map out a better way to handle problems that arise. Consider a team approach, job sharing, or other ways to share responsibilities at work. At home, let your hus-

the skin to reduce swelling.

Have a nightcap of E. Keep a supply of vitamin E gel capsules in the refrigerator. Before heading for bed, open up one capsule for each foot and rub in its cool, healing gel. "Vitamin E is a vital skin vitamin that really seems to help with swelling and achy joints," says Dr. Stone.

If none of these remedies helps, or if your bunions seem to be getting bigger and more painful, see a podiatrist. You may need corrective surgery to realign the big toe joint and restore normal function.

Helpful Hint

Make sure that the widest part of your foot corresponds to the widest part of your shoe. To check if the shoe is roomy enough for you, make sure that you can wiggle your toes freely inside the shoe. ■

band and kids know that you expect everyone to help around the house. If you're taking care of an ailing parent, insist that your siblings help out, or consider home care services for the elderly.

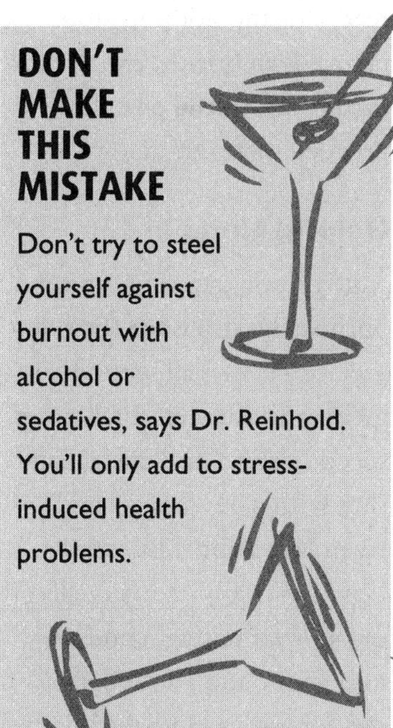

DON'T MAKE THIS MISTAKE

Don't try to steel yourself against burnout with alcohol or sedatives, says Dr. Reinhold. You'll only add to stress-induced health problems.

Slow down—or stop. "If you have a tendency toward burnout, you probably try to do too much too fast," says Dr. Reinhold. "'Let me think about it and get back to you' are 10 lifesaving words you need to use often." Or, learn to say no without feeling guilty. (For more tips on how to manage overwork, see page 327.)

Take minibreaks. Since overwork is the first step toward burnout, it's essential for women to schedule regular respites from the daily grind, says Lynne McClure, Ph.D., owner of a management consulting firm in Phoenix. "If you can't afford the time or money for a long vacation, try to schedule at least a few days off."

Helpful Hints

If you're burned out because you're bored with your job or no longer find it satisfying, ask to exchange part of your job with a coworker, become a mentor to a new employee, or transfer to another project or part of the company, suggests Dr. Reinhold.

Sometimes burnout is easily remedied, and sometimes it's not. Consult a counselor if, despite your efforts for relief, you feel hopelessly exhausted—especially if feelings of depression linger for more than 2 weeks, or if a sense of being burned out interferes with your ability to do your job, interact socially, or function in other ways. ■

Burns

Skin-Saving Strategies from a Top Chef

After 12 years in the kitchen, Katy Sparks, executive chef of Quilty's, a busy restaurant in the heart of New York City, knows how to dodge a burn. She has learned the hard way.

"Cooking in restaurants is about speed and precision—beginners tend to burn themselves quite a bit," says Sparks during a break between the lunch and dinner crowds. "The worst burn I ever got was a nasty grease burn on my face. But I was lucky—it healed nicely."

Home cooks are more likely to burn their hands than their faces. But you can learn a lot about preventing kitchen burns from Sparks—with added advice from J. Crit Harley, M.D., a behavioral medicine specialist and former emergency room physician in Hendersonville, North Carolina. Here's how.

• To avoid grease splatter burns **when you brown foods** like chicken breasts in a pan of hot oil, gently place food in the pan. "Never drop food into a pan—you're more likely to get splattered that way," says Sparks. "You just can't move your hand fast enough to avoid the splatter."

• **When removing a hot uncovered pot or pan of food from the stove,** hold it away from your body, tipped away slightly, so that any splashes are directed away from you, says Sparks.

• **Stock plenty of oven mitts** and potholders within easy reach of the stove. Teflon-coated fabrics with a good grip are best, says Dr. Harley. Toss out any that are frayed or worn or that have burn holes.

• Before you remove hot dishes from the oven, stove top, or microwave, **make sure you have plenty of counter space** on which to set them. "Too often, we're pulling a hot meat dish with gravy out of the oven and there's no room for it on the counter," says Dr. Harley. "Before we know it, the hot gravy is splashing around like a tidal wave."

• Slow down. The more hurried you are, the more likely you are to not pay attention and set yourself up for a kitchen burn. Before you reach for the hot pot, stop, take a deep breath, exhale, and **focus only on the pot**. Then proceed, says Dr. Harley.

Helpful Hints

If you do get a superficial burn without blisters (first degree or very small second degree), you can get quick relief, speed healing, and avoid scarring with aloe vera gel and lavender essential oil, says David Winston, a nationally recognized herbalist and ethnobotanist and a founder of the American Herbalist's Guild. **Keep a vial of lavender**

DON'T MAKE THIS MISTAKE

Never spread butter or margarine on a burn. While a cool, solid fat may feel soothing, butter and margarine contain salt, which draws water out of cells, causing them to collapse—which slows down the healing process. Slathering a burn with butter or margarine can also accelerate bacteria growth and lead to infection, warns Dr. Harley.

oil and an aloe plant on the counter or windowsill. In addition to relieving pain, the aloe-lavender combination reduces inflammation, redness, and swelling and might protect burns from infection.

Mix a couple spoonfuls of fresh aloe gel—scooped right out of a broken leaf of the plant—with a drop of lavender oil and apply as frequently as needed. You can keep the mixture in a glass or ceramic dish covered with plastic wrap in the refrigerator for as long as you need it. ■

Bursitis and Tendinitis

Ice + Spice for Shoulder Pain

Yow! Those 18 holes of golf a day you played on your vacation sure were fun. Too bad your shoulder feels like you beat it with your nine iron. What's up?

"You probably have either bursitis or tendinitis," says Lynne Nicolson, M.D., chief of physical medicine and rehabilitation at Sunnyview Rehabilitation Center in Schenectady, New York. One is an inflammation of the bursa, or fluid-filled sacs that absorb the shock of any forceful movement. The other is an inflammation of any tendon that connects muscle to bone.

Any effort that repeatedly stresses the same joint—say, painting your bedroom, washing all the windows in your house, or raking leaves for hours—can trigger bursitis or tendinitis, especially if you're out of shape or don't stretch regularly.

"You probably can't tell which one you have—the pain is similar for bursitis and tendinitis, and they can both be caused by overuse," says Dr. Nicolson. "And it really ››

FREE UP A FROZEN SHOULDER

Pain may make you shy away from moving your shoulder, but it's very important to keep it mobile. If you move it less and less, muscles and tendons will contract and the joint will stiffen, making it difficult to move, even after the inflammation subsides. To prevent "frozen shoulder," gently use your arm every day, even if it hurts to move it. "If it's too painful to use the muscles, use the unaffected arm to move the affected arm," suggests Dr. Nicolson.

doesn't matter which you have—the treatment is the same for both." If symptoms do not respond to the suggestions below or get worse after 3 to 4 days, see your doctor, especially if you can't move your shoulder.

- Stop what you're doing.
- Apply cold packs—15 to 20 minutes on, every 4 to 6 hours—for the first 24 to 36 hours. (A bag of ice cubes wrapped in cloth will do.)
- Perform range-of-motion exercises in a hot tub, bathtub, whirlpool, or swimming pool. Let the limb float, and let the buoyancy of the water move it gently, without pushing.
- If you still feel stiff, and there is no swelling, apply a heating pad.

A CURE FOR MOUSE SHOULDER

Using a computer for hours at a time, day after day (or night after night) can leave you with "mouse shoulder"—bursitis-like pain in the shoulder of whatever hand you use to manipulate your computer mouse.

"The problem comes from using a computer mouse that is located too high, too low, or at a poor angle," explains Dr. Lee. "Use a desk and chair designed for computer use, not the dining room table." Ideally, the mouse should be lower than your elbow and on the same level of your keyboard, if possible, which will allow your shoulders to remain relaxed and comfortable.

Other Natural Remedies

Used with standard treatments—such as ice, range-of-motion exercise, and painkillers—alternative remedies can speed relief, says Alison Lee, M.D., acupuncturist, specialist in pain management, and medical director of the Barefoot Doctors in Ann Arbor, Michigan.

Here's what else you can try at home.

- Rub the area with Tiger Balm, a Chinese massage cream scented with menthol, one or two times a day or as needed. Look for Tiger Balm in health food stores or pharmacies.
- If you can't find Tiger Balm, make a paste of water and tumeric powder (a spice used in curry dishes). Rub it on the shoulder that hurts one or two times a day or as needed.
- Add a tablespoon or two of flaxseed oil to your salad dressing. Omega-3 fatty acids in flaxseed oil reduce inflammation. This is most appropriate if you have recurring bursitis or tendinitis. ■

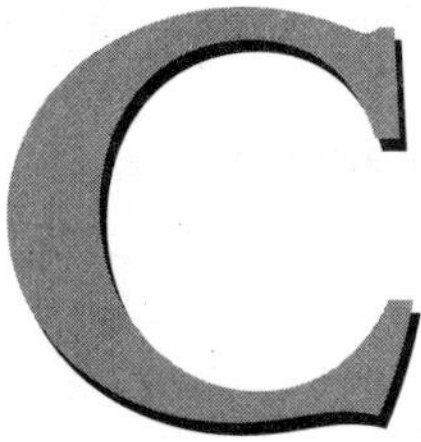

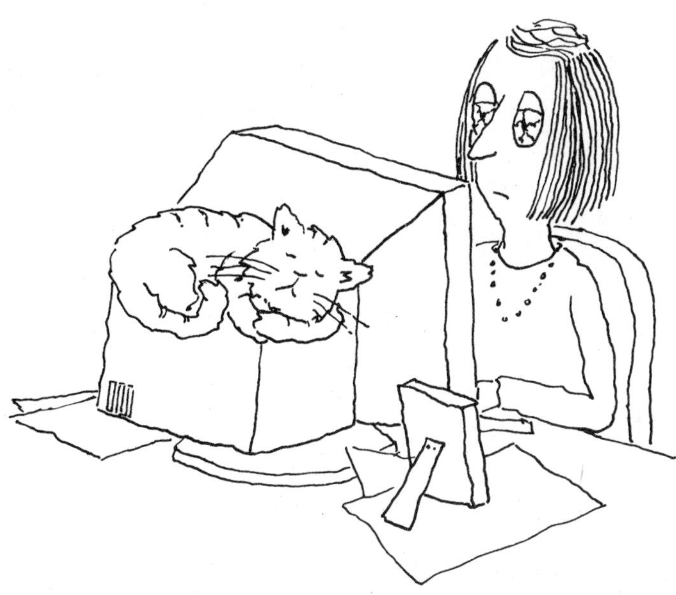

Spending hours at a computer, at home or at work,
can leave your eyes itchy, red, and dried out.
For instant relief, see page 98.

Caffeine

Five Hidden Benefits of Drinking Coffee

Sometimes it seems the only difference between medical researchers and the rest of us is that they need lots of studies to know what we could have told them in the first place. As stimulants go, coffee is a great pick-me-up.

And consumed in moderation, it won't hurt you. "Of the hundreds of studies of caffeine, 90 percent are positive—that is, there's no hint of lasting damage," says Manfred Kroger, Ph.D., professor of food science at Pennsylvania State University in University Park. The 85 to 120 milligrams of caffeine in an 8-ounce cup of coffee (36 to 54 milligrams for a can of soda) can benefit you in several ways.

1. It gives you a mental edge. Coffee's wake-up call tests out just as well in the lab as at the breakfast table. In one study conducted by researchers at Johns Hopkins University in Baltimore, for example, volunteers felt more awake, confidant, and eager to work each time they were given caffeine. Other studies show that as little as ⅓ cup of coffee—just a few sips—helps you perform math or read more quickly. "Alertness and mental skills go together," Dr. Kroger says. "After a cup of coffee, I can do crossword puzzles better and faster because I'm more alert."

2. It helps you exercise. Need a little help getting through that 6:00 P.M. aerobics class? Caffeine also appears to help your muscles burn their fuel stores more efficiently and contract more intensely. That's why Olympic officials limit caffeine consumption by competitors—it gives them an unfair advantage.

3. It reduces your risk of gallstones. A large, long-term study at Harvard University discovered that men who drank 2 to 3 cups of regular coffee per day had a 40 percent lower risk of developing gallstone disease than the coffee abstainers. Since women are even more prone to gallstones than men, the benefits could very well be even higher for women.

4. It relieves pain. Headache? Try coffee. Caffeine is added to some over-the-counter pain relievers because combining caffeine with aspirin, acetaminophen (such as Excedrin Extra Strength or Anacin) or ››

DON'T MAKE THIS MISTAKE

Just because 2 cups of coffee help you stay alert doesn't mean that you'll be twice as sharp with 4. "Too much caffeine has a negative effect," Dr. Kroger says. More than a cup or 2 a day (3, tops) for some people contributes to sleeplessness, to say nothing of the notorious (and very real) "coffee nerves." "Overindulge, and you'll be able to do less instead of more. My best advice," says Dr. Kroger, "is to know your limits."

ibuprofen (Advil, Motrin) makes the active ingredient work better. Some research even shows that caffeine alone reduces pain, perhaps by slightly decreasing bloodflow in the head.

5. It's a great no-cal dessert option. Assuming you enjoy its natural taste, unaltered by cream and sugar, coffee offers a virtually calorieless way to sip dessert. "Coffee enhances socialization," Dr. Kroger says. "That's why people gather at the coffee urn. It's part of American and European culture." If you don't care for it black, try something brewed with flavored coffee beans, or have a fat-free milk latte.

Helpful Hint

A cup of coffee is mostly water, but caffeine is a diuretic—it stimulates urination, so you'll lose about half of that fluid in a few hours. To stay ahead of the hydration game, drink at least one extra glass of water for every cup of coffee (or any other caffeinated beverage). ■

Calcium

Handy Ways to Build Bone Even If You Don't Drink Milk by the Glass

Calcium is a mineral that means different things to different people," says Barbara Dixon,R.D., a nutrition educator in Baton Rouge, Louisiana. "If you want to stand up tall at age 75, calcium is your insurance policy to do just that. If you have high blood pressure, calcium can bring it down and keep it down," says Dixon.

Did you know that calcium is also needed for a normal heartbeat, nerve and muscle function, blood clotting, and a healthy immune system? Pretty impressive list of benefits, wouldn't you say?

Unfortunately, most women don't drink the three to four glasses of milk a day to get the 1,000 to 1,200 milligrams of calcium necessary for optimum health. You're more likely to avoid it altogether if it doesn't taste good, you're lactose intolerant, or you believe that milk just doesn't go with any of your meals—except maybe breakfast. You'll be happy to know that you don't have to drink milk by the glass to get your daily calcium needs. Here are a whole host of ways to get more of the calcium you need if you don't drink milk by the glass.

More Than 400 Milligrams

Rolaids: 550 milligrams per tablet

Viactiv soft calcium chews: 500 milligrams per chew

Edy's fat-free frozen yogurt: 450 milligrams per ½-cup serving; 900 milligrams per cup

Tums: 400 milligrams per 2 tablets

Calcium supplements: 400 milligrams calcium carbonate; 380 milligrams dicalcium phosphate; 210 milligrams calcium citrate

Calcium-fortified Total cereal with fat-free milk: 400 milligrams per ¾-cup serving of Total with ½ cup of fat-free milk

200–400 Milligrams

Alba dairy shake mix: Chocolate, vanilla, and strawberry; 350 milligrams per 8-ounce serving when prepared with water, 500 milligrams when prepared with half water and half fat-free milk

Calcium-fortified orange juice: 300 to 350 milligrams per 8-ounce serving

Breakfast smoothie: In a blender, combine 1 cup of fat-free or low-fat milk, ½ cup of frozen banana slices, 1 tablespoon of peanut butter, ¼ teaspoon of ground cinnamon, ½ teaspoon of vanilla extract, and sweetened cocoa powder (optional). Blend all ingredients until creamy (300 milligrams per 8-ounce serving).

Silk Soy Milk: Chocolate, vanilla, or plain; 300 milligrams per 1 cup

Kelloggs calcium-fortified Eggo waffles: 300 milligrams per serving (two waffles)

Healthy Choice cheese French bread pizza: 250 milligrams for 1 pizza (1 serving)

Café latte or café mocha with fat-free milk: Small: 237 milligrams; medium: 316 milligrams; large: 395 milligrams.

Low-fat or fat-free yogurt: 200 to 350 milligrams per 8-ounce serving

Up to 300 Milligrams

Fat-free or reduced-fat cheese: 200 to 300 milligrams per two 1-ounce slices

DON'T MAKE THIS MISTAKE

If you take supplements as your primary source of calcium, take 400 IU of vitamin D and 300 milligrams of magnesium daily to ensure calcium absorption.

Calcium-fortified Light and Lively cottage cheese: 200 milligrams per ½-cup serving

Kelloggs calcium-fortified Nutri-Grain bars: 200 milligrams per bar

Campbell's Healthy Request condensed cream-based soups prepared with fat-free milk: 170 to 300 milligrams per 1-cup serving of Cream of Mushroom, Cream of Celery, Cream of Broccoli, or Cream of Chicken

Fat-free instant pudding mix prepared with fat-free milk: 150 milligrams per ½-cup serving

Fat-free tapioca pudding mix prepared with fat-free milk: 150 milligrams per ½-cup serving

Campbell's Plus Ready-to-Serve Soups: 100 milligrams per 1-cup serving of Hearty Minestrone, Roasted Vegetables with Barley and Wild Rice, Tomato Garden Vegetables, or Pasta and Vegetables

Rice pudding: 80 milligrams per ½-cup serving ■

Calorie Counting

A Simple Formula for Dieters Who Hate Math

Which would you rather do: count calories or watch the grass grow?

If you chose the latter, you're probably not alone.

"Calorie counting isn't much fun," says Linda Eck Clemens, R.D., Ed.D., professor of consumer science and education at the University of Memphis. "It's boring and limiting because it places the emphasis on what you can't eat."

There's no way to get around it, though: If you want to lose weight, you have to be aware of how many calories you consume and expend. It's the scientific basis for maintaining or losing weight.

Here's a simple three-step plan, calculated for your body weight.

1. To figure out how many calories a day your body uses at your present weight: Divide your current weight by 2.2 (to convert pounds to kilograms). Then, multiply your weight in kilograms by 30 (the amount of calories you need per pound of body weight). If you're 160 pounds, you weigh 72.7 kilograms. Multiply 72.7 by 30, and you arrive at 2,182 calories. Eat more, and you'll gain weight. Eat less, and you'll lose weight. Eat neither more nor less, and you'll stay the same.

2. To figure out how many calories a day you should eat to lose weight: Multiply your weight (in kilograms) by 25. So if you weigh 160 pounds, to lose about 1½ pounds a week, you'd need to consume 1,817 calories, or 365 fewer calories per day.

Carpal Tunnel Syndrome

Tame the Tingling with Yoga

What do computer operators, race car drivers, and mail sorters share in common? All are prone to wrist pain known as carpal tunnel syndrome (CTS).

CTS is a debilitating condition caused by irritated, swollen tendons pressing against both blood vessels and a major nerve that leads from the arm into the fingers. Bloodflow is reduced, and the squeezed nerve causes pain, tingling, or even burning sensations in the hand, fingers, and thumb. Repetitive motions of the hands and wrists, such as tapping computer keys for hours and other activities that could overwork the hands and wrists, may cause CTS.

Traditional remedies range from prescription drugs and over-the-counter pain medications to surgery. But Marian Garfinkel, Ph.D., has uncovered a new solution: yoga.

"Yoga is about getting the mind and body to work as one in the present moment. It teaches you how to strengthen, stretch, and promote flexibility in joints, including your wrists," says Dr. Garfinkel, guest lecturer at the Medical College of Pennsylvania (MCP) Hahnemann University in Philadelphia and senior Iyengar yoga teacher.

Dr. Garfinkel directed a study involving 42 men and women with CTS, who used yoga postures to increase grip

3. To figure out how many calories a day you actually consume: For 2 weeks, keep a log of everything you eat and add up the calories. (What you eat standing up, on the run, or on the fly counts, too.) To determine your daily average, divide your total caloric total by 14. If it's considerably higher than the total in step 2, cut out enough food to bring it down to that number.

A good rule of thumb: Cut 250 calories a day to lose ½ pound a week, or 500 calories a day to lose a pound a week. And don't try to lose more than 2 pounds per week.

Helpful Hints

Most of your calories should come from grains, fruits, and vegetables. No more than 30 percent of your calories should come from fat.

If you eat a lot of restaurant meals, be careful. When Dr. Clemens studied the eating habits of 129 women, she found that those who ate out 6 to 13 times a week consumed nearly 300 more calories per day than those who at out 5 times a week or less. "Make sure you're not giving yourself permission to overeat every time you go out," she says. "A lot of people do."

Since exercise uses up calories, it's easier to cut several hundred calories a day without feeling famished. "If you exercise more, you can eat more," Dr. Clemens says. ■

DON'T MAKE THIS MISTAKE

Never "guesstimate" your calorie intake. Studies show that even well-intentioned dieters almost always underestimate.

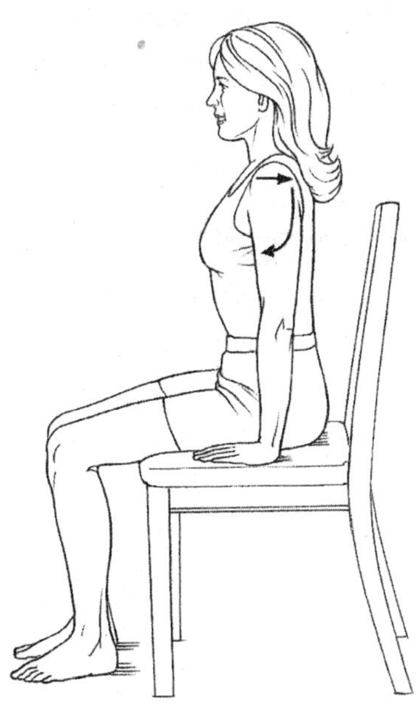

strength while reducing pain. Each of these postures takes about 20 seconds to perform, and can yield positive results. In all of these poses, be sure to keep your shoulders down and away from your ears.

To increase strength and flexibility in your wrists, try these yoga positions.

Shoulder stretch (*left*). Sit in a chair and press your hands into the seat, palm side down. Press your shoulder blades into your back and move your shoulders back and down slowly for 20 seconds. Take care not to tense your shoulders, neck, or face. Relax and repeat. ››

TINGLING? CHECK IT OUT

If you experience persistent tingling in your fingers, don't attempt yoga without first seeing your doctor. You may have an advanced form of CTS that requires more serious attention.

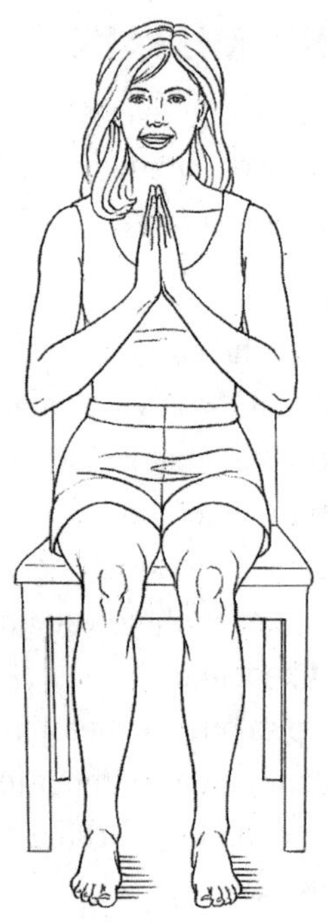

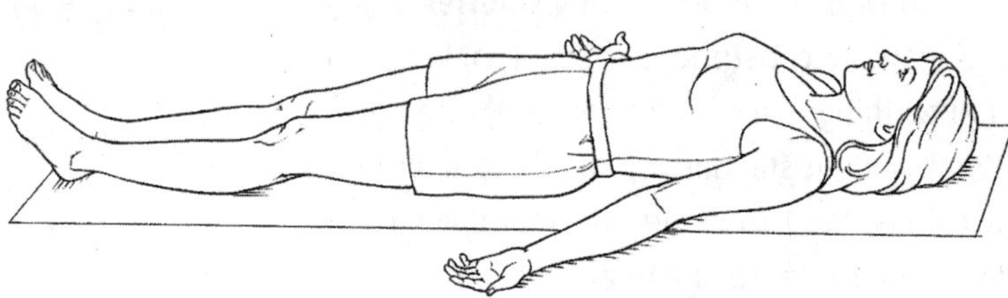

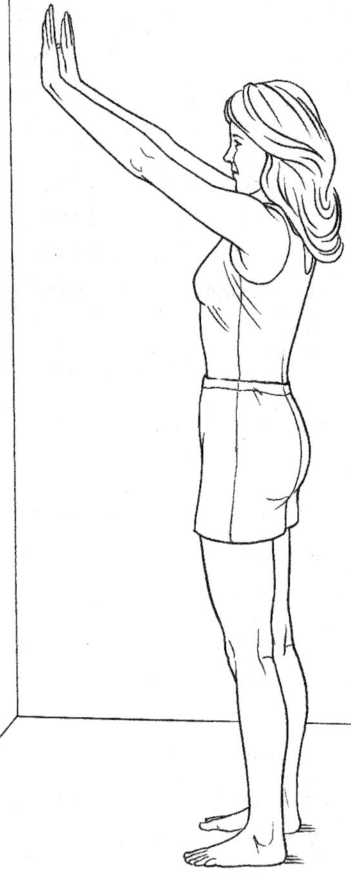

Prayer position (*above*). Sit in a chair. Press the palms and fingers of both hands together in a prayer position. Hold for 20 seconds, then release and press again. Finally, with palms still pressed together, stretch your fingers to increase the distance between them. Hold for 20 seconds and relax. Repeat.

Ceiling reach (*right*). Stand up and stretch your arms and fingers forward and up with your open palms facing the wall directly in front of you. Keep your fingers together and your elbows locked. Keeping your arms straight, continue to slowly stretch your fingers toward the ceiling while keeping your palms facing the wall. Hold for 20 seconds and repeat.

Relaxation pose (*above*). For this final position, lie flat on your back. Keep both arms slightly away from your thighs. Palms should be up, heels together with your feet in a V-position. Close your eyes. Breathe softly, inhaling and exhaling through your nose. Remain in this position for 10 minutes or longer. Bend your legs and roll over on your side to get up.

Helpful Hints

When performing yoga, avoid holding your breath. Inhaling softly and quietly will help you relax and remain focused. ■

Car Safety

Never Do This When You Drive

Tracy Fantaccione is a good example of what not *to do while driving a car. Like a lot of busy women, the 40-year-old marketing consultant from Boca Raton, Florida, talks on her cellular phone. She drives fast. She cranks up the rock music blaring from her car radio. She used to eat a slice of gooey pizza and a salad. She read the newspaper. And, until she poked her eye, she applied eyeliner—while driving on the interstate.*

Fantaccione is lucky, very lucky. Despite her bad driving habits, she has never had an accident. But she has had plenty of near hits.

Fantaccione is all too typical of a growing phenomenon among women (and men) who seem to do anything in their cars but keep their full attention on their driving, putting themselves and others at risk. Don't take these risks.

"Cars used to be designed to take us from here to there," says Carole Guzzetta, director of the National Safety Belt Coalition and former chief of the consumer division for the National Highway Traffic Safety Administration in Washington, D.C. "Now, they've become offices on wheels with portable phones, faxes, laptops, and even small television sets. All these gadgets distract us from driving. And it takes just a split second for a crash to happen."

Safety experts offer these strategies to help you steer clear of accidents.

• Don't balance coffee mugs and sodas on the dashboard or between your knees. Instead, use beverage containers with lids and tapered bottoms that fit in cup holders.

• Avoid fumbling with a map or trying to decipher instructions scribbled on a scrap of paper while driving. Instead, print directions to your destination in large block letters on full-size papers taped to the dashboard in front of you. That way, you can keep both hands on the steering wheel and your eyes on the road. If you get lost or miss a turn, pull over.

• Eat before you start out, not while you drive. On long trips, eat during rest stops.

DON'T MAKE THIS MISTAKE

Never make or take calls on your car or cellular phone while driving. If you're running late, pull over to call ahead. Make business calls on food and rest breaks. You'll also be able to pay more attention to your phone conversation while the car is in park.

Other things you should never do in your car include smoking, changing CDs or audiocassettes, touching up your lipstick or mascara, and polishing your nails. And of course, never drink and drive.

Helpful Hint

Take a look around at other drivers. Ask yourself, "What if the driver ahead of me suddenly decides to turn right without signaling? Or the truck driver next to me swerves into my lane?" Always plan an escape route to prepare for the unexpected. You can't do that if you're on the phone, eating, or applying makeup at the wheel. ■

Cataracts

Cool Ways to Protect Your Eyes from Cloudy Vision

If you're in the habit of donning sunglasses every time you step outdoors, you're already taking an important step in protecting your eyesight for years to come. (And you'll look cool, too.)

Two out of three women over the age of 60 develop cataracts, spots in the lens that tend to develop over time. Initially, these spots don't interfere with vision—you could have minuscule cataracts now and not even know it. With time, however, they can expand, fogging your eyesight as though you were looking through a gauze veil. You wouldn't see blues and violets as well, and oncoming car headlights would create glare.

Cataracts can be caused by a blow to the eye. And to some degree, cataracts are part of the normal aging process. But years of exposure to sunlight can also cause cataracts on the front of the lens, says Sheila West, Ph.D., professor of ophthalmology at the Wilmer Eye Institute at Johns Hopkins University in Baltimore. Evidently, ultraviolet-B (IVB) rays—the same rays that burn unprotected skin—may damage proteins or DNA in the lens of your eyes, possibly similar to the way they damage protein or DNA in your skin.

The effects are cumulative, says Dr. West. In one study of men and women age 65 and older (prime candidates for cataracts), she found that the more time your eyes are exposed to sunlight over your lifetime, your higher the risk of cataracts.

You don't have to live in the dark to prevent cataracts and save your sight. Simply protect your eyes outdoors, whether at work or play. Here's how.

Wear plastic sunglasses anytime you're in the sun. They don't have to be expensive or dark, says Dr. West. Plastic sunglasses (plastic blocks more of the UVB rays than glass) on the market block up to 100 percent of the UVB rays, she says.

Add a wide-brimmed hat or baseball-style cap. It's one more way to decrease sunlight exposure, says Dr. West.

Don't light up. Experts aren't sure why, but heavy smokers are three times as likely to develop cataracts as those who don't smoke.

Swallow some vitamin C. Studies show that supplementing with vitamin C may reduce the risk of cataract development by as much as 77 percent. Most doctors recommend a daily vitamin C supplement of 200 to 500 milligrams.

Helpful Hint

If you wear contact lenses, ask your optometrist or eye care practitioner for contacts with built-in UVB protection. (Most contact lenses have that protection these days.) ■

Cellulite

The One and Only Remedy

We've wrapped it, massaged it, creamed it, and squeezed it. We've tried to starve it out and sweat it out. Still, we just can't get it out.

For decades, the beauty industry has been tantalizing us with magic potions and lotions to help smooth out the unsightly age- and fat-producing dimpled look on our buttocks and thighs known as cellulite. Some women have even resorted to painful and costly liposuction. All for very modest and very temporary results at best.

Now it appears that a "near cure" is on the horizon—if you're willing to pay the price in time and money.

The treatment is call Endermologie, which has been popular in Europe for more than a decade but hit the shores of the United States only a few years ago.

The intense, massagelike treatment involves a device that lifts and works the skin to stretch, relax, and smooth the connective tissue between fat and skin. The result is a diminished look in the quilted appearance of the skin. The rub is that it takes twice-weekly sessions for at least 10 weeks at $100 a pop to get smooth-skin results that last—at best—for only 3 to 4 months. It also includes religious attention to "lifestyle maintenance," which means eating only low-fat foods, drinking a lot of water, and exercising every day.

While it doesn't claim to melt away cellulite, it can smooth out the rough appearance. In fact, suspicious researchers at Vanderbilt University's School of Medicine in Nashville put it to the test using 20 Yucatan minipigs (chosen for their skin's likeness to that of humans) as guinea pigs. After going through 20 Endermologie treatments on one side of their bodies, skin biopsies revealed "what appeared to be new collagen deposited horizontally in the deepest layer of skin tissue," says David Adcock, M.D., one of the researchers. This could be why women are seeing positive results.

"I think Endermologie treatments are a wonderful pampering experience," says Deborah S. Sarnoff, M.D., a dermatologist and assistant clinical professor at New York University Medical Center, who has performed the treatments in her office with "nice results."

"You get a deep massage; you feel good. Women feel like they have more energy, and it's a tool to help them make lifestyle changes and lose weight," says Dr. Sarnoff.

Despite the cost and dedication involved, interest in the technique is taking hold. "Many women believe that if they have the money to splurge, and this is something they really want to do, they make up their minds to do it, and they pamper themselves," says Dr. Sarnoff.

What cost vanity? You have the answer. ■

Cesarean Delivery

Heal Your Whole Body, Not Just the Incision

Whether planned or performed as an emergency, delivering by cesarean section can leave you hurting, physically and emotionally.

"Cesarean section is major abdominal surgery, and it takes at least 6 to 8 weeks to recover," says Margaret Malnory, R.N., clinical nurse specialist for women and children at All Saints Healthcare in Racine, Wisconsin, nurse researcher at the University of Wisconsin Medical School in Madison, and a former labor and delivery room nurse. "In addition to the trauma of surgery, your body starts making that physical and hormonal transition from being pregnant to not being pregnant, and you have to take care of your new baby. That's quite a load on the mother."

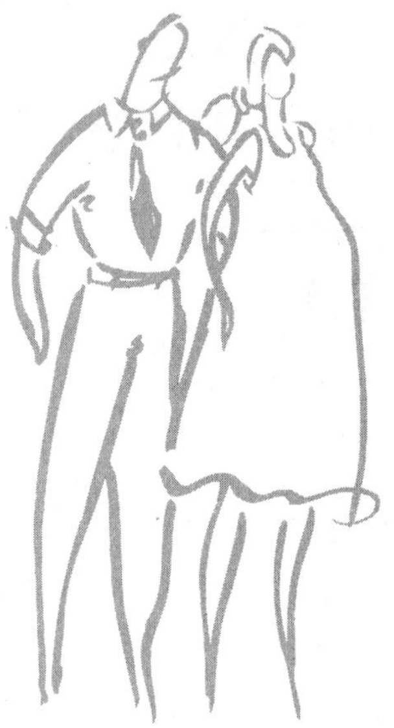

For the most part, your doctor will monitor the healing of your abdominal in-

Chapped Lips

Smooth Lips Sail Ships

Betsy Alison, 40, of Newport, Rhode Island, is a world-class yachtswoman. Winner of more than 20 world and national yacht-racing titles, her efforts have landed her a mantle full of yachting trophies—and a world-class case of chapped lips.

"For a competitive sailor, chapped lips are an occupational hazard," says Alison, five times named Rolex Yachtswoman of the Year. "I'm out on the water for about 9 hours a day, 80 days a year. Sun, wind, and salt air dry out my lips. And as a crew member, I'm always talking and licking my lips," she says. "My lips get so chapped that they blister on the *inside*."

To protect her lips from sun and wind, Alison looks for lip balm with sunscreen, with an SPF of no less than 30, which is about the highest you'll find. (Look for Blistex Ultra Protection and Chapstick Ultra).

And that's a good start, says Michael Jacobs, M.D., a physician on Martha's Vineyard, Massachusetts, and a yachtsman himself. He recommends lip balms with an SPF of at least 15, in tube or stick form (such as Blistex Lip Tone and Chapstick Sunblock 15).

cision during the first several weeks after the delivery. But at-home recovery is pretty much left up to you, along with all of your new responsibilities. That can be exhausting and stressful.

If you were supposed to have a vaginal birth but ended up with an emergency C-section, you may come away feeling disappointed and discouraged, says Malnory. "It's reasonable to have these feelings, even up to a year afterward. You're mourning over something you didn't get to experience."

To speed recovery, take these steps.

Tame the pain. This is a very important part of the recovery, says Malnory. "If you don't get your pain under control and stay on top of it, your body will expend more energy trying to cope with the pain so you can function. You'll delay healing and won't be able to care for your baby to the best of your ability." So take acetaminophen, ibuprofen, or medication prescribed on a regular schedule.

Power up on protein. Your incision requires extra calories and proper nutrition to heal correctly. Eat foods high in protein such as poultry, eggs, milk, cheese, yogurt, legumes, and peanut butter on toast, says Malnory. Unless ››

DON'T MAKE THIS MISTAKE

Delving into household chores too soon after a cesarean delivery will delay your recovery. Get as much help as possible from family and friends to assist with cooking, cleaning, laundry, and grocery shopping. Your focus should be on you and your baby.

Opt for lip balm with aloe. Aloe helps heal irritated skin by promoting cell growth and enhancing the healing process.

Apply liberally. Circle your lips with the balm until every nook and cranny is covered, says Dr. Jacobs. And, go over your lips a couple of times.

Reapply every 2 hours. "I put on lip balm at least 8 to 10 times a day—probably more," says Alison.

Take it everywhere you go. You don't want to get caught feeling like your lips are starting to chap but not being able do anything about it. Dr. Jacobs recommends buying several tubes or sticks of your favorite lip balm and tucking them anyplace you might need them—purse, gym bag, car console, desk drawers, or your coat pocket.

Helpful Hint

To refresh lips that are dry due to wind or icy weather, remove any lipstick or lip balm by gently blotting with a tissue. Then wet a plain black or green tea bag with warm (not hot) water and apply it to your lips for several minutes. Blot your lips to dry.

"The tannic acid in the tea tightens the skin and helps your lips retain moisture," says Frank Yurasek, an acupuncturist and homeopathic physician at the Alternative Medicine Clinic in Chicago. Repeat with fresh tea bags several times a day, if you like. And be sure to reapply lip balm between treatments. ■

you've been told otherwise, choose low-fat versions when possible, and aim for three servings a day, even if you're breastfeeding.

Choose to snooze. Sleep when the baby sleeps. Keep a bassinet in your room or have your spouse bring the baby to you at night for feedings so you don't keep getting out of bed. "Women make the mistake of writing thank you cards or entertaining visitors when the baby is napping. You should be doing whatever you can to conserve your energy," says Malnory.

Limit exercise. No matter how anxious you are to shed your baby fat, dance aerobics will have to be put on hold. In fact, you shouldn't do any exercise until your incision is healed and your energy is back. "Ambulation helps keep your bowels moving and gets rid of excess fluids that you've accumulated during pregnancy," says Malnory. "Your doctor will probably want you up and walking as soon as possible, but hold off on more strenuous exercise for at least 4 weeks." ■

Chicken Soup

Power Up Your #1 Cold Fighter

You've heard of the Bard of Stratford-upon-Avon. Now meet the Bard of Chicken Soup.

He's Irwin Ziment, M.D., professor and chief of medicine at Olive View–UCLA Medical Center in Sylmar, California, an expert in respiratory pharmacology.

To Dr. Ziment, chicken soup is rich not only in medicinal value but also in poetry.

"Chicken soup is comforting, warm, and reminiscent of the traditions of one's upbringing," he says. "It has the same appeal as a nursery rhyme."

So primal is this appeal that even a whiff of chicken soup can instantly transport you back to the days when you stayed home from school and Mom lovingly nursed you back to health.

Scientists now know that chicken soup contains cysteine, an amino acid that imparts that wonderfully piquant, chicken-soup flavor. It also has numerous health benefits.

"Cysteine is an antioxidant that also has a quite remarkable ability to reduce the viscosity, or stickiness, of phlegm," Dr. Ziment says.

An oft-cited study at Mount Sinai Medical Center in Miami Beach showed that drinking hot chicken soup unclogs nasal passages better than drinking hot water. And a researcher at the University of Nebraska Medical Center in Omaha carried out a laboratory study on chicken soup and found that it has properties that could reduce the inflammation associated with colds and flu.

Problem is, chicken soup contains too little cysteine to pack a therapeutic punch. As prepared in most kitchens, it has benefits that are more psychological than physiological. To become a truly effective medicine, chicken soup needs assistance.

"It has to be very spicy," Dr. Ziment says.

When chicken soup is prepared with hot spices, its benefits are magnified. Extremely spicy chicken soup stimulates the alimentary tract in the mouth, throat, and stomach. This increases the secretion of watery fluids in the respiratory tract, which makes phlegm easier to cough or blow out.

Dr. Ziment's work with patients has convinced him that chicken soup is at least as effective as any over-the-counter expectorant remedy used in coughs and colds. Here are his recommendations for transforming ordinary chicken soup into a potent expectorant.

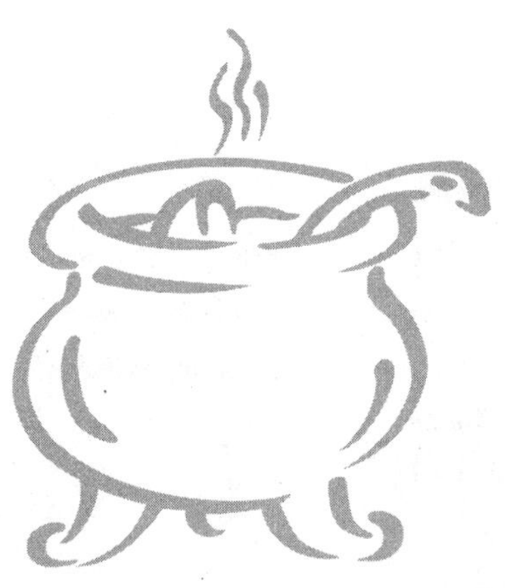

Start with a clear broth. It doesn't matter if it's made from scratch or poured from a can. Forget the noodles and veggies. "If you include them, it becomes a food instead of a drug," Dr. Ziment says.

Spice it until your nose runs. Use the hottest spices you can stand, such as garlic, ginger, horseradish, hot-pepper sauce, or curry powder. "Go to the point where it's almost impossible to tolerate, then back away," Dr. Ziment says. If you start to cough or choke, add some cooling herbs such as basil or mint.

Drink it hot. "You could drink it cold, but heat potentiates the action," says Dr. Ziment.

Treat it like cold syrup. "Use as little as a teaspoonful or as much as a cupful and take it three or four times a day," Dr. Ziment says. "It may be the only remedy you need in treating the typical cold." Drink the soup for 3 to 4 days. If your cough or cold doesn't get better after 2 days—or if it gets worse—consult your doctor, especially if you have heart or lung disease.

DON'T MAKE THIS MISTAKE

Combining willow bark with alcohol can cause stomach irritation.

Helpful Hint

Although spicy chicken soup relieves congestion, it won't do anything for headaches and body aches. If you're reluctant to use synthetic pain relievers, try adding a bit of willow bark to the soup. Willow bark contains natural aspirin. Add 1 to 3 grams of dried bark or 1 to 3 milliliters of tincture to your soup. Do this up to three times a day. Do not take willow bark if you need to avoid aspirin, especially if you are taking blood-thinning medication such as warfarin (Coumadin) because its active ingredient is related to aspirin. It may interact with barbiturates or sedatives such as aprobarbital (Amytal) or alprazolam (Xanax). ■

Chile Peppers

The Condiment That Heals

"Instead of jogging, I eat enchiladas topped with red chile sauce for lunch," jokes Paul Bosland, Ph.D., professor at New Mexico State University in Las Cruces and director of the Chile Pepper Institute. In response to the heat that the peppers produce, your body produces endorphins, the same feel-good and pain-protection brain chemicals stimulated by exercise, he explains.

The active ingredient in chiles is capsaicin (pronounced cap-SAY-I-sin). From serranos to jalapeños, chiles are also rich in vitamin C and beta-carotene. Research shows that these powerful little pods can assist your health in more ways than one: Chiles (or dishes made with them) can:

- Break up the congestion of a stuffy nose by opening sinuses and nasal passages.
- Relieve coughs and bronchitis.
- Soothe toothaches and sore throats.
- Help move food through your system.

Chiles may also:

- Lower bad (LDL) cholesterol, decreasing risk of stroke, high blood pressure, and heart disease.
- Help thin the blood, possibly preventing blood clots that lead to heart attack and stroke.
- Cure fungal infections.

When applied to the skin, over-the-counter topical creams containing capsaicin help relieve the pain of osteoarthritis, rheumatoid arthritis, phantom limb pain, nerve pain, psoriasis, even cluster headaches. Rub it on, it burns, and whatever was hurting before stops hurting.

"Capsaicin desensitizes the nerve endings responsive to heat or chemical stimulation," explains Robert LaMotte, Ph.D., professor of anesthesiology and neurobiology at Yale University School of Medicine.

DON'T MAKE THIS MISTAKE

Dr. Bosland doesn't recommend rubbing chiles directly on the skin. "Creams contain controlled amounts of capsaicin and heat. Jalapeños and other peppers vary in how much capsaicin they contain and how much heat they produce. If you use too much, you can blister your skin."

Helpful Hint

Be careful to wash your hands well after preparing chile peppers or using capsaicin cream. It can be painful and irritating to the eyes. ■

FIGHT FIRE WITH ICE CREAM

If you sample a chile pepper that's too hot for your taste, *don't* reach for a glass of water. The active ingredient in chile peppers isn't water-soluble, so it won't have much effect, says Dr. Bosland. For similar reasons, forget beer or margaritas. The best fire fighters, in order:

Best: Any milk product (milk, sour cream, ice cream)

Second best: Sweets (sugar, honey)

Third: Carbohydrates (breads, crackers)

Chocolate

17 Gotta-Have-It Guilt-Free Treats

Blame Christopher Columbus for your chocolate cravings. When he discovered cocoa beans in the Caribbean, he and his presumably all-male crew hated the taste. But back home, the women went wild.

Five centuries later, chocolate suppliers still can't keep up with demand. A mere mouthful of chocolate triggers a rush of feel-good brain chemicals like endorphins and serotonin. Eighteenth century physicians prescribed chocolate to remedy broken hearts and chronic illnesses. More recently, a study of Harvard University graduates found that chocolate- and other candy-eaters live nearly 1 year longer than those who abstain. Researchers speculated that antioxidants in the chocolate may have been responsible.

Here are 17 ways to satisfy your chocolate cravings without expanding your waistline. These goodies all have less than 200 calories and no more than 7 grams of fat. (The boldface ones come with a bonus of extra vitamins and minerals.)

1. Two Snackwell's Mint Creme cookies: (110 calories, 3.5 grams of fat)

2. Two Snackwell's Caramel Delights cookies (140 calories, 4 grams of fat)

3. Three Girl Scout Thin Mint cookies (105 calories, 6 grams of fat)

4. Three Chips Ahoy! Reduced-Fat Chocolate Chip Cookies (140 calories, 5 grams of fat)

5. One Pepperidge Farm Chocolate Chunk Reduced-Fat Cookie (110 calories, 4.5 grams of fat)

6. Two Pepperidge Farm Orange Milano Cookies (130 calories, 7 grams of fat)

7. Three Nabisco Reduced-Fat Oreo Cookies (130 calories, 3.5 grams of fat)

8. 15 Quaker Mini Chocolate Crunch Rice Cakes (162 calories, 1 gram of fat)

9. One Snackwell's individually wrapped Fudge Brownie (130 calories, 2 grams of fat)

10. One Fudgsicle fat-free frozen bar (60 calories, 0 grams of fat)

11. Gold-Star Chocolate Treats

12. One glass (8 ounces) **Hershey's fat-free chocolate milk** (150 calories, 0 grams of fat)

13. One carton (8 ounces) **Light Dannon White Chocolate Raspberry Nonfat Yogurt** (120 calories, 0 grams of fat)

14. One container (4 ounces) **Jell-O Fat-Free Chocolate Pudding Snack** (100 calories, 0 grams of fat)

15. One package (1.58 ounces) **Raisinets** chocolate-covered raisins (185 calories, 7 grams of fat)

16. ½ cup **Ben and Jerry's Devil's Food low-fat chocolate sorbet** (160 calories, 2 grams of fat)

17. ½ cup **Healthy Choice Cherry Chocolate Chunk Low-Fat Ice Cream** (110 calories, 2 grams of fat) ■

Chromium

Do You Really Need a Supplement? It Depends

Ads for chromium picolinate—a widely sold chromium supplement—offer a variety of potential benefits, from helping ease diabetes and lowering your cholesterol to losing weight and building muscle endurance.

Some claims for chromium supplements have considerable merit, some do not. This micronutrient plays a big role in metabolism of carbohydrates and fats. Without it, your blood sugar would go haywire.

Although chromium is widely available, if you eat a lot of refined foods, you may not be getting the Daily Value of 120 micrograms. The richest sources are whole grains, nuts, cheeses, broccoli, and brewer's yeast So if you include those in your daily diet, your chromium will add up.

There's solid proof that people with diabetes benefit from extra chromium.

Chromium and insulin tag team blood glucose,

Clutter

Divide and Conquer Paperwork and Paraphernalia

Kim Stewart, a child psychologist and mother of 4-year-old triplets, has learned how to hold back the avalanche of toys, clothes, crayons, and papers that, if untended, could engulf her St. Louis home.

The kids' stuff is neatly stored in bins, boxes, and baskets around the home. Dr. Stewart and her husband, Jim, each have a desk to hold their grown-up debris, and all the mail goes into a predesignated pile.

"If you keep on top of it, it doesn't get overwhelming," Dr. Stewart says.

Dr. Stewart has the right idea, says Deniece Schofield, author of Confessions of an Organized Homemaker *and* Confessions of a Happily Organized Family. *Clear plastic boxes allow the family to see what's inside without rifling through them to find what they need. Plus, the kids are learning at an early age that they have a role in keeping the home tidy.*

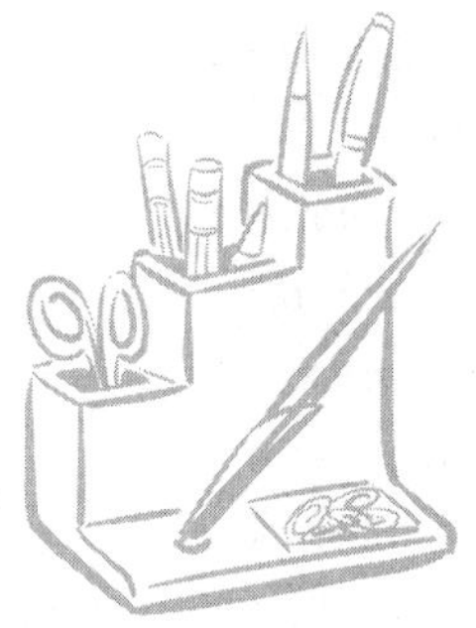

You, too, will find it easier to keep your home neat if you stop clutter from accumulating, says Schofield. Here's how.

Give everything a home. Every item under your roof, from your keys to the mail to the Scotch tape, belongs in a specific place. When you see something out of place, take a moment to put it away immediately.

normalizing your sugar levels by helping cells store glucose and release energy. The problem for women with diabetes is that they lose chromium in their urine. As a result, insulin doesn't work and glucose runs amuck. Chromium supplements help them regain control, says Richard Anderson, Ph.D., lead scientist in the nutrient requirements and functions laboratory at the U.S. Department of Agriculture Beltsville Human Nutrition Research Center in Maryland.

Under a doctor's supervision, women with diabetes should take about 400 to 600 micrograms of chromium picolinate a day, recommends Dr. Anderson. Your blood glucose levels should be monitored regularly so that, if necessary, your doctor can adjust your medication requirements. ■

DON'T MAKE THIS MISTAKE

If you're trying to lose weight, don't bother picking up a bottle of chromium picolinate. Numerous studies have shown that it is ineffective for losing weight, increasing muscle, or improving strength. Also, there's little evidence that it lowers cholesterol.

Rank all your household items from A to D, from most frequently used to least. Then keep A and B items handy, stow C items out of sight, and throw out D items. Take your kitchen, for example: Things you use every day or once a week, like salt and pepper shakers, measuring cups, and potato mashers, would be A's and B's—store them in easy-to-reach places. Seasonal or special occasion items, like oversized serving platters, novelty cake pans, and corn-on-the-cob holders, are C items—store them in the basement. Sell what you never use at a yard sale or give it to charity. Throw out D-grade odds and ends like warped cookie sheets and orphaned container lids.

Many women (and men) complain that they don't have enough storage space, when in fact, much of the space they do have is filled with objects they never use, Schofield points out.

Teach by example. Don't nag your family if they leave things out of place. Instead, quietly fix the problem and make sure they see where the item should go. Eventually, they'll get the hint and do it themselves.

Dr. Stewart says that her organizational plan has already rubbed off on her kids—they comment whenever they notice that their toys are put away in the wrong box.

Helpful Hint

Tackle chores one at a time. Whether it's cleaning the fridge or clearing off the dining-room table, don't start the second chore until you've finished the first. Otherwise, you'll leave clutter strewn all around your workplace. ■

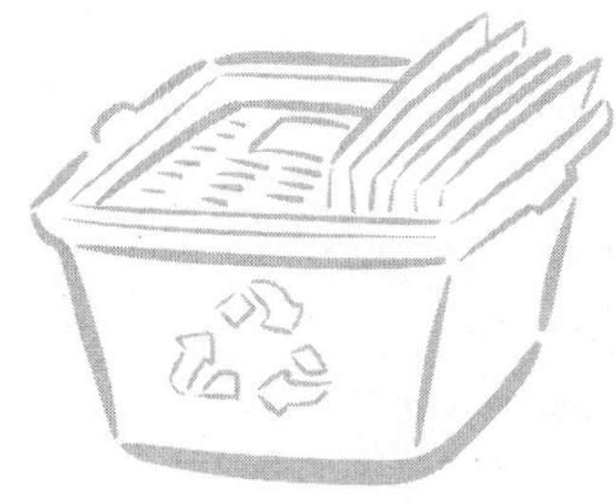

Cold Hands and Feet

Toasty Tips from Mt. Everest

Men and women alike have climbed the world's highest mountains, pushing themselves to their limits, admiring our planet from lofty peaks, and telling thrilling tales for the rest of their lives.

In the process, they get really cold hands and feet.

Two doctors who have tromped through high-altitude snow from Alaska to the Himalayas offer a flurry of hints on keeping your fingers and toes warm under any circumstances.

Keep your center warm. "Mountaineers have an old saying: If your feet are cold, put on a hat," says Ken Zafren, M.D., an emergency physician and medical director for the Denali National Park Mountaineering Rangers in Anchorage. But it works: When you get cold, your brain instinctively diverts heat away from your feet and hands and toward your vital organs. By holding in your body heat with a hat—and ample clothing on your arms, legs, and torso—your body will have more warmth to share with your hands and feet.

Wear mittens, not gloves. Mittens will keep your hands warmer than gloves. To understand why, just look at a penguin. This Antarctic bird is smooth and round, with thin flippers and short legs, so penguin bodies have less surface area to lose heat, says Ken Kamler, M.D., a New York City physician and regular visitor to Mount Everest. (He treated some of the climbers imperiled on the well-publicized Everest expedition in 1996, which was covered in the Imax documentary *Everest* and recounted in the best-selling book, *Into Thin Air.*) Similarly, when you wear mittens, your fingers huddle together in one group and put off less heat than they would if each were in its own glove finger.

Wear glove liners underneath your mittens. Two layers keep you warmer than

ONE LAYER IS BETTER THAN TWO

Wearing an extra pair of thick socks can do more harm than good: If your boots fit too tightly, crowding your feet, they'll constrict your bloodflow, and your feet will get cold more quickly. You'll also lose the pocket of warm air in your shoes that surrounds your feet, much like the layer of warm water inside a scuba diver's wet suit.

SPICE UP YOUR FEET

Some outdoor enthusiasts borrow a warming technique right out of the kitchen, says Dr. Zafren. They sprinkle red pepper into their socks. This increases bloodflow to the feet and makes them warmer.

If you want to try this, be careful: Add a small amount of ground red pepper or pepper flakes to talc or cornstarch and sprinkle it into your socks. Gradually add more pepper until you find an amount that adds heat to your feet, but doesn't hurt them.

one and give you protection if you need to remove your mittens for any reason, like taking pictures. For really harsh weather, Dr. Zafren recommends waterproof and windproof covers that you slip on over your mittens for added protection.

Wear sock liners. Dr. Kamler suggests that you wear a pair of polypropylene (a synthetic) socks underneath wool socks.

Helpful Hint

If you have Raynaud's phenomenon, your hands and feet will tend to become extra numb or painful even when exposed to mildly chilly temperatures. So you'll need to wear gloves and warm socks more often than usual—or avoid the cold altogether, Dr. Zafren says. ■

Colds

The 2-Day Cure

Cold germs are everywhere: Your hands. Other people's hands. And they travel, via handshakes, doorknobs—and of course, sneezes.

Your best defense against cold viruses: fighting back hard and fast before a full-scale war erupts.

"By taking action at the very first sign of symptoms, you can stop your cold dead in its tracks in as little as 2 days," says Toni Bark, M.D., a homeopathic physician and medical director of Center for the Healing Arts in Glencoe, Illinois. Here is Dr. Bark's six-step action plan for getting rid of a cold in 2 days.

DON'T MAKE THIS MISTAKE

Avoid taking aspirin, acetaminophen, or ibuprofen to bring down a low-grade fever or to relieve symptoms. The fever will fight the virus and shorten the duration of the cold. If you have a fever of 101°F or above for more than a couple of days, chances are you don't have a cold, but maybe the flu or another illness, which may warrant medical attention, says Dr. Bark.

1. At the first sign of a sniffle, sip hot chicken soup twice a day. If you're a vegetarian, try miso soup or vegetable broth. Avoid soups with MSG or hydrolyzed vegetable protein, Dr. Bark cautions. Add one or two crushed or chopped garlic cloves and a pinch of red pepper flakes or powder—as much as you can stand—per bowl. Studies show that chicken soup and garlic have strong antiviral properties, says Dr. Bark. The red pepper will open up your sinuses and loosen congestion.

2. If you have a sore throat, **suck on three to five zinc lozenges** containing 5 to 15 milligrams of zinc gluconate throughout the day. Zinc is thought to stop the virus from multiplying.

3. Sip herbal tea laced with echinacea or astragalus (also known as *huang qi*) every 1 to 2 hours throughout ›› the day. To make the tea, place 1 to 2 dropperfuls of echinacea or astragalus extract (or tincture) into a cup of ginger or chamomile tea. Echinacea and astragalus stimulate the immune system and can shorten the life span of the virus. (Skip this step if you're pregnant.)

4. Take 2,000 to 3,000 milligrams of vitamin C in divided doses during the day. Vitamin C jump-starts your immune system by arming white blood cells with the right ammunition to fight off the cold. It also acts as an antihistamine to help dry up watery eyes and a runny nose. (Don't take vitamin C and zinc at the same time. Vitamin C binds with zinc, making the zinc less effective. Take the vitamin C first, or wait ½ hour after the lozenge has disappeared. And be aware that excess vitamin C may cause diarrhea in some people.)

5. Soak in a hot bath for 20 to 30 minutes while sipping on some hot herbal tea or hot garlicky chicken soup. The hot bath and the hot liquid will temporarily heat up your body, elevating your white blood cell count to fend off the virus. (Avoid soaking in a hot bath if you already have a fever of 102°F or above, or if you're pregnant. The hot water could boost your fever dangerously high, and—in the case of pregnancy—could harm your baby.)

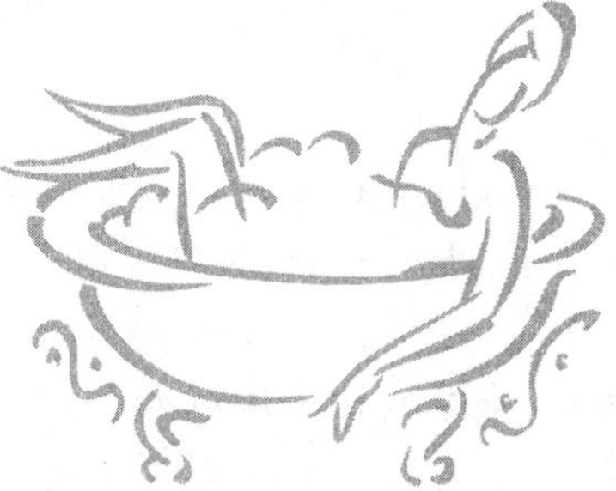

6. After your bath, slip into some warm pajamas and hop into bed. Sip on some more hot garlicky soup or herbal tea. Then go to sleep. You'll feel 80 percent better the next morning. ■

Cold Sores and Canker Sores

A Smorgasbord of (Practically) Overnight Cures

If you're patient, those annoying mouth sores will go away on their own in a week to 10 days. But who can be patient when the inside of your mouth is a torture chamber, or your lip sports an open sore?

Better to act fast with natural home remedies. "Use natural substances as soon as you feel symptoms," says Donald Brown, N.D., a naturopathic physician in Maplewood, New Jersey. "Start early, and you can decrease the severity and speed up the healing time."

Cold Sores

Caused by a herpes virus, 90 percent of us will get cold sores on our lips or in our mouths at least once. Almost half us will endure one or more repeat episodes. If you have a cold or canker sore, there are several natural ways to speed healing.

Lemon balm. Extracts of this perennial herb have antiviral properties. Applied to the sore, it can reduce pain and speed healing. Look for a topical ointment with extract of lemon balm. It's sold under the brand name Herpilyn. Apply the cream two to four times daily for up to 10 days.

Licorice. Licorice-containing gels have anti-inflammatory and anti-viral properties that combat cold sores. Begin using the gel at the first signs of a cold sore and continue until the cold sore has healed. This product, called Licrogel, is only available through your doctor.

Lysine. This amino acid supplement may halve your recovery time, according to one small study. Dr. Brown recommends swallowing 1,000 milligrams a day, backed up by 2,000 to 3,000 milligrams of vitamin C, to bolster your immune system, until your cold sore is gone. (If taking this much vitamin C gives you diarrhea, cut back.)

Helpful Hints: Found in seeds, nuts, peas, and chocolate, the amino acid arginine fuels the herpes virus responsible for cold sores. Lysine is most effective against cold sores if you limit foods rich in arginine.

IS YOUR TOOTHPASTE GIVING YOU GRIEF?

It's rare, but in some women, sodium lauryl sulfate, a detergent used in some toothpastes, triggers canker sores. If you're bothered by frequent canker sores, look for brands (such as Rembrandt Whitening Toothpaste for Canker Sore Prevention or Biotene) that omit this ingredient.

You may also find it helpful to try a special toothpaste (such as Colgate Total) that includes triclosan, an antimicrobial agent that helps control canker sores.

If cold sore outbreaks recur frequently, ask your doctor about the antiviral drug acyclovir (Zovirax). Used daily, it may prevent cold sore outbreaks.

Sun exposure (along with fatigue, emotional stress, and other infections) can lead to a herpes outbreak. So use a sunscreen around your mouth and a lip balm with sunblock. If you have an open sore, don't use the lip balm directly on your lips or the skin around the outside border, or you'll spread the virus. Instead, apply it with a cotton swab.

Canker Sores

Even more vexing than cold sores, these are crater-shaped sores that appear inside your cheeks or along your gums or tongue. The list of foods that might trigger canker sores could fill a deli menu, though acidic foods like citrus fruits, tomatoes, and wine are the likeliest suspects. "Keep track of what you eat in a food diary so you can figure out your personal triggers," says Cherilyn Sheets, D.D.S., a dentist in Newport Beach, California. Once the trigger's pulled, however, try one of these natural remedies.

Paste on licorice. De-glycerizinized licorice (DGL) works best, Dr. Brown says. Buy DGL powder from a health food store and mix with a little water to form a paste. Then let it disperse in your mouth. Repeat this three or four times daily. Do this until your canker sores go away.

Do not use licorice if you have diabetes, high blood ››

pressure, liver or kidney disorders, or low potassium levels.

Apply a wet tea bag. There's pain relief in the nerve-dulling tannins of black tea. Just hold a wet bag to the spot where it hurts.

Stick on E butter. John Heinerman, Ph.D., director of the Anthropological Research Center in Salt Lake City, who has studied folk remedies for years, suggests this: Put a little peanut butter on a quarter-size piece of white bread. Empty the contents of a vitamin E oil capsule over it, press the whole thing against the sore and leave it there a while. "The peanut butter helps it stick, and the vitamin E helps the canker sores heal faster," Dr. Heinerman says.

It's a good idea to get clearance from your doctor before taking more than 400 IU. One

Comfort Foods

Satisfy Your Soul without Packing On the Pounds

How comforting it would be if "comfort foods" fulfilled a basic nutritional need. We could all rest easier if scientists proved that chocoholics crave chocolate because of the phosphorus it supplies, or that ice-cream fiends need more calcium.

Sorry. It just isn't true.

"There's no real evidence for the so-called wisdom of the body." says Adam Drewnowski, Ph.D., director of the nutritional sciences program at the University of Washington in Seattle. "With the exception of salt, people do not seek out foods that their diets are missing."

After studying women who craved sweets and fats, Dr. Drewnowski concluded that comfort foods serve only one basic function: stress relief. Certain foods stimulate the brain's opiate receptors, areas that trigger pleasant feelings. When Dr. Drewnowski gave the women an opiate-blocking drug, he found that their cravings melted like an M&M on a hot sidewalk.

So does that mean you have to spend your life as a comfort-food junkie unless you go on opiate-blocking drugs?

Hardly, says psychologist Doreen Virtue, Ph.D., author of *Constant Craving.*

Early in her career, Dr. Virtue was a drug and alcohol counselor who noticed that different personality types leaned toward different addictive substances. Later, after specializing in eating disorders, she wondered if the same applied to comfort-food addicts.

"There were the same sort of patterns," she says. "The women (and men) who craved ice cream were very different from the people who craved popcorn."

Her clients had just one thing in common: a link between comfort and food that was established in childhood. "As Mom is handing you a cookie, she's smiling and praising you, so you get those warm feelings that tell you, 'Gosh, Mom really approves of me and I'm an okay person,'" Dr. Virtue says.

study using low-dose (70 IU per day) supplements showed increased risk of hemorrhagic stroke.

Dab on myrrh. Buy tinctures of this ancient herb at a health food store and dab a few drops onto your sores two or three times a day until your sore has healed. Myrrh's astringent, or tightening, qualities will ease the pain.

Helpful Hints

When you apply anything directly on a sore in your mouth, you'll get the best results if you dry the area around it first and avoid eating or drinking afterward.

If nothing seems to help, ask your doctor or dentist about amlexanox (Aphthasol), a prescription drug for treating canker sores. ■

Watching thousands of television commercials taught her clients that it was okay to medicate themselves with food. So as adults, they turned to particular foods to "treat" particular emotional woes. When they found that higher and higher "doses" were required to achieve the desired effect, they turned to Dr. Virtue for help.

Dr. Virtue identified the psychological characteristics of comfort-food abusers and devised healthful ways to help them feel comforted. See if you recognize yourself in the following categories.

The chocoholic. *Problem:* You need more love. Chocolate contains chemicals that make you feel as if you're in love. *Fix:* Make a low-calorie shake with ginger ale, ice, and chocolate extract. To lift your spirits, take a whiff of fresh coffee; pleasant scents stimulate a nerve in the body that triggers wakefulness.

The ice-cream fiend. *Problem:* You're depressed. Dairy foods contain chemicals that pull you out of the dumps. *Fix:* Write down your feelings in a journal. "Studies show that journaling boosts your mood and is correlated with high mental health."

The chip head. *Problem:* You're stressed, possibly because of a high-pressure job. Eating popcorn, pretzels, chips, and other salty, crunchy snacks is calming because you're gnawing out of anger, anxiety, and frustration. *Fix:* Gnaw on carrots, celery, broccoli, or cauliflower dipped in a low-calorie, fat-free salad dressing.

The sweet tooth. *Problem:* You're bored, so you gobble candy and other sugary snacks to make you feel more alive. *Fix:* Find a neighborhood fruit stand that sells fresh apples, peaches, and watermelon. The sugars in candy and in fruit are similar in that they are both nutritive sweeteners, and they provide similar amounts of energy. "At first, women think that fruit won't satisfy them, but that's because they've been eating poor-quality, store-bought fruit," Dr. Virtue says. "If they spend the extra money to get high-quality fruit, they won't consider it a compromise." ■

Computer Addiction

Rediscover Real People, Real Hobbies—And Real Life

In normal time, an hour seems like an hour. Sit down at the computer, and time seems to fly by at the speed of light. Hours spent shopping, chatting, and exploring online can feel like just a few minutes.

"I call it terminal time warp," says Kimberly Young, Psy.D., a psychology professor at the University of Pittsburgh at Bradford, founder of the Center for On-Line Addiction and author of Caught in the Net. *Absorbed in the computer screen, a heavy user may neglect her children, abandon her other hobbies, and ignore her husband and longtime friends. Dr. Young counsels hundreds of women trying to wean themselves off 10 hours a day spent online.*

Computer addiction isn't an epidemic. One online survey (admittedly a self-selected group) suggests that about 6 percent of the more than 17,000 men and women who responded considered themselves addicted. Many reported losing their inhibitions while online, as well as losing track of time and feeling a loss of control. Experts theorize that Internet addicts may be trying to fill an emptiness or avoid a problem in their lives, such as boredom or loneliness. Women commonly turn to chat groups, where they can share their burdens and joys with other computer users.

"Instant intimacies can develop on line," says Dr. Young. "What might take months or years in real life can take days or weeks online, because the anonymity enables people to feel more open."

Both Dr. Young and Maressa Hecht Orzack, Ph.D., founder and coordinator of the computer service at McLean Hospital, a teaching hospital for Harvard Medical School near Boston, say that overcoming Internet addiction is like coping with a food addiction. Computer use is so common that most women can't completely stop using computers any more than they can quit eating, so the goal is to learn moderation.

Here's how.

Get your information from the real world. If you need to know the news, weather forecasts, or movie listings, pick up a newspaper or turn on the television instead of heading for the Internet. You'll have one less opportunity to become glued to your computer.

Play hard to get. If you overuse certain functions of the Internet, place obstacles in your way to make them harder to start. For example, if you're drawn to the chat groups, remove the program that allows you to participate or bury it deep into your computer so you have to issue several commands or mouse clicks to open it, Dr. Orzack suggests. If you can't stop buying items from Web auctions, install a filtering program that won't let you access the troublesome sites.

Mark your calendar. Each week, budget a certain amount of time that you can spend on the Internet. Set each session an hour or two before an event

10 SYMPTOMS OF COMPUTER ADDICTION

Not sure if the Net has snared you? Computer addicts display most or all of these signs, according to Dr. Young. You may be hooked if:

1. You can't control the time you spend online to the point that you skip meals or rarely sleep.
2. You lie about the time you spend on the computer to close friends and family.
3. The computer gains an inflated status in your life.
4. You constantly daydream about chat rooms or e-mails when away from your computer.
5. Your credit cards are maxed out from purchasing items online, especially online auction Web sites.
6. When you feel sad or depressed, you turn to your computer pals instead of friends or family members.
7. You waver between feeling joyful and guilty when online.
8. Your computer time interferes with your job or home responsibilities.
9. You take on an anonymous online persona that conflicts with your morals and values.
10. You get angry or depressed when power failures or other glitches abruptly bounce you off-line.

If five or more of these signs describe you, you may be seriously addicted to life online, according to Dr. Young. If you find it difficult to limit the time you spend on your computer using the tips suggested here, ask your friends, family, or a counselor for help.

that you absolutely cannot miss so you'll be forced to leave the computer at a certain time, Dr. Young recommends.

Give yourself a ring. Set an alarm clock to signal the end of your session and place it where you'll have to move away from the computer to turn it off.

Take measure of your real life. Think about what your needs are that the Internet is satisfying, and confront these issues away from the keyboard. If you're drawn to an attractive-sounding man whose e-mail messages are more romantic than a conversation with your husband, for example, you need to work on communication with your real-life mate.

If you're a stay-at-home mom escaping the stress of caring for a toddler, or an empty nester feeling lonely, look for a real-life support group that can share your concerns or a volunteer organization that offers companionship and puts your spare time to good use.

Never give out your real name, your phone number, or your address when you're online. Relationships with people you meet online call for the same kind of precautions as meeting people in the real world. ■

Computer Eyestrain

Comfort Tactics for Keyboard Jockeys

As a bookkeeper, Dawn Caddell of Wilmington, Delaware, stares at numbers on a flickering computer screen day after day. And for years, she was also unknowingly staring in the face of one of the greatest occupational hazards of modern times: computer eyestrain.

Eye and vision problems are the most frequently reported health care problem among men and women who work on computers. That's because computer users tend to blink less than usual while they work, which leads to itchy, burning, dried-out eyes, says Robert Abel Jr., M.D., clinical professor of ophthalmology at Thomas Jefferson University in Philadelphia and author of The Eye Care Revolution. *The computer also forces us to focus our eyes more than usual, which can cause headaches, light sensitivity, or blurred or double vision.*

Caddell got lucky: She realized that moving her monitor screen closer kept her from straining her eyes. And while finding the right distance between you and your computer is a good first step for curing eyestrain, Dr. Abel says there's plenty more you can do.

Keep your distance. "Fifteen inches away is good for some people. Twenty-four inches away is good for another," says Dr Abel. Experiment with a couple of different distances until you find one that allows you to clearly see what's on the screen without having to squint or crane your neck forward.

Follow the 30-30 rule. To avoid eye dryness, take a 30-second break every 30 minutes. When you do, try this exercise: Hold your head still and move your eyes around the room for a few seconds. Then move your head around, and keep your eyes fixed. Finally, look as far away as you can, down the hall or out the window, and think about letting your eyes relax.

Make more moisture. Put a humidifier or even a large potted plant in your office to increase the moisture in the room. That will help keep your eyes moist and will compensate for less-frequent blinking.

Drink five to six glasses of water. Not only will this help keep your eyes more lubricated but it also will force you to take bathroom breaks, and therefore time away from the computer.

Cut out any glare on your computer screen. Reposition either the screen or the lights in your office, or keep the windows covered, or use a filter for the top of the screen.

DON'T MAKE THIS MISTAKE

Turning up the lights will put an added strain on your eyes. It's best to keep the lights low to avoid glare.

Helpful Hint

Taking a daily dose of 100 to 500 milligrams of docosahexaenoic acid (DHA), an omega-3 fatty acid (fish oil), can help relieve dry eyes, says Dr. Abel. DHA is available in softgel capsules, often in combination with eicosapentaenoic acid (EPA). ■

Congestion

Do the Pepper-Mill Twist

If you have a stuffy nose or congested lungs, you could take over-the-counter decongestants or antihistamines. But you might end up trading one kind of discomfort for another. Sound familiar? If so, Angela Stengler, N.D., a naturopathic physician in San Diego, recommends the following natural un-stuffers.

Black pepper. Some restaurants use pepper grinders the size of Seattle's Space Needle. If you're feeling stuffy, let the waiter twist until his arm hurts when he points the pepper grinder at your salad. Black pepper dilates blood vessels in the nose, stimulating secretions that drain sinuses.

A polite sprinkle won't get the job done. "You definitely need more of a medicinal food dose—up to 2 teaspoons," says Dr. Stengler.

Red pepper. If you can take the heat, red pepper (cayenne) is even better than black. The capsaicin that makes it hot also acts as a natural anti-inflammatory.

The easiest way to take red pepper is to put it in food. Again, you need 2 teaspoons of it to get the effect. That may bite a little, but "it's a safe, easy, and inexpensive way to relieve congestion," says Dr. Stengler.

If you have a really stuffy nose or you can't stomach all that red pepper, you could try taking up to three 450-milligram capsules of red pepper spread throughout the day, she adds.

Horseradish. This root is so potent that some people can drain their sinuses by just smelling it. For the rest of us, the best way to use it is simply to eat some prepared horseradish, sold in the dairy section of most supermarkets. A quarter of a teaspoon should do the trick. Wasabi, a form of Japanese horseradish typically used on sushi, works just fine also, Dr. Stengler says. Powdered wasabi is sold in supermarkets.

Basil. A digestive herb, basil is also a natural expectorant that helps relieve chest ››

TREAT YOURSELF TO A EUCALYPTUS STEAMBATH

Breathing steam into your nose and lungs is a wonderful way to ease congestion. Adding eucalyptus leaves to steaming hot water works especially well, says Dr. Stengler.

Unless you have a eucalyptus wreath somewhere around your house and are willing to sacrifice a few leaves, your best bet is to buy a small vial of the essential oil at a health food store. Boil lots of water in your biggest pot, remove it from the stove, and add just a few drops of the eucalyptus oil (it's very strong). Hold a large towel over your head and lower your face slowly, 12 inches away from the water, so you don't scald yourself.

Breathe in the steam alternately through your mouth and nose for 10 to 15 minutes. If you're still congested after a week or two, discontinue the steam treatments and consult your doctor.

congestion. Dry or fresh, basil can be sprinkled into hot tea or broth or added to sauces or soups to taste.

Helpful Hint

Chicken soup has been shown to slow phlegm production. The fragrant steam helps unclog your nasal passages. It's a comfortable way to get down needed nutrients at a time when you're probably not too keen on eating. Adding garlic and onions—both antivirals—fights the infection. And it's the perfect vehicle for those congestion-relieving kitchen spices. If adding more than one ruins the flavor for you, just use cayenne. "Cayenne works well, so try just that first," says Dr. Stengler. ■

Constipation

Unclog a Sluggish Bowel with This Three-Ingredient Formula

Who says there are no magic formulas in medicine? Here's a constipation remedy that almost always works: Eat 25 grams of fiber, drink 64 ounces of water, walk for 30 minutes. Repeat daily.

"Do all three, and the results are remarkable," says Ernestine Hambrick, M.D., a retired colon and rectal surgeon in Chicago. No skimping, though. Each of the three components are equally essential.

25 Grams of Fiber

Fiber from food absorbs fluid in your digestive tract to create a soft bulk that stimulates the colon to move things along. Many women fall way short on fiber, an invitation to constipation. Yet getting your 25 grams quota is easy.

The morning fix. High-fiber cereals can have 7 grams or more of fiber per serving. Choose whole grain cereal, sprinkle in a generous portion of raisins, and you're nearly halfway to your 25 grams before 9:00 A.M.

Have five servings of fruits and vegetables a day. Count 'em up: Fruit with breakfast—1. A salad at lunch—2. An apple as an afternoon snack—3. Two vegetables with dinner—4 and 5. Ta-dah!

Choose whole wheat bread over white. And opt for rye crispbread or whole wheat crackers over chips or cheese curls.

The bran shower. Pure milled bran doesn't taste like much, but if you add 2 to 3 teaspoons of it to your favorite cereal, stir it into apple sauce with cinnamon, or juice it up with fruit in the morning, you'll get a fair amount of fiber—3 grams—without tasting it.

Oat bran makes some women a little *more* constipated. (No one is really sure why the two brans behave differently in people.) If that's you, use wheat bran, suggests Dr. Hambrick.

64 Ounces of Water

The magic formula won't work unless you drink eight 8-ounce glasses of water a day, in order to give fiber something to absorb.

Spread it out. Get in the habit of drinking a glass of water every 2 hours, Dr. Hambrick suggests. Have the first at 8 in the morning, the last at 10 at night, and you've done your eight.

Add a twist. A little lemon or lime juice with ice turns a humdrum glass of water into a refreshing beverage.

Juice counts. Clean, calorie-less, cost-free water is your healthiest choice for hydration. But you can substitute juice for a glass or two, if you like.

Carry water "to go." Carry a 32-ounce bottle of water around with you. It's socially acceptable and a great way to fill half your water quota a little at a time.

Double up at mealtime. Lunch and dinner are good times to drink your liquids; the sodium in your food helps you retain the fluid better. Drink two 8-ounce glasses at each, and you're halfway to 64 ounces.

30 Minutes of Walking

Physical activity puts the water and fiber into action.

"When you're active and walking briskly for ½ hour each day, things move through your system much better," Dr. Hambrick says. ■

Contact Lens Problems

To Save Your Sight, Act Fast

Ann Wieczorowski, voice teacher and classical singer in Washington, D.C., inserted her soft contact lenses after taking a shower, as usual. But this time, her eyes burned and reddened. She quickly removed the lenses, but the redness didn't go away. "Both eyes stung terribly," says Wieczorowski, "It happened fast and quickly got worse. I thought I was going to go blind."

She rinsed her eyes thoroughly, to no avail. She called her optometrist, who sent her to an ophthalmologist. The ophthalmologist figured that she must have transferred something—probably soap—from her fingers to the lenses. He gave Wieczorowski a prescription for the ensuing infection, which helped tremendously. But it was a few days before she could wear contact lenses again. "It was scary," says Wieczorowski. "You don't realize how much you value your sight until you go through something like that."

Wieczorowski's experience was not unusual, says her optometrist, Barbara Anan, O.D., in Washington, D.C. Residue from anything you've handled—soap, hand lotion, jalapeño peppers—causes burning (although not rinsing off lens cleaning solution thoroughly is the most common problem). "The cleaning solution can affect the cornea where the lens sits and cause temporary irritation and possibly an infection," explains Dr. Anan. Your eyes hurt, burn, redden, swell, itch, and tear—and you panic. ››

For women, eye makeup can cause problems, too. Mascara, for example, can flake off and scratch the sensitive cornea, explains Dr. Anan. Hairspray leaves sticky residue on your lens and tends to build up over time, muddying your vision, creating a "goo" that interferes with your eye's natural lubrication, or even triggering an allergic reaction.

A contact lens problem can be a real emergency; if your cornea is damaged, you can lose your sight in the eye. If you experience any kind of discomfort from contact lenses, immediately take out the lens, then flush your eye with saline solution if you wear soft lenses and have saline on hand. If you have hard lenses, use tap water or, preferably, eyewash (like Collyrium), says Dr. Anan. Do not reinsert the lens until the redness and tearing are gone. If irritation persists after rinsing your eyes, you might need medical attention. Ask your optometrist or ophthalmologist—she'll either ask you to go to her office or a hospital emergency room.

To prevent future problems, Dr. Anan offers these tips.

DON'T MAKE THIS MISTAKE

Never use saliva to wet or clean your lenses—it carries impurities and may cause infection. "If you can't clean the lens properly, with rinsing solution, take the lens out and leave it out," says Dr. Anan. And if you need to use eyedrops, use only drops specifically formulated for use with contact lenses. Otherwise, remove your lenses before applying drops. Also, never reinsert a lens that's chipped or torn.

- Use mascara formulated for contact lens wearers—it's less likely to flake. And put eyeliner only on the outside of your eyelid.
- Throw out mascara after 3 months—the tube is a great environment for bacteria.
- Choose makeup that washes off without makeup-remover cream, which can leave a film on your eye, or use an eye-makeup remover specially made for contact lens users, like Almay or L'Oreal.
- Never share eye makeup with anyone.
- Always wash your hands well after handling substances that might irritate your eyes, and rinse off soap thoroughly.
- Close your eyes when you spray your hair. Back away several steps before opening your eyes.
- You shouldn't wear your lenses if you're getting your hair dyed and never if you're getting your eyebrows dyed.
- Always keep a bottle of sterile saline solution handy—in the car, at work, in your gym bag—anywhere else you might need to clean your lenses.

Helpful Hint

Ask your lens provider, "If I ever have an emergency, what should I do and whom should I contact?" Then, post the information plainly, so you can read it without your lenses. Also, put a note in your wallet that you wear contact lenses and that, in case of an emergency, they should be removed. Parents should tell the school nurse if their children wear contact lenses, for the same reason. ■

Corns and Calluses

Give Your Shoes the Squeeze Test

Picture a construction worker's hands, covered with thick calluses. "The same thing happens to the skin on your feet," says Stephen Conti, M.D, professor at the University of Pittsburgh School of Medicine and an orthopedic surgeon specializing in foot and ankle care. "Skin thickens in response to frequent pressure of any kind, forming corns or calluses."

Squeeze your toes together with shoes that are too narrow—common with women's footwear—and you get corns between your toes or on the outsides of your big and little toes, says Dr. Conti. Pound the bottom of your foot against the sole of your shoe, and you get calluses, especially if there is some kind of subtle problem with the way you walk. Both corns and calluses are thickened skin, caused by pressure.

Foot specialists recommend these remedies.

Pad the pain. Over-the-counter unmedicated corn pads attach to the corn with adhesive, and with an opening for your corn to peek through, redistributing pressure from the corn onto nearby skin.

Scrape gently. When your feet are moist from a shower, use a pumice stone to gently scrape down corns and calluses, recommends Ellen Sobel, D.P.M., Ph.D., associate professor of orthopedic science at New York College of Podiatric Medicine. Just scrape enough to get the callus off. Don't scrape too far. If the area bleeds or is close to bleeding or feels sensitive, you've gone too far. And don't cut them with scissors or nail clippers—you may cut too deep. If the calluses are very heavy or painful, have a podiatrist shave them down.

Helpful Hints

If you continue to wear shoes that caused the problem, your corns and calluses will come back. Obviously, if your shoes are too tight, get rid of them and buy a larger size.

To find out if your shoes are too tight, give them the squeeze test: With your shoe on, stand with your full weight on that foot. Ask your spouse or a friend to squeeze the shoe at the site where your corn is. "If you cannot budge the leather, regardless of how soft it might be when your foot is not in the shoe, it will perpetuate your corn," says Thomas M. Novella, D.P.M., adjunct professor of orthopedic science at the New York College of Podiatric Medicine, who has ››

SKIP THE CORN PADS

Medicated corn pads, available in drugstores, erode the corn with a tissue-dissolving chemical. These are dangerous if left on the skin for too long, especially between the toes, warns Dr. Novella. Avoid them, especially if your circulation is poor due to diabetes or other problems.

treated thousands of dancers and recreational athletes.

You can also find relief for calluses with soft pads or insoles or simply by wearing a softer-soled shoe, Dr. Novella recommends. If this isn't enough, you may need custom orthotics, in-shoe devices that redirect or redistribute weight so that more of your foot bears your body weight, minimizing pressure at any one point. ■

Coughing Fits

Send Your Hacking Packing

In the middle of a performance of Shostakovich's Fifth Symphony, the musical director for the New York Philharmonic orchestra abruptly put down his baton and walked off the stage.

He didn't like what he was hearing—from the audience, not the orchestra. Too many people were coughing—endlessly.

It probably wasn't any fun for the people coughing, either. A hacking fit is your body's natural attempt to clear airborne irritants and mucous buildup from your airways. Your body's trying to expel the offending material, with no concern for orchestra conductors, librarians, fellow theater patrons or others who value quiet.

If you've tried cough drops and you're still hacking—or you don't have any cough drops handy—try these emergency measures instead.

Catch your breath. Take in a breath and exhale it, then take another and hold your breath for a few moments. Now take quick breaths in and out through your nose for a minute. Rest for a few minutes and repeat, increasing the time you take the short breaths through your nose.

Some people tend to cough more in stressful situations, so a breathing technique like this may help keep you calm and less likely to cough, says Gary Gross, M.D., clinical professor of medicine at the University of Texas Southwestern Medical School in Dallas.

Coat your throat. "If you suck on hard candy, because you're coating the back of your throat where some of the cough receptors are, that seems to suppress a cough," Dr. Gross says.

So if you're heading to an event where silence is a virtue, stow some unwrapped hard candies—so you won't have to rattle the cellophane wrappers—in a plastic sandwich bag in your purse. The flavor doesn't seem to matter, so pick your favorite.

Water it down. If you can, slip out to the water fountain for a few sips of water. It'll help loosen and remove mucus from the back of your throat, where it would trigger the cough reflex, Dr. Gross says.

Helpful Hint

If you have a chronic cough you can't get rid of, whether it's productive or dry, check it out with your doctor. A constant cough can signal any number of problems, including asthma, tuberculosis, and acid reflux disease. ■

Coworker Conflict

Sharpen Your Diplomacy Skills

During her 20-plus years as a business consultant in Mountain View, California, Marilyn Manning, Ph.D., has seen so many sticky workplace situations that she could open a glue factory.

Particularly difficult to resolve, she says, are conflicts arising between workers on the same rung of the corporate ladder. They'd rather not complain to a supervisor about a coworker's backbiting or gum cracking, but they don't have the savvy to settle it themselves.

For many women, confronting a coworker goes against their grain.

"We feel that we have to be friends with everybody and we have to be nice," says Dr. Manning, co-author of Leadership Skills for Women. *"Part of female conditioning in the workplace is to not raise your voice, to not show anger. Some women are afraid that if they express emotions, they might cry."*

Taking a walk around the building is a healthy way to let off steam—in the short term. But the problem will still be there when you get back. If you can't bear to ignore the problem, you can deal with it—smartly, says Dr. Manning. Here's how.

Wait it out. Give yourself time to calm down, however long it takes. Calm down, collect your thoughts, and consider your strategy, says Dr. Manning.

Narrow your list of grievances. Even if everything the other person does bothers you, focus on the most important one.

Address the problem calmly and rationally. Say the problem is noise. Suppose you work near someone who's seemingly incapable of talking, laughing, or even sneezing quietly. She's so distracting that you wish she had a volume-control knob. You've tried subtle tactics—like shushing or glaring. They don't work.

Address the coworker calmly, at a time when she's not rushed. Ask if she has a few minutes to speak privately.

Explain how her action affects your work. For example, tell the coworker in conciliatory tones, "I have difficulty concentrating on my work because there's a lot of background noise. I'd like to request that you be aware it affects my productivity and I'd like to ask if we could work something out."

Offer to contribute to the solution. Say, "What could I do to make this work?" For example, if shushing ››

DON'T MAKE THIS MISTAKE

Many a career has been self-sabotaged by a memo or e-mail fired off in the heat of the moment. Dr. Manning cites the advice that Abraham Lincoln once gave a subordinate who had written but not sent a poison-pen letter: "It's a good letter and you had a good time writing it and feel better. Now, burn it."

annoys your coworker as much as her high-decibel conversation bothers you, offer a humorous, win-win solution: no more shushing if she'll agree to tone it down when you give a time-out signal.

Helpful Hint

If you must vent about a coworker conflict, find a sympathetic ear outside the office. Confiding workplace woes to another coworker can set you up for trouble. If your relationship with a colleague sours, he or she can use your complaints against you. "A high percentage of people who are not speaking or who have serious conflicts are former friends," Dr. Manning says. ■

Cranberries and Blueberries

The Fruits That Give Bacteria the Boot

In the early 1900s, women tried some unusual health remedies, such as guzzling water enriched with radioactive radium to restore youthful vigor, wearing electrified belts to cure nerve problems, and drinking cranberry juice to prevent urinary tract infections.

The first two remedies are long gone, joining others on the long list of bad ideas. But the cranberry juice cure, it seems, is here to stay. In the 1920s, medical theorists believed that when women drank cranberry juice, their urine became more acidic and unfriendly to bacteria.

A century or so later, doctors still recommend cranberry juice for women prone to urinary tract infections, or UTIs. And now we know exactly how it works.

As bacteria climb up into the urinary tract, tiny fingerlike attachments latch on to the walls of the urethra and bladder, says Amy B. Howell, Ph.D., a research scientist at the Rutgers University Blueberry Cranberry Research Center in Chatsworth, New Jersey.

Once bacteria dig in, they give off toxins responsible for lower-back pain, frequent or burning urination, and in severe cases, fever—symptoms that may signal an infection.

Dr. Howell and her colleagues discovered that cranberries (and blueberries) contain chemicals called condensed tannins that coat the bacteria's attachments like nonstick Teflon, so the germs lose their grip. Instead, they slide through the urinary tract and are flushed out of your body with urine.

Once the bacteria gain a firm foothold in your system, the chemicals in the berries are not as effective, Dr. Howell says. So if you already have a full-blown UTI, it's a good idea to see your doctor. But if you're prone to repeat infections or feel one coming on, make sure you eat or drink one of the following every day.

• 10 ounces of cranberry-juice cocktail. Make sure the

DON'T MAKE THIS MISTAKE

Cranberry capsules may or may not work, says Dr. Howell, because they may not contain enough of the active antiadherence ingredients. If you do try the capsules, make sure the label says they are guaranteed to contain these natural compounds. Follow label instructions.

label says it contains at least 25 percent cranberry juice. You won't be able to find pure cranberry juice, and if you did, you wouldn't want to drink it—it's too sour and acidic. The juice works whether it's sweetened with sugar or artificial sweeteners, says Dr. Howell.

• ½ cup of dried cranberries or blueberries or cranberry sauce

• 1 cup of fresh blueberries

Helpful Hint

In a pinch, eating a slice of blueberry pie can stand in for fresh blueberries. Baking doesn't damage the antibacterial chemicals. ■

Crash Dieting

Are You Losing Too Much Weight Too Fast? For Best Results, Eat *More*

Technically, crash dieting is usually defined as eating fewer than 1,200 calories a day to lose weight. In practice, any drastic restriction in what you eat—like existing on cabbage soup, fruit juices, or some other fad diet—may also constitute crash dieting.

"It can mean anything people want it to mean," says Susan Yanovski, M.D., director of the Obesity and Eating Disorders Program at the National Institute of Diabetes and Digestive and Kidney Diseases in Rockville, Maryland.

Diet books are often built around crash diets. Although such books take different approaches, they usually call for a daily calorie intake below 1,200 calories, which experts say is dangerous and ineffective. Crash diets tend to force you into a starvation mode and put you at an increased risk of everything from bad breath, hair loss, and menstrual irregularity to low blood pressure, gall bladder attacks, and sudden death.

Usually, for naught.

"The weight loss on crash diets—especially carbohydrate-restricted diets—is mostly water," says Judith S. Stern, Sc.D., professor of nutrition and internal medicine at the University of California at Davis. "As soon as you put a little carbohydrate back in ›› your diet, you'll gain the water weight back."

If you lose any tissue at all, it's usually the tissue you most want to keep—muscle—and very little fat. On a crash diet, even the heart muscle can atrophy, or shrink.

"Muscle is metabolically active," Dr. Stern says. "It burns up calories. What you really want to get rid of is fat."

So if you want to lose weight, give crash diets the heave-ho and adopt a more sensible plan.

Be realistic. Chances are that you didn't gain that extra weight in a week, so you can't expect to take it off in a week.

Shoot for a 1 percent loss per week. Most women should stick with a well-balanced diet that cuts 250 to 500 calories per day, which should result in a weight loss of ½ to 1 pound per week. Otherwise healthy yet seriously overweight women should aim to lose no more than 1 percent of their body weight per week, says Dr.

Criticism

Help Your Husband without Nagging Him to Death

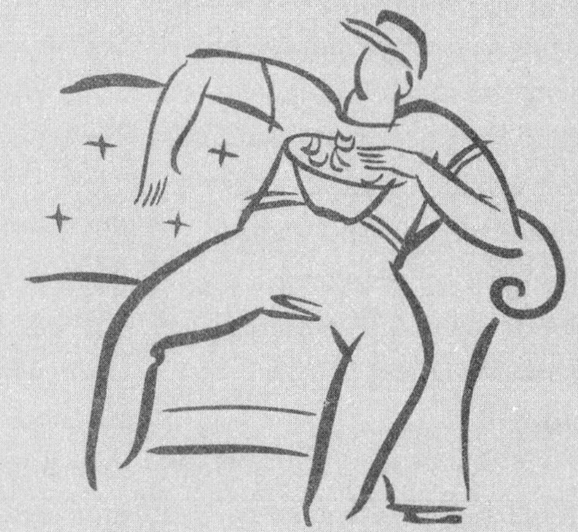

Criticizing someone you love is bad for their health.

"People who feel criticized by their families have higher levels of hostility and depression, which are linked to unhealthy behavior," says Kevin Fiscella, M.D., associate professor of family medicine at the University of Rochester in New York who has studied the effects of criticism. "It doesn't matter what you criticize them about—things are going to get worse."

The next time you find yourself admonishing your husband (or anyone else) to stop smoking, start exercising, eat healthier, lose weight (or all four), try these tactics instead, suggests Dr. Fiscella.

Couch any suggestions in terms of concern, love, and appreciation. "Keep in mind that while he may resist on the surface, most people do wish they were healthier," Dr. Fiscella says.

Approach him when things are going well. If you time your comments when the two of you are feeling connected, he's going to be more receptive.

Choose the right words. "Part of the trick is learning to not say what you want to say," Dr. Fis-

Stern. If you weight 220 pounds, for example, your shouldn't try to lose more than 2.2 pounds a week.

Work up a sweat. Regular exercise, especially strength training, will keep you from losing too much muscle mass, an inherent risk in any weight-loss program. ■

PLOYS TO IGNORE

Crash diet promoters often bolster their claims with quotes from individuals who have bona fide weight loss credentials. Don't be fooled: Few experts genuinely endorse any form of crash dieting.

Also, be wary of claims that crash diets can help jump-start a weight-loss plan. Experts say that the only suitable candidates for diets that are very low in calories are obese people who have dangerously high cholesterol and/or high blood pressure. Even then, they must be supervised by a medical professional.

cella says. "If you want to be helpful, you need to control your words." Here are his recommended conversation starters.

"Have you ever wished you were in better shape?" In other words, ask about his views on the subject instead of laying yours on him. The idea, of course, is to get *him* to say something like, "Yeah, I really should start exercising." He may not act on it right away, but the seed he plants himself is far more fertile.

"Is there anything I can do to help?" If he does recognize the possibility of change, your best follow-up is to offer general support, rather than preemptive instructions or advice.

"I'm really scared about what smoking might be doing to your health." "I" statements have a much better chance of getting through than "you" statements such as "You really should stop smoking," which he'll translate as "You're weak and stupid."

"Hey, I just read about a new smoking cessation technique that works better than anything else." Then casually show him the article. Sometimes information, neutrally presented, can get somebody to at least think about behavior changes.

Wouldn't it be fun to play some tennis (take a bike ride, go hiking, whatever)?" Suggest that the two of you begin doing some physical activity together—as fun, not duty. Pick one you think he likes. Exercise is often a good starting point for other healthy changes.

Be patient. "Most lifestyle behaviors are very difficult to change," Dr. Fiscella says. ■

DON'T GLOAT

Setting a "good example" can sometimes backfire. That's because calling attention to your own good habits can come off as holier-than-thou. The last thing any man wants to hear is "I exercise every day, so why can't you?" If you exercise, continue to work out. Just don't be self-righteous about it.

Crow's-Feet and Lip Lines

Wrinkle Creams for Sensitive Skin

Many women enthusiastically try popular anti-wrinkle creams containing alpha hydroxy acids (AHAs), hoping to smooth creeping crow's-feet and laugh lines. AHAs such as glycolic and lactic acid work in two ways: They exfoliate your skin, removing dull, dead surface cells, and they retain moisture, puffing out fine lines.

Many women enjoy the results and use AHAs with no problem. But some women with sensitive skin find them too harsh.

You can avoid the stinging, burning, and irritation sometimes associated with "anti-aging" creams. The trick is choosing the right one—and then using the right amount, says Leslie S. Baumann, M.D., a dermatologist and director of cosmetic surgery at the University of Miami.

- Buy an AHA cream with a weaker concentration—5 percent instead of 10 percent—formulated for sensitive skin.

Cubicle Rage

Make Peace with Your Office Space

For decades, psychologists have known that rats confined to close quarters become angry, depressed, and rageful. Working in a cubicle can make you edgy, too.

"Creating ratlike cubicles for human beings was about the dumbest thing workplace engineers could have done," says Barbara Reinhold, Ph.D., a career consultant, associate professor of psychology at Smith College, in Northampton, Massachusetts, and author of Toxic Work.

Paradoxically, cubicle work is both claustrophic and open. Workers are hemmed in by partitions, yet have no protection from noise. This is problematic for women, whose private telephone calls to spouses, pharmacists, and ob-gyn specialists and the like will be easily overheard by coworkers.

Although any cubicle worker can lose it, female workers seldom express their rage by packing a Colt .45.

"Women tend to lose it quietly," Dr. Reinhold says. "They often don't get to the *Thelma and Louise* stage."

Instead, they typically take out their frustrations on themselves and their families, says Lynne McClure, Ph.D., author of *Risky Business: Managing Employee Violence in the Workplace*, in Mesa, Arizona.

Some become sad and tearful and eat too many cupcakes. Others become hostile and withdrawn and snap at their husbands and children.

Although working in a cubicle makes you feel like you're the only one trying to concentrate in a roomful of channel flippers, you can break out of the box.

Here are some suggestions.

- Ask for permission to work one day a week at home. It'll give you some measure of control over your

• Look for beta hydroxy acids (BHAs). Like AHAs, BHAs reduce the appearance of fine lines and wrinkles by exfoliating your skin. They're less irritating than AHAs, and they have an added benefit: Derived from an ingredient similar to aspirin—salicylic acid—they also act as an anti-inflammatory. That virtually guarantees less redness and burning. Products containing BHAs are available in department stores nationwide and in higher strengths by prescription.

Regardless of whether you select a wrinkle cream with AHAs or BHAs, use only a dollop the size of a pea for your whole face, every other day or every 2 days, says Dr. Baumann. ■

DON'T MAKE THIS MISTAKE

Regardless of what type of skin you have, never apply a wrinkle cream to your eyelids or lips—the skin there is thinner and at greater risk of irritation. And never go outside without a lotion or cream with an SPF of 15 or higher, to prevent premature skin aging.

work week. For best results, make sure you can explain to your boss how your new schedule would improve your job performance.

• Go outdoors or into a vacant office when you can. "When you're stuck in a cubicle, you need to take a break whenever you can, even if it's only 2 to 3 minutes at a time," says Dr. McClure.

• If you can afford it, buy a cell phone and leave your cubicle to make private calls, even if you have to step outside.

• Personalize your office with items like vacation or family photos. This will make it feel like your own space instead of a sterile, impersonal area. Also, the items you use can help make you feel comfortable or more at home.

Helpful Hint

On the way home from work, mentally close the door on your cubicle, even if it doesn't have one. "Every mile you go, picture it closing at work and opening at home," Dr. McClure says. "And when you get home, take 10 to 15 minutes to change your clothes, relax, and shift your mind-set." ■

CONTROL YOUR BLOOD PRESSURE WITH POTTED PLANTS

It's normal for blood pressure to rise as you work at your desk. Working in close proximity to coworkers can be especially stressful. The antidote? Potted plants.

In a study of computer workers at Washington State University in Pullman, those who occupied work stations with plants that shielded them from view showed significantly smaller increases in blood pressure as they worked than those not shielded by plants.

Cuts

Slice Bagels (and Other Foods) Safely

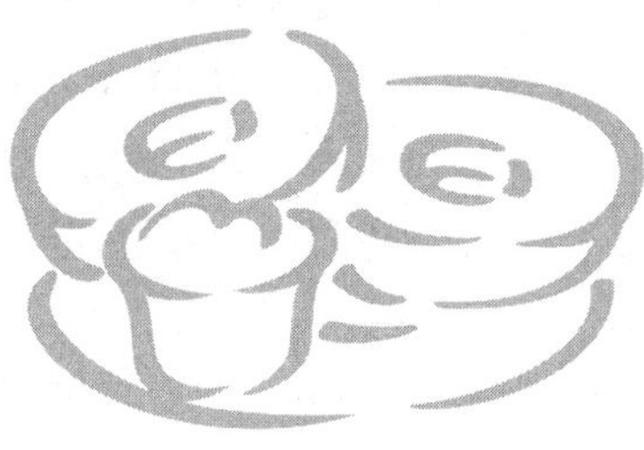

Emergency room physicians across the country have reported an unusual rise in the number of people they treat for wounds sustained trying to cut bagels. In fact, kitchen accidents—including slicing bagels—are common causes of cuts among women.

"Bagel-cutting injuries are one of the more underreported accidents of our times," says Elaine Josephson, M.D., attending emergency department physician at St. Luke's–Roosevelt Hospital Center in New York City and a spokesperson for the American College of Emergency Physicians. "Most people—men and women alike—have trouble cutting things that are round." That includes bagels as well as apples, onions, carrots, and the like.

Here's how to cut a bagel (and other round foods).

Place a bagel on its side to halve it. That's safer than balancing it precariously on its rounded edge. (Or, consider using a bagel slicer.)

Square it off. Once you make the first cut through an apple, onion or other round food, lay the food on the newly created flat side. Then continue to slice, quarter, or dice the food.

Use a serrated knife. A knife with tiny teeth along the edge can dig in more easily, reducing the chance that the knife will slip off the bagel, apple, or other food you're cutting.

Don't hold the knife in a death grip. Instead, grasp the handle between your thumb and forefinger. Allow the rest of your fingers to lie naturally along the handle's curve. Your grip should be firm, without being too tight.

Always cut away from you. Lightly grasp the food in the other hand and cut away from you in sawing-motion strokes that are slow and steady.

Helpful Hint

Soft or fresh bagels are easier to cut and less susceptible to slippage than hard bagels. ■

FIRST-AID FOR BAGEL INJURIES

If you accidentally cut yourself slicing a bagel (or anything else):

- Wash the cut immediately with soap (preferably antibacterial) and water to prevent infection.
- Apply pressure with a clean towel to stop any bleeding.
- If the cut appears open or does not stop bleeding within several minutes of applied pressure, go to the emergency room, pronto. You may need stitches or some other form of closure for the wound.
- If the cut isn't open and the bleeding has stopped, clean and dry the wound. Then apply an antibacterial ointment and cover the entire cut with an adhesive bandage to keep out dirt and protect the wound from further injury. Cleanse the wound and change the dressing daily until it's healed.

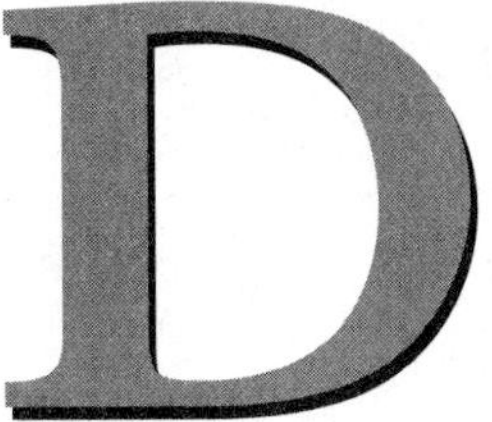

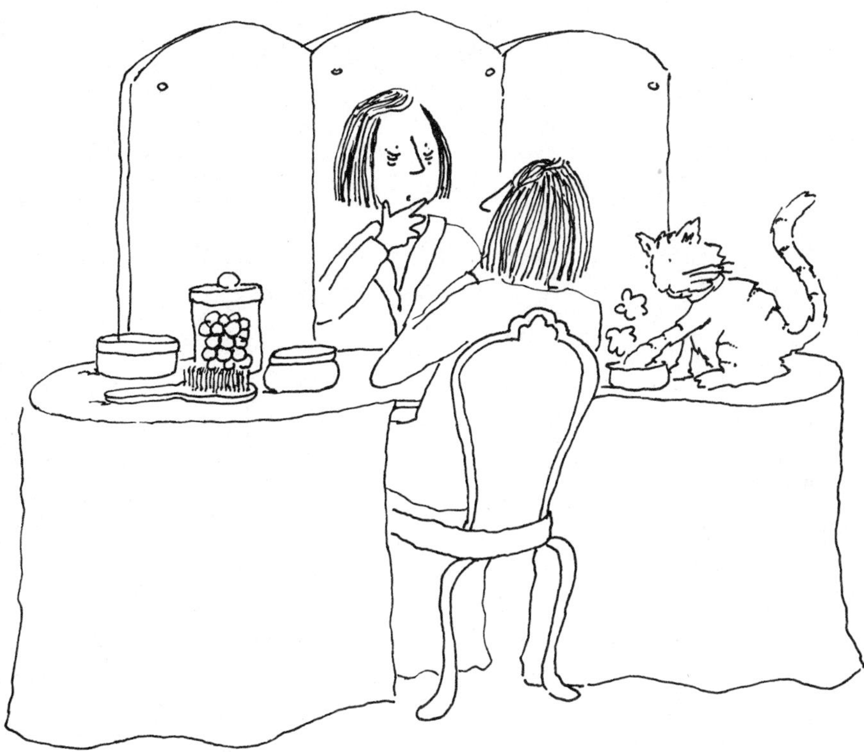

Using the wrong kind of concealer for dark under-eye circles can leave you looking worse, not better.

For inside tips, see page 116.

Dandruff

The 7-Day Flake-Fighting Formula

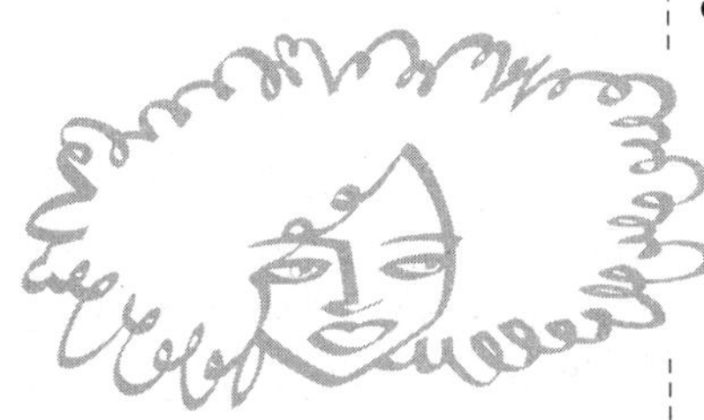

The skin you have on your body now isn't the same skin you were wearing a month ago. Sure, you still look the same. But the cells on the surface of your skin die off every 28 days, replaced by identical new cells. Normally, this constant turnover goes unnoticed. With dandruff, however, the cells on your scalp clump together and collect on your shoulders.

No one is sure why dandruff occurs, says Janet Hickman, M.D., a dermatologist at Dermatology Consultants and vice president, associate medical director, and dandruff researcher at the Education and Research Foundation, both in Lynchburg, Virginia. However, a certain kind of yeast commonly found on the scalp, Pityrosporum ovale, *seems to irritate some women's skin more than others, causing the skin cells to cling together in flakes as they fall away. And for many women, dandruff seems to worsen in times of stress. If you have dandruff, you've probably already discovered that regular shampoo doesn't help, even if you wash your hair daily. Dandruff shampoos carry any one of five active ingredients: ketoconazole, which once was a prescription-only medication; coal tar; zinc pyrithione; selenium sulfide; and salicylic acid. The first four ingredients fight the yeast, while salicylic acid works more to break up the clumps and release them from your scalp, Dr Hickman says.*

Dandruff shampoo seems to help for a while, but then the problem returns. That's because over time, your scalp develops a resistance to antidandruff agents. Here's what dermatologists recommend.

Mix and match. If you see the problem returning, switch to a shampoo that contains a different active ingredient.

If that doesn't work, use a shampoo with ketoconazole twice a week and a different type of dandruff shampoo the other 5 days, recommends Robert Brodell, M.D., professor of internal medicine in the dermatology department at Northeastern Ohio Universities College of Medicine in Warren.

Rub it in. Whichever shampoo you use, rub it vigorously into your scalp with your fingertips and leave it in for about 3 minutes before rinsing it out. While you're waiting to rinse, you can wash the rest of your body.

Seek help when needed. See your doctor if you have any hair loss along with the dandruff or if you don't see an improvement after 3 weeks of dandruff shampooing, Dr. Hickman advises. You could possibly have seborrheic dermatitis or another condition, which calls for a different approach. ■

DON'T MAKE THIS MISTAKE

Try to avoid very stiff hair sprays that may leave dry, flaky residue buildup that mimics dandruff.

Dark Under-Eye Circles

A Cure for Raccoon Eyes

Most women blame lack of sleep for under-eye circles. But insomnia has little to do with it.

"You can be the healthiest, most well-rested woman in the world and still have under-eye circles," says Ly-Le Tran, M.D., vice president of corporate scientific affairs for L'Oreal in Clark, New Jersey.

What's more, the skin isn't really dark—it just looks that way. Blood passing through vessels just underneath the skin surface create a red or purplish shadow.

Not everyone has dark circles. People from Mediterranean and Middle Eastern areas have naturally hyper-pigmented skin around their eyes. "Some women (and men) are just born with more prominent vascular structures than others," says Dr. Tran. Second, fair skin is more transparent, so if you're fair, your blood vessels are more visible. Third, as you age, your skin gets thinner, so blood vessels are more noticeable.

Any type of allergy can cause the blood vessels under your eyes to dilate and become more noticeable. Allergies can also lead to puffiness under your eyes, accentuating dark circles.

If dark circles are hereditary, the only permanent solution is either a chemical peel or laser treatments to remove the veins (both medical procedures). With a chemical peel, the dermatologist puts a mild acid on your skin that causes a minor burn—somewhat like a rug burn. The new skin will be thicker and will better hide the blood

Deadlines

Finish Any Job on Time

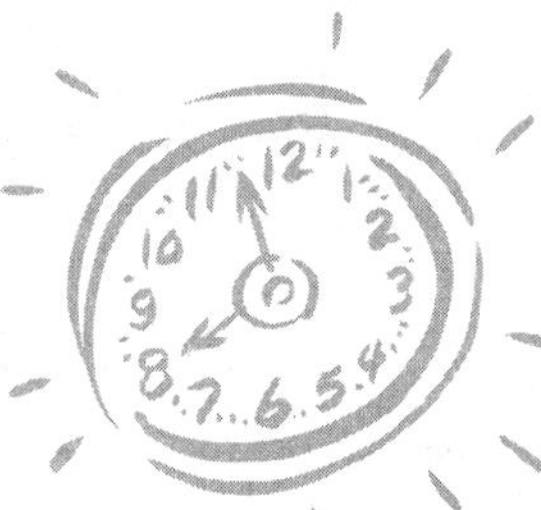

When Egyptologists finally get around to deciphering all the hieroglyphs, they're sure to find one that roughly translates as, "You want this pyramid finished by the end of the month? I'm out of stone blocks. You have to give me a little more time."

It'll just be further proof that deadlines—and the excuses for not meeting them—have bedeviled humankind since antiquity.

For today's pyramid builders—women pulling shifts at home and in the workplace—meeting deadlines can be a real challenge. A child's illness, a burst pipe, or some other household emergency can place even the most dedicated employee hopelessly behind schedule.

Experts offer these tips for meeting and (if necessary) renegotiating deadlines.

Set realistic expectations for yourself. Whatever the scope of the project, be sure that you understand the level of quality that's expected. "Usually, we set our standards too high," says Marilyn Manning, Ph.D., a business consultant in Mountain View, California. "Dead-

vessels. A laser, too, creates a mild burn, but it may or may not be as effective.

For a temporary but less expensive fix, you can do what a lot of women do for dark circles—hide them. To avoid ending up with white circles in their place, follow this advice from Nicole Harris, a makeup artist from Kenneth's Salon in New York City.

- Select a concealer cream that's one shade lighter than your own skin tone, no lighter.
- Use the edge of a damp sponge wedge or your fingertips to apply concealer.
- Apply from the inner corner of your eye (by your nose) to about halfway across at the center of your eye.
- Blend well by patting the margins down into your cheek area.
- Always set concealer with a light dusting of translucent powder.

DON'T MAKE THESE MISTAKES

Don't extend concealer toward the outer corner of your eyes—it will cake into little laugh lines. Also, if you have puffy bags under your eyes, don't use concealer there. The lighter color will only accent the puffiness. Instead, choose a color that matches your natural skin tone.

Helpful Hint

You can use concealer with foundation makeup. Apply concealer first, then foundation. Be sure to pat the second layer into place under your eyes. "If you stroke it, you'll erase the foundation," says Harris. "And if you leave little finger or sponge prints, you're using too much concealer." ■

SHOW NO FEAR

With a deadline looming overhead like a hungry T-Rex, it's normal to feel panicky. But keep it to yourself. "When you share your panic, you're looking for empathy, understanding, and pity," Dr. Manning says. "It can give the impression that you're not organized, that you get stressed easily, and that you lack competence—signals that you don't want to send."

lines become unmanageable when there are certain points of ambiguity."

Develop a strategic plan. Make a realistic estimate of how long it will take to complete the project and how many resources you'll need. Rank your tasks in order of importance and tackle the most crucial ones first. If you break each task into manageable chunks, the project will seem much less daunting.

Float a trial balloon. Well in advance of your deadline, give your boss an outline or rough draft of your work. If you're on track, great. If not, you can spare yourself a lot of grief. "Often, it's not that we have problems meeting the deadline, but we meet it with our version of the assignment," Dr. Manning says. "If it doesn't meet our boss's expectation, we're faced with the panic of trying to quickly revise it."

Build in check points. In team-oriented workplaces, ❯❯

a project's success depends on the cooperation of many people. If any one of them drops the ball, the project suffers. If you're a project manager, you need to build checkpoints into the schedule. "Think of the worst-case scenario and build in steps to avoid it," Dr. Manning says.

Call in reinforcements. If it appears that you or your team can't meet a deadline, ask for additional resources. "You may be able to get temporary help for a few hours a week to help complete the project," says Dr. Manning.

Suppose you've taken all these precautions and your boss throws yet another assignment on your plate that's due first thing in the morning. How do you bargain for more time?

"Very carefully," says career consultant Barbara Reinhold, Ed.D., in Northampton, Massachusetts. Instead of saying no, Dr. Reinhold recommends saying something like this: "I'm working on this other project for tomorrow and I'd like to know which one you want me to do." "That's very different from saying you're overworked and can't do it," she says. ■

Dental Floss

Houseclean Your Teeth in 60 Seconds

Denise Barton can let dirty dishes sit in the sink.

She can let the laundry go.

She can even let the grass grow unmowed in the yard of her home in North Andover, Massachusetts.

But would this 44-year-old working mother of two go to bed at night without flossing?

"Never!" she says with a smile. "I have 3 years and $20,000 in orthodontic bills tied up in these teeth. I'm not going to lose them now."

Dentists wish that more women were like Barton. The prospect of the country's 60 million aging baby boomers losing their grins to gum disease is nothing to laugh at—particularly when the cure may be as simple as 24 inches of waxed string.

"Flossing is the only way to remove plaque from the sides of your teeth," says David L. Cochran, D.D.S., chair of the research, science, and therapy committee of the American Academy of Periodontology. "Once you get into the flossing habit, it feels so good that you won't want to stop. It's a cleanliness thing."

And a lifesaver.

"It seems clear that gum disease, far from being just an oral health problem, actually represents a significant health risk to millions of people," says Robert Genco, D.D.S., editor in chief of the *Journal of Periodontology*.

Blame it on bacteria. Your mouth is home to more than 300 different species of bacteria. While they're useful in digestion, the bacteria wreck havoc on the teeth. Food particles that lodge in the tiny spaces between teeth are a breeding ground for these bacteria. Brushing alone can't get rid of them. Left to multiply, the bacteria form a film on the teeth called plaque, which inflames the gums and leads to a painful condition called gingivitis. Without proper care to treat the inflamed tissue, the gums and bone are weakened, and tooth loss results.

The problem isn't just in your head. Gum disease has been linked to many health ills throughout the body. Those rogue bacteria enter into the bloodstream through damaged gums and can attack the heart valves and attach themselves to blood vessels, aggravating fatty buildup. Individuals with periodontal disease are twice as likely to get heart disease as those with healthy gums. The bacteria also can cause infections in people with chronic illnesses like diabetes or lung conditions.

Women should be particularly mindful of their teeth during pregnancy because hormone changes during childbearing tend to increase the incidence of gum disease, which has been linked with premature births.

"Flossing is simple. It only takes a minute," says Dr. Cochran. Use about 2 feet of floss wrapped around your middle fingers. Holding the floss between your thumb and forefinger, gently guide the floss between adjacent teeth, down to the opening just above the gumline. Arc the floss in a C-shape around a tooth and rub up and down. Repeat for every tooth with a new section of floss.

Helpful Hint

If you don't like sticking your fingers in your mouth, pick up a wishbone-shaped floss holder at your local pharmacy. It works almost as well as the string-on-a-roll type. And it could save you a lifetime of smiles. ■

Depression

St. John's Wort to the Rescue

If you've tried Prozac or some other prescription antidepressant but don't like the side effects (lower sexual desire being one), you might want to consider St. John's wort.

St. John's wort has gotten a lot of publicity over the years as "natural" Prozac. Studies have found that St. John's wort alleviates mild to moderate depression as effectively as prescription antidepressants. Scientists aren't sure how St. John's wort works but speculate that it increases levels of the mood-elevating chemical serotonin. Its active ingredient hypericin is believed responsible for the herb's antidepressant effects, but research indicates that St. John's wort may contain many active ingredients.

"It's not just one molecule with one effect, as with synthetic drugs," says Harold Bloomfield, M.D., author of *Hypericum and Depression.* "St. John's wort has many active ingredients, and they all work together."

Widely used to relieve depression in European countries, St. John's wort has some definite advantages over synthetic drugs. It's not addictive, causes no withdrawal symptoms, and can be safely ›› mixed with alcohol. Nor does it produce the side effects commonly associated with antidepressant drugs, such as nausea, gastrointestinal distress, and lowered sex drive.

"Prescription antidepressants aren't necessary to treat mild depression," says Dr. Bloomfield.

"St. John's wort is the first thing I prescribe for depression," says Hyla Cass, M.D., assistant clinical professor of psychiatry at the University of California at Los Angeles School of Medicine. "It may not help every woman, but it's unlikely ever to hurt anyone."

If your doctor has ruled out serious depression, you may want to give St. John's wort a

DON'T MAKE THIS MISTAKE

If you're already taking an antidepressant, don't suddenly stop taking it and switch to St. John's wort. Nor should you add the herb to your regimen. Instead, with your doctor's guidance, taper your antidepressant use, while gradually increasing your intake of St. John's wort. "The longer someone has been on an antidepressant like Prozac, the more slowly you have to wean them off," says Dr. Bloomfield.

Diabetes

Six Ways to Control Blood Sugar (None of Which Involve Needles)

If you have diabetes, chances are your doctor has already given you plenty of advice designed to avoid "complications" like heart attack, stroke, and nerve disease: Get as close as possible to your desirable weight. Exercise at least 20 minutes a day, 3 days a week, Reduce the amount of fat you consume to no more than 30 percent of total calories (and the saturated fat to 10 percent). And if you're on insulin, monitor your blood sugar levels carefully.

In addition, these lesser-known but very promising strategies may also help. (If you want to try these strategies and you're on insulin, work with your doctor—your dosage may need to be changed.)

1. Eat a teaspoon of psyllium seed with each meal. A plant fiber best known for preventing constipation, psyllium may also lower elevated blood sugar levels, according to one study. It's readily available in powdered form at supermarkets and health food stores. Dissolve a teaspoon in a cup of water before each meal—or add it to cereals, soups, fruit juices, or smoothies.

2. Try alpha-lipoic acid. German research shows that this ultra-powerful antioxidant will reduce blood sugar levels and improve your cholesterol counts. But most remarkably, try. Here's what you need to know.

Take just what you need, and no more. Doctors who prescribe St. John's wort usually suggest 300 milligrams three times a day. Look for products with 0.3 percent extract of the chemical hypericin.

The best dose, says Dr. Cass, "is the lowest one that produces results." She suggests starting with the recommended dose, then tapering after a few months to find the optimum dose. Some people will find that they can eventually stop taking the herb completely without symptoms recurring.

Take it with food. Some women experience nausea the first few days, which usually vanishes when the herb is taken with food.

Wear sunscreen, wraparound sunglasses, and a hat if you go outdoors. Evidence suggests that St. John's wort may increase sensitivity to the sun if you're light-skinned.

Helpful Hint

Don't expect instant results. "Like prescription antidepressants, St. John's wort often takes 3 to 4 weeks before it kicks in," explains Dr. Bloomfield. ■

alpha-lipoic acid may reduce nerve numbness and pain caused by diabetic neuropathy, a form of nerve damage that can lead to loss of vision or kidney problems. Sometimes called thioctic acid, alpha-lipoic acid is available in capsules. The effective dose is 600 milligrams a day, says Aaron Vinik, M.D., Ph.D., director of research at the Strelitz Diabetes Institute in Norfolk, Virginia.

3. Swallow a baby aspirin every day. Aspirin reduces heart attack risk by discouraging blood cells called platelets from sticking together in the arteries. Amazingly, it's even more effective for those with diabetes than for those without diabetes. That's good news, since diabetic women are the only population group in which the incidence of heart attack has been going up in recent years. "No one with diabetes should go without a baby aspirin on a daily basis," says Dr. Vinik. Ask your doctor how much aspirin is right for you.

4. Take 5 to 10 tablets of brewer's yeast daily. Gamma-linolenic acid is the hot new kid on the diabetes-control block. This fatty acid makes it easier for your body to build nerve tissue. Benefit: less of the nerve damage that causes trouble for women with diabetes. It's perfectly safe, though some complain of a bit of heartburn or dyspepsia. Doctors who prescribe it recommend 4,000 milligrams daily. Brewer's yeast tablets contain either 400 or 800 milligrams of gamma-linolenic acid, says Dr. Vinik. (Don't use gamma-linolenic acid supplements without the supervision of a physician if you are taking aspirin or anticoagulants—blood thinners—regularly, have a seizure disorder, or are taking epilepsy medication such as phenothiazines.)

5. Ask about supplements of vitamins E and C. Studies suggest that supplements of both antioxidants can help. ››

In one study, men with diabetes and women who had started to show signs of complications had lower levels of these nutrients than those who were free of problems. Other studies have shown that taking 800 IU a day of vitamin E may reduce high blood sugar levels. Another small study showed that a bit more—900 IU a day—can improve nerve function in those with type 2 (non-insulin-dependent) diabetes. Daily doses of 500 milligrams of vitamin C may help reduce the amount of blood sugar that binds to proteins, which contributes to complications. Men and women with type 1 (insulin-dependent) diabetes appear to have difficulty absorbing vitamin C, so they may need more. (If you have diabetes, get your doctor's okay before trying this.)

6. Get enough chromium. Since chromium helps make your cells receptive to insulin, make sure that you get your Daily Value of 120 micrograms. Since it's hard to get that much from your diet, a multivitamin/mineral supplement may be a good idea. ■

Diarrhea

Nurse Your Bowels Back to Normal

If you have diarrhea, it's probably little comfort to know that loose, watery bowels are your body's way of flushing out bacteria or other nasty stuff that can make you sick all over. You're miserable and want this dubious healing experience to be over a.s.a.p.

Don't *reach for the antidiarrheal medicine.*

"Yes, diarrhea is an embarrassing nuisance, and I can understand that women want relief," says Barbara Harland, Ph.D., professor in the department of nutritional sciences at Howard University College of Pharmacy, Nursing, and Allied Health Sciences in Washington, D.C. "But it's better if you can bring your body back to normal without medication." Here's how.

Drink up. Talk about counterintuitive. Your problem can only be described as "excess liquidity," yet doctors recommend more fluids? Absolutely, because diarrhea dehydrates. So drink at least eight glasses of water a day with diarrhea, just as you would for its opposite, constipation.

Eat some Jell-O. If eight glasses of water is more than you can get down, try other forms of water, including flavored gelatin dessert, ice chips, clear broth, flat soda, or Popsicles. Avoid caffeinated drinks (which flush fluid from your body) and diet soda or anything else with sorbitol (an artificial sweetener that retains fluid in the intestine). Both make diarrhea worse.

Raid your kids' medicine cabinet. Electrolyte replacement drinks for children, like Pedialyte or Lytren, can also help adults replace potassium or other electrolytes lost in fluid. Or have a sports drink like Gatorade or All Sport, diluted one-to-one with water.

Eat something bland. Your body needs calories to fortify itself. The trick is to find food that doesn't stimulate much intestinal action. Until you're better, bland is best: clear soups,

DON'T MAKE THIS MISTAKE

If you have diarrhea, drink liquids, but avoid apple juice, prune juice, and cranberry juice. They make diarrhea worse.

boiled vegetables, bananas, a baked potato without the skin, rice, and white toast. A lean cut of meat is okay, but in general, avoid fatty foods like French fries and cheeseburgers.

Munch on salted crackers. They're bland, and they replace some sodium chloride, another electrolyte in lost fluid.

Forget fiber for now. In the long run, bulk-forming fiber is just what your plumbing needs. But right now, you want to give your bowels a rest. So steer clear of the high-fiber stuff like bran flakes or raw vegetables.

Try yogurt, but not milk. Consuming dairy products is usually not a good idea if you have diarrhea. But a cup of yogurt a day may bring relief if your diarrhea stems from an infection. It helps restore the balance of good and bad bacteria in your digestive tract.

Don't expect instantaneous results. If you have diarrhea, it will probably take 2 to 3 days to get back to normal. If you must medicate, Imodium A-D, Pepto-Bismol, and Kaopectate can be effective and soothing to an irritated bowel, says Donna Bliss, R.N., Ph.D., assistant professor of nursing at the University of Minnesota in Minneapolis. Follow label instructions.

If diarrhea lasts more than 3 days, you have rectal bleeding, or you are alternating between constipation and diarrhea, see a doctor to rule out irritable bowel syndrome or other conditions that call for a different approach.

Helpful Hint

If diarrhea accompanies menstrual cramps at period time, try ibuprofen as your pain reliever of choice. It may tame diarrhea the same way it takes care of the cramps—by controlling production of prostaglandins, lipids that generate pain. ■

Diet Pills

An Expensive Way to Lose a Little Weight

Weight loss drugs have a shaky history. In the early 1900s, the first diet pills contained arsenic and strychnine. After World War II, amphetamine-based diet pills left countless women edgy, addicted, and still overweight. The FDA asked a manufacturer to voluntarily withdraw the "fen" part of the fen-phen combination after it was linked with heart valve abnormalities.

Still, the quest for the perfect diet pill continues. The FDA has approved two new prescription weight loss drugs: sibutramine, which acts on the brain's neurotransmitters to dull the appetite, and orlistat, which blocks the absorption of about one-third of dietary fat. Five other FDA-approved prescription weight loss drugs are available for short-term ❯❯

use: methamphetamine, diethylpropion, benzphetamine, mazindol, and phendimetrazine.

They're intended for people who are at least 20 percent above their ideal weight—that is, for women who should weigh 125 pounds, for example, but weigh 150 or more. Yet the drugs have modest effects.

"In general, women who take prescription weight loss drugs lose between 5 and 10 percent of their initial body weight," says Susan Yanovski, M.D., director of the obesity and eating disorders program at the National Institute of Diabetes and Digestive and Kidney Diseases in Rockville, Maryland. If you weigh 150 pounds, that's a loss of 7½ to 15 pounds. If you weigh 200 pounds, it's a loss of 10 to 20 pounds. So the drugs aren't likely to turn a Kate Smith into a Kate Moss.

"They can help women lose enough weight to have health benefits, such as lower cholesterol and lower blood pressure, however," says Dr. Yanovski.

If you're thinking about trying prescription weight loss drugs, consider the following:

You have to take them indefinitely. It's like taking a drug for any chronic health condition, like diabetes, high blood pressure, or depression.

Long-term safety is unknown. Although sibutramine and orlistat have been approved for long-term use,

"NATURAL" DIET AIDS: LEAVE THEM ON THE SHELF

Take a close look at so-called natural fat burners sold on television and in magazine ads, and you'll discover all manner of odd combinations. A few include chitosan (made from lobster shells and crab shells), conjugated linoleic acid (a mixture of polyunsaturated fats found in the gut of cattle), and cellasene, a mixture of herbs, lecithin, and fish oil.

In truth, the only way these diet aids work is if you exercise vigorously while listening to 30-minute infomercials for the products. Studies show that they're only marginally effective.

Worse, some can have dangerous side effects. Phenylpropanolamine—sold over the counter in drugstores and supermarkets—has been associated with stroke, seizure, heart attack, and even death. Nevertheless, it has been approved for weight loss by the FDA. Others have not: The FDA has banned 111 ingredients from being used as weight loss aids, including caffeine, guar gum, and spirulina, a species of blue-green algae.

Beware of any products claiming to absorb or burn fat. They don't work. Products to avoid that have not been approved by the FDA for use as over-the-counter weight loss drugs include:

- Diet patches (worn on the skin)
- Fat blockers (purported to physically absorb fat and interfere with fat you eat)
- Starch blockers (promise to block starch digestion)
- Magnet pill (allegedly flush fat out of the body)
- Magic roots from the Orient (such as glucomannan)

Some of these can cause dangerous intestinal obstructions; others may cause nausea, vomiting, diarrhea, and stomach pain.

there's no data on their safety and effectiveness for more than a year or two.

Side effects can be serious (and embarrassing). Sibutramine increases blood pressure—a distinct disadvantage if you have high blood pressure to begin with. Orlistat blocks the absorption of fat-soluble vitamins and can cause oily stools, spotting, and an inability to control bowel movements.

Nondrug approaches may work better. You could lose weight with no side effects or risk to your health by eating less food and getting more exercise. ■

Distractions

Lessons in Concentration from a Lady Pool Shark

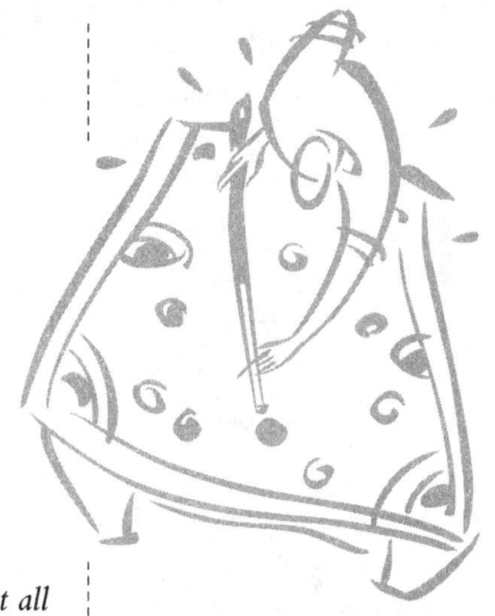

When Ewa Mataya Laurance, world champion billiards player, needs to focus on her game, what does she do? Anyone who can perform such a precise, accurate task under extreme pressure, with crowds staring and television cameras in her face, must have a few tricks up her sleeve.

"I've trained myself to focus on the task at hand and block out all other distractions," says Laurance, who lives in Charlotte, North Carolina. "I used to practice playing pool with my young daughter in the room with me. Learning to focus with her there made it a cinch to concentrate during competition."

Also, Laurance notes that she never plays pool for fun. "I do something else for recreation, so that whenever I play pool, I'm very serious, and I never let my concentration down at any time."

Experts heartily endorse Mataya Laurance's approach.

"Learning how to focus and setting boundaries are the keys to blocking out distractions," says Carol Goldberg, Ph.D., clinical psychologist and president of Getting Ahead Programs, a New York–based corporation conducting workshops on stress management, health, and wellness. Her suggestions:

- Make a time for play and a time for work and set clear boundaries between them.
- Write out a schedule for your day so that you can refer to it whenever you find yourself getting distracted.
- Set up times when you will be available to others, and be firm about saying no to interruptions.
- Break large projects into specific small amounts of time. "If you tell yourself that you'll work on something for precisely 1 hour and then take a break, you'll find it easier to focus than if the task seems like it will drag on inde- ››

terminately," says Dr. Goldberg.

• Make a list of what you need to do and when you'll do it, and reward yourself when you stick to it. Dr. Goldberg advises that for short tasks, try challenging yourself to complete them all the way through without stopping to do something else.

• Keep your desk or workspace clean and organized so that you won't have to search for items that you need, and you won't be distracted by clutter.

• Use meditation as a means of becoming more focused. "If you meditate regularly, you will actually become better at concentrating in all areas of your life," says Dr. Goldberg.

• Try to find something enjoyable about each task. "If you're doing something that you don't enjoy, you'll look for distractions," Dr. Goldberg says.

Helpful Hint

As with any other skills, concentration improves with practice. Just like Laurance, you must practice staying focused, says Dr. Goldberg. Realize that you can make that phone call later, and focus on the task at hand. After enough practice, you will be better at it. ■

Diverticular Disease

Take Time for Breakfast—Your Colon Will Thank You

Few diseases are more confusing than diverticulosis and diverticulitis. They're not exactly the same thing.

Diverticula are small "outpouchings" or "outpocketings" in the colon that seem to be caused by a low-fiber diet. The presence of these outpouchings (diverticulosis) is quite common—and they're more likely to occur as you get older—although you may not even know you have them unless they become inflamed and burst (diverticulitis). This is rare, but devastating. Leaking intestinal pockets cause fever, abdominal pain, even abscess.

Most women diagnosed with diverticulosis are well over age 60 and will not develop problems. In fact, only 10 to 25 percent of men or women with diverticulosis develop diverticulitis.

"Even when problems do occur, they're not always severe," says Patricia Roberts, M.D., staff surgeon at the Lahey Clinic in Burlington, Massachusetts. The most severe diverticulitis attacks may require emergency surgery for perforated bowel, for example. But most people have mild symptoms, such as tenderness around the left lower abdomen, cramps, and constipation, which can be managed with a high-fiber diet and antibiotics during bouts of fever.

Considered a medical curiosity when first identified in the early 1700s, diverticula became commonplace shortly after our Western diet started relying on white flour, refined sugar, and red meat, and we started eating less fiber.

"A high-fiber diet keeps the bowel open," says Marshall Sparberg, M.D., professor of medicine at Northwestern University Medical School in Chicago. Fiber absorbs water, softening stools and increasing bulk so that stools pass through quickly, reducing pressure on diverticula.

Women may be particularly susceptible because they are too busy to take the time for a decent breakfast and bowel movement, says Dr. Sparberg. "The bowel is most active in the morning, so eat a good high-fiber breakfast, drink something hot, and take the time for a good bowel movement," he advises.

To keep your colon free of diverticular trouble, Dr. Sparberg recommends these dietary strategies.

• Try to eat about 25 grams of fiber per day. Eat more high-fiber foods like bran, oats, and other foods that absorb liquid to make bulk.

• If you can't eat enough fiber, take Metamucil (psyllium husk fiber) or Citrucel (made from a cellulose material).

• Drink lots of liquids because fiber combines with liquid, forming soft, bulky stools that pass through more quickly and easily. This is especially important if you're taking Metamucil or Citrucel, which must be taken with plenty of water.

• To prevent an attack of diverticulitis, avoid nuts and seeds because they may plug up the diverticula (smooth peanut butter is okay). ■

DON'T MAKE THIS MISTAKE

If you have lower abdominal pain and fever together, get medical attention without delay. "People with diverticulitis may think they have stomach flu and not get it treated soon enough, and it develops into an abscess," says Dr. Sparberg. If you get treated quickly, you may only need a liquid diet and antibiotics. If you wait until it's severe, you may need hospitalization.

Dizziness and Vertigo

Be Your Own Detective

As a kid, you and your playmates probably enjoyed making yourselves dizzy, turning cartwheels on a grassy lawn or hopping on a carnival ride.

But when you feel off-kilter for no apparent reason, the fun stops. Vertigo, a sensation of spinning, and dizziness, which is a vague woozy feeling, can interfere with your ability to work or even get out of bed in the morning.

Trying to find out why you are dizzy can be a long, drawn-out process. If your sense of balance starts to go awry, pay a visit to your family doctor, who may refer you to an ear, nose, and throat specialist. The following information may help pinpoint the cause of your trouble.

You begin to feel woozy a week or so after having a head cold, but your hearing is fine.

You may have viral labyrinthitis. Your labyrinths are tiny canals in your inner ear that control your sense of balance, and when they become irritated—say, from a virus—they can send you reeling, says Mohamed Hamid, M.D., Ph.D., medical director of the Cleveland Hearing and Balance Center in Ohio.

Though this usually goes away on its own within 6 weeks, your doctor may give you exercises to help restore your sense of balance. ››

You can't hear well, you have ringing in the ears, and you experience vertigo for 30 minutes to 8 hours.

You may have Ménière's disease, characterized by a buildup of fluid in the labyrinths in the inner ear.

Cutting down on dietary salt, learning how to reduce your stress, and getting plenty of sleep may help, Dr. Hamid says. So can reducing use of water pills or steroids, with your doctor's consent.

Vertigo comes and goes quickly and is brought on when you suddenly move your head a certain way. You may feel it when you roll over in bed or tip your head back for a shampoo at the hairdresser.

The full name of this ailment is enough to make your head spin: benign paroxysmal positional vertigo (BPPV).

It's caused by tiny particles in your inner ear that migrate out of their normal position. A doctor or therapist familiar with this condition can cure it by directing you through a simple treatment in which you move your head and body to shift the particles back into place.

You feel dizzy for weeks after returning from a cruise.

You may be feeling the residual effects of a motion sickness condition dubbed mal de debarquement (MDD). Some people stay sick for weeks after getting off a cruise ship, and women are three times more likely to become dizzy from movements in traveling than men, Dr. Hamid says.

Treatment for motion sickness involves antinausea medications (when it's at its worst) and at-home exercises to train your eyes, inner ears, and body to work together so that they don't send conflicting signals to your brain. Your health care provider can teach you.

You feel faint or lightheaded upon standing up.

Most likely, your blood pressure was disrupted, Dr. Hamid says. Your doctor may prescribe medication or advise you to change your diet. ■

Doctor Visits

Make Every Minute Count

When we buy real estate, we live by the mantra "location, location, location." In medicine, start chanting "preparation, preparation, preparation."

The reason is simple: "The economics of medical practice prompt physicians to see as many patients as possible in as little time possible," says Lila Wallis, M.D., clinical professor of medicine at Weill Medical College of Cornell University, an attending physician at New York Presbyterian Hospital, both in New York City, and author of The Whole Woman. *"Consequently, doctors are rushed."*

Here's what you can do to make the most of your next doctor visit.

When You Make the Appointment

Schedule regular checkups as early as possible. Some doctors are booked 6 months in advance, says Leslie Frankel, M.D., an obstetrician and gynecologist at G.C.S.F. ObGyn Associates in the Philadelphia area. "Some of Dr. Frankel's patients call the first day of the month for an appointment 6 months out," says her scheduling manager, Debbie Kelble.

Briefly tell the scheduling person what your issues are. "They can help determine how much time you need," says Margaret Houston, M.D., a family practice physician with the Mayo Clinic in Rochester, Minnesota.

To avoid a long wait when you arrive, try to get the first appointment of the day. Or, call just before your appointment to find out if the doctor is behind schedule.

Before the Visit

List your symptoms. "If you have several, rank your symptoms in importance," says Dr. Houston.

Do some background research. If you're not sure what symptoms are most important, read up on them. "In a sense, a woman has to take charge, using the physician as a consultant," says Dr. Wallis. That doesn't mean you should diagnose yourself, but you do need to learn about your body and its problems.

Don't inundate your doctor with pages downloaded from the Internet. Instead, summarize what you've learned.

Jot down any over-the-counter or prescription medicine you're taking, along with how often and how much of it you take each day. It's also important to make note of any herbs, vitamins, or natural supplements you might be using.

Write down your questions. Focus on your biggest concerns. "Ask yourself, 'What worries me most?'" says Dr. Wallis. "Is it failing memory, which runs in my family? Is it breast cancer?" You don't want to leave the doctor's office with big concerns still looming.

During the Visit

Get right to the point. If your biggest concern is dizziness, for instance, don't start talking about the gallbladder surgery you had last year.

Present your complaints chronologically. For instance, if your first symptom of dizziness started 2 months ago, then got worse a month ago, then became a constant problem in the last week, say so. If you lost your balance and fell in the last 2 days, say so.

Let the doctor know what, if anything, you've done to try to remedy the condition. Tell her if you've changed your diet in any way or taken any vitamins, herbs, or over-the-counter remedies, for instance, and what effect they have had on your symptoms.

Be frank. If you fear you have a drinking problem or worry about your mental health, say so.

Take notes while the doctor talks. If you are seeing a specialist or feel stressed about your health, bring a friend or relative with you to take notes and offer support. Then, summarize what the doctor has told you to make sure you understand the advice.

Helpful Hint

To get the attention you need, it's important to find a good doctor, then continue to see her regularly. "If you wait 5 years for a checkup, you'll have a million questions that will never get answered," says Dr. Houston. ■

Drowsiness

A Pilot's Secrets for Staying Alert

Patrice Washington can't afford to snooze on the job. As a pilot for United Parcel Service who flies nights from coast to coast—sometimes for 15 hours at a time—her life depends on staying alert.

Chances are, nodding off while you're at work isn't a life-threatening situation, but it could be a job-threatening one. To stay alert and energized throughout the day, Washington and Wayne F. Kendall Jr., M.D., an aeromedical advisor for Aviation and Preventive Medicine Associates in Palmer Lake, Colorado, offer these tried-and-true tips straight from the cockpit.

DON'T MAKE THIS MISTAKE

If you feel sluggish and weary every day for no reason, don't hesitate to see your doctor. You may be suffering from sleep apnea (a treatable yet often undiagnosed condition in which breathing actually stops during sleep, depriving your brain of oxygen). Or you may want to rule out hypothyroidism or other serious medical conditions.

Lighten up. Inside the cockpit, airplane pilots switch on lights that mimic daylight. And that wakes them up quickly, says Dr. Kendall.

So if you have a window in your office, peel back the blinds and let in the sunshine. Or, add some lamps and equip them with bulbs no dimmer than 90 watts.

Chill out. Most pilots like to keep their cockpits at about 72°F, says Dr. Kendall. It's been found to be the perfect temperature for alertness.

Got a warm office? Open those windows or ask management to turn down the thermostat to a more comfortable temperature. "You'll be amazed how fast you wake up in a cool environment," says Washington.

Chew the fat. When their eyelids get heavy, pilots are taught to strike up conversations that require some thought, says Dr. Kendall. "It's like the instructor who catches you dozing off in the classroom and then suddenly asks you a question. You automatically wake up."

Your office fix: If you're about to fall asleep, take the opportunity to problem-solve with coworkers or make a quick call to a friend.

Fuel up. Foods high in fiber and low in fat boost your energy and keep it steady throughout the day. Heavy meals, on the other hand, weigh you down and make you sleepy, says Washington.

If you find yourself dozing after breakfast or lunch, consider switching to what pilots eat: hot or cold cereals with fat-free milk, bagels with peanut butter, 100 percent fruit juice, and whole fruits for breakfast. Eat soups, salads, low-fat lunchmeats on whole wheat bread, grilled chicken, fish, and vegetables for lunch and dinner.

Work that body. During 2-hour layovers, some pilots jog, walk, or do stretching exercises. "This gets the blood circulating and gives you the extra energy you need to continue your day," says Washington.

And for you? Go for a 30-minute jog or walk with coworkers or do some light weight training. Chained to your desk? Then stand up, walk around your office, and do some stretching exercises, starting from your neck down to your toes.

Catch some Zzzs. Between flights, some pilots find a quiet lounge and hit the hay. "Taking naps makes a huge difference in your ability to fly a plane later that night," says Washington.

If you have an office lounge with a sofa and a door you can close, lie down and take a 30- to 40-minute nap on your lunch hour. But no longer. "Once you sleep past 40 minutes, your body enters a deeper stage of sleep, and you'll end up feeling sluggish instead of refreshed for the rest of the day," says Dr. Kendall. ■

Drug Interactions

Keeping Peace with Your Internal Pharmacy

Did you know that anyone who's taking a prescription diuretic shouldn't suck on too many licorice cough drops? (Licorice can lead to fluid retention, counteracting the effect of the drug.) Or if you're taking a blood-thinning medication for high blood pressure, you can't take aspirin, which can thin the blood even further? Or that antacids can interfere with certain drugs prescribed for heart disease, such as captopril (Capoten) and broad-spectrum antibiotics like tetracycline?

Even if you take good care of yourself, sooner or later you're likely to use medication of some kind, be it an over-the-counter drug or a prescription medicine. Used individually, a drug may work they way it's supposed to. Combined with other drugs, it may not work, or may have unintended effects. Here's what Candy Tsourounis, Pharm.D., assistant clinical professor in the department of clinical pharmacy at the University of California, San Francisco, recommends to prevent problems.

Make a list and check it twice. Always keep an updated list of every health-related remedy you're using, no matter how minor it seems. Include prescription and over-the-counter drugs (even ones you use on your skin or eyes), vitamins, herbs, and other supplements. Take your list with you every time you visit your doctor and pharmacist, and ask if the new medicine will interact with any of the others.

Always use the same pharmacy to fill your prescriptions. The pharmacist will have a file of your past prescriptions and will be better able to notice if a newly prescribed drug could interact with one you're already taking. If a chain pharmacy has several locations in your town, ask whether their computers are linked and can share ›› your prescription history before you visit more than one of them.

Grill your pharmacist. Ask what the medicine is supposed to do, how long you should take it, what side effects to watch for and, of course, if it interacts with any of the products you're already using. "This is important—if the pharmacist doesn't have time to answer your questions, find one who does," says Dr. Tsourounis.

Read the label and any pamphlets or printouts that come with the drug. Ask about any discrepancies between what you read and what your doctor or pharmacist has told you about the drug.

Look before you swallow. If you've been taking a drug for awhile and it suddenly looks different after you get a refill, call the pharmacy to check that it's the right medication, Dr. Tsourounis suggests.

Follow the same rules on the Net. If you fill a prescription from a pharmacy Web site on the Internet, be sure that the business has a licensed and registered pharmacist who can answer any questions about your medications.

Helpful Hint

Always ask the pharmacist if you should take the drug prescribed on a full or empty stomach, or if you should avoid alcohol or grapefruit juice, all of which can affect how the drug works in your body. ■

Dry Eyes

A No-Mess Way to Apply Eyedrops

One way to take care of your dry-eye problem might be to buy a weeper like The Bridges of Madison County *on video and view the film over and over. Fortunately, there's a home remedy far less threatening to your sanity.*

Which is a good thing, because dry eyes—common in women over age 40—is a bigger problem than it sounds. When your eyes are constantly gritty, burning or even teary (an overcompensation), getting through the day can be a painful ordeal. Depending on the cause, dry eyes can even threaten your vision, if left untreated.

"Most women can deal with dry eyes on their own, though," says Monica L. Monica, M.D., Ph.D., an ophthalmologist in New Orleans. Over-the-counter lubricating eyedrops may be all you need, she says. They create the tear film that your eyes should be creating on their own, but aren't.

Dr. Monica offers the following tips to turn you into a master moistener, even if your wear eye makeup.

Make a pocket. Use a finger to lower your bottom lid. That creates a nice pocket to receive the drops. Look up as you fill the pocket.

Hit the corner. If you can't master the pocket approach, try aiming for the corner of your eye rather than the middle. You're less likely to get a runover.

Shut your eyes. Once the drops reach their destination, close your eyes and keep them closed for about 10 seconds. That keeps the drops in place

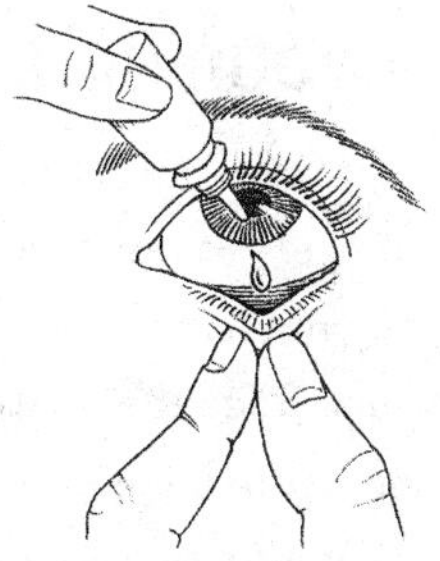

better than blinking does.

Get horizontal. Some women find that they can take a steadier aim if they apply drops while lying down.

Try a gel. Lubrication in ointment form is usually used at bedtime, since it can blur your vision for a while. But GenTeal now makes a minimum-blur gel that many find much easier to get into the eye pocket than drops. Plus, the gel lasts longer.

Take a tip. Put a dab of the gel at the end of a cotton swab for easier application. Just make sure it doesn't soak into the cotton, since you don't want any fibers in your eye. Or you can use your clean pinky finger.

Time it. Apply drops before you put on your makeup whenever possible.

Practice. No matter how clumsy you are at first, you will get better with practice, says Dr. Monica.

Helpful Hint

Keep drops handy and use them in situations that tend to dry out your eyes.

• Working at a computer. You don't blink enough when you're staring at that screen.

• Flying. Pressurized cabins are notoriously desiccating.

• Skiing. The air is thinner and drier at higher elevations.

• Taking antihistamines. They can also dry your eyes.

• Sleeping with a fan running in your bedroom.

• Driving with the air vent of your car blasting your face. ■

DON'T MAKE THIS MISTAKE

Antiredness drops can dry your eyes more. Buy artificial tears instead. And check the label for a "PF" indicating that the drops are free of preservatives, which can irritate your eyes or trigger allergies.

Dry Hair

Try Jojoba (and Stay Away from the Grill!)

"Very few people are born with dry hair," says Diana Bihova, M.D., a dermatologist in New York City and author of Beauty from the Inside Out. *But over time, exposure to sun, wind, chlorinated water, chemicals—and even overzealous shampooing—can leave your hair dry.*

"Women often think that the solution to dry hair is to buy a more expensive shampoo or conditioner," says Dr. Bihova. "But it's not always the answer."

To restore natural moisture to dry, lifeless hair, here's what Dr. Bihova recommends.

• Shampoo every other day (or once a day, if you must), but never twice a day. Shampooing less frequently will give the oils in your scalp a ❯❯

chance to moisturize your hair naturally.

• Use a mild shampoo, such as baby shampoo.

• Use moderately warm water when shampooing your hair. "Hot water can dry it out," says Dr. Bihova.

• Use a shampoo for chemically treated hair if your hair is permed or colored.

• Use a "daily" conditioner every other day. Apply conditioner only to the ends, where your hair is most likely to have been worn down through shampooing, brushing, and blow-drying.

If your hair is still dry, deep-condition once a week. Rub jojoba oil throughout your hair. Then wrap a towel around your head to keep your hair warm and covered. Keep it on for 20 to 30 minutes, then remove and shampoo. Jojoba oil acts as a humectant moisturizer, drawing moisture in from the atmosphere. It's available at your local health food store.

• Let your hair air-dry whenever possible.

• If you must use a blow-dryer, set the heat on a low or cool setting and hold the dryer at least 6 inches—or even better, an arm's length—from your head.

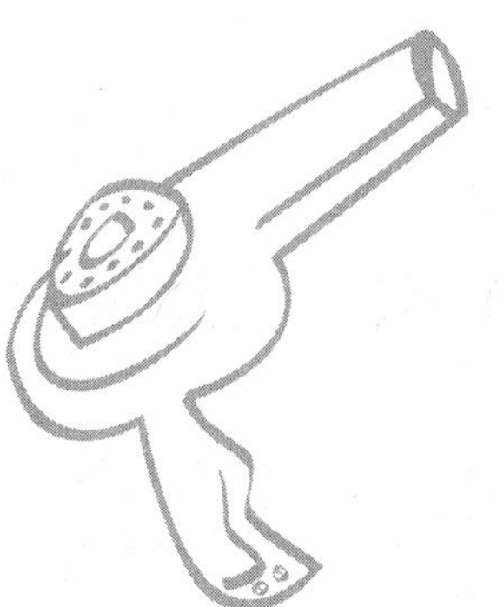

HAIR SPRAY THAT WON'T DRY YOUR HAIR

Looking for an alternative to chemical hair sprays? Try this all-natural blend: Simply chop up one lemon or orange. Put it in a pot with 2 cups of water and boil with the lid off until half the liquid evaporates. Then cool, strain the pits and pulp, place the mixture in a spray bottle, and add 1 ounce of rubbing alcohol. If it's too sticky, just add water. It will keep for up to 2 weeks outside the refrigerator.

Helpful Hint

Try supplementing your diet with black currant oil or evening primrose oil, both of which promote healthy hair and skin. Take one 500-milligram tablet twice a day. You should see improvement in 6 to 8 weeks. Then cut the dose in half. ■

DON'T MAKE THIS MISTAKE

Hair spray is flammable. If you use any kind of hair spray—aerosol or pump—make sure you don't light a match, cigarette, or candle near your hair. Same goes if you stand too close to a grill when you light the burner. The alcohol or propellants in the spray could ignite.

E–F

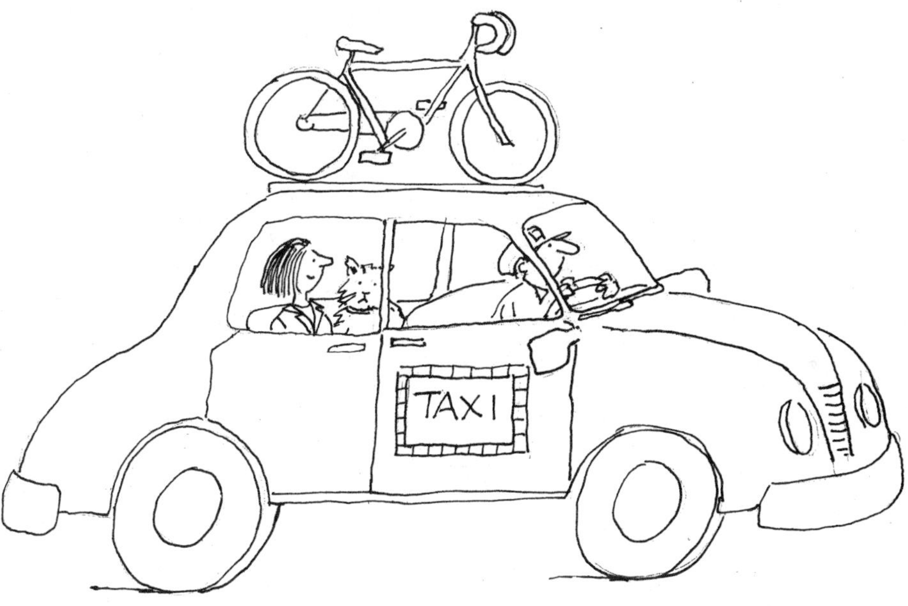

You don't have to leave home to get more exercise.
Find out how on page 142.

Earaches and Ear Infections

Antibiotics Aren't Always the Answer

You've taken your children to their pediatrician for earaches countless times. Now you're the one in pain. Everything sounds muffled. Your ear feels full. And it hurts.

Ear infections—and the accompanying earaches—occur when fluid builds up inside your middle ear (behind the eardrum), usually due to colds or allergies. Unable to drain through the eustachian tube, a narrow canal that connects your middle ear with the back of your nose, the fluid presses against your eardrum, creating the pressure and pain of an earache. The trapped mucus may then become infected.

Children get frequent earaches because their eustachian tube is horizontal, making it more difficult for fluids to drain from the ear, explains Mary Ann Block, D.O., medical director of the Block Center in Hurst, Texas, and author of No More Antibiotics: Preventing and Treating Children's Ear and Respiratory Infections the Natural Way. *By the time we're adults, the eustachian tube is more vertical, so our ears are less prone to infection.*

Concerned about hearing loss and the spread of infection, many doctors routinely prescribe antibiotics for ear infections. But antibiotics work only for bacterial infections, not ones caused by viruses. And, you may be able to avoid getting ear infections altogether by changing your diet.

DON'T MAKE THESE MISTAKES

Once you start taking an antibiotic, take the full course, even if you feel better. Otherwise, the infection will return full force. Also, see your doctor if your ear pain is severe; is accompanied by drainage, discharge, or a fever of 102°F; or persists for 48 hours despite treatment. And see a doctor immediately if you have a sudden change in hearing, become dizzy, can't concentrate, or notice weakness in your facial muscles on the same side as your affected ear.

"The simplest thing you can do is stop eating dairy products, whether you have a known allergy to dairy or not," advises Dr. Block, who says that **allergies to ice cream, cheese, yogurt, and other cow's-milk products can be the root of ear problems.** Eat any food to which you're allergic, and your sinuses and eustachian tube can become inflamed and swollen. Fluid can't drain, mucus accumulates, and soon your ear is aching and infected.

If you already have an ear infection, then taking an antibiotic may be in order. But you can also take these steps to soothe the pain and promote healing.

Turn to herbs. Robert Ivker, D.O, assistant clinical professor in the department of family medicine and clinical instructor in the department of otolaryngology at the University of Colorado School of ››

Medicine in Denver and author of *Sinus Survival: The Holistic Medical Treatment for Allergies, Asthma, Bronchitis, Colds, and Sinusitis,* recommends an herbal mix of garlic and mullein to kill bacteria, and St. John's wort to reduce inflammation. (Omit the St. John's if you're taking antidepressants of any kind).

Here's his recipe: Combine two parts garlic oil, one part liquid mullein, and one part St. John's wort extract (all available at health food stores) in a small dropper bottle. Warm the mixture by running the bottle under warm water. Place 2 or 3 drops in your affected ear, then loosely plug the ear with cotton. Repeat two or three times daily.

Reach for medicinal eucalyptus. Medicinal eucalyptus oil relieves inflammation in your mucus membranes. Directing the oil away from your face, spritz a tissue with two sprays and inhale the aroma for 30 seconds as needed throughout the day for up to 2 weeks.

Try hot and cold. Wet a washcloth with very warm water and hold it against your outer ear for 3 minutes. Remove the hot compress and apply a cold, damp washcloth to the same ear for 30 sec-

Echinacea

A Cornucopia of Uses

You don't have to be an herbal expert to know the value of echinacea. Few herbs have achieved the stature of the humble purple coneflower, long regarded as the best natural cold fighter around.

In fact, so strong is echinacea's cold-combating reputation, it has quite overshadowed this versatile herb's other useful properties.

"Echinacea is an invaluable part of my herbal pharmacy," says Mark Stengler, N.D., a naturopathic physician in San Diego and author of *Natural Physician: Your Guide for Common Ailments.* "I consider echinacea a mainstay for treating infectious diseases and enhancing immunity."

Echinacea works in numerous ways to boost your immune system, increase white blood cell production, and reduce fevers and inflammation.

Helpful Hints

Although nine species of echinacea exist, only two—*Echinacea angustifolia* and *Echinacea purpurea*—are used medicinally. When selecting echinacea teas, tinctures, or capsules, make sure that one, or both, of these species are used.

Don't use echinacea if you're allergic to closely related plants such as ragweed, asters, and chrysanthemums.

Active ingredients called alkylamides in the plant's roots and leaves are believed to activate production of interferon and properdin, two proteins known for fighting bacteria and viruses.

Beyond treating colds, echinacea can help make symptoms subside for:

Canker sores. Combat mouth sores by squeezing 1 or 2 dropperfuls of echinacea tincture into an 8-ounce glass of water. Swish the liquid in your mouth, rinse, and spit. Finish the entire glass and repeat a few times a day until the sore goes away.

onds. Continue alternating hot and cold washcloths until the pain is relieved—usually a few minutes.

Steam. In a middle ear infection, thick mucus gets caught in your ear, Dr. Ivker explains. Steam can open your nasal passages and thin the mucus so it can drain. Boil a pot of water and, keeping your face at least 12 inches from the pot, inhale for 20 minutes three times daily.

Chew gum with xylitol. This natural sweetener, often found in "sugar-free" gum, reduces the growth of the bacteria that leads to ear infections, says Dr. Block. One study found that children who chewed xylitol gum got 40 percent fewer ear infections than children who chewed regular gum. But adults can benefit, too.

Helpful Hint

If you get recurrent ear infections (and you don't fly frequently or scuba dive, both of which involve changes in air pressure that can contribute to ear problems), see an ear, nose, and throat specialist to ensure there's nothing structurally wrong with your ear. ■

Ear infections. Fend off chronic ear infections by drinking an 8-ounce glass of water containing 1 dropperful of echinacea tincture hourly whenever you feel soreness and tenderness in the ear. If pus is present, an infection may have caused your eardrum to rupture. See your doctor before using echinacea.

Pinkeye. For minor inflammation of the membrane that lines the inside of the eyelid and outside lining of the eyeball, take two echinacea capsules (250 milligrams each) or 60 drops three times daily until the infection clears up. Pinkeye can be highly contagious, so be sure to see a doctor for a proper diagnosis before taking the herb.

Gingivitis. Lightly cover your gums with echinacea tincture before you head for bed and leave it on overnight. Use it for 2 to 3 weeks. Echinacea has a mild anti-inflammatory effect.

Urinary tract infections. Most UTIs are caused by a bacteria, so tap the antibacterial actions of echinacea by taking two capsules (250 milligrams each) or 60 drops three times daily for at least 10 days, or until the infection is cured.

Warts. Echinacea's antiviral properties can do battle against the virus that causes common warts. Take two capsules (250 milligrams each) or 30 drops twice daily for 3 to 4 weeks. ■

WHEN *NOT* TO TAKE ECHINACEA

Many women rely on echinacea to prevent or shorten the course of a cold. This herb stimulates the immune system to fight off the infection. "But if you have lupus, multiple sclerosis, tuberculosis, AIDS, or other autoimmune disease, the herb may fuel the condition, so it may progress more rapidly, warns Teresa Bailey Klepser, Pharm.D., assistant professor in the department of internal medicine at the University of Iowa in Iowa City.

Eczema

Alternative Remedies for a Stubborn Rash

Sometimes, nothing you do for eczema seems to work. Or it gets worse. Your skin itches. You scratch. It itches more. You scratch harder. You develop flaky, red skin that still itches. You apply a moisturizer. Painful, itchy blisters pop up. You slather on even more lotion, to no avail.

Frustrated, you ask your doctor for help. She prescribes a steroid cream. It works—for a while. But when you stop using it, the problem returns. Now what?

It's time for Plan B.

"Herbalists prefer to address the problem that lies beneath the skin condition rather than the symptoms," says Douglas Schar, a London-based herbalist specializing in disease-preventing herbal medicines. Eczema shows up on the neck, face, legs, and on the inner folds of your elbows, knees, and wrists. But the problem is usually more than just skin deep.

The underlying cause is often an unsuspected food allergy. Dairy products, eggs, soy, wheat, and peanuts are common triggers. But any kind of allergy can cause the immune system to go into overdrive, attack the body, and produce the rash of eczema (also called atopic dermatitis).

Moisturizing lotions may soothe the discomfort. But you have to find out what you're allergic to and avoid it. Avoiding scented laundry detergent, fragranced soaps, rough clothing, dust, pollen, and exposure to dry, cold air can help. But you probably knew that already. Here's what else you can try.

Sip Oregon grape tea. Oregon grape root, available at health food stores, acts as an antihistamine, anti-inflammatory, antifungal. Schar highly recommends this herb for skin problems.

Add 1 tablespoon of the dried root to 1 cup of boiling water. Boil it for 10 minutes. Strain and drink it every morning. (For added benefit and to improve the flavor, add a handful of dried chamomile.) Be patient: This tonic may take a year or more to completely clear your skin, but you may see improvement in 3 to 6 months.

Eat more salmon, mackerel, and tuna. These fish contain omega-3's and other essential fatty acids, which go a long way toward preventing allergies and inflammation, says William D. Nelson, N.D., a naturopathic physician in private practice in Colorado Springs, Colorado. Most people with eczema don't get enough essential fatty acids, which sets them up for conditions such as eczema.

Add the right fat. To control an allergic rash due to eczema and relieve inflamed skin, take ½ tablespoon every day of either flaxseed oil, borage oil, evening primrose oil, or oil with omega-3's. If you prefer to take oil in capsule form, aim for 3,000 to 5,000 milligrams. Do not take borage oil if you are pregnant or breastfeeding. It may cause headaches, indigestion, nausea, and softening of stools.

Give zinc a chance. Zinc helps skin heal, especially if you've scratched yourself raw. Take 46 to 60 milligrams a day in three divided doses with meals. *Doses above 20 milligrams per day must be taken under medical supervision.* ■

Endometriosis

Put an End to Excruciating Pain with Vitamins, Acupuncture, and More

Ask any woman who has endometriosis, "What's the worst thing about the disease?" and chances are she'll say, "The pain. The debilitating pain."

With endometriosis, fragments of the uterine lining—the endometrium—grow outside the uterus into the abdomen and on the ovaries. It can cause painful menstrual cramping; irregular, profuse bleeding; pelvic pain; diarrhea; or painful bowel movements around the time of menstruation.

Your doctor will probably prescribe hormonal drugs, oral contraceptives, or possibly even surgery to put and end to the misery. Complementing medical treatment with natural remedies can bring more complete relief. In a survey of 2,300 women conducted by the Endometriosis Association, a national support group, nearly two-thirds used alternative treatments such as dietary changes, vitamin or mineral supplements, herbs, or acupuncture to help ease pain or other symptoms.

"Natural remedies are a wonderful addition to a woman's endometriosis drug treatment program," says Deborah A. Metzger, M.D., Ph.D., medical director at Helena Women's Health in Palo Alto, California, a medical practice that combines conventional and alternative medicine to treat female reproductive problems. "These natural remedies target the immune system, which plays a major role in controlling pain and the progression of the disease."

Here's a look at some of the nondrug options that helped the women surveyed.

Dietary changes. Sixty percent of the women had less pain after they eliminated meat, dairy products, coffee, and other caffeinated beverages from their diets and added foods and supplements rich in omega-3 fatty acids: salmon, tuna, mackerel, evening primrose oil, and flaxseed oil. Omega-3 fatty acids counteract prostaglandins (hormones produced in many parts of the body, including endometrial tissue) that cause the uterine contractions that lead to cramps.

Vitamins and minerals. Fifty-five percent of the women discovered that taking vitamin B-complex, calcium, and magnesium helped alleviate symptoms. These nutrients act as smooth muscle relaxants—that is, they relieve cramps and even PMS symptoms, says Dr. Metzger. She recommends a daily regimen of 1,200 to 1,500 milli- ››

grams of calcium, 200 milligrams of magnesium, and a B-complex tablet or capsule to be taken indefinitely.

Acupuncture and acupressure. Fifty-six percent of the women got relief from having thin needles (acupuncture) or firm pressure (acupressure) applied to specific points on their bodies. If you'd like to try acupuncture, see an acupuncturist who's certified by the National Certification Commission for Acupuncture and Oriental Medicine, Department 0595, Washington, D.C. 20073-0595. They will provide referrals for a small fee. Or you can access their Web site at www.nccaom.org.

PRESS HERE TO STOP ENDOMETRIAL PAIN

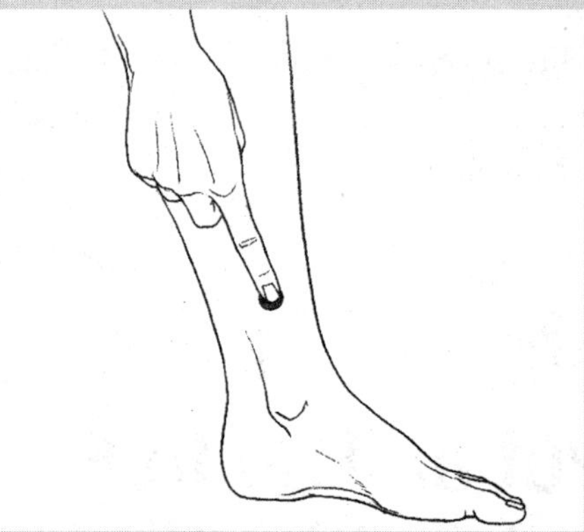

The next time it feels as though a sword is lodged in your uterus, try acupressure.

The point that's said to ease painful cramping is located on the inside of your leg, about 2 inches up from your ankle. Apply firm downward pressure on the point for 1 to 2 minutes; repeat on the other leg.

Helpful Hints

For painful cramps, make a tea using cramp bark tincture, available at health food stores and often recommended by herbalists. Put $\frac{1}{4}$ to $\frac{1}{2}$ teaspoon of the tincture in a cup of tea, and drink up to 4 cups a day. (It's a good idea to consult your doctor before taking herbs for endometriosis, as they can interfere with some medications.) ■

Exercise

Cures for the "No Active Ingredients" Lifestyle

Reams of studies show that women who keep active are more successful at losing unwanted pounds—and keeping them off—than women who are inactive for whatever reason. Many sit at computers all day. Or they hate to do aerobics. Or they simply don't have time to go to a gym every day.

Working out to loud music in a gym is one way to exercise. But it's not the only way to exercise.

"You don't necessarily have to put on a silly outfit and drive somewhere to exercise," says Jill Braverman-Panza, M.D., chair of the American Medical Women's Association subcommittee on eating disorders and an internist, bariatric physician, and pharmacist in Albany, New York. "For example, you can park at the far end of the lot and walk to the store or office building. You'll lose weight, and your car won't get dinged."

If your lifestyle has "no active ingredients," here are some ways Dr. Braverman-Panza suggests to get more exercise, simply by making a few changes in your daily routine. Using the following examples as a guide, give yourself points for building exercise into your day. Subtract points for missed opportunities. Aim for at least 25 points a week, focusing on the boldface activities.

If you work at a computer, get up and walk around for 5 minutes, once an hour. (+1 point)

When you talk on the telephone, pace back and forth. (+2 points)

Phone your neighbor and ask her to go for a walk after supper. (+4 points)

Join a walking club. (+5 points)

Play Frisbee with your dog. (+2 points)

Play Frisbee with your kids. (+3 points)

Play Frisbee with coworkers at lunchtime. (+4 points)

Use your Frisbee as a pizza pan. (-5 points)

Wash your car. (+3 points)

Drive to a car wash. (0 points)

Rake leaves. (+2 points)

Walk across the street and rake your neighbor's leaves. (+3 points)

Clear leaves with a hose or leaf blower. (-5 points)

Make homemade bread by hand. (+2 points)

Make homemade bread with a bread machine. (-2 points)

Take an aerobics class that's in your office building. (+6 points)

Take the elevator to the aerobics class in your building. (-2 points)

Wash all the windows in your house. (+5 points)

Hire someone to wash all the windows in your house. (-5 points)

Watch reruns of *Seinfeld.* (0 points)

Watch reruns of *Seinfeld* while you refinish furniture. (+3 points)

Read the morning paper. (0 points)

Read the morning paper while you ride your stationary bike. (+4 points)

As you ride your stationary bike, consult the paper for notices for upcoming charity walks or 5-K races you can enter. (+5 points)

Listen to National Public Radio. (0 points)

Listen to National Public Radio while you mop the kitchen floor. (+4 points)

Listen to the Ramones as you mop the floor. (+5 points)

Lop off a piece of apple pie as you settle down to watch the evening news. (-5 points)

Bake an apple pie from scratch. (+1 point)

Pick apples at a pick-your-own orchard. (+6 points)

Take your family canoeing, hiking, or cross-country skiing. (+10 points)

Take your family to a video arcade. (-5 points)

Take your family out to an all-you-can-eat buffet. (-10 points)

Rent an exercise video—and use it. (+5 points)

Rent *Titanic.* (-5 points) ■

Facial Hair

Which Hair Removal Method Is Safest for You?

Women aren't supposed to have mustaches. But let's face it—many do. If you sprout a lone, coarse hair on your chin, it's no big deal. Pluck it. But a smooth growth of fuzz on your upper lip can be embarrassing.

"Nothing is stopping women from shaving," says Victor Newcomer, M.D., professor of dermatology at the University of California, Los Angeles, UCLA School of Medicine. Shaving facial hair doesn't leave stubble. It doesn't grow back faster or coarser. Once a week would do it. And no one needs to know. After all, it works fine for your legs.

"Nevertheless, some women find shaving facial hair makes them feel too masculine," he says. That leaves old standbys—like plucking, waxing, bleaching, chemical depilatories, and electrolysis—plus new options like laser removal and something called sugaring. Here's Dr. Newcomer's advice.

Plucking is painful, tedious, and time-consuming.

Best for: Brows only. Desensitize with an ice pack for 15 seconds before you begin.

Bleaching disguises the hair, drawing less attention to the area. But the hair remains.

Best for: Light mustaches, not heavy growth.

Waxing pulls hair out by the roots and is mildly to moderately painful, depending on your tolerance.

Best for: Light fuzz.

Helpful Hints: Prewaxed plastic strips aren't as painful to use as warm wax that hardens as it cools. A variation, known as sugaring, coats hair with a paste of sugar and wax—it's easier to pull off than wax and less traumatizing to the skin. Both the prewaxed plastic strips and kits for sugaring are available at drug and beauty supply stores.

Chemical depilatories are creams that dissolve hair. Leave the cream on for 10 minutes, then wipe it off.

Best for: Skin that's not easily irritated. (Chemicals can irritate sensitive skin.)

Helpful Hints: Do not apply to sunburned or broken skin. Look for creams with hair-growth inhibitors and fruit enzymes—ingredients that interfere with the protein that lets hair grow—so that hair grows back less quickly. Apply aloe if your skin is irritated after use. And next time, choose a method that's easier on your skin.

Electrolysis is the only permanent hair-removal option. You can't do it yourself; it's

DON'T MAKE THIS MISTAKE

Don't use wax or have laser treatments to remove hair if you take Accutane or use Retin-A or Renova, medications used for acne or wrinkles—they make skin more sensitive. And avoid sun exposure. Wax can remove skin along with the hair, and sun exposure makes skin more vulnerable to laser burns.

performed in a salon or hair-removal office by inserting a probe into each individual hair follicle and passing an electric current through it. Removing all the hair on your upper lip may take several sessions.

Best for: Women allergic to bleaches, depilatories, or wax, or anyone who wants to remove facial hair permanently.

Helpful Hint: If done improperly, electrolysis can leave scars, so choose a highly experienced technician. The technician should be a member of a state or national electrolysis association and be a Certified Professional Electrolysist (CPE).

Lasers send a beam of concentrated light into the hair follicle, damaging it so that hair falls out. Unlike electrolysis, laser hair removal isn't permanent—hair grows back in 3 to 9 months, but you'll need fewer sessions.

Best for: Women with pale skin and dark, coarse hair. (Lasers zap pigment as well as hair, so if you're dark-complexioned, you could end up with light spots.)

Helpful Hints: A dermatologist is apt to be better trained at laser hair removal than a spa attendant. Always have a test area done first. And if you have excess hair, check with your doctor to rule out a hormone imbalance. ■

Fast Food

Reduce Drive-Thru Distress

The stress of ordering fast food may do more to raise your cholesterol than a ½-pound burger and supersize order of french fries.

A study at Duke University found that calm women tended to have lower cholesterol than women who frequently lashed out at others in hostility. And when you keep your aggravation in check, you'll also probably get better service, says Donald Smith, former restaurant owner, fast-food industry executive and professor emeritus of restaurant management at Washington State University in Pullman.

If you're in a hurry, things are probably just as hectic on the other side of the counter. And they may be new at their jobs, notes Smith.

Here's how to navigate the fast-food system with less hassle so you'll leave a happier customer—and maybe with lower cholesterol.

Choose your specialty. If you want chicken, go to a restaurant that specializes in chicken, not a chain that tries to offer some of everything. The places that focus on one style of food, from chicken to Mexican items, will be best organized to serve it faster.

Double your pleasure. Head for drive-thru restaurants that have two windows—one for a cashier to take your money, and another for a worker to hand you your food. They're faster than chains where one person handles both. Your journey may also go quicker if there are two menus in the drive-thru ›› area so you can plan your order early in the line.

Take notes. Keep a pad of paper and pen handy in the glove box. If you're heading for the drive-thru with a carload of kids, jot down their orders while in line so you can read them in an organized fashion to the attendant.

Order in order. The fast-food worker will probably enter your request into her computer in the order of sandwiches, side items, and sodas. Giving it to her in that order makes her job easier.

Speak up. The speaker systems for ordering at fast-food restaurants often turn voices into scratchy babble. Speak directly into the microphone in a slow, steady manner so the attendant has a better chance of getting your order right.

Step inside. If you see a line of cars at the drive-thru—particularly if one is packed with customers—park your car and order inside. You'll almost always get faster service, Smith says.

Helpful Hint

Ironically, if you visit the restaurant near the busy time, you may get your food quicker than during slack periods. Many chains toss out unsold items every few minutes, so at a slow time, they may have to make your meal from scratch. The best time to order lunch, for example, is close to 11:30 A.M. or 1:30 P.M. ■

Fat-Free Foods

Why You're Eating Less Fat but Not Losing Weight

Q: How big is a serving of fat-free cookies?

A: One box.

A favorite joke among dietitians, this reflects how most of us eat. It's so easy to gobble large quantities of fat-free foods while adding 1,200 calories to your diet. (In truth, one serving is 1 or 2 cookies, whether they're regular or fat-free.)

Nine out of 10 women eat some kind of fat-free food, be it milk, salad dressings, sauces, mayonnaise, cheese, yogurt, sour cream, margarine, potato chips, crackers, meat, ice cream, frozen desserts, or baked goods. Fat-free facsimiles have taken over supermarket shelves and freezer cases.

"Ironically, the only place you can find an old-fashioned, full-fat yogurt made from whole milk is in a health food store," says Barbara Rolls, Ph.D., director of the Laboratory for the Study of Human Ingestive Behavior at Pennsylvania State University in University Park and coauthor of the book *Volumetrics*.

For foods to qualify as fat-free, the FDA requires these products to contain no more than 0.5 gram of fat per serving. Low-fat foods have a bit more—3 grams per serving. Reduced-fat foods are harder to pin down—the only guide-

DON'T MAKE THESE MISTAKES

A "fat-free" label can foster the illusion that you have calories in the bank. During one of her studies, Dr. Rolls gave one group of women low-fat yogurt and another group high-fat yogurt, but neither group knew that the yogurts contained the same number of calories. Afterward, the low-fat group ate a significantly heavier lunch. "They equated the low-fat label with low calories and gave themselves license to eat more lunch," Dr. Rolls says.

Also, eating fat-free snacks and desserts isn't a substitute for getting more exercise and featuring fruits, vegetables, and whole grains in your diet to control your weight and protect against heart disease and cancer. Think of them as an added resource, not the mainstay of your diet.

line is that they contain at least 25 percent less fat than the regular versions.

Although eating such foods can reduce fat consumption, it doesn't always reduce waistlines. Some low-fat peanut butters, puddings, nondairy creamers, and cookies contain just as many calories as the high-fat versions. What manufacturers omit in fat, they make up for in sugar, fat substitutes, and other ingredients—all of which have calories.

Still, Dr. Rolls believes that, used correctly, fat-free (and low- or reduced-fat) foods have a place in your diet. Here's the smart way to incorporate fat-free foods into your diet.

Count calories, not fat grams. "Women got so caught up in counting fat grams that they've ignored calories," says Dr. Rolls. "If you're trying to lose weight, it's your total intake of calories that counts, regardless of where they came from."

Concentrate on "big" foods with few calories. Nutritionists call it calorie density: two slices of whole wheat bread have as many calories as a fat-free piece of candy, but it's bigger and full of fiber, leaving you feeling fuller and satisfied, so you don't eat six or seven rolls. Go for "low caloric density" foods over dense foods like cookies and ice cream.

Compare Nutrition Facts labels. Unless the fat-free version contains fewer calories than the full-fat version, there's no advantage for weight loss. You might as well eat the real thing.

Eat the same quantity. If you're accustomed to using 2 tablespoons of full-fat salad dressing, use 2 tablespoons of the fat-free version. Extra helpings are self-defeating. Same goes for eating the whole box of fat-free cookies.

Go easy on snacks. Eating fat-free foods at mealtimes isn't an excuse for eating more snacks at other times. You'll make up for the calories saved, and then some.

Helpful Hint

If you find fat-free foods too bland, you may instinctively compensate by eating more in an effort to feel satisfied. You may be better off eating low- or reduced-fat food instead. ■

Fatigue

Mealtime Makeovers for the Energy You Need

Fatigue has reached epidemic levels. Millions of women are tired. For some, the reasons are obvious—too much to do, too little time, and not enough sleep. For others, the cause is more elusive. Their doctors tell them they're healthy. But they feel like they're running in quicksand. What's up?

Their fat intake, probably.

"A high-fat diet can make you feel sluggish and weighted down because the body has to work harder to digest fat," says Franca Alphin, R.D., administrative director at the Duke University Diet and Fitness Center in Durham, North Carolina. "Plus, your brain and muscles won't get the energy they need to function optimally."

Take Connie Bissonnette, 58, a lab technician in St. Paul, Minnesota. Raised in a meat and potatoes–loving family, she breakfasted on scrambled eggs, bacon, and toast slathered with butter. For lunch? Pizza. Then steak or fried food for dinner. And she regularly snacked on candy bars and ice cream.

Problem was, Connie felt that she needed a nap to get through the day. Concerned about her chronic fatigue, her son Jeff, an exercise physiologist, convinced her to make a small change in her diet: substitute jelly for butter on her morning toast. She felt a little better. Then she began to bake food instead of frying, cook lean chicken and turkey instead of beef, eat eggs without the yolks, and buy low-fat salad dressings. And she ate more fruits and vegetables. Connie's new eating habits also helped her lose 37 pounds. Before long, Connie felt more energetic than ever before

It's no wonder, says Alphin. "Women who eat low-fat, nutrient-dense foods have so much more energy, because the carbohydrates, vitamins, and minerals needed to keep their brains alert and their muscles energized are abundant," says Alphin.

If, like Connie, your diet is high in fat and low in energy-boosting foods, consider these mealtime makeovers. Then watch your energy soar.

Balance your breakfast. Grabbing a bagel to eat on the run isn't a bad idea. But if it's energy you want, start your day with ½ cup of Kellogg's Raisin Bran or All-Bran cereal with fat-free milk and a piece of fruit, or an egg-white omelet with vegetables, a slice of toast with jam, a piece of fruit, and 1 cup of fat-free milk. Both are perfect carbohydrate-protein combinations.

DON'T MAKE THESE MISTAKES

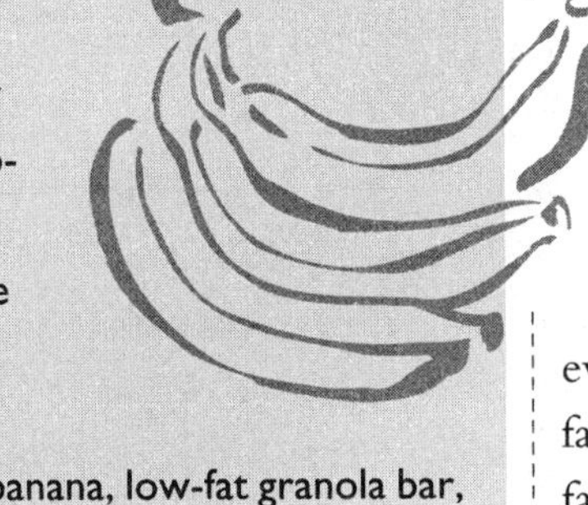

If you're in desperate need of an energy boost, don't reach for candy or a chocolate bar. Your blood sugar levels will spike, then crash. So you'll get the surge of energy you wanted—but only for an hour or so. Then you'll start feeling fatigued all over again. Your best bets: a banana, low-fat granola bar, or three or four graham crackers.

Add some protein to your lunchtime carbs. Foods high in carbohydrates, such as pasta, breads, and potatoes, increase levels of the brain chemical serotonin if they are eaten without any protein. Serotonin can improve your mood but can also cause drowsiness. Instead, eating some protein at lunchtime will prevent the increase in serotonin while activating the energizing brain chemicals dopamine and norepinephrine, says Judith Wurtman, Ph.D., director of the Triad Weight Management Center/McLean Hospital in Belmont, Massachussetts.

For a real power lunch, try some of the following protein-packed favorites.

- A mixed green salad filled with chicken or tuna, kidney or garbanzo beans, and low-fat dressing. Add a roll or ½ a whole wheat pita
- 3 ounces of sliced turkey, chicken, or lean roast beef on whole wheat bread, topped with low-fat mayonnaise, lettuce, and tomato; serve with 8 ounces of fat-free milk
- 1 cup of minestrone soup and a baked potato topped with broccoli or other vegetables and ½ cup of cottage cheese; substitute a sweet potato for the white potato for added fiber if you like

Make your evening meal low-fat. If you want to sustain your energy well into the evening hours, aim for a low-fat supper. Remember, high-fat foods will weigh you down and tire you out.

Here are some low-fat dinner ideas.

Choice 1

- 4 to 5 ounces of baked salmon, orange roughy, trout or other fish
- 1 cup of brown rice or couscous
- 2 cups of steamed mixed vegetables

Choice 2

- 4 to 5 ounces of grilled or baked skinless chicken
- A baked white or sweet potato or 1 cup of pasta salad
- 2 cups of grilled vegetables

Choice 3

- Vegetarian chili made with soy crumbles
- A tossed green salad with low-fat dressing
- One slice of whole wheat bread ■

Fat Substitutes

Don't Go Hog Wild

A nation-wide epidemic of fat phobia spurred food manufacturers to develop fat substitutes—faux fats that mimic the creaminess of fat without the calories and cholesterol. First came fat-free salad dressings, followed by fat-free cheese, frozen desserts, baked goods, and potato chips.

Most fat substitutes (such as Oatrim, made from crushed oats) are carbohydrate-based. A few (like Simplesse) are protein-based. Others (such as Benefat) are fat-based. So they aren't calorie-free.

Are these fat substitutes safe? And can they help you control your weight? It depends on whom you ask—and how you use them.

The best known and most controversial fat substitute is olestra, a synthetic product made by chemically combining sugar with vegetable oil. In 1996, the Food and Drug Administration approved the use of olestra in snacks, but required a label notice warning that olestra can cause abdominal cramping, loose stools, and the inhibited absorption of some vitamins and minerals. Yet studies in which neither the people eating the chips nor the researchers noting their reactions knew who was getting the olestra chips or the full-fat chips have shown that olestra chips are no more likely than regular chips to cause stomach upsets.

During its passage through the gastrointestinal tract, olestra captures fat-soluble vitamins and carotenoids (nutrients related to beta-carotene, which your body converts to vitamin A). To help make up for the loss, the FDA requires olestra's manufacturer to add extra vitamin A, D, E, and K to its products, but doesn't require additional carotenoids.

That worries olestra critics such as Joan Gussow, Ed.D., professor emeritus in nutrition and education at Columbia University Teacher's College and one of a few members who voted against olestra on an FDA advisory panel.

"I'm not sure they're safe, and I'm pretty sure they're not going to be effective," Dr. Gussow says of fat substitutes. She's concerned that fat substitutes could alter the body's hunger response. "They deceive the tastebuds," she says. "If your body is being told lies all the time, you can no longer rely on instinct to control hunger."

You could end up eating more fat substitutes *and* real fats, says Dr. Gussow. "For example, we've had sugar substitutes for years, yet sugar consumption has continued to rise."

Since the FDA has designated most fat substitutes as "generally recognized as safe," it appears that fat substitutes are here to stay.

Fat substitutes can help you control your weight, if and only if you use them intelligently, says Barbara Rolls, Ph.D., professor of nutrition at Pennsylvania State University in University Park.

Use them as substitutes, not additions to your diet. If

you customarily eat regular potato chips or baked goods, try the low-fat version. But don't start eating snacks or baked goods just because they're fat-free. "You shouldn't be adding these things to your diet because you think they have a special property that's going to help you lose weight," advises Dr. Rolls.

Compare labels. Make sure the low-fat version is lower in calories than the regular version. Reduced-fat Skippy peanut butter, for instance, contains just as many calories as the full-fat version.

Ease into it. "If you're trying something you've never tried before, don't eat too much of it," Dr. Rolls says. "Any kind of food can upset your stomach if you're not used to it."

Helpful Hint

To avoid potential side effects of fat substitutes, try other ways to reduce the fat in foods. Use nonstick spray, experiment with seasonings, or just use less fat in recipes. In baking recipes, use applesauce or prune puree to replace up to 50 percent of the fat. "Anything that reduces fat content can be regarded as a fat substitute," Dr. Rolls says. ■

Fever

Herbal Combos That Break a Sweat

A slightly elevated fever is nothing to be afraid of. An increase of a few degrees above normal—99.9° to 102°F or so—is actually good for you. Invading organisms grow more slowly at a raised body temperature. So when a virus or bacterial infection infiltrates your body, white blood cells—your body's front line of immune defense—release endogenous pyrogens, substances that trigger your brain to raise your internal temperature, causing a fever.

"Your body knows what it's doing," says Helen Healy, N.D., a naturopathic physician and director of the Wellspring Naturopathic Clinic in St. Paul, Minnesota. "It creates the fever to generate a better immune response and get rid of whatever ails you once and for all."

Still, it's tempting to bring out the offensive weapons. Over-the-counter pain relievers—aspirin, ibuprofen, or acetaminophen—will temporarily bring down your fever. "But if you take a drug to suppress the fever, it makes you more vulnerable to any other toxins produced by the bacteria or virus," Dr. Healy says. "Instead, work with *the fever." Here's how.*

DON'T MAKE THIS MISTAKE

If your fever reaches 103°F or higher or persists for more than 72 hours, call your doctor. Same goes if you have a severe headache or stiff neck, you're coughing up discolored phlegm, or have pain while urinating along with the fever.

Slow down. "Call in sick and get somebody else to help the kids with their homework," Dr. Healy says. "A woman with a fever needs a break."

Get into bed. Your body can't heal if you're banging away at a keyboard, talking on the phone, and fielding ›› questions from your kids or coworkers—all at the same time. "When you have a fever, anytime is bedtime," Dr. Healy says.

Pamper yourself. Make yourself comfortable. Prepare a soothing cup of tea or broth. Better yet, let somebody else make it for you.

Load up on water, sports drinks, chicken soup, broth, and other fluids. That spaced-out feeling you get when you're home with a fever isn't from watching endless game shows, talk shows, soap operas, and reruns of 1970s sitcoms. A fever severely dehydrates your brain and your body, so make a special effort to drink eight or more 8-ounce glasses of water a day.

Sweat It Out with Herbal Tea

Elder and yarrow induce perspiration, helping a fever do its work. Combined with echinacea, a proven infection-fighter, these herbs will help your fever go away faster. Dr. Healy recommends the following regimen. Use small amounts of dried flowers of elder and yarrow, and cut-and-

Fiber

The World's Most Powerful Weight Loss Aid

Okay, so it doesn't have much sex appeal. But if there's one food factor that really delivers, it's fiber. It can help lower blood cholesterol, stabilize blood sugar in women with diabetes, and prevent ills of the gastrointestinal tract—constipation, diarrhea, hemorrhoids, diverticulosis, even colon cancer. There's also evidence that a high-fiber diet may help protect against breast cancer.

"Fiber is great," says Carla Wolper, R.D., a registered dietitian at St. Luke's–Roosevelt Hospital Center in the obesity research center in New York City. As the indigestible part of plants, fiber isn't absorbed by the body. It travels pretty much intact from the stomach to the intestines. There, it soaks up water like a sponge, softening and bulking up the stool so it moves through the gastrointestinal tract quickly and efficiently. This not only alleviates many bowel disturbances but it also prevents harmful, cancer-causing substances from camping out and getting a stronghold. Fiber's amazing cholesterol-lowering effect is achieved in the same process. While absorbing water in the intestines, fiber also sucks up bile, a fluid secreted by the liver that aids digestion. To make more bile, the liver pilfers cholesterol from the bloodstream. Happily, the result is lower blood cholesterol.

If that's not enough to win you over, consider this: Fiber has been called the most powerful weight loss aid in the world. That's because **high-fiber foods make you feel full on fewer calories.**

Now, do we have your attention?

Good, because few women get the recommended 20 to 35 grams of fiber per day—the amount studies suggest for blanket health protec-

sifted echinacea root, available at health food stores.

• Put a teaspoon of the echinacea in 1 cup of water, boil for a few minutes, and simmer for 10 to 15 minutes more. Strain and put aside.

• Mix equal amounts of the elder and yarrow flowers, then steep a teaspoonful of that blend in a cup of hot water for 10 minutes.

• Combine the teas and reheat (but do not boil), then pour into a large mug. Add honey and take this toddy to bed.

• Bundle yourself up with a hot-water bottle at your feet and sip the tea until it's gone. Then go to sleep.

"This tea breaks the fever because you'll just plain sweat it out," says Dr. Healy. (Discontinue using elderflower if you experience vomiting or severe diarrhea. People who are allergic to ragweed, asters, and chrysanthemums or who have tuberculosis or an autoimmune condition such as lupus or multiple sclerosis should not use echinacea because it stimulates the immune system.) ■

DON'T MAKE THIS MISTAKE

Don't rely solely on fiber supplements to meet your recommended daily requirements. You'll miss out on a whole slew of disease-fighting vitamins and minerals available only in food. And don't forget to drink lots of water, at least eight 8-ounce glasses a day, while eating a high-fiber diet and/or taking fiber supplements. If you run dry, you risk becoming constipated or experiencing other unpleasant gastrointestinal disturbances like gas or a more serious complication like a bowel obstruction.

tion. Indeed, most of us get half that amount or less. Yet fiber is extremely easy to access. Just look to fruits, vegetables, legumes (beans and peas), and whole grains like oats and whole wheat. Or, for an extra boost, supplement with a granulated fiber product like wheat bran or psyllium.

Not surprisingly, some breakfast cereals top the charts for fiber content. One-third cup of Kellogg's All-Bran Bran Buds packs a whopping 13 grams. One-half cup of Kellogg's All-Bran contains 10 grams. **A 1-cup serving of Kellogg's Raisin Bran has 8 grams.** Following is a dozen more sources of fiber that can help you get closer to meeting your daily needs.

- Black beans: 7.5 grams per ½ cup
- Dried figs: 6.9 grams for 3
- Dried pears: 6.5 grams in 5 halves
- Kidney beans: 6.5 grams per ½ cup
- Artichoke: 6.5 grams in 1 medium
- Lentil soup: 5.6 grams per 1 cup
- Baked potato with skin: 4.8 grams
- Raspberries: 4.2 grams per ½ cup
- Split pea soup: 4 grams per 1 cup
- Blackberries: 3.8 grams per ½ cup
- Apple with peel: 3.7 grams
- Baked sweet potato: 3.4 grams ■

Fiber Supplements

When It Comes to Colon Helpers, Easy-Does-It Is Best

It's like a mantra among nutrition experts: Eat 20 to 35 grams of fiber a day to keep your bowel contents moving along, help protect yourself against cancer and heart disease, and feel satisfied and lose weight. If you're doing everything you can to get your quota—choosing the highest-fiber cereals and crackers you can find, eating whole grains over white, and piling enough fruits and vegetables on your plate to sink a Chilean freighter—fiber supplements can help you fill the gap.

One way to measure your intake is to count grams. Another is to count bowel movements.

"If you don't have at least two bowel movements a day, and you find it difficult to add more fruits, vegetables, whole grains, or beans to your diet, then you need a fiber supplement," says Robert Charm, M.D., gastroenterologist and clinical professor of gastroenterology and internal medicine at the University of California, Davis. Otherwise, high fiber foods are your best source.

That's because fiber supplements won't provide the additional benefits of vitamins, minerals, antioxidants, and other disease-fighting phytochemicals that you'll find in whole fruits, grains, and other unrefined foods. Made from seeds, gums, or other plant residue and sold in supermarkets, pharmacies, and health food stores, fiber supplements are available as either tablets (such as oat bran and calcium polycarbophil), capsules (such as pectin, glucomannan and guar gum), or powders (such as psyllium and methylcellulose).

So which fiber supplement is right for you? It depends on what you need.

If your pipes are running a little slow:

Women who have only one bowel movement a day or every 2 days need to pick up a supplement containing soluble fiber, like psyllium or pectin, says Dr. Charm. This intestinal cleanser softens your stools. And while it's there, fiber helps lower cholesterol and cholesterol building blocks—decreasing your risk for heart disease.

If you're haven't had a bowel movement for a week:

You need an insoluble fiber such as wheat bran or flaxseed, says Dr. Charm. These laxatives soften stools and also prod your bowels to get them and their contents moving—relieving constipation.

Your bowels are regular, but you know you don't get all the dietary fiber you need.

DON'T MAKE THESE MISTAKES

High-fiber meals, along with fiber supplements, can lower absorption of some medications. If you're taking medications, talk to your doctor or pharmacist before adding fiber supplements to your diet. Also, don't take fiber supplements if you have trouble swallowing or if you've been diagnosed with a gastrointestinal disorder, such as diverticulitis, ulcerative colitis, or Crohn's disease.

Look for a supplement that contains both soluble and insoluble fibers. In addition to their individual benefits, together these dietary wonder twins carry fat, estrogens, and cancer-causing compounds out of your body, which may decrease your risk for breast and colon cancer.

Adjust the Dose

If you decide to take a fiber supplement, start with one dose an hour after you eat dinner, recommends Dr. Charm. This should cause a bowel movement by morning.

If you're waking up in the middle of the night to go:

You're taking too much. Simply cut the dosage in half the next night.

If after 2 days you don't get any results:

Try taking an extra dose about an hour before or after breakfast.

If you can't bear to drink the stuff or can't swallow large pills:

Just mix a powdered fiber supplement with orange or apple juice instead of water. And drink them immediately—some fibers form gels if they sit in liquid too long. Be sure to drink plenty of water when you take any fiber supplement, advises Dr. Charm. He recommends at least eight 8-ounce glasses a day.

Helpful Hint

If you're trying to lose weight, take your fiber supplement 15 minutes before you eat. This will make you feel full, so you may eat fewer calories. ■

Fibromyalgia

Help for Women Who Are Tired of Being in Pain

You hurt. All the time. Your muscles ache. You have tender, painful spots from head to toe. Your doctor has ruled out rheumatoid arthritis and multiple sclerosis.

You're told you have fibromyalgia, also called fibrositis and trigger point syndrome, typified by overall aching and specific areas of severe pain, often accompanied by disrupted sleep. Experts don't yet know what causes fibromyalgia, and there are no tests to confirm diagnosis.

If you're like a lot of women with fibromyalgia, you've tried everything—chiropractic adjustments, massage, deep muscle therapy, ultrasound, and supplements, says David Flemming, M.D., who combines psychology and rehabilitation at the Center for Integrated Therapy in Chicago. Treatment is a matter of trial and error: No single treatment works for everyone. Here are some promising options.

Hypnosis. When hypnosis is used as part of a comprehensive program including rest, exercise, and specific treatments, great improvement and even remission can result, says Dr. Flemming. Specialized forms of hypnosis are sometimes needed, the same used to treat post traumatic stress disorder and multiple personality disorder, although this does not mean that fibromyalgia is necessarily associated with these problems. Psychologists who have experience in treating these conditions are equipped to train women in self-hypnosis for ›› fibromyalgia. It's well worth the try: Women with fibromyalgia often respond exceptionally well to hypnosis.

Thyroid hormones. "In many cases, pain and other symptoms of fibromyalgia resemble underactive thyroid conditions, and treatment with thyroid hormones of some kind can bring dramatic relief," says Dr. Flemming.

"We've been amazed at how well this has worked for some people," he says. A thyroid blood test can determine which, if any, thyroid hormones you may need.

Antidepressants. Your physician may recommend antidepressant medication, not because you're depressed, but because low doses will help you sleep and function better.

What You Can Do for Yourself

As for self-help measures, the number one recommendation is daily aerobic exercise.

Forget it, you say? Who wants to exercise when your muscles ache? Yes, exercise will hurt while you're doing it, when you're done, and possibly the next day at first. Do it anyway, says Urscia Mahring, D.C., a chiropractor at Back to Health in Alexandria, Virginia, and member of the American Chiropractic Association. It may never be the most pleasant part of your day, but exercise will help relieve pain, increase endurance, and raise your pain tolerance so you can make it through the day.

Exercise is vital to improvement, but overexercising will make the condition worse, warns Dr. Flemming. Begin with range-of-movement exercise only, preferably in a pool. Then progress to light aerobic exercise such as walking, biking, and swimming. Flexibility exercises and stretching are also very important. Avoid strength training and other rigorous exercise. Swimming or other water exercise may be your best bet. However, cold water can be too chilly if you're cold-sensitive, says Dr. Mahring. Try to find a comfortably heated pool.

If you can afford it, hire a personal trainer for a few sessions who will consult with your doctor and slowly get you started in an exercise program that's progressive yet manageable for your pain level.

Dr. Mahring instructs her patients with fibromyalgia: "Whatever strategy will make you successful—an exercise buddy, a trainer, a friend nagging you—whatever it takes, you have to get up and do it."

HELP IS AVAILABLE

If you have fibromyalgia, trying to go it alone can be tough and frustrating. Check your local newspaper, or search http://supportwork.org, the national online support group directory compiled by SupportWorks, a nonprofit organization based in Charlotte, North Carolina, to find a local fibromyalgia support group in your area.

Helpful Hint

For best results, be sure you're seeing a rheumatologist who specializes in the treatment of fibromyalgia. ■

Fish

Cook Fish like a Pro—Every Time

Eating fish twice a week or more can go a long way toward protecting your health: Fish contain omega-3 fatty acids—a type of fat that prevents heart disease, may fight breast and colon cancer, and possibly even protect women from depression.

Salmon, mackerel, sardines, herring, anchovies, rainbow trout, bluefish, and white albacore tuna are high in eicosapentaenoic acid (EPA) and docosahexaenoic acid (DHA). These fats may do you a world of good: They appear to raise levels of high-density lipoprotein (HDL) cholesterol, the "good" cholesterol that helps keep fatty sludge from depositing in your arteries.

Omega-3's may help make women not only healthier but also happier. In a study of depression rated in several countries, scientists found that the more fish people eat, the less they seem to experience depression.

Milder fish, like haddock and cod, are lower in fat, so they are naturally lower in omega-3's. But they're still a respectable source of protein and other nutrients.

For lunch, a tuna salad sandwich will fill the bill. But for dinner, you probably want something more elegant. Yet a lot of women are intimidated by the prospect of shopping for fish and worry that they'll cook it wrong and ruin dinner.

"Relax," says Claud Mann, a certified professional chef and fish expert. "Buying and cooking fish needn't send you into a panic."

Take a whiff. "A really great fish market should smell like a salty ocean breeze when you walk in, not a beached whale," says Mann. "If you are repelled by the odor, shop elsewhere. You can also ask the clerk for a sniff of the fish you're interested in buying."

DON'T MAKE THESE MISTAKES

Quickly defrosting fish in the microwave is a nuclear mistake. It'll lose moisture and dry out. Defrosting under water will make the fish mushy. The best way to defrost fish is slowly in the refrigerator. A large fish will take 24 hours.

Look for ice. Fillets and steaks should set on top of ice; whole fish should be covered by it. They should never sit in pools of ice water or their own juice—that makes fish mushy.

Don't let a "previously frozen" sign detour you. By the time fish is brought off the boat, sold to a wholesaler, and passed on to your supermarket, it may have been out of the water, sitting in refrigeration, for 10 days or more. Frozen fish, on the other hand, are exposed to polar temperatures minutes after they're caught. With this quick-freezing process, no damaging ice crystals form in the flesh of the fish, so when it defrosts, it'll still have great texture and a lot of moisture, perhaps ›› more than fish that's never been frozen.

Buy fish last. "Instead of picking up your fillet first and strolling around the market for 45 minutes, get it right before you're ready to check out, as if it were ice cream," recommends Mann.

Always buy fish the same day you eat it. Seafood doesn't stay fresh in your refrigerator more than a day.

Helpful Hint: For a whole fish, figure 8 to 12 ounces per person. With a steak or fillet, figure about 6 ounces per person.

Cook It Fast, Cook It Right

Once you get fish home from the store, follow these tips for preparing perfect fish every time.

Take your fish out of the refrigerator 15 to 20 minutes before you're ready to cook it. A cold piece of fish might shrink and, consequently, stick to a hot pan.

Allow 8 minutes per inch. The conventional guidelines is 10 minutes per inch. But when you take it out of the oven or off the stove, it continues cooking for another 2 minutes. Skin side up or skin side down? It doesn't matter which side of a fillet you start cooking on. You have to cook it for an equal amount of time on both sides.

Keep a close eye on your catch. Fish can go from cooked to perfection to overdone in a matter of minutes. If you've never cooked fish before, sauté or grill it so you can watch it. When fish is done, it should look slightly flaky on the outside and milky and opaque in the center, not solid white—that's overcooked. ■

BEYOND TUNA: A BEGINNER'S GUIDE TO FISH

Fish expert Claud Mann says that one key to cooking fish like a pro is choosing the right cooking method. His guidelines for beginners:

Low-fat: cod, flounder, haddock, grouper, blue gill, turbo, snapper, whiting, orange roughy, bass, trout

Best for: poaching, sautéing, fish cakes

Usually not good for: stews, chowders, grilling, broiling, baking

These lean fish fall apart easily. If you want to use them in a stew or chowder, sauté them separately and add them to the pot minutes before you serve. If they sit in liquid too long, these fish flake into tiny pieces—leaving your dinner guests wondering, "Where's the grouper?"

Moderate fat: salmon, swordfish, pompano, albacore tuna, monkfish, shark

Best for: grilling, broiling, sautéing, stir-frying, stewing, steaming

Usually not good for: poaching

"These are great starter fish," says Mann. "They're not as delicate as lower-fat fish, so they won't break apart as easily during cooking."

High-fat: mackerel, shad, blue fish

Best for: grilling, broiling, roasting, stewing, cat food

Usually not good for: first-time fish eaters.

"Don't start with any of these fish," says Mann. "They are as high in ocean flavor as they are in fat."

Flat Hair

Volumizing Tips from the "Big Hair" State

Here in Texas, a lot of women like 'big hair,'" says Sherri Jordan, a hair stylist in Houston. But it's far from easy to maintain even moderate lift, especially if your hair is fine or flat.

"I should know," says Jordon, "because my hair is fine and flat."

In 20 years of styling her own hair, and that of thousands of other Texas women, Jordan has learned a few tricks that help fine, flat hair. Here are some of her best.

Towel your hair until it's 70 to 80 percent dry before styling it. Then turn your head upside down and use the blow-dryer on the hair closest to your scalp until it is almost damp. This will help your hair stand up—or, as Jordan says, "give it a little poof." To add more fullness, lift sections of hair with a round brush and aim the dryer 2 to 4 inches from your head.

Roll it up, shake it out. Velcro rollers won't add much fullness to hair that tends to lie flat. Instead, use heated electric rollers. Leave rollers in for 5 to 10 minutes, take them out, and shake out your hair.

Use a moisturizing conditioner two or three times a week. "Women with fine hair often don't use a conditioner because they think it will make their hair flatter," says Jordan. And too much conditioner can weight down fine hair. "But if you put a tiny touch of moisturizing conditioner on, it will help your hair block out the humidity in the air, which can make hair go flat."

Get a new cut. Work with your stylist to find the cut that works best for you. A little layering can give your hair a huge lift, for example. So can a short style, which is often more flattering than long hair if your hair is fine. A medium bob that goes around the face and curves under the jawline can pump up the hair and give it personality.

Finally, "if all else fails," says Jordan, "try a permanent body wave." Having your perm properly wrapped and timed is the key to a good-looking perm, so a salon perm is your best bet.

DON'T MAKE THIS MISTAKE

"Women with fine, flat hair often use a lot of hair spray, thinking that more is better," says Jordon. "But in fact, too much spray can weigh down your hair and make it more flat." Instead, try a light spritz of a bionutrient styling spray. They tend to be light and airy. Bionutrient sprays contain panthenol (a B vitamin) and organic proteins. They help condition your hair and protect it from environmental and styling damage.

Helpful Hint

Carry hair clips with you, and if your hair goes flat while you are out of the house, you can camouflage the damage. Simply pull it back, twist it around, and pin it up. If you have short hair, comb it behind your ears and flatten it. "The trick is to make it look intentional," she says. ■

Flavonoids

Fill Your Shopping Cart with These Heart Helpers

Take a random sampling of foods from your local supermarket—grapes, oranges, apples, onions, cherries, tomatoes, beans, nuts. Throw in a box of tea and a bar of dark chocolate. Open a bottle of merlot.

Next, take a slice of each food—skin included—and a splash of the wine. Look at everything under a microscope. What will you find? Flavonoids—4,000 different substances found in varying combinations in a wide range of fruits, vegetables, tea, and wine.

Flavonoids are much more than a botanical curiosity—they protect your heart in three important ways, explains Sheri Zidenberg-Cherr, Ph.D., researcher and antioxidant specialist at the University of California, Davis. They prevent LDL cholesterol and platelets, two of a blood clot's essential building blocks, from sticking to arteries; they neutralize cell-damaging free radicals; and they reduce inflammation in blood vessels.

Scientists group flavonoids into five different groups—catechins, flavanones, flavonols, anthocyanidins, and caffeic acid. Eating just one type of flavonoid won't provide all three benefits. Different ones perform different tasks, and some are better at their jobs than others. For example, quercetin and catechins (found in apples, onions, and tea) are best at preventing LDL dams from forming in your blood vessels. But when you want to keep sticky platelets off artery walls, catechins can't help you—quercetin's your flavonoid.

Scientists are still sorting out which flavonoids do what, but two things are clear: Many flavonoids are beneficial, and these ticker protectors are easy to find. You can get all you need simply by eating a variety of fruits and vegetables each day.

To be sure your shopping cart contains foods that supply flavonoids of all types, include these items are on your grocery list.

Catechins: Apples, chocolate, any kind of grapes, tea

Flavanones: Citrus fruits

Flavonols (quercetin and polyphenols): Apples, all kinds of grapes, olives, onions, tea

Anthocyanidins: Cherries, any kind of grapes, strawberries

Caffeic Acid: Apples, cherries, coffee, any kind of grapes, olives, plums, tomatoes

Helpful Hints

Red wine contains three kinds of flavonoids—catechins, flavonols, and caffeic acid—and is a richer source of these antioxidants than white. That's because grape skins—home to flavonoids—are kept in the barrel during fermentation of red wine, but not white.

In apples, flavonoids are concentrated in the skin, so don't peel before eating. (But do wash thoroughly.) ■

Flaxseed

A Salad Oil That Prevents Cancer

Breast cancer. Blindness. Even heart disease. Is it possible that a handful of flaxseed each day can help prevent all three?

Those are some mighty big claims for such a tiny seed. But this underappreciated herb contains a unique combination of health protectors: lignans, omega-3 fatty acids, and fiber. And it's this trio that's making experts take a second look at the disease-fighting power of flax.

In your body, flaxseed functions as an intestinal housekeeper, decluttering your arteries of cholesterol and scooping up cancer-causing compounds and lowering your risk of heart disease, stroke, and colon cancer in the course of a day's work. It even clears clogged colons and helps prevent diverticulosis.

Flaxseed is also rich in alpha-linolenic acid, a member of the omega-3 family of heart-healthy fatty acids otherwise found in cold-water fish like mackerel. Not only do these specialized fats lower your odds of a heart attack. They also help prevent macular degeneration and cataracts, as well as help control inflammation—easing psoriasis, rheumatoid arthritis, ulcerative colitis, allergies, and asthma.

And then there are lignans. Created by plants such as flax, these estrogen-like fibers are thought to prevent your body from "fertilizing" tumor cells, thereby lowering your risk for breast cancer. You'll find these cancer-deterring plant estrogens in soy products, too. But flax—and especially flaxseed oil—is a more concentrated source. In fact, "flaxseed oil has 100 times more lignans than any other plant," says Mitchell Gaynor, M.D., author of *Dr. Gaynor's Cancer Prevention Program* and director of medical oncology at Cornell University's Strang Cancer Prevention Center in New York.

DON'T MAKE THIS MISTAKE

Linseed oil sold at hardware stores is a form of flax oil, but you don't want to drink it—it's meant for softening baseball mitts and polishing wood. You want food-grade flaxseed oil instead.

Flaxseed, flaxmeal, and flaxseed oil are available at health food stores and some supermarkets. How much you need in order to reap its benefits depends on what form you use.

Flaxseed: Dr. Gaynor recommends 1 to 2 tablespoons daily. Toss it on top of your salad, bake it on top of bread, or mix it with dried fruit for a mid-afternoon snack.

Flaxmeal: Dr. Gaynor recommends 3 grams daily—that's about ½ tablespoon. Add it to bread dough, health shakes, and smoothies. Or, sprinkle it on oatmeal or breakfast cereal.

Flax oil: The usual dosage is 1 to 3 teaspoons daily, drizzled on salad—like olive oil—or mixed in yogurt (it adds a nutty flavor). ››

HOW FRESH IS THAT FLAXSEED OIL, ANYWAY?

Like a fine wine, there are certain things to look for in a bottle of flaxseed oil, according to Jerry Hickey, R.Ph., coauthor of *Dr. Gaynor's Cancer Prevention Program* and chairman of the Society of Natural Pharmacy. Here's how to ensure that you're getting the best oil available.

- Shop at busy stores with high shelf turnover and, therefore, fresher flax.
- Buy only products that are refrigerated; flax oil is unstable in heat.
- Choose a bottle that's nitrogen-packed, which means that the air has been sucked out of the container. Flax oxidizes when exposed to air, causing it to spoil faster.
- Look for oils labeled "high lignan." Flaxseed and flax meal all contain breast cancer–stunting lignans, but some flax oils don't.
- To avoid flax treated with pesticides, look for products labeled "organic," which are widely available. When you get home, taste it. Flaxseed oil shouldn't taste strong. If it does, it's rancid, and you won't get the oil's health benefits. Return the bottle.

Helpful Hints

To preserve flaxseed oil's healthful goodness and nutty flavor, never cook with it. Heat quickly oxidizes flax oil, causing it to go rancid. Also, flax in all its forms—seed, meal, and oil—spoils quickly. So keep all three refrigerated in air-tight containers. Toss after 4 weeks. ■

Flu

Save the Day with These Antiviral Powerhouses

Every year, the flu virus steals an entire week out of millions of women's lives. If you're one of them, you don't have to resign yourself to days of misery. You can do more than you realize to fight back.

Start by not *fighting it. Follow the good old-fashioned advice and make sure you get plenty of rest and lots of fluids.*

Here's what you can try. (Since flu can strike suddenly and leave you too exhausted to leave the house, it's best to have these flu fighters on hand during flu season.)

Echinacea. Known as purple coneflower, this herb enhances general immunity, stimulates the body's antiviral substance, interferon, and has been shown in test-tube studies to fight the influenza virus. Studies show that taking echinacea as a tincture or extract when symptoms first appear can help you recover from the flu more quickly, says Linda B. White, M.D., coauthor of *Kids, Herbs, and Health.*

Experts believe that echi-

nacea is best used to nip respiratory illnesses in the bud, Dr. White says. She offers the following dosage suggestions. *For tincture:* ¼ teaspoon four times daily of an extract labeled "1:5 strength." Dilute the tincture in a little fruit juice or herbal tea to improve the taste, she suggests. *For capsules:* 1,500 to 2,500 milligrams daily. Since it stimulates the immune system, do not use echinacea if you have an autoimmune condition such as lupus, tuberculosis, or multiple sclerosis. Do not use if you are allergic to plants in the daisy family, such as chamomile and marigold.

Elderberry. This herb has been found to inhibit types A and B influenza viruses. In one study, 90 percent of those given elderberry experienced a complete cure in 2 to 3 days, versus at least 6 days for those taking a placebo. The study used Sambucol (a standardized extract of elderberry in syrup form), and adults took 4 tablespoons daily for 3 days. **The compounds found in elderberry inhibit the enzyme that flu viruses use to penetrate cell membranes,** says Dr. White. You can take elderberry as a syrup, tea, tincture, or in capsules or lozenges. Many elderberry products contain other natural ingredients, so follow package instructions.

Garlic. Not only does garlic boost immunity in general but it has also been shown to inhibit the type B influenza virus. Some of its active ingredients are eliminated through the lungs, right where we need them to target infections. Garlic also promotes expectoration, helping you cough up mucus. Add it to meals, or take supplements, advises Dr. White. **Some herbalists suggest eating about six fresh cloves of garlic a day when you are sick.** A painless way to do this is to blend three garlic cloves into ½ cup of carrot juice and drink it down. If you prefer to swallow a pill, take capsules containing 3,000 to 4,000 micrograms of allicin (one of the active ingredients in garlic) every day.

Licorice root. This sweet-and-savory tasting herb inhibits the growth of flu viruses. According to Dr. White, it fights them by sparking the body's production of antiviral interferon and helps prevent virus cells from multiplying. It also soothes inflamed respiratory linings and helps expectorate mucus. You can take licorice in tea (it blends well with other cold and flu herbs), tincture (20 to 30 drops three times a day), or capsules (up to six 400- to 500-milligram capsules daily). Its best for short-term use, so don't use it daily for more than 4 to 6 weeks. Don't use licorice at all if you have high blood pressure, liver or kidney disease, diabetes, or low blood potassium levels. ››

SIP THIS FLU-BUSTER TEA

Dr. White suggests sipping this tea when you're under the weather: Blend equal parts of dried peppermint leaves, lemon balm leaves, elderflowers or berries, and yarrow leaves or flowers. Steep 1 to 2 teaspoons of the mix into a 4-ounce cup of just-boiled water for 5 to 10 minutes. Strain and drink while warm. If you have the chills, add a dash of powdered ginger to the tea to get your blood flowing and warm you up, she adds.

To prevent flu germs from making their way into your body, remember to wash your hands often, and don't rub your eyes or bite your fingernails. "The vast majority of cases of the flu are transmitted by hand," says Anton J. Kuzel, M.D., vice chairman of the department of family practice at Virginia Commonwealth University's Medical College campus in Richmond.

Helpful Hints

Certain antibacterial and antiviral drugs, such as Relenza, Symmetrel, and Flumadine, are available to combat the flu and help relieve symptoms earlier; see your doctor for a prescription. Try to get to your doctor as soon as you feel the telltale flu symptoms coming on, says Peter Gross, M.D., chair of the department of internal Medicine at Hackensack University Medical Center in New Jersey. That's especially true if your flu symptoms include a high fever, severe cough, chest pain, severe shortness of breath, or confusion, or if you have a headache even after you have taken a painkiller for it, or if you have a weakened immune system or a chronic autoimmune disease.

Get a flu shot every year before flu season. Flu shots are generally recommended for anyone over age 65 or for people with conditions such as diabetes, asthma, or other chronic heart or lung problems. **But doctors now recommend that people of all ages get a flu shot.** Getting your shot is a minor pain, but it's nearly 90 percent effective in preventing flu types A and B, which kill as many as 50,000 people in the typical epidemic year, according to the Centers for Disease Control and Prevention. At the very least, it will save you from using up your vacation days in bed with the flu.

Can't stomach needles? **Ask your doctor about the new flu vaccine that's delivered via drops or spray to the nose,** suggests Dr. Gross. ■

Flyaway Hair

Emergency Tactics for Out-of-Control Static

As a hairstylist in the Windy City, Amy Everett of Chicago has seen her fair share of flyaway hair.

"Actually, the wind has nothing to do with it," says Everett. Sure, it will mess up your do. But what really causes flyaway hair—hair that fiercely resists staying where you want it—is dry air and the lack of humidity that often comes with cold temperatures.

Everett has styled the hair of many celebrities who have visited Chicago—including Sarah Ferguson, the Duchess of York; former First Lady Barbara Bush; and fashion maven Gloria Vanderbilt. She's perfected ways to tame the most seemingly untamable hair. Her secret: Restore moisture to the hair. Here's how.

Stop blow-drying your hair when it still feels a little cold. Stop when it no longer feels wet or heavy, but before it's completely dry.

Blow-dry from the scalp out. Flip your hair over and get most of the moisture out of the

Food Allergies

Watch Out for Hidden Ingredients

Having a food allergy complicates food shopping. Besides scrutinizing food labels for fat grams, calories, fiber, and sodium, you have to identify ingredients that could trigger annoying or possibly even life-threatening reactions.

"The problem is that whatever you're allergic to—milk, wheat, soy, eggs—has many pseudonyms, and to avoid trouble, you have to be able to recognize them," says Daryl R. Altman, M.D., director of Allergy Information Services in Baldwin, New York.

The next time you shop for groceries, play detective. The chart on page 166 can help.

DON'T MAKE THIS MISTAKE

Never assume that a food is safe to eat after reading its label once. Food manufacturers, especially makers of processed foods, can frequently change what they use to make a food, says Dr. Altman. So it's best to read the label every time you buy the product.

Identifying a true food allergy requires a thorough medical history and tests with food extracts. Once a food allergy has been diagnosed, the only treatment is to avoid the food completely. For some highly sensitive women, even minute quantities of an allergen can cause a reaction, says Anne Muñoz-Furlong, president and founder of the Food Allergy Network, a nonprofit organization based in Fairfax, Virginia. Yet the FDA does ››

roots, then stand and work on the outside layers. This helps you avoid overdrying the outside layers, which are most susceptible to becoming flyaway.

Spray lightly with a spray-on conditioner, also known as a moisture mist. "Women with fine hair are afraid to use a conditioner. They think it will weigh it down," says Everett. But fine hair especially needs moisture to remain manageable.

Go easy on the spray. Many women are tempted to use too much hair spray to control flyaway hair. It's fine to use it when your hair becomes unruly, but keep it light, says Everett.

Helpful Hints

If your hair becomes flyaway while you are away from home, simply wet your hands and run them through your hair. This will restore moisture and control, especially if your hair is short.

In an emergency, try Static Guard. "The same stuff you use to remove static from your slip or skirts will work on your hair," says Everett. "Don't spray it directly on your hair, though. Spray it on your brush, then brush it through your hair." ■

not always require "trace ingredients" to be listed on food labels. So she advises women with food allergies to avoid foods with vaguely listed ingredients such as "natural flavors," or to call the manufacturer and ask if it contains the food to which they are allergic.

The Food Allergy Network publishes a newsletter to keep readers with allergies up-to-date on hidden sources of allergenic ingredients. For a sample, send your request with a self-addressed stamped envelope to the Food Allergy Network at 10400 Eaton Place, Suite 107, Fairfax, VA 22030-2208. ■

DECODE FOOD LABELS

If you have food allergies, learn what ingredients derived from the foods cause trouble for you, starting with this list, provided by the Food Allergy Network. It doesn't include all possible food allergens, though, and manufacturers may also use other terms for these foods. For more information, contact the manufacturer directly. You'll find the phone number on many labels.

Food	Label Terms
Corn	buretose, cerulose, dextrin, grits, hydrolyzed vegetable protein, lactic acid, sorbitol, vegetable gum, vegetable starch
Eggs	albumin, egg lecithin, egg powder, egg solids, egg whites, globulin, livetin, lysozyme (used in Europe), ovalbumin, ovomucin, ovomucoid, ovovitellin
Milk	calcium caseinate, casein hydrolysate, caseinate, curds, lactalbumin, lactoglobulin, rennet casein, whey
Soy	hydrolyzed vegetable protein, lecithin, natural flavoring, soy flour, textured vegetable protein (tvp), tofu, vegetable broth, vegetable gum, vegetable oil, vegetable starch, hydrolyzed vegetable protein
Wheat	aestivum, farina, galvanized starch, gluten, hydrogenated starch hydrolysates, hydrolyzed vegetable protein, modified food starch, modified starch, natural flavoring, semolina, spelt, vegetable gum, vegetable starch

Food Cravings

Balance Your Six Tastes

If you're in the habit of driving across town at midnight to buy a pint of rocky road ice cream, odds are you don't just like *rocky road. You probably* crave *it.*

"Women tell me that when they eat a food they crave, it's like someone else's hand is scooping ice cream into their mouths—they're in a trance," says Doreen Virtue, Ph.D., a psychologist and eating disorders specialist in Newport Beach, California.

According to one survey, 97 percent of women (versus 68 percent of men) have experienced that gotta-have-it feeling for a particular food.

No one knows exactly why women have food cravings. Some experts blame female hormones for the pickles-and-ice-cream syndrome that often develops during pregnancy.

Others blame the socialization process that makes food an "acceptable" female addiction.

If food cravings strike only occasionally and don't cause bingeing, there's little cause for alarm. But **if you're regularly devouring entire containers of ice cream, something may be out of whack.**

To thwart such cravings, the standard advice is to drink water, take a walk, and ask yourself if there's a hidden reason why you "need" that entire 1-pound bag of M&M's. If that doesn't work, many experts say it's okay to surrender to a craving as long as you exercise strict portion control.

Not everyone thinks these tactics make sense. **The best way to control food cravings is to eat a daily diet incorporating the six essential tastes: sweet, sour, salty, bitter, astringent, and pungent,** says Nancy Lonsdorf, M.D., medical director of the Maharishi Ayurveda Medical Center in Rockville, Maryland, and coauthor of *A Woman's Best Medicine.*

DON'T MAKE THIS MISTAKE

If this diet works for you, don't revert to your former eating habits. "If you start grabbing junk food, eating on the run, and doing all the wrong things again, the cravings will return," Dr. Lonsdorf says.

"Our diet in the West is heavy on sweet, sour, and salty tastes," says Dr. Lonsdorf, an adherent of Ayurvedic medicine, which originated in India. "When you eat too much of them, you gain weight, feel sluggish, and get sinus congestion, aches, pains, and stiffness."

Here are Dr. Lonsdorf's suggestions for correcting the imbalance, based on Ayurvedic principles.

Get bitter. Eat more kale, spinach, and broccoli. "Dark green leafy and bitter vegetables stimulate the liver's ability to detoxify the body," Dr. Lonsdorf says.

Pucker up. Eat more chickpeas, lentils, and pinto beans—or any other food that makes your mouth go dry. "If you feed yourself a balance of tastes, including astringent foods, it will keep your body feeling happy so that it doesn't send you these craving signals," Dr. Lonsdorf says.

Spice up your life. Eat more jalapeño peppers and hot spices such as black pepper, cumin, or ginger. "Pungent foods help you digest food properly," Dr. Lonsdorf says.

Helpful Hint

If you can't include all six tastes with every meal, at least try to include them with lunch. "You'll probably notice that your late-afternoon and nighttime cravings subside," Dr. Lonsdorf says.

One woman who followed this diet stopped craving chocolate and started craving kale. "Maybe the bitter in the chocolate was the only bitter her body knew," Dr. Lonsdorf says. **"Many women may be craving chocolate because they've never eaten green leafy vegetables."** ■

Forgetfulness

Memory Helpers for the Overwrought

Among life's little miseries, few are as exasperating as forgetfulness.

If you've ever blanked out while trying to remember a name or wandered around a parking lot searching for your "lost" car, you may begin to wonder if you've lost your marbles.

If you have only an occasional memory lapse, don't sweat it, says brain researcher Gary Small, M.D., of the UCLA Medical School, who has studied brain function and memory in men and women. "Most busy women have such problems," Dr. Small says. "They're what I call the walking forgetful."

Research shows that brain function is enhanced by exercise, a balanced diet, and getting enough sleep. But beyond these commonsense approaches, there a number of steps you can take to sharpen your memory.

Play the name game. When you're introduced to someone, it's easier to remember her first name if you repeat it during the conversation. To remember her last name, spell it out to yourself. Look for a physical characteristic to associate the name with the face. With difficult names, associate a visual image with each syllable (for example, a Raggedy Ann doll with the syllable "an"). "If I can picture it, it's easier to remember," Dr. Small says.

Treat yourself to an "executive" parking spot. Any available spot will do, at work or at the mall, as long as it's the same spot each time. Your brain likes routine. "So much of daily memory and daily functioning depends on repeated learning," Dr. Small says. That's why women may have temporary memory lapses when they move to a new job in a new city—you have to learn so many things you used to take for granted.

Keep written and mental lists. If you're taking medications, use a chart, calendar, or weekly pill box. If you're trying to remember what you need at the supermarket, cluster the items by food group. "Instead of trying to remember 9 separate items, think of them as three fruits, three vegetables and three cereals," Dr. Small says. Or, just write it down.

DON'T MAKE THIS MISTAKE

If your memory seems to be failing steadily, don't hesitate to consult your doctor. Many treatable conditions can cause forgetfulness, among them depression, drug side effects, and thyroid disorders. Your doctor can determine whether or not you have age-related memory impairment or something more serious.

If memory lapses are affecting your ability to function, you may be at higher risk of developing Alzheimer's disease. The earlier you're diagnosed, the earlier you can begin treatment. Estrogen replacement therapy, for example, may delay or prevent Alzheimer's disease," Dr. Small says.

Consider vitamin E. A large national study conducted by Columbia University College of Physicians and Surgeons found that when treated daily with 2,000 IU of vitamin E, Alzheimer's patients had slowed functional decline. **Although researchers have not yet proven that vitamin E will prevent Alzheimer's or delay its onset, it is possible that the antioxidant effects of vitamin E may have a preventive advantage.**

Because it is generally nontoxic and inexpensive, Dr. Small recommends it to his Alzheimer's patients at doses between 1,200 and 2,000 IU a day (taking amounts over 400 IU should be discussed with your doctor). If you don't have Alzheimer's but are worried about getting it, 800 IU would be preferable. However, if you want to simply keep your memory sharp, try including foods rich in antioxidants, like blueberries and strawberries, in your diet every day, says Dr. Small. They're high in vitamin E.

Helpful Hint

The more you challenge your brain, the better it'll perform. Any kind of mental exercise, such as working crossword puzzles, can help improve your memory. "Just be sure it's something you enjoy," Dr. Small says. "If you don't enjoy it, it's going to be a drag." ■

Forgiveness

Who, What, Where, When, How, and Why to Let Go of Hurtful Wrongs

Imagine a long steel chain wrapped around your ankle, dragging behind you everywhere you go. Weighing you down. Holding you back.

Now imagine the freedom you'd feel removing that chain—link by rusty link. That's what happens when you forgive. All the energy you spent being angry, bitter, and resentful suddenly reappears, providing an opportunity for emotional and physical healing to begin. And none too soon: Keeping these emotions bottled up inside you for months—or years—puts you at a higher risk for developing high blood pressure, heart disease, stroke, depression, or even cancer, says Norma Dearing, director of prayer ministry at the Christian Healing Ministries in Jacksonville, Florida.

In other words, "When you forgive, you're not letting the person who wronged you off the hook, you're really letting yourself off the hook," says Reverend Linda Shaheerah Beatty, an ordained minister at Transforming Love Community Church in Detroit. "Forgiveness is letting go; it's discovering what hurt us and healing those hurts." ››

Here is a step-by-step guide to who, what, where, when, and how to forgive.

Who should you forgive? No matter how many people have hurt you, it's important to forgive everyone, even if they've never apologized, says Reverend Beatty. "Most of the time, when people hurt us, they are acting out pain that they've endured in their lives. We just end up getting the brunt of it, because we're in the line of fire," she says.

What should you forgive? Betrayal, gossip, infidelity, broken promises—even verbal and physical abuse. These offenses—and the people who committed them—may seem impossible to forgive at first, especially if you've lived with the pain for years. Just try to be patient and ask for divine help in the forgiving process. It may take longer for you to forgive an unfaithful husband than a gossiping friend. But that's okay. Once you start dealing with your past hurts, and decide to release yourself from the anger, the guilt, and the shame, you'll begin to heal, says Dearing.

Where to say "I forgive you." Face-to-face is probably best, says Reverend Beatty. "You can look into that person's eyes and soul. The true essence of you is going to speak even louder than your words. And if that doesn't work, you can always write a letter. They can read it over and over again, and they won't be able to add anything to your words," she says.

A phone call can work well, too—but before deciding, consider the situation and the person you're forgiving.

When do you say "I forgive you?" The best time to speak to someone is when you're not angry. It's always best to deal with your anger first, then approach the other person once you've calmed down. A good way to alleviate anger is to talk to a close friend about the situation. Getting it off your chest not only reduces tension but may also give you new insight, says Reverend Beatty.

Frostbite

Signals You Should Never Ignore

Anyone who has read *Into Thin Air,* Jon Krakauer's best-selling account of mountain climbers who disastrously braved Mount Everest, probably remembers the author's graphic description of the severe frostbite suffered by fellow climber Beck Weathers: patches of skin frozen into ink-black patches.

Unless you're thinking of signing up for a similar conquest, you're not likely to suffer frostbite nearly that severe. But you do need to watch out for subtler signs of mild or moderate frostbite if you're outdoors in the cold for, say, a football game or a day of skiing in weather below 32°F, especially if it's windy. Here's how to save your skin, according to Eric A. Weiss, M.D., an emergency physician at Stanford University Medical Center.

DON'T MAKE THIS MISTAKE

There are lots of misconceptions about the definitions of forgiveness. Here's what forgiveness is not.

- Forgiveness is not condoning abusive behavior.
- Forgiveness is not conditional—"I'll forgive you if you change."
- Forgiveness is not reconciliation (though reconciliation can be a step in forgiveness).
- Forgiveness is not denying that something happened.
- Forgiveness is not forgetting.
- Forgiveness is not saying "Everything is okay now" or "I'm completely okay now."

How to say "I forgive you." When confronting someone you want to forgive, explain how their actions or words made you feel. Use phrases like "I felt hurt when you . . ." or "I felt betrayed when you. . . ." The "I" phrases take the blame off the other person and focus on your feelings, says Reverend Beatty.

You can also write daily forgiveness affirmations on paper that say something like "I forgive so-and-so for . . ." or "I forgive myself for. . . ."

Helpful Hint

If you like to pray, make a list of all the people you haven't forgiven and the hurtful things they've done to you, suggests Dearing.

Give each person her own separate, but small, sheet of paper. You could also verbally state what everyone has done as you pile the sheets of paper in your hands. Put your hands together, and hold them up to God. Then, turn them over and release the papers and all of that pain and hurt to the Lord, asking him to take away the anger, resentment, and bitterness that you have in your heart. Then burn or throw away the papers. ■

Do you feel tingling in your toes, fingers, nose, or ears? If yes, most likely you have "frostnip," a superficial form of frostbite. Get out of the cold. Warm your toes on a friend's bare stomach. Failing that, stick your hands in your armpits or groin. You can also hold a cloth against whatever parts are cold. If feeling returns in 30 minutes, you should be all right.

Is your skin stiff, and does it have a white, waxy appearance? If yes, you have frostbite. Don't rub the skin, or you will damage the tissues. Instead, soak your hand or foot in warm water (dishwashing temperature, 102° to 104°F) for 45 minutes. Never expose it to direct heat, like a heating pad or fireplace heat. Take aspirin or ibuprofen for the pain and see a doctor right away.

Do not thaw out a frostbitten extremity if there is a chance that it will refreeze. Instead, wait until you're somewhere where it will not refreeze.

Helpful Hint

If you're going out into the bitter cold, make sure that every inch of skin is covered, including your nose. Buy the warmest gloves—or even better, mittens—and socks you can find, plus a face mask (available at sporting goods stores). ■

Fruit

Top Picks from the Produce Bin

Imagine tickling your tastebuds with a bowl of perfectly ripe, gloriously scented strawberries. Ummm. What could be better?

Not much—and not just for the pleasure of eating them. Strawberries and other fruits are super foods that deliver untold health perks in every bite. Full of fiber and bursting with secret ingredients, including thousands of compounds called phytochemicals as well as antioxidant nutrients, fruit offers protection against heart disease, stroke, and many different types of cancer.

Some fruits, like purple grapes, are rich in plant pigments called flavonoids that have powerful antioxidant abilities to prevent cell damage from what scientists call free radicals—naturally occurring substances that damage (oxidize) body tissues and blood fats, leading to cancer and coronary artery disease. Many fruits, like cantaloupe and mangoes, are rich in beta-carotene and vitamin C, two other potent antioxidants that boost immunity and guard against disease, says Jennifer K. Nelson, R.D., director of clinical dietetics in the division of endocrinology, metabolism, and internal medicine at the Mayo Clinic in Rochester, Minnesota.

DON'T MAKE THIS MISTAKE

Don't substitute drinking fruit juices for eating whole fruit. Stripped of their valuable fiber, fruit juices are concentrated sources of sugar and calories.

According to experts at the National Cancer Institute, you should eat up to five servings of fruit each day. Unfortunately, many of us aren't eating that amount and, therefore, aren't getting the nutrients needed for optimal health.

All fruits are healthy, say experts, so one fruit is as good as the next. If you're not accustomed to eating fruit, start with these five, for maximum eating pleasure and nutrient density.

- Papaya: Half a fruit packs 94 milligrams of vitamin C.
- Cantaloupe: 1 cup cubed has 67 milligrams of vitamin C; ½ cantaloupe yields 5 milligrams of beta-carotene, about one-third of the daily amount recommended by experts.
- Mango: One contains 57 milligrams of vitamin C and 5 milligrams of beta-carotene.
- Strawberries: ½ cup has 42 milligrams of vitamin C and is a good source of flavonoids.
- Cranberries: These are flavonoid-rich and a good source of an antioxidant that shows promise against cancer. ■

G

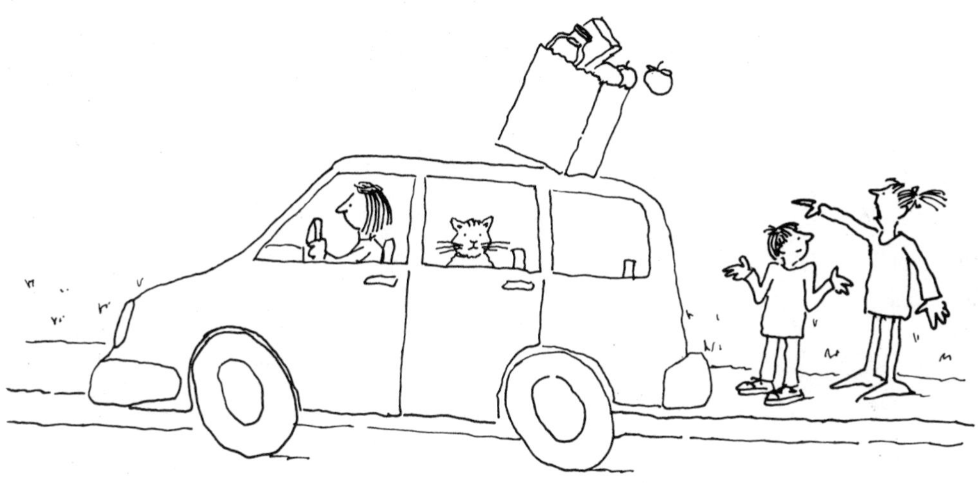

Forgetful? Remember to take your ginkgo,
a natural tonic for the aging brain.
For details, see page 182.

Gallbladder Problems

Secrets to a Stone-Free Life

Like some children and all movie audiences, gallstones are at their best when they're silent. Many of the estimated 16 to 20 million Americans (typically female, middle-age, and overweight) with gallstones don't experience symptoms and may not even be aware of their condition.

They're the lucky ones. The stones (usually accumulations of cholesterol) nest in your gallbladder, a small organ near your liver whose job it is to store the bile that the liver makes for digestion. After a meal, when it's time for the bile to go to work, the gallbladder contracts to secrete it. That's when those stones can hurt.

The only way to get rid of stones you already have is to have your gallbladder removed (a safe and common surgical procedure). But you can discourage more stones—or, better yet, prevent the first one from forming. "We know a lot about what lifestyle changes may reduce the risk of gallstones forming to begin with," says Joanne Donovan, M.D., Ph.D., a gastroenterologist at the Boston Veterans Administration Medical Center and assistant professor of medicine at Harvard Medical School. Here's what to do.

WHAT'S GOOD FOR YOUR GALLBLADDER MAY BE BAD FOR YOUR LIVER

Besides protecting your heart, moderate alcohol consumption may help prevent gallstones—provided you don't have liver problems. If you do, the risks outweigh the benefits.

Lose weight slowly. Crash diets create gallstones. "Rapid weight loss is the major contributor to gallstone disease," Dr. Donovan says. "Even a few weeks of starving yourself can do it." Skipping breakfast often or frequent fasting have the same effect because your gallbladder isn't contracting often enough to flush itself.

But lose it. Being overweight interferes with proper gallbladder functioning and can lead to stones. So if you're carrying around extra pounds, your goal is to get rid of them—just not all at once. One to 2 pounds a week is a safe weight loss pace.

And keep it off. Yo-yo dieting—which doctors call weight cycling—is another road to Stonesville. "Women who go up and down in weight are at higher risk than women who stay at any given weight," Dr. Donovan says.

Eat less fat and more vegetables. That's a good way to keep your weight down, of course. But beyond that, studies keep showing that people who eat more vegetables and less fat have less gallstone disease.

Get your exercise. Whether it's because of its weight loss benefits or for other reasons, regular moderate exercise reduces your risk of gallstones. One study tells the story: One out of three cases of gallstone disease in men could be prevented by ››

30 minutes of endurance-type training five times a week. "We have no reason to think that this isn't true for women as well," Dr. Donovan says.

Keep taking that daily aspirin. If you've been prescribed a daily aspirin to prevent heart attack, your gallbladder may benefit, too. "Daily aspirin may interrupt the pathways to gallstone formation," Dr. Donovan says.

Helpful Hint

While taking lots of extra vitamin C won't prevent gallstones, some research suggests that not getting enough increases the likelihood of stone formation. So make sure you get your Daily Value—60 milligrams—of C (the amount in 4½ ounces of orange juice). ■

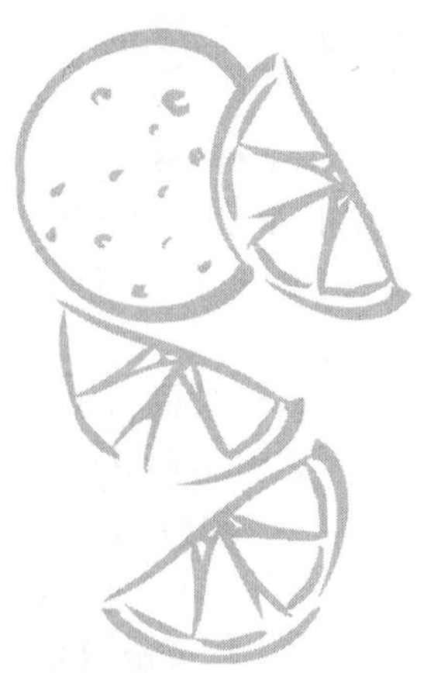

Garlic

Get All the Benefits (without Bad Breath!)

What do builders of the ancient Egyptian pyramids, Roman gladiators, and residents of Gilroy, California, have in common? All hail the taste and medicinal benefits of garlic.

Historians tell of pyramid builders who went on strike when deprived of their daily rations of garlic. Roman gladiators believed that garlic (which they knew as Allium sativum*) gave them greater strength, so much so that they would eat cloves before big stadium matches. Gilroy residents, proud of living in the country's garlic capital, honor this stinking bulb at the annual garlic festival held each July.*

And if any herb is worth raising a...er...stink about, it's garlic. It's been said to help prevent or treat the common cold, earaches, toothaches, yeast infections, some types of cancers, high cholesterol, and high blood pressure.

The real power in this plant comes from allicin, garlic's active chemical ingredient. Allicin has been proven as an antibacterial, antimicrobial, antifungal, and antioxidant agent. It's also responsible for garlic's pungent odor, says Mark Stengler, N.D., a naturopathic physician in San Diego—and a devoted garlic fan.

Forget the proverbial apple—most garlic proponents say that eating a clove of fresh garlic a day is the route to better health. But then you'd have no friends—none that would want to get within 10 feet of you, anyway. So here are some other ways to get your daily intake of garlic:

Daily garlic supplements. Cut the odor without sacrificing the medicinal help by taking Kwai or Kyolic pills (both have been scientifically proven to lower cholesterol levels). Garlic pills coated with enteric improve the absorption of allicin, cut odor, and dissolve quickly in the intestines.

Pickled garlic cloves. If you detest the taste of raw cloves, try this pickled garlic recipe. In a bowl, mix ¼ cup each of apple cider vinegar, honey, water, and soy sauce. Pour these ingredients into a glass pint jar. Then add enough peeled garlic cloves so they are bathed in liquid. Tighten the lid and store in the refrigerator for 2 weeks to marinate. Then, keep your immune system bolstered by eating one or two pickled cloves a day, either alone or with crackers or bread. Pickled garlic tastes deliciously sweet, salty, and sour, but the garlic odor may still prevail on your breath. Counter it by eating a few fresh sprigs of parsley or fennel seeds.

Chop or mash cloves. No chewing is necessary if you simply chop or mash raw garlic cloves and mix with food throughout the day.

DON'T MAKE THIS MISTAKE

Garlic thins your blood, which helps prevent dangerous blood clots. But you shouldn't take garlic supplements or eat large amounts of garlic (more than two cloves per day) without your doctor's approval if you take regular doses of aspirin, warfarin (Coumadin), or other blood-thinning drugs, since you may bleed too easily. For the same reason, do not eat large amounts of garlic before undergoing surgery, including dental surgery.

Helpful Hints

Cutting or crushing garlic 10 to 15 minutes before heating allows time for the active ingredients to form, making the most of its healing power. If you're not fond of garlic's strong flavor, you may enjoy elephant garlic, a member of the leek family that looks like oversized garlic. Available in supermarkets, it smells like garlic but tastes milder. "Flavor-wise, elephant garlic is mild, more like leeks or yellow onions," says Patsy Ross, vice president of marketing for Christopher Ranch, the largest garlic producer in the country, located in—of course—Gilroy, California. Because of its mild, almost bland taste, Ross says many people slice elephant garlic and use it raw in salads and sandwiches or cook it lightly and add it to other foods. Although elephant garlic doesn't contain allicin, one study showed that it may reduce the risk for some types of cancer, presumably due to sulfur compounds it contains. ■

Gastroesophageal Reflux

Keep Acid in Its Place

Gastroesophageal reflux disease (GERD) is a ghastly sounding name for what amounts to faulty internal traffic control. Stomach acid goes the wrong way (up) on what's supposed to be a one-way street—your esophagus. That results in heartburn, which is a simple way to describe the discomfort of this acid regurgitation.

Occasional heartburn can be handled with herbs or antacids. Frequent episodes deserve medical attention. Over-the-counter medicines such as Tagamet or Pepcid AC, known as histamine 2 (H2) blockers, can also help prevent GERD-induced heartburn. But you can also avoid ›› trouble simply by watching what you eat—and how you eat it.

Steer Clear of Known Offenders

Certain foods are more problematic than others. Here's what to avoid.

Bacon double cheeseburgers. "More than anything else, fat really seems to predispose you to acid reflux," says Stuart Spechler, M.D., professor of internal medicine at the University of Texas Southwestern Medical Center in Dallas. Any kind of animal fats may cause trouble.

Chocolate. There's something about the chemical makeup of the chocolate itself that weakens the sphincter muscles at the bottom of the esophagus. So it's no friend to women with GERD. "Avoid fatty foods and chocolate, and you're going a long way toward taking care of the problem," Dr. Spechler says.

DON'T MAKE THIS MISTAKE

Elevating the head of your bed on 4-inch to 6-inch blocks or bricks enables gravity to help keep down acid. Don't try to prop yourself up with an extra pillow or two, however. To help prevent heartburn, you need your whole body at a slight incline as you sleep, not just your head and shoulders.

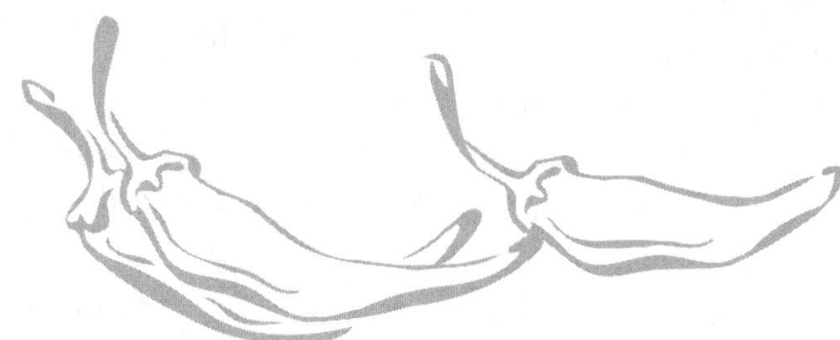

Vegetable oil. Eastern medicine categorizes both foods and conditions according to four major elements—earth, wind, fire, and water. "Hyperacidity is a fiery condition," says David Frawley, O.M.D., doctor of oriental medicine and director of the American Institute of Vedic Studies in Sante Fe, New Mexico. "In the scheme of things, some vegetables oils are considered 'hot', others 'cool.'" Cooling oils include coconut, sunflower and safflower oils, and ghee, which is clarified butter. So women experiencing hyperacidity may fare better if they use sunflower and safflower oil, while avoiding other vegetable oils (considered "hot").

Spicy foods. More often, "hot food" brings to mind chiles, paprika, cayenne, and the like. To avoid heartburn, these, too, should be used very sparingly, advises Dr. Frawley. Instead, use two spices that actually help control acidity. One is turmeric, an excellent cooking spice that's used in curry and stimulates digestion to prevent acid buildup. Another is cilantro (or coriander leaf), which is common in Mexican food—it counteracts the acidic effect of chiles by reducing gas.

Citrus fruits and yogurt. While otherwise healthful, oranges, grapefruit, pineapple, and other acidic fruits kick up trouble for women prone to reflux. So can yogurt.

Helpful Hint

Anecdotal evidence suggests that many women are most vulnerable to acidity during menstruation. According to

Eastern medicine, health problems are categorized according to five different principles, or humors: fire, earth, metal, water, and wood. The female reproductive and blood systems are related to the humor fire, and acidity is a feature of fire. Take extra care to avoid offending foods at that time.

Other Tactics That Help

Be regular. Skipping meals is no solution to reflux because your stomach secretes acid regularly even when you eat irregularly. "If you feel hungry, you ought to put something in your stomach," Dr. Frawley says.

Think small. Eating more smaller meals is safer than eating fewer big ones, Dr. Frawley says.

Dine early. The later you eat, the weaker your digestion because Eastern medicine believes your digestive fire peaks about noon, says Dr. Frawley. He suggests not eating less than 3 hours before you retire.

Sit up. Lying down after a meal only makes it easier for the acid to rise up into your esophagus. ■

Gift-Giving Angst

The New Rules of Gift Exchanges

Twenty or so Novembers ago, Charles Langham of Charlottesville, Virginia, and his coworkers were making plans for the upcoming holidays. Like most of us, they expected to receive a lot of gifts they didn't ask for and spend money on gifts other people didn't want. So they formed SCROOGE—the Society to Curtail Ridiculous, Outrageous, and Ostentatious Gift Exchanges.

SCROOGE publishes an annual newsletter before Christmas. But its message—keep presents simple and affordable—can apply to gift-giving all year. Here's how.

In General

If you have a talent for making crafts, artwork, or other goodies, give them as gifts. Your friends may remember these longer than they would store-bought presents, Langham says.

Think quality, not quantity. If you have a certain amount of money to spend for a gift, buy something that's small yet nice as opposed to an object that's sizable but cheap-looking, recommends Maria Everding, founder of the Etiquette Institute in St. Louis and author of *Panache That Pays*.

Pay with cash, not credit. That way, you're apt to think a little longer about the money you're about to spend, and you won't be as stunned when the credit-card bill arrives.

Set guidelines—and stick to them. Whether they involve your family, friends, or coworkers, setting ground rules avoids awkward situations, suggests Everding. ››

DON'T MAKE THIS MISTAKE

Always wrap your gift nicely, even if the store puts it in an attractive bag. "Otherwise, you're saying, 'Hey, I don't think too much of you—here's a bag with a gift on the inside,'" says Everding.

End-of-the-Year Holidays

Set a dollar limit. SCROOGE suggests 1 percent of your gross annual pay be spent on all your holiday gifts. If you make $30,000 a year, for example, consider limiting yourself to $300 of gift-wrapped cheer.

Draw names. If you exchange gifts with your extended family, do what many large families traditionally do: Draw names so that each person buys a gift for one person instead for everyone, Everding suggests.

Weddings

Bring or send a gift only if you attend the wedding. Otherwise, you shouldn't feel obligated to send a present, Everding says.

At Work

Rarely, if ever, give your boss an individual gift. It may make your coworkers think you're trying to curry favor, plus it can make your relationship with the boss awkward.

If you must give a gift, several employees should contribute to it, Everding says. Make a donation to a charity in your boss's name or take her out to lunch.

If you're a supervisor, refrain from giving gifts to employees. If gifts to staff are customary in your workplace, stick with something impersonal, like a gift certificate to a restaurant or the movies.

Celebrate collectively. To stanch the stream of dollars that you spend on coworkers' birthdays, suggest that your office hold a simple monthly party for everyone whose birthday falls in that month.

Helpful Hint

If you're invited to someone's home, you should bring a small gift, such as a bottle of wine or box of chocolates, for your host or hostess. It's not intended to be opened and consumed while you're there.

If your host or hostess doesn't drink or needs to avoid sweets, flowers or other fancy foods (like gourmet olive oil) are safe choices. ■

Ginger

Settle Your Stomach with Spice

Before refrigerators, ginger was used as a preservative, to prevent food from spoiling. Today, women can depend on this spice as a nondrug remedy for nausea and other ailments.

"Ginger offers many gifts—it's a tonic, a circulatory stimulant, a digestive stimulant, and an immune system booster," says Douglas Schar, DipPhyt., MCPP, a practicing medical herbalist in London.

Like a doctor on call inside your body, ginger instinctively knows to go where it is most needed. Ginger's medicinal qualities are housed in the rhizome, the underground stem of the plant often mistaken for a root.

Ginger is best known for relieving motion sickness and nausea. It is what herbalists call a carminative, which means that it settles the intestine. But this spice may also come to the aid for tension headaches, high cholesterol, arthritic pain, diarrhea induced by food poisoning, menstrual cramps, and flatulence.

Two of ginger's key active compounds, gingerols and shogaols, soothe stomach upsets and gassy buildups by improving digestive organ secretions, and reduce gas by relaxing the intestinal wall muscles. But no one is sure how ginger helps other conditions.

"Ginger's active oils get absorbed in the stomach and travel through the bloodstream to where they need to go," says Schar. "Sometimes, when you take ginger, you may feel flushed." That's because ginger causes the blood vessels to dilate.

You can take ginger up to three times a day. To get the most medicinal value from various forms of ginger, Schar offers these guidelines.

DON'T MAKE THIS MISTAKE

Ginger ale isn't a substitute for the real thing. "It's basically liquid sugar, with little or no true ginger," says Schar. "You'd be much better off, health-wise, eating a piece of crystallized ginger candy." Look for it in Asian food markets, health food stores, and specialty food shops.

DRY HEAVES? TRY GINGER TEA

Ginger works wonders for motion sickness, but that's not the only digestive disorder this medicinal root eases. It also may soothe dry heaves, including nausea associated with chemotherapy.

To maximize ginger's antinausea benefits and create a perfect cup of ginger tea, follow these directions from Varro Tyler, Sc.D., Ph.D., dean emeritus of Purdue University School of Pharmacy and Pharmacal Sciences in West Lafayette, Indiana, and author of *The Honest Herbal.*

- Grate 1 teaspoon of fresh or jarred gingerroot.
- Place ginger in 1 cup of boiled water and cover. (Covering the cup prevents the nausea-easing ingredients from evaporating.) Steep about 15 minutes.
- If you prefer sweet tea, add a teaspoon or two of honey.

Drink a cup any time you feel queasy, says Dr. Tyler. Ginger doesn't interact with chemo treatments.

Fresh rhizome: Grate ½ teaspoon of fresh ginger and stir into an 8-ounce glass of water or orange juice, up to three tims a day.

Capsules: Take one 250-milligram capsule up to three times a day.

Infused tea: Pour a cup of boiling water over 1 teaspoon of fresh grated ginger and let it infuse for 5 minutes. Drink up to 3 cups a day.

Tincture (also known as standardized extract): Place 30 drops of ginger tincture into an 8-ounce glass of water and drink up to three times a day.

Ginger is very safe. The only side effects—heartburn and mild allergic reaction—occur only rarely, says Angela Stengler, N.D., a naturopathic physician in San Diego. But ginger may increase bile secretion, so if you have gallstones, check with your doctor before taking it.

Helpful Hints

Choose ginger supplements that contain 100 percent pure ginger, says Schar. That way, you're guaranteed to be getting the active compounds. ■

Ginkgo Biloba

A Tonic for Your Brain

Ginkgo biloba trees grow in the congested, polluted streets of New York City as easily as the spacious landscapes of Sumter, South Carolina.

In fact, ginkgo reigns as the oldest tree species on the planet. Scientists have discovered that it is highly resistant to pollution, pesticides, and insects.

"During prehistoric days, volcanoes and toxic substances in the air wiped out some species, but not the ginkgo tree," says Georges Halpern, M.D., Ph.D., professor emeritus of medicine at the University of California, Davis, and author of *Ginkgo: A Practical Guide.* "Today, even air pollution is no match for the ginkgo tree."

What's more, ginkgo can help *you* survive. The active compounds extracted from its leaves act as a natural tonic for the aging brain, helping protect against conditions often associated with growing older, like forgetfulness, poor concentration, blood clots, macular degeneration, tinnitus, and poor circulation.

Scientists aren't sure exactly how ginkgo works, but its benefits are well-documented. **Ginkgo protects blood vessels of the brain, keeping them young.** It also helps some areas of the brain, probably those associated with memory, function better.

Ginseng

The Right Type for the Right Problem

Siberian ginseng. Asian ginseng. American ginseng. What's the difference? And should you care?

"Ginseng varieties are like distant cousins—related, but with distinct personalities," says Mark Stengler, N.D., a naturopathic physician in San Diego and author of The Natural Physician: Your Guide for Common Ailments. *"It's important to select the right type for your health needs." He offers these tips to sort it all out.*

American ginseng *(Panax quinquefolium)*: Herbalists consider the root of this species cooling by nature and recommend it to tame hot flashes and night sweats and relieve chronic chest congestion. Grown primarily in Wisconsin, this ginseng caters to the needs of asthmatics with dry coughs. In the Orient, it's imported and valued as an overall energy or body tonic. For best results, take one or two capsules (100 milligrams each) or 30 to 60 drops of tincture three times daily, suggests Dr. Stengler.

Asian ginseng, also known as Korean or Chinese ginseng (*Panax ginseng*): Warming by nature, the Asian form is considered to be the strongest of all ginsengs, according to herbalists and naturopathic physicians. This type of ginseng helps maintain stamina and mental sharpness and, surprisingly, treats chronic diar-

"Think of ginkgo as giving your brain a tune-up," says Dr. Halpern. "Because it improves bloodflow, which delivers more nutrients and oxygen to the brain, ginkgo helps your brain run better."

With your brain operating on all cylinders, you are apt to think more clearly, and you're less likely to forget where you left your car keys. Dr. Halpern recommends taking 120 to 160 milligrams of ginkgo tablets or capsules a day in divided doses (don't exceed 240 milligrams). For optimal results, select standardized extract tablets that contain 24 percent ginkgoflavoglycosides and 6 percent terpenelactones, the two groups of active chemicals found in ginkgo leaves.

DON'T MAKE THIS MISTAKE

If you're taking aspirin or an anticoagulant (blood-thinning) medication, check with your physician before using ginkgo. Combining ginkgo with these bloodthinners may interfere with the body's ability to clot and stop bleeding. This is especially key for women who bleed heavily during menstruation. Also, don't use ginkgo with antidepressant MAO inhibitor drugs or nonsteroidal anti-inflammatory medications.

Helpful Hint

Be patient. Ginkgo takes time to build up in your body. Expect to wait 6 to 8 weeks before you notice any benefits. ■

rhea. Dr. Stengler recommends taking two capsules (500 milligrams total) twice a day for these conditions.

If taken with caffeine, American and Asian ginsengs may cause irritability. Also, don't use either type of ginseng if you have high blood pressure.

Siberian ginseng *(Eleutherococcus senticosus)*: Valued by natural medicine experts for its versatility, Siberian ginseng is often recommended for people new to using herbal medicines. Less expensive and a bit weaker than the other ginsengs, Siberian is easily tolerated by most people and seems to help guard against physical and mental stress. The most common form of ginseng sold in the United States, it's grown here, not in Siberia. Dr. Stengler recommends taking one capsule (250 milligrams) or 30 drops of tincture two or three times daily.

Helpful Hints

All three types of ginseng are believed to support the adrenal glands (which secrete hormones needed to cope with stress) and improve energy levels. **So any one of them can help when you're worn out,** exhausted, or stressed. But they're best used as preventive medicine, says Dr. Stengler.

Most ginseng products vary in concentration and potency, so read label instructions carefully. For Siberian ginseng, select a standardized extract product containing 0.3 to 0.8 percent eleutherosides for highest quality. For the other type of ginsengs, look for products specifying that they contain ginsenosides.

Finally, **be patient.** Ginseng must be taken daily over several weeks in order to have a beneficial effect. ■

Grapes

Enjoy the Health Benefits of Wine without the Alcohol

Red wine is extolled for its ability to protect your heart. Researchers credit flavonoids, special compounds found in wine, with preventing artery-clogging platelets from sticking to your blood vessels—sort of a Teflon coating for your blood vessels. Flavonoids have strong antioxidant properties and appear to neutralize cell-damaging free radicals, a by-product of metabolism, which may protect against chronic illnesses like heart disease and some forms of cancer.

But drinking wine isn't the only way to reap these benefits. Next time you're shopping, just pick up a bottle of grape juice or a bunch of grapes.

"Fresh grapes are the original source of the beneficial compounds associated with grape products, including wine," says Courtney Romano, R.D., a registered dietitian in Kirkland, Washington, and nutrition consultant for the California Table Grape Commission.

Each tiny grape may hold more than 1,000 different flavonoids. Research into grape compounds is fairly new, but one study found that drinking Concord grape juice reduced platelet activity as much as 50 percent in men and women, which should decrease the incidence of dangerous blood clots that can lead to heart attack or stroke. Another study found that purple grape juice helps arteries respond to increased bloodflow, slowing the processes that help LDL, a cholesterol component that contributes to the buildup of fatty plaque in arteries.

Research also suggests that some flavonoids in grapes may lower your risk of breast and other cancers.

Some of the protective substances in grapes are concentrated in the skin, stems, and seeds. So you will get more of these from red wine, purple and red grapes, and juice than white grapes or juice.

"It makes sense to include daily consumption of purple or red grape juice as part of a diet high in fruits and vegetables and low in saturated fat," says John Folts, Ph.D., at the Coronary Thrombosis Research and Prevention Laboratory at the University of Wisconsin Medical School in Madison.

Here are some ways to work more grapes into your daily diet, even if you don't (or can't) drink wine.

- Reach for grape juice instead of soda.
- Make an alcohol-free spritzer with grape juice, seltzer water, and ice.
- Buy alcohol-free red or blush wine.
- Make a quick parfait of grapes and fat-free vanilla-flavored yogurt.
- Serve grapes Mediterranean style—as an after-dinner dessert with a sliver or two of goat cheese.
- Add grapes to tuna, chicken, or Caesar salad.
- Next time you crave something sweet, reach for grapes instead of a candy bar. Or try them frozen. ■

Green Tea

Cancer Prevention in a Bag

According to Chinese folklore, Emperor Sh'eng Nung discovered green tea accidentally. Sometime around 2737 B.C., the emperor was relaxing under a tree while nearby, a small cauldron of water boiled over an open fire. A gentle breeze blew a few leaves into the boiling water. Intrigued by its aroma, the emperor poured himself a cup, took a sip, and smiled.

Green tea is made from unfermented leaves of the tea plant, Camellia sinensis. *During harvesting, the leaves are handled gently and heated. It tastes a lot like black tea, but somewhat milder and less bitter.*

Green tea is consumed by one-fifth of all tea drinkers in the world (including many in China). It's also the national beverage in Japan. This tea is proving to be worth the sip. Not only does a cup of green tea contain half the caffeine of coffee, but drinking 1 to 2 cups a day may reduce your risk for cancer.

"No one knows exactly how the ingredients in green tea may protect against cancer," says Douglas Schar, DipPhyt., MCPP, a practicing medical herbalist in London. "We do know that cultures that drink green tea have much lower incidents of cancer."

HOW TO BREW A PERFECT CUP OF GREEN TEA

To maximize the medicinal benefits of green tea, bring water to a boil, then pour it over a tea bag in a cup. Let it stand for about 3 minutes, no longer. As tea sits, compounds called tannins become more concentrated and make the tea taste more bitter. (Eighty percent of antioxidants in green tea are released within 5 minutes of brewing, according to a USDA/Tufts University study. Letting tea sit any longer is marginally beneficial.)

Don't add milk to the tea. Milk proteins neutralize the antioxidants in tea. (Honey is okay.)

Scientists believe that green tea may get some cancer-fighting punch from antioxidant polyphenols called catechins. Inside the body, catechins not only lower harmful LDL cholesterol levels but also act like a sheriff's posse when it comes to free radicals. They round up free radicals (unstable molecules that can damage cells), which when left alone, contribute to cancer cell growth.

Researchers at the University of Kansas found that catechins were 100 times more effective than vitamin C and 25 times stronger than vitamin E in blocking the cell mutations that cause cancer. In Japan, a survey of 472 women with breast cancer found that women who drank green tea before they were diagnosed were less likely to have their cancer spread to their lymph nodes. The cancer was also less likely to return. In Shanghai, China, men and women who drank green tea had lower risks of stomach cancer than non–green tea drinkers.

One cup of brewed green tea provides the same ››

amount of antioxidants as one to two servings of vegetables. It also contains 1.6 times more of these cancer-protection antioxidant chemicals than an 8-ounce glass of orange juice, says Ronald Prior, D.Ph., Ph.D., research scientist for the USDA's Human Nutrition Center on Aging at Tufts University in Boston. So if you can't always manage to eat the 5 daily servings of fruits and vegetables recommended by experts for cancer protection, drinking green tea can help fill in the gap. Keep some bags of green tea handy at work and on the road. ■

Grief

Emotional Pain Relievers for Women

Dealing with the loss of a loved one is never easy, but some experts say it can be especially difficult for women.

"Women often have an especially hard time working though grief because they are so focused on supporting others that they put their own needs and feelings aside," says James Campbell, Ph.D., professor of philosophy at Rochester Institute of Technology in New York. "But grieving is good—and necessary."

"The most important thing you can do to cope with grief is to embrace it, not resist it," says Dr. Campbell. "By allowing grief to go on, it resolves itself."

Grieving is painful. Experts offer these strategies to help you work through grief constructively.

Surround yourself with people to support you, but know that oftentimes, family members are not the best people to do this. Your family may be so close to you that it pains them too much to see you suffer, says Dr. Campbell. Consequently, they unconsciously send you messages that they want you to stop, when what you need to do is continue grieving. A friend who is slightly removed from the loss may be a greater support.

Communicate with the deceased, in your own way, to help resolve some of your feelings. If you've lost your husband or another loved one, write him an honest letter telling him how you feel without him—even if that means writing an angry letter expressing your sense of betrayal that he left you. Or, go to his burial site and talk to him or bring him something that he used to enjoy. "One woman I counseled used to visit her son's grave and pour cans of Coca-Cola onto the ground while she talked to him. It was always his favorite beverage, and it made her feel close to him to give it to him," says Dr. Campbell.

Be prepared to go back into the grieving state from time to time, especially on holidays or anniversaries. Just don't run away from the memory of the deceased, says

Dr. Campbell. You will miss him especially during these times, so make him part of the holiday by talking about him with others, sharing favorite stories, or looking at photos. You may want to light a candle for the deceased and keep it present as a way of having him there.

Do kind deeds for others, like working in a soup kitchen. It will help distract you in a positive way, says Dr. Campbell. "By doing something kind for other people, you will feel that you are helping ease someone else's pain, which can also help ease your own."

Affirm life. Go for walks, go to movies, enjoy your favorite foods and hobbies. Continue to eat right and exercise, care for yourself, and be attentive to yourself, says Christina M. Puchalski, M.D., assistant professor of medicine at the Center to Improve Care of the Dying at George Washington University Medical Center in Washington, D.C., and director of education at the National Institute for Healthcare Research.

COPING WITH THE LOSS OF A PET

Pets are part of the family. So it's only natural that when you lose a pet, it can hurt just as much as if you lost a human companion. "It's important not to minimize this pain," says Susan Phillips Cohen, a doctor of social work and director of counseling at the Animal Medical Center in New York City. "Allow yourself to grieve the loss of a pet just as you would the loss of a family member or good friend."

Dr. Cohen suggests the following tactics for recovering from the loss of a pet.

Hold a small memorial service for your pet. Invite friends and family if you like, and visit the pet's grave or spread his ashes while reading poetry or sharing memories.

Make something that will help you remember your pet. Needlepoint or paint a picture of him, frame your favorite photo of him and drape his collar over the corner of it, plant a tree, write a poem, or keep a journal of your reflections about him.

Talk about it. Don't feel silly or self-conscious about sitting down with a friend and discussing how the loss has affected you.

Join a pet loss support group. There, you can work through your feelings of loss in an understanding environment. Ask your vet about groups in your area.

Listen to your heart when considering replacing your pet. For some, a new pet helps their healing process, especially if the pet was a very large part of their daily routine.

Lavish attention on your other pets, if you have them. "There is no doubt that animals grieve when their companions are gone," says Dr. Cohen. Your remaining pets will need comforting, and spending time with them can help you to heal as well.

Practice your faith. "Men and women who have a spiritual belief tend to cope better with grief," says Dr. Puchalski.

Do something to memorialize your loved one, whatever that may mean to you. Plant a tree as a ›› remembrance, write a poem, paint a picture, or keep a journal of your feelings and memories of the deceased, says Dr. Puchalski.

Meditate or practice yoga. These relaxation methods have extremely calming effects and can help you feel emotionally and spiritually in touch with the person you've lost.

Grieving takes a very long time. Don't rush back to work or to all of your regular daily activities before you are ready, says Dr. Campbell. If you don't seem to be moving through the grief, however, you should see a counselor. If you aren't sure, you might consider asking a trusted friend if it seems to them that you are having an especially difficult time coping.

Helpful Hint

Joining an activist group related to the loss of your loved one, such as a cancer society or anti-drunk-driving group, will help you grieve by creating some good from your loss, says Dr. Campbell. ■

H

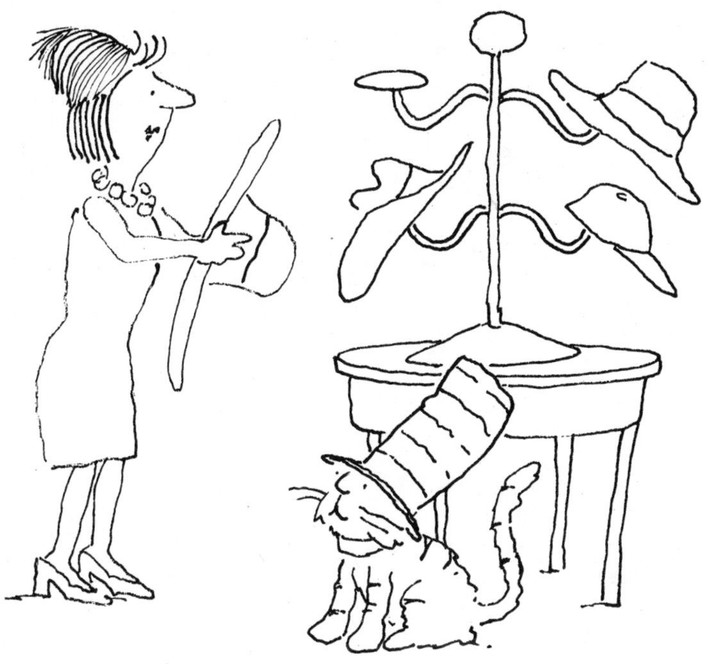

No one ever died of "hat hair."
But choosing the right hat can prevent unflattering dents and static. See page 194.

Hair Straighteners

A Natural Alternative to Chemical Relaxers

While millions of women regularly get perms to curl their naturally straight locks, others long to smooth out naturally curly or kinky hair. But unless you're careful, chemical straighteners (also called hair relaxers) can leave your hair thin, brittle, or dull.

"Trying to straighten hair that's naturally curly or kinky is complicated—and potentially dangerous," says Pamela Ferrell, co-owner of Cornrows & Co. Salon in Washington, D.C. She compares it to overcooking pasta.

"If you cook pasta too long, it will turn to mush, and there is nothing you can do to get it back," says Ferrell, who has styled the hair of singer Diana Ross, among other African American women who've come to her to have their hair naturally styled. "It's the same thing with relaxing the hair: Overdo it, and you permanently damage the hair."

Ferrell's advice: Avoid relaxers. Some contain sodium hydroxide (a caustic soda lye) or ammonium thioglycolate, both of which can dissolve the hair if left on too long.

Instead, use a blow-dryer with a comb attachment every time you shampoo your hair. "This will straighten your hair just as much as a relaxer, without the damage," says Ferrell. Here's how.

- After shampooing, comb your hair into 6 to 15 sections, depending on how thick and long it is.
- Pin the sections in loose twists on top of your head.
- Then, starting at the nape, untwist one section at a time, stretch the ends outward, blow-drying the ends first and then the hair close to the scalp. Angle the blow-dryer away from your scalp to avoid burning.

Helpful Hint

Use a conditioning or moisturizing shampoo. "Kinky, textured hair needs a shampoo that cleans your hair but does not strip it of its oils," says Ferrell. ■

DON'T MAKE THESE MISTAKES

- If styling techniques don't achieve the effect you want and you decide to try a chemical relaxer anyway, **leave it on for no more than 5 minutes.** Use it no more than three times a year. Apply it only to new-growth hair and never to hair that has been previously relaxed.
- Many women tend to avoid frequent shampooing to preserve their hair style. But it is important to **shampoo at least once a week in the winter and twice a week in the summer.** Otherwise, unhealthy bacterial agents may develop and lead to hair and scalp problems.
- If your hair has become overprocessed from chemical relaxers, **wait for an inch of new growth, then cut it short to the new growth.** Or braid it, which will allow your hair to rest without too much combing, which might cause the processed hair to break.

Hand Washing

Tune Up and Turn On the Water

What's the single most important action you can take to protect your health?

Wash your hands often, especially after using the bathroom and before handling food or beverages.

A rushed restroom rinse after leaving the toilet stall doesn't come close to getting rid of bacteria that can make you sick or spread infections to others, says Don Beckstead, M.D., associate program director of Allegheny Family Physicians in Altoona, Pennsylvania. "Most people don't wash their hands long enough or thoroughly enough," he says.

To be sure you're washing thoroughly, experts at the International Food Safety Council suggest you sing "Happy Birthday" twice while soaping up. It should take about 20 seconds—long enough to kill most germs.

Use a nickel-size dollop of soap, says Dr. Beckstead. Then wash from your fingernails to your

Hangovers

No Guaranteed Cures for Morning-After Misery

As former bartender and shift manager at Pat O'Brien's pub in New Orleans, Lisa Lovelace has heard—even tried—outlandish remedies to cure a hangover. The Bourbon Street bar attracts Mardi Gras celebrants seeking the bar's world-famous Hurricane drink, a 24-ounce sweet but potent beverage packed with 4 ounces of rum.

She's been in the booze business long enough to know that an instant hangover cure does not exist. Doctors agree.

"The only 100 percent guaranteed cure for hangovers is to not drink in excess," says Joel Meshulam, M.D., an internist and hangover treatment expert at Mercy Medical Center in Baltimore. Alcohol acts as a toxin to your liver, nervous system, and kidneys, and in excess, leaves you with a hammering headache, a nauseated stomach, and a mouth so dry that your tongue feels like a dead mouse.

Don't buy into the "hair of the dog" myth. Greeting the morning with a Bloody Mary—or another drink—may appear to mask your misery for the time being. But it only adds more alcohol to your system. Your body needs time—and lots of water—to help those symptoms subside.

"If someone ever did market a hangover capsule, it would have to be mighty big and full of water, because that's what really helps rehydrate your body after a night of drinking alcohol," says Dr. Meshulam.

If you drink but want to skip the hangover, Dr. Meshulam offers these do's and don'ts.

Stick with one kind of drink,

wrists in comfortably hot running water, rubbing vigorously.

"Pay special attention to these much-forgotten places: between fingers (including the webbing) and under and around fingernails," says Dr. Beckstead. "If you don't want to remove your rings, slide them up a little, wash, then slide them back down." Rinse thoroughly.

If you're in a public restroom, grab a paper towel before you wash your hands so that you don't have to touch the towel dispenser after you've washed, says Dr. Beckstead. Also, use a paper towel to turn off the faucet. Dry your hands thoroughly—moisture breeds germs. Then use a new paper towel to open the door of the bathroom when you're ready to exit.

Helpful Hint

Carry a trial-size bottle of an instant hand sanitizer, such as Purell or Suave, to use when there are no hand-washing facilities after using a portable toilet or before handling food. Rub a dollop into your hands for about 15 seconds. It will kill 99.9 percent of germs—without water or towels. ■

and have only two. Beer is safer than wine, rum, or whiskey—a 12-ounce glass of beer typically contains 5 percent alcohol, compared with a 5-ounce glass of wine (12 percent alcohol) or a shot (1½ ounces) of rum or whiskey (40 percent alcohol).

Alternate a full glass of water with every alcoholic drink. You'll reduce your alcohol intake while replenishing your body of needed fluids.

Drink an alcohol-free nightcap. Dr. Meshulam suggests a sports drink such as Gatorade or All Sport that contains potassium and other minerals your body loses when your kidneys are working overtime. And it wouldn't hurt to take a B-complex vitamin, including thiamin, at bedtime, says Dr. Meshulam, to replace B vitamins depleted by alcohol.

If you overdo it anyway and feel sick, don't fight the urge to vomit. It's the fastest way to rid the body of unwanted toxins.

Helpful Hint

Select vodka or sake over bourbon, rum, or cognac. While the evidence is only anecdotal, clear distilled beverages like vodka and sake don't contain toxic impurities called congeners commonly found in other, dark forms of alcohol like bourbon, rum, or cognac, and are considered less vicious. ■

DON'T MAKE THIS MISTAKE

Never take over-the-counter medications containing acetaminophen (the key ingredient in Tylenol) for a pounding hangover headache. Heavy alcohol combined with acetaminophen can cause serious liver damage, according to one study. Also, aspirin or ibuprofen combined with alcohol and taken to relieve discomfort can cause internal bleeding in someone with gastritis, says Clarita E. Herrara, M.D., clinical instructor in primary care at the New York Medical College in Valhalla.

Hat Hair

Keep Your Head Warm, Dry—And Looking Good

"Wear a hat." It's standard advice for avoiding hypothermia, frostbitten ears, and sunburn. Problem is, when you return indoors and take off your hat, you have a serious case of hat hair—packed flat against your head, out of control with static, comically indented, or all three.

When your hair is constricted under a hat, your scalp gives off body heat, generating moisture, which reactivates whatever styling products may be in your hair, causing your hair to reshape itself, says New York City hair stylist Aidan Harty.

"If you're a model on a photo shoot and show up with hat hair, a photographer may just cut off whatever sticks up or put on Static Guard to keep it down," says Harty. For the rest of us, he and hairstylist Carlo Cantavero of Greenwich, Connecticut, offer more reasonable solutions.

Avoid knit and wool hats. They form a vacuum that grabs the hair and leaves it looking helter-skelter. Choose fabrics such as corduroy or felt, possibly with ear flaps for extra warmth. Or opt for ear muffs. (But remember, they won't keep body heat from escaping through the top of your head.)

Wrap your head in a silk scarf. If warmth isn't an issue and you're just trying to keep your hair tidy in the wind, go for a scarf. Scarves exert less pressure than hats and keep hair from tangling.

Hay Fever

Relief without Medicine—Or Drowsiness

Wouldn't it be great to go through spring and fall without the sneezy, drippy, stuffy, puffy, and tired feeling brought on by hay fever? Wouldn't it be even better to do it without resorting to medications that can make you feel even lousier and drowsier?

Natural remedies offer an effective alternative. In fact, medications treat only the symptoms, but alternative methods can stop the underlying problem, says David Edelberg, M.D., assistant professor of medicine at Rush Medical College, section chief of holistic medicine at Illinois Masonic Medical Center and Grant Hospital, all in Chicago, and founder of the American WholeHealth Centers in Chicago, Boston, Denver, and Bethesda, Maryland.

He recommends this daily hay fever–season ritual to keep you clear of symptoms.

Drink 3 cups of elderflower tea. Elderflower is an herb that helps control inflammation of nasal passages. You'll find elderflower tea bags in health food stores.

Rub 3 to 4 drops each of Roman chamomile and lavender essential oils into 1 ounce of vegetable oil and massage it onto your back and chest. These oils work like an anti-inflammatory to reduce swelling and dry up your runny nose.

Wear a straw hat. A straw hat has enough ventilation to allow air in, which will keep your scalp from perspiring in warm weather. It also leaves extra room so your hair doesn't get compressed at the crown.

If you have long hair, just give your hair a good brushing. In most cases, that will make it go back to its original shape.

Pull your hair back in a ponytail. "It keeps everything neat and in one spot," says Harty. Then, when you take off your hat, take down your ponytail, too. You'll still have volume, and your hair won't have moved all over the place. If it's still unsightly, brush it back and put it in a scrunchie or bun.

If your hair is short, brush it back, put it behind your ears, and spray it into place.

GO LIGHTLY ON SPRAYS AND GELS

Women often put more spray and gel in their hair in winter, hoping that it will help keep the shape of the hair under the weight of a hat. But the more substances you put on your hair, the more likely you are to get an extreme case of hat hair because all those chemicals will become reactivated under the hat.

Helpful Hints

Use a conditioner after you shampoo. Hats tend to cause static, an electrical charge that makes hair fly up, up, and away. Moisturizing conditioners will help keep it calm. And always have hair spray in your purse for when you take off your hat. ■

Take 250 milligrams of stinging nettle three times a day. Studies show that this herb provides substantial relief from all hay fever symptoms. In some women with allergies, however, stinging nettle can actually make symptoms worse. If you notice problems, take only one dose a day, or stop taking it.

These herbs can be used with conventional medication, says Dr. Edelberg. Of course, if you're already taking prescription medication, Dr. Edelberg says you should not discontinue use without getting your doctor's okay.

Helpful Hints

If you are very clogged, place a few drops of eucalyptus or pine essential oil in boiling water and inhale the steam. Be careful not to get too close, as you don't want to burn your face. It'll help open up clogged nasal passages, which will relieve any sinus pressure.

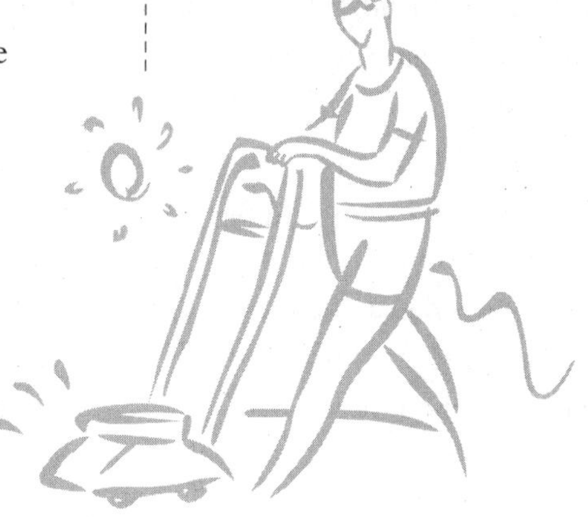

If you are mildly congested, just put a few drops into a relaxing bath. You can also put a few drops into a handkerchief and inhale as needed. ■

Headaches

Block Rebound Pain and Save Your Kidneys

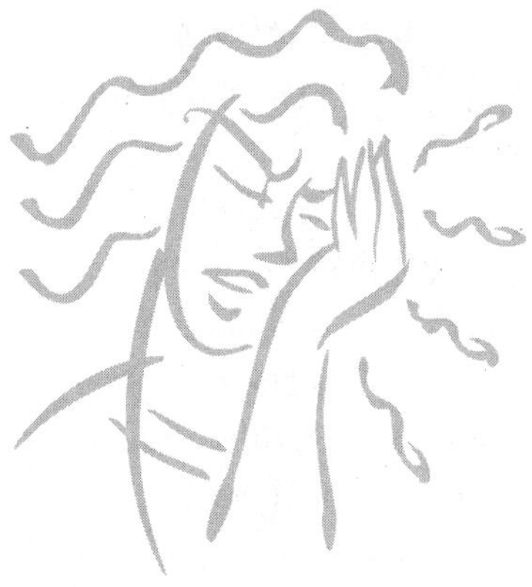

The head pounding begins. An aspirin tames the throb, but a few hours later, the headache returns. Your first instinct might be to reach for aspirin again, but you may be unwittingly setting yourself up for an endless cycle of headaches.

Aspirin and other over-the-counter analgesics work by shrinking the blood vessels around your brain, easing the pain and pressure of tension headaches. But if you use these painkillers again and again, you may be exposing yourself to "rebound" headaches. After your painkiller wears off, the blood vessels can expand again, causing the pain to return and triggering the need to take even more over-the-counter pain medications.

"Headaches become more frequent and come back as soon as the pain reliever wears off. Eventually, the pain reliever no longer works," says Kevin Sherin, M.D., clinical associate professor in family medicine at the University of Illinois in Chicago.

The next time a headache strikes, follow these natural remedies from Dr. Sherin. They should provide relief within 10 to 20 minutes—and with no rebound effect. If your headache is severe and remains unrelieved for 24 hours, see your doctor.

Take matters into your own hands. Gently massage your temples and forehead by making small circles with your fingertips. Press against the tense area and rub with a circular motion. Do this for a few minutes, or until you sense your headache subsiding. You can also massage the back of your neck, at the base of your skull.

Try a neck stretch. Relax tense muscles by first placing your right palm against the right side of your head and slowly and gently pressing so that your head tilts toward your left shoulder. Pause and hold for 10 to 20 seconds. Then return your head to a forward-facing position. Repeat the same steps, using your left hand against the left side of your head. Repeat the right and left movements until the pain subsides.

Dab on peppermint oil. Fend off head pain by mixing a few drops of peppermint oil with a few drops of vegetable oil. Then gently massage the blend on your forehead and both temples. The menthol in peppermint oil acts as a natural analgesic, stimulating then relaxing the nerves causing the headache.

Lay on the lavender. Place 5 drops of lavender essential oil in a bowl containing 1 cup of cold water. Swish a washcloth in the bowl and wring it out. Then lie down and close your eyes in a quiet room. Place the washcloth over your forehead and eyes to subside the pain. Allow about 20 minutes for the full effect. Lavender relaxes you and calms your nerves.

Go for hot and cold. Soak in a hot tub while placing an ice pack on your head. The cold ice shrinks blood vessels pressing on nerve endings in your head. The warm bath helps your muscles to relax.

Bag the pain. Contracted muscles at the base of the skull often cause tension headaches. Put a bag of ice on these muscles at the back of the neck. It may hurt a bit at first, but the cold will work to reduce the size of the aching blood vessels. ■

SAVE YOUR KIDNEYS

Rebound headaches aren't the only reason to use over-the-counter painkillers sparingly. Over time and in large doses, these analgesic medications can damage your liver and kidneys or cause bleeding in your digestive tract, says Dr. Sherin. Anyone with known kidney disease should avoid taking over-the-counter painkillers daily, even at standard doses.

Hearing Loss and Tinnitus

Tips for Rock-and-Roll Fans (and Everyone Else)

No matter how fond you are of the hair on your head, it's probably not as important to your well-being as the hair you have in *your head. You can't shampoo, condition, brush, or style these hairs, found deep in your inner ears, but you should treat them with care.*

These microscopic hairs, which live on cells in your inner ear, vibrate when sound waves enter your ears, creating electrical signals that your brain can understand as music, voices, and other sounds.

Noises that are too loud can bend or break the hairs, causing the cells to "leak" random electrical impulses to your brain as noise. This noise produces degrees of hearing loss or a ringing in the ears, a condition known as tinnitus. The damage accumulates over your lifetime and eventually can ruin your hearing. Talk about your bad hair days!

As a rule of thumb, prolonged exposure to any noise louder than 65 to 70 decibels—about as loud as a typical conversation—can damage your ears. **Anything louder than, say, the sound of a lawn mower, at 85 decibels, forces you to shout and can damage your hearing,** says Marshall Chasin, an ››

DON'T MAKE THIS MISTAKE

If you have tinnitus, try to avoid loud noises, aspirin, caffeine, and excessive alcohol. They can all make the ringing louder.

audiologist with the Musicians Clinics of Canada in Toronto.

Even if you sat next to the amplifier at too many Duran Duran concerts way back in the early 1980s, you can still take steps to prevent further harm to your hearing.

Say hmmm to loud noises. If you know you're about to hear a quick, loud noise that you can't avoid, hum to yourself throughout it, Chasin says. Humming activates a tiny muscle in your middle ear, which helps protect you from the noise for about 10 seconds at a time, he says. Drummers sometimes do this as they crash cymbals.

Let your ears rest. You should give your ears about 16 hours of relative quiet after each cacophony that you endure so they can recuperate, Chasin says. If you vacuum the rugs in the morning, for example, don't mow the lawn in the afternoon (or better yet, find someone else to do it for you.)

Muffle your ears. Jack Vernon, D.Ph., Ph.D., professor emeritus of otolaryngology at Oregon Health Sciences University in Portland and a founder of the country's first tinnitus clinic, advises his patients to don ear protection before firing up the vacuum cleaner or using other noisy equipment. Look for either foam-filled safety ear muffs that cover the entire ear to form an air seal or earplugs made of silicone or other material designed to reduce noise by as much as 15 to 30 decibels.

In his woodworking shop, Dr. Vernon has a pair of ear muffs hanging from each power tool.

Leave the room after turning on the dishwasher or clothes washer and dryer.

Wear your hair down to there. When your hair hangs over your ears, it helps block out some noise, thereby giving your ears a little protection, Chasin says. ■

SOLUTIONS FOR TINNITUS

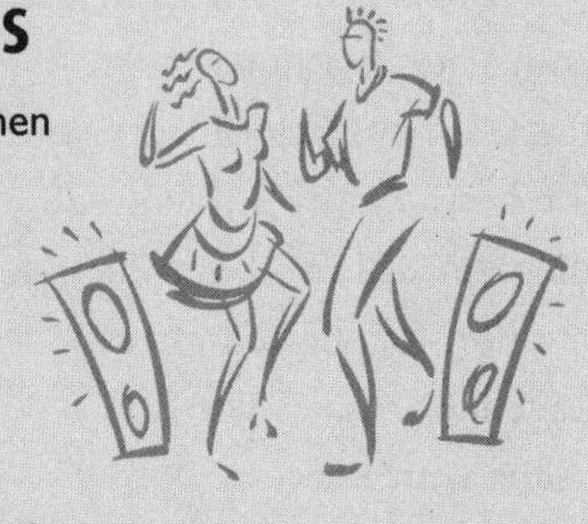

If you're one of the millions of women who experience tinnitus—a sometimes-maddening ringing in the ears that can be caused by too much loud noise—here's how to silence the sounds inside you.

Sleep soundly. You may find that your internal noise bothers you most at night, when your surroundings are quieter.

Steady background noise can cover it up. Run an electric fan in your room or tune a radio between stations for some low static (use FM radio, not AM, for a smoother level of static).

Mask it. If your tinnitus bothers you during the day, you can wear an adjustable device built into a hearing aid called a tinnitus masker that produces a low level of pleasant noise to mask your buzzing, says Dr. Vernon.

Retrain yourself. Ask your doctor about tinnitus retraining therapy, which involves wearing sound-producing devices in your ears for several hours a day, combined with counseling sessions, says Chasin. After a year or so, many people find that they can ignore their own tinnitus sounds without help.

Heartburn

Squelch Post-Meal Acidity with Sticky Herbs (Not Marshmallow Chicks)

The afterglow of a fine meal might include amiable conversation, a pleasant walk, and perhaps even a little romance—none of which is likely if you feel as though battery acid is sloshing around your upper chest and lower throat.

With post-meal heartburn, that's exactly what's going on—stomach acid, not battery acid, is sneaking up your esophagus. Recurrent heartburn—occurring once a week or more—can be a sign of gastroesophageal reflux, which has its own set of solutions (see page 177.) Occasional heartburn is more likely an aftereffect of eating too much or the wrong food (or both).

Antacids contain magnesium or aluminum compounds and usually provide temporary relief. In some people, they cause diarrhea. So you may need an alternative.

"Certain herbs are very good for countering acidity," says David Frawley, O.M.D., a doctor of Oriental medicine and director of the American Institute of Vedic Studies in Santa Fe, New Mexico. "As a bonus, they're good general tonics for women—they are nutritious and build energy reserves." Here's what to try.

Marshmallow. Herbs like marshmallow root are known as demulcents—they soften, cool, and protect your mucous membranes—just what you need when your esophagus is burning up with acid. Buy powdered marshmallow root at a health food store—it's easier than making a tea and works just as well. Just stir a teaspoon of the powder into a cup of water. It's a little gooey for an after-dinner libation, but that's what gives it its beneficial effect. Don't take it at the same time as any medication, as it may slow the absorption.

IN A PINCH, CHEW GUM

How about a stick of gum for dessert?

Chewing gum increases the flow of acid-neutralizing saliva (which is alkaline). It also stimulates your esophageal muscles to contract, helping keep the acid down. "If you have mild to moderate heartburn, chewing gum can tide you over," says Dr. Spechler. (If peppermint or spearmint makes your heartburn worse, try another flavor.)

Slippery elm. Yet another demulcent, slippery elm yields a gelatinous liquid when you stir a teaspoon of the powder into a cup of water. It doesn't taste any better than marshmallow, so you might want to add a little sugar. (With sticky herbs, sugar works better than honey, says Dr. Frawley.)

Marshmallow and slippery elm are all available in capsule form at health food stores. Not only are the capsules easier to take but they're also a better choice for those who find that any fluids sometimes make their heartburn worse. ››

Dill, fennel, or anise seeds. You can buy these at supermarkets and health food stores. Steep a tablespoon in 8 ounces of water. For heartburn, the trick is to drink 1 to 2 cups of this tea by the spoonful—one every few minutes—until your symptoms subside (but don't use fennel tea for more than 6 weeks).

Helpful Hint

If you don't have any other heartburn relief on hand, drink plenty of water for temporary relief, suggests Stuart Spechler, M.D., professor of internal medicine at the University of Texas Southwestern Medical Center in Dallas. It'll dilute the acid as well as wash it out of your esophagus. ■

DON'T MAKE THIS MISTAKE

Ginger or peppermint tea might make your heartburn worse. Skip it and use the recommended herbs instead.

Heart Disease

Double Your Protection with Vitamin E and Aspirin

Those humble little aspirins you thought were only good to dull your headaches are such valuable weapons against heart attacks that even some doctors are popping them daily. And when you team up aspirin with another common item on your shelf—vitamin E—you've got an anti–heart attack combo that's about as safe, cheap, and simple as it is effective.

Aspirin helps prevent heart attacks by discouraging blood cells known as platelets from sticking together. This is great for women, because heart attacks experienced by women are more likely caused by blood clots than by blocked arteries, which usually trigger heart attacks in men.

How much aspirin will your doctor recommend? It depends.

If you've been diagnosed with coronary heart disease but have not had a heart attack: You may reduce your chances of a heart attack by a third by taking aspirin regularly. "Women with coronary disease should be taking an aspirin every day," says Nanette Wenger, M.D., professor of medicine (cardiology) at Emory University School of Medicine and chief of cardiology at Grady Memorial Hospital in Atlanta.

If you've had a heart attack: Taking anywhere from

WHAT ELSE YOU SHOULD DO

Vitamin E and aspirin won't cancel out the harmful effects of a heart-hostile lifestyle. You still need to exercise, lose excess weight, limit your intake of saturated fat (found in meat, dairy products, and baked goods), control your blood pressure, lose excess pounds, control diabetes, not smoke, and learn smart ways to weather the effects of stress.

50 milligrams (a baby aspirin) to one adult aspirin (325 milligrams) daily may prevent another one.

If you're having a heart attack: Taking a 325-milligram adult aspirin right away may improve your survival chances by 25 percent. (If it's coated, chew it for more rapid results.) Yale researchers found that one reason top hospitals save more heart attack patients may be that they're more forthcoming with the aspirin.

If you don't have coronary heart disease, but do have risk factors such as diabetes or high cholesterol: Follow your doctor's recommendation. A woman without heart disease or multiple risk factors runs such a low risk of heart attack that it's not worth risking minor or unlikely complications of taking aspirin, like stomach irritation, bleeding or, rarely, hemorrhagic stroke.

HEART ATTACK PREVENTION IN A GLASS

If you're at risk for a heart attack, your doctor may prescribe daily aspirin and vitamin E supplements. If so, consider washing them down with tea. When researchers considered the coffee- and tea-drinking habits of several hundred men and women, regular tea drinkers had about half the heart attack risk of those not drinking tea. (Coffee consumption had no effect on the risk of heart attacks.)

The tea in question is black tea. It's rich in flavonoids, natural antioxidants that the researchers suspect may account for tea's apparent heart benefits.

Moderate tea drinking—1 to 2 cups a day—won't do you any harm and may do your heart a world of good, says Howard Sesso, Sc.D., the Harvard Medical School epidemiologist who led the study.

Vitamin E

While aspirin inhibits clotting, vitamin E appears to discourage cholesterol from oxydizing into its artery-clogging form. Vitamin E is a star-quality antioxidant that may reduce your chances of heart attack by 33 percent—or even as much as 77 percent if you've already experienced angina or other signs of heart disease. Combined with aspirin, your protection is virtually doubled.

Include foods rich in E in your diet. Consuming almonds, peanuts, olive oil, sunflower seeds, and wheat germ can help you get 100 IU a day, the minimum needed for protection, according to research.

Consider supplements. If you already have heart disease, you may need more vitamin E. Golden capsules of vitamin E can help you reach higher intakes—up to 800 IU, the amount needed to help prevent heart attacks. Discuss this with your doctor first, though: One study using low-dose supplements showed increased risk of hemorrhagic stroke. ■

Hemorrhoids

A Simple Remedy for Desk-Job Derriere

Thank the Greeks for hemorrhoids. The rectal trouble that your grandmother referred to as piles comes from *haimorroides*, the Greek word for "flowing with blood." When you have hemorrhoids, the veins around the anus become swollen, irritated, and inflamed, causing itching, pain, and rectal bleeding. Hemorrhoids can occur inside the anal canal or protrude outside the anal opening.

Prolonged sitting, constipation, and irritating foods like strong spices, coffee, and alcohol can all contribute to hemorrhoids. Anything you can do to avoid the basic causes will help. Standard advice includes eating plenty of fiber and drinking eight glasses of water daily (which you should do anyway). **Pregnant women are especially susceptible to hemorrhoids.**

Hepatitis C

Herbal Help for Liver Trouble from a Nurse Who Knows

Long Island nurse Gina Pollichino was receiving transfusions of a blood product to treat an immune disorder she'd had since birth. After getting a tainted dose, she came down with the hepatitis C virus.

This type of hepatitis is scary, because there is no sure cure, and at best, it will remain dormant for decades. As it lingers, it's hard on the liver, and it can lead to liver damage (cirrhosis) and liver cancer. The first symptoms often are similar to signs of flu, such as joint pain and fatigue. But by the time you start to feel symptoms, your liver may already be damaged. Some who get the virus will be able to beat it with medications such as interferon.

Pollichino is among a growing number of people who are coping with this illness. In the late 1980s and early 1990s, as AIDS news played out on televisions in living rooms across the country, hepatitis C was sneaking in through the basement window.

Hepatitis C is transmitted by contaminated blood or intravenous use of illegal drugs. So you should get checked for hepatitis C if you had a transfusion of blood or a blood product before 1992. You should also get checked if you've ever taken illegal drugs with a needle or snorted cocaine, even once long ago.

For Pollichino, an R.N., hepatitis C started off unusually fierce but has reverted to a more normal, smoldering level. She runs a local support group for others with hepatitis C for the American Liver Foundation. Here's some of the advice she offers, along with other expert tips.

Take it easy. You may tire more easily than normal, especially if you're on interferon.

If you already have hemorrhoids, relief can be as close as your nearest pharmacy, says Betzy Bancroft, a professional member of the American Herbalists Guild in Washington, New Jersey.

Pick up a bottle of witch hazel, a soothing yet astringent liquid that is extracted from the witch hazel shrub. "Witch hazel is a natural astringent that helps shrink and tighten swollen tissues and soothe inflamed, itchy areas," says Bancroft.

Apply witch hazel in whatever way you find most convenient:

- Soak cotton balls in witch hazel and **dab onto the inflamed area several times a day,** or whenever symptoms occur.
- Pour about a pint of witch hazel into a bathtub filled with a couple of inches of warm water and **soak for at least 15 minutes.**
- Instead of using dry toilet paper, which can be abrasive, **moisten toilet paper with witch hazel** before wiping after a bowel movement. ■

Learn to tackle only the important things you need to do and not feel guilty about the things you can't.

Get all the rest you can. Since insomnia is sometimes an effect of the disease, make time for a nap if you need one.

Pamper your liver. Among its other important chores, your liver disarms poisons and ushers them out of your body. As a result, you must give up alcohol and quit smoking, since these put an unnecessary strain on the organ. And eliminate painkillers with acetaminophen, which can be hard on the liver.

Try an herbal boost. Pollichino takes milk thistle, an herb that can help repair liver damage, according to published studies. A substance in the plant's seedlike fruit—silymarin—can both slow the damage and help your liver recover from it, says Varro Tyler, Sc.D., Ph.D., herbal expert; distinguished professor emeritus of pharmacognosy at Purdue University in West Lafayette, Indiana; and author of *Tyler's Honest Herbal.* Look for capsules, tablets, or soft gels containing 150 milligrams of milk-thistle extract standardized to contain 70 percent silymarin. Take one capsule three times a day.

According to herbalists, **other herbs that may help your liver include dandelion root and the Chinese plant schizandra.** Both are available in capsule form at many health food and herbal stores. The standardized capsule extract of dandelion root is 500 milligrams and should be taken twice a day. Schizandra is found in 100-milligram capsules standardized to contain 9 percent schizandris and should also be taken twice a day, according to David Edelberg, M.D., assistant professor of medicine at Rush Medical College, section chief of holistic medicine at Illinois Masonic Medical Center and Grant Hospital, all in Chicago, and founder of the American WholeHealth Centers in Chicago, Boston, Denver, and Bethesda, Maryland. "I also recommend a potent antioxidant called alpha lipoic acid, available in 100-milligram capsules, to be taken twice a day," says Dr. Edelberg.

Eat right and exercise. While exercise and proper nutrition are important for ›› everyone, they're especially vital for people with hepatitis C because they help fight fatigue, Pollichino says. So try to exercise several times a week, even if that means just going for a walk. And pay attention to what you eat—aim for regular meals and nutritious foods.

These lifestyle changes are your best defense. "More and more studies are emerging to show that when people with hepatitis C really take care of themselves by eating a healthy diet, taking appropriate supplements, reducing their stress, and eliminating alcohol, drugs, cigarette smoke, and foods with lots of additives and preservatives, they dramatically reduce their chances of developing cirrhosis of the liver and liver cancer," says Dr. Edelberg.

Helpful Hint

Join a hepatitis support group. You can pick up more hints for coping with the illness and share suggestions of your own, says Pollichino. To locate a group near you, contact the American Liver Foundation at 1-800-GO LIVER or write to them at 75 Maiden Lane, 6th floor, Suite 603, New York, NY 10038-4810. ■

Herbal Diet Aids

"Natural" Weight Loss Pills to Avoid

"Lose weight NATURALLY!"

"Boost your metabolism with HERBS!"

"Whittle your waist—WITHOUT EXERCISE!"

Herbal diet aids sound *like the perfect weight loss solution. Should you try them? Definitely not.*

"If there were a really good, safe, clinically proven herbal weight loss product out there, I'd be the first to recommend it," says Gail Mahady, R.Ph., Ph.D., a University of Illinois–Chicago pharmacognosist and registered pharmacist who has researched medicinal plants. "But that's not the case."

Too often, women assume that "natural" means "safe," especially when it comes to diet aids. Sometimes, herbal ingredients can be just as strong as their man-made counterparts, not milder. "The combination of ephedrine alkaloids (ephedrine, pseudoephedrine, methylephedrine, norephedrine, and norpseudoephedrine) you get in some herbal diet aids is just as potent as, if not more potent than, the single-ingredient over-the-counter decongestant products that contain synthetic pseudoephedrine or ephedrine," says Bill J. Gurley, Ph.D., a pharmaceutical scientist at the University of Arkansas for Medical Sciences in Little Rock.

Here, from potentially dangerous to simply ineffective, is a rundown on the herbs most often touted for their supposed weight loss properties.

Ma huang: Also known as *Ephedra sinica*, ma huang acts as a cardiac stimulant, raising your heart rate and blood pressure. It can also affect your central nervous system, making you anxious, nervous, and talkative. All this makes ephedra a risky proposition for women with heart problems, high blood pressure, diabetes, or an overactive thyroid. Women taking MAO inhibitor antidepressants should also avoid this herb.

Make no mistake about it: Ephedra works like a powerful

drug because it is a powerful drug; **more than 1,000 adverse events such as seizures and even deaths associated with the herb have been reported to the FDA.** You can easily take too much. What's more, drinking coffee or other caffeinated beverages while taking ephedra increases its stimulant effects. "Plus, the amount of botanical ephedrine found in ma huang supplements can "vary dramatically from bottle to bottle," Dr. Gurley says. "You really have no idea of how much of the active ingredient, ephedrine, you're taking."

Guarana: Derived from the seeds of a tropical plant, guarana (*Paullinia cupana*) supplies as much caffeine as coffee—and sometimes more. One 455-milligram capsule of guarana, for example, contains 100 milligrams of caffeine—about what you'd get in a cup of coffee. As with coffee, taking guarana speeds up your metabolism slightly. But **in large doses, it can also trigger anxiety, insomnia, stomach upset, and other side effects associated with drinking a lot of coffee.**

Guarana is often sold as part of herbal combinations containing ma huang, accentuating the harmful effects of that herb. Guarana contains exceptionally high concentrations of tannins, and long-term use may increase the likelihood of cancer. Experts warn that women who are sensitive to caffeine, who are prone to anxiety, who have high blood pressure, or who have heart disease should avoid guarana.

Senna: Often found in so-called diet teas, senna (either *Folium sennae* or *Fructus sennae*) is a stimulant laxative, which may explain its reputation for weight loss. But all you're losing is water, Dr. Mahady says. **"You'll lose it one day and gain it back the very next day."** Senna also can cause diarrhea, which can upset the balance of electrolytes and fluid in your body and lead to heart problems. And the herb can create rebound constipation, where your muscles are dependent on its laxative effects. So senna can be both ineffective *and* dangerous for weight loss.

St. John's wort: This herb (*Hypericum perforatum*) mimics the effect of some antidepressants by increasing the amount of serotonin in the brain and decreasing hunger, *theoretically* causing weight loss. In reality, says Dr. Mahady, "Antidepressants can actually cause weight gain, because when you feel better, you may be more likely to eat more. When you're depressed, you probably eat less."

Garcinia cambogia: At one time, well-respected herbalists thought this herb held great promise for dieters. But garcinia, also known as hydroxycitric acid, actually has little effect on weight loss, according to one study. **Men and women who took garcinia three times a day lost the same amount of weight (6 to 9 pounds) as others who ate the same diet but did not take garcinia.** Those results didn't surprise researcher Joseph R. Vasselli, Ph.D., a biopsychologist at the Obesity Research Center at St. Luke's-Roosevelt Hospital in New York City. Garcinia works by blocking fat synthesis in the liver, but fat synthesis occurs only if you get less than 10 percent of your daily calories from fat. "Anyone who can do that has no problem controlling their body fat," Dr. Vasselli says. Therefore, there's no need for garcinia. ■

Herbal Supplements

Herbs and Drugs That Don't Mix

In supermarkets and pharmacies everywhere, herbal supplements share shelf space with vitamins, minerals, laxatives, eyedrops, and other over-the-counter health products. It seems you can find herbs touted for just about every health problem known to women, from PMS and weight loss to depression and memory loss.

More and more research supports the benefits of herbal medicine—the key word being medicine. *So more women are turning to herbal supplements. But suppose you're already taking prescription medicine?*

Unless you're careful, mixing herbal medicine with prescription medicine can be dangerous, says Marie Mulligan, M.D., clinical researcher at Kaiser Permanente in Santa Rosa, California. Some herbs and drugs interact, making your prescription medicine more potent or less effective. And some herbs can make certain medical conditions worse. Experts warn about the following situations.

DON'T MAKE THIS MISTAKE

Don't take medicinal herbs if you are pregnant or nursing.

Surgery. Your doctor may advise you to avoid aspirin and ibuprofen for 2 weeks before surgery because they interfere with your blood's ability to clot and increase bleeding, says Dr. Mulligan. But supplements of garlic, ginkgo, and feverfew (among others) can also increase bleeding. (So can vitamin E.) Talk to your physician or anaesthesiologist about any supplements you're taking well in advance of surgery.

Hiccups

Five Cures You Never Heard Of

Throw a fit in the office, and you'll be labeled a troublemaker. But if your diaphragm throws a fit, you've got hiccups.

And if you're like most people, you've tried everything from holding your breath and gulping down water to burping or swallowing in mid hic—even putting sugar under your tongue. But to no avail.

Next time, skip the folk remedies. Here are six scientifically sound—but little known—cures that experts recommend for instant results.

1. With your index finger and thumb, firmly squeeze the sides of your nose where the bone ends and the cartilage begins. That's your gallbladder acupressure point. When you pinch that spot, you'll stimulate your digestive juices, which can stop those hiccups, says David J. Nickel, O.M.D., a doctor of Oriental medicine and licensed acupuncturist in Santa Monica, California.

2. Lift your uvula (that fleshy punching bag in the back of your throat) with the back of a cold spoon. This will stimulate nerve endings in your throat that will send signals to your diaphragm or other muscles involved in respiration

Blood thinners. Do not combine the blood thinner warfarin (Coumadin) with blood-thinning herbs like garlic and ginkgo. Like aspirin, they can make the warfarin more potent and increase the risk for bleeding, says Teresa Bailey Klepser, Pharm.D., assistant clinical professor in the department of family medicine at the University of Iowa, in Iowa City. For that matter, don't take ginkgo and aspirin together, either. "Some people who've done this have had internal organ bleeding and bleeding in the brain," says Dr. Klepser.

SEPARATE SOY AND THYROID MEDICATION

Mounting evidence suggests that soy (including supplements with isoflavones, the estrogen-like active ingredient in soy) may relieve discomfort associated with menopause. But when taken at the same time as thyroid hormones, soy may interfere with the absorption of the medication. "Separate them by 2 to 3 hours," says Dr. Mulligan. Foods that are high in isoflavones, including many soy products like tofu and soy milk, may also be a potential problem, especially foods that are high in soy protein, since it is associated with isoflavone content. Look for the words *isolated soy protein, soy protein isolate,* or *textured soy protein* on the labels.

Helpful Hint

Tell your physician and pharmacist about every herb and supplement that you're taking or considering. Otherwise, you may do more harm than good. And if you have an adverse reaction to an herb, stop taking it and alert your doctor. ■

and interrupt the hiccup cycle, says James H. Lewis, M.D., professor of medicine in the division of gastroenterology at Georgetown University Medical Center in Washington, D.C. This may make you gag, and in this circumstance, that is a good sign. Gagging may also interrupt and end the hiccup cycle, says Dr. Lewis.

3. Swallow a glob of peanut butter. This will also tantalize those nerve endings in your throat and may end the hiccup attack, says Dr. Lewis.

4. Stick an index finger in each ear and plug your nose with your pinkies. This is an ancient cure dating back hundreds of years. The theory is that you'll disrupt your normal respiration and break the cycle, says Dr. Lewis.

WHEN NOTHING HELPS

Hiccups usually last for only a couple of minutes. But don't ignore them if they last for more than 48 hours or recur for a month or more. Chronic hiccups may indicate that you have a more serious medical problem.

5. Press your pinky. Firmly squeeze the middle joint of your pinky finger while exhaling for 5 seconds. Let off the pressure while inhaling for 5 seconds, then exhale for 5 seconds while squeezing your pinky again. Repeat for about 2 minutes, or until your hiccups stop, says Dr. Nickel. ■

High Blood Pressure

Two-at-a-Time Nondrug Strategies

Thanks to estrogen, high blood pressure (or hypertension) hits women later in life than men. Not that protection from the female hormone is ironclad. Women can—and do—develop high blood pressure before estrogen production wanes at menopause.

If your blood pressure is normal, congratulations. If it's between 120/80 and 150/95, relax—literally. You can take advantage of some surprisingly simple ways to get the pressure down without medications.

"If you're borderline hypertensive, there's a lot you can do to either prevent the need for drugs or reduce the amount of drugs you have to take," says Thomas Pickering, M.D., Ph.D., cardiologist and professor of medicine at New York Hospital–Cornell Medical Center and author of Good News about High Blood Pressure.

For best results, try the following teams of pressure-reducing tips.

Eat more fish + less fat. In a study conducted in Australia, overweight men and women who ate 4 ounces of fish a day dropped 6 blood pressure points in 4 months. But those who ate fish *and* cut back on dietary fat got extra blood pressure–lowering benefits. For women who have elevated blood pressure, Dr. Pickering recommends three to seven fish meals a week—more than the usual twice-a-week directive.

Cook with garlic + basil. A cornerstone of Mediterranean cuisine, garlic has a documented blood pressure–lowering effect. Try to eat a clove or two each day. Fresh basil leaves also help keep blood pressure in check. Think pesto.

Load up on fiber + shun processed wheat. Dietary fiber has clear cardiovascular benefits. Processed wheat, on the other hand, creates an insulin surge, which triggers a rise in blood pressure for several hours. One study at Tulane University in New Orleans found that subjects with the highest blood insulin levels were three times more likely to have high blood pressure. So substitute fiber-rich unprocessed whole grain bread for that white bread.

Consume potassium + magnesium + calcium. All three minerals help keep your blood pressure down. Even better, choose food sources over capsules. "Getting these minerals in combination naturally from food has more of an effect than taking them indi-

QUIET, PLEASE, I'M TRYING TO LOWER MY BLOOD PRESSURE

Austrian researchers monitoring 118 workers spotted a consistent 4-point increase in blood pressure among men and women working in a noisy factory. Blood pressure inched upward even if the noise was incurred in short bursts. To counter the effect of noise on *your* blood pressure, avoid it wherever possible. Shut out lawn mower and traffic noises, wear ear protectors when working with loud machinery, and tone down the volume on your radio or CD player.

vidually as supplements," says Dr. Pickering. This could mean a difference of 3 to 4 points.

For potassium, eat four to five daily servings of fruits and vegetables, especially cantaloupe, baked potatoes, bananas, citrus fruits, and tomatoes. You'll find the highest amounts of magnesium in almonds and pumpkin seeds. Low-fat or fat-free dairy products like milk and yogurt provide ample calcium, but so do calcium-fortified orange juice, soy milk, and waffles.

Move it + lose it. A morning bout of 30 minutes of daily aerobic exercise will help lower your blood pressure for most of the day. Do it regularly, and the benefits will be permanent. Overweight? Losing weight in and of itself will lower your blood pressure. Better yet, the combination of losing weight and getting regular exercise can pare your pressure by 20 points.

Reduce stress + add quiet activity. Stress raises blood pressure, so eliminate what you can. For example, ask for more authority on the job; the resulting sense of control reduces stress. Insist on clarity about whom you report to; trying to please too many bosses is stressful. Then manage the stress that's left by using relaxation techniques. In one 3-month study, 20 minutes a day of meditation lowered study participants' blood pressure by 11 points. Others find success with breathing exercises, nature walks, or even watching tropical fish. ■

High Cholesterol

Five Foods That Lower Your Count

Like most women, you hear a lot about what not *to eat to lower cholesterol—namely, food from animal sources. Meat, dairy products, and lard are the main sources of saturated fats and the only sources of dietary cholesterol. Together, saturated fat and cholesterol raise levels of cholesterol in your blood, forming a waxy slug that chokes off your coronary arteries, jeopardizing your heart's ability to function well (or at all).*

But there's more to cholesterol control than avoiding high-fat foods. Researchers have unveiled five interesting (and delicious) cholesterol-lowering foods that can help you put a little offense in the defense of your heart. Every 1 percent reduction in total cholesterol reduces your risk of heart disease by 2 percent. So eating each of the following foods can make a big difference.

1. APPLES

What they do: One study done at the University of California, Davis, found that eating apples or drinking apple juice can reduce the oxidation (and hence the harm) of bad LDL cholesterol by as much as 38 percent.

Why they work: The good guys here might be phenols, the same plant-based antioxidants that make red wine one of the more pleasant heart-healthy beverages. (The difference is that you can knock back as much apple juice as you want and still drive your kids to soccer practice.) ››

2. WALNUTS

What they do: When researchers analyzed a walnut-producing region of France, they found that people who consumed the most walnuts and walnut oil had the highest levels of HDL cholesterol, a protective form of cholesterol that carries more harmful LDL cholesterol out of the body. That's especially important for women, who tend to have lower levels of HDL than men as they get older.

Why they work: The oil in walnuts consists overwhelmingly of polyunsaturated (63 percent) and monounsaturated (23 percent) fats, with very little of the harmful saturated fat. This could be protective, according to the French researchers.

3. BEANS

What they do: Open a big can of beans, season with herbs and spices, add chopped vegetables instead of lard or bacon, and eat a cup a day. Your cholesterol may drop as much as 10 percent in 6 weeks.

Why they work: Beans—any kind of beans—are fiber-rich and a good source of folate, a B vitamin that researchers from the Dutch Heart Foundation found helps lower cholesterol.

4. GARLIC

What it does: Some—but not all—studies show that

Hives

Remedies That Won't Put You to Sleep

Almost everything under the sun—including the sun—can cause those itchy, burning welts on your skin known as hives. You can get them from food, bug bites, medicines, cold water, an infection—you get the idea.

Regardless of the instigator, **the common denominator for any outbreak of hives is histamine,** a chemical your body releases when exposed to allergens. Histamine dilates blood vessels, among other reactions, and also triggers hives.

Your first instinct may be to take an antihistamine, such as Benadryl, says Dee Anna Glaser, M.D., associate professor of dermatology at St. Louis University School of Medicine. **In most cases, an antihistamine will bring you relief. But it can also make you really drowsy**—a major annoyance at anytime but bedtime. It can be dangerous if you need to drive, and counterproductive if you're trying to work.

Avoiding what triggers your hives whenever possible makes sense. Otherwise, David Edelberg, M.D., assistant professor of medicine at Rush Medical College, section chief of holistic medicine at Illinois Masonic Medical Center and Grant Hospital, all in Chicago, and founder of the American WholeHealth Centers in Chicago, Boston, Denver, and Bethesda, Maryland, recommends combining these natural remedies that won't put you to sleep.

taking daily garlic powder tablets standardized to 5 milligrams of the principal active ingredient allicin can lower your cholesterol levels by 11 percent. (Since garlic thins the blood, you shouldn't take garlic supplements if you're taking blood sugar control medication or anticoagulants or if you're facing surgery.)

Why it works: Since not all studies showed an improvement in cholesterol levels, no one is sure how it might work. But it will improve your overall blood circulation. So try a clove or two a day in food, recommends Irene Gavras, M.D., clinical professor of medicine at Boston University School of Medicine.

5. CHEERIOS

What they do: Researchers from the University of Minnesota Heart Prevention Clinic fed half their subjects cornflakes for 6 weeks and the others Cheerios, made from oats. Compared with cornflakes, the Cheerios gang showed a 3.8 percent cholesterol reduction.

Why they work: Soluble fiber is a proven cholesterol reducer, and oats are loaded with it. "Soluble fiber is good, whether it's in oatmeal or Cheerios," says Dr. Gavras. ■

DON'T MAKE THIS MISTAKE

If you have hives around your eyes or mouth or if you have trouble breathing, don't delay: Go to an emergency room immediately. You may be having a life-threatening allergic reaction.

• Take 1,000 milligrams of vitamin C three times a day. At this dose, vitamin C can work like an antihistamine. **Excess vitamin C may cause diarrhea in some people. If that happens, reduce your dosage.**

• Take 300 to 500 milligrams of quercetin three times a day. A natural anti-inflammatory sold at health food stores, quercetin is a bioflavonoid derived from plants and believed to help fight allergic reactions.

• Take 1,000 milligrams of fish oil in capsule form three times a day. Fish oil has anti-inflammatory properties that can help reduce hives.

• Supplement your diet with three 500-milligram doses a day of pantothenic acid, a B vitamin. Pantothenic acid will stimulate your adrenal gland into producing your own anti-inflammatory, called cortisol.

Helpful Hint

If you're prone to allergies and have had hives before, you may want to ask your doctor if you should carry an emergency kit that contains an epinephrine injection. Epinephrine is a hormone that instantly aborts a full-blown allergy attack in progress. ■

Holiday Stress

When "Good Enough" Is Great

For years, Nancy Loving Tubesing, Ed.D., went into what she calls pre-holiday psychosis just before Christmas.

Striving for a "perfect" holiday, she obsessed over every task—baking cookies, sending out cards, making handmade gifts for everyone, decorating the house, staging family get-togethers. It left her stressed and exhausted.

"Women have traditionally borne the responsibility for making holidays happen," says Dr. Tubesing, coauthor of Kicking Your Holiday Stress Habits.

Eventually, Dr. Tubesing realized that the holidays didn't have to make her as nutty as a fruitcake. An uncomplicated Christmas can be as joyous—maybe more so—as one that's top-heavy with elaborate plans and details.

Here's how to make your holidays less stressful and more joyous.

List all your holiday expectations. Include everything—gifts, food, entertaining, rituals. "Writing everything down gives you a baseline," says Dr. Tubesing. "And after seeing it all written down, you may even laugh at your unrealistic expectations."

Decide what's most meaningful to you. "For me, it's the candlelight service on Christmas Eve," says Dr. Tubesing. "Focus on your top three."

Eliminate what you find most stressful. If something leaves you anxious instead of joyful, cross it off. Dr. Tubesing no longer makes handmade gifts for everyone, for example.

Reassess your list every year. Families change with every wedding, divorce, birth, and death. Over the years, holiday needs change. Get out your list around Halloween and eliminate or replace former traditions, as needed.

Simplify. Just because you've always spent hours stringing popcorn and cranberries for the tree doesn't mean you have to continue if it's become a chore, for example. Reevaluate your Christmas card list. Include short personal compliments instead of an elaborate brag letter. Bake one kind of cookie—and only one kind—with someone who truly enjoys the ritual.

Spread out the joy. Instead of a huge feast and gift fest, consider seeing your family in small doses, or even holding family get-togethers after December. "This is especially helpful if the holidays are

DON'T MAKE THIS MISTAKE

"In the guise of taking responsibility and being a self-sacrificing provider, women often take control of the holidays and don't let anyone else in on the process," Dr. Tubesing says. "That's a danger." If your husband and kids feel excluded, let them do the next Christmas their way.

fraught with painful memories."

Reach out to others. Set aside chores to spend time with your kids. Patch up a relationship with an estranged friend. And don't forget the wider community. "Deny yourself a treat so somebody else can have a treat," Dr. Tubesing says. "Instead of having a big roast beef, turkey, or ham, eat a rice-and-vegetable stir-fry and use the savings to buy something wonderful for the food bank." ■

Hormone Replacement Therapy

Find the Mix That Works Best for You

You probably know that replacing estrogen and other hormones that dwindle after menopause can help alleviate the symptoms of menopause while protecting your heart and bones. The benefits are well-documented: Most women experience a major reduction in hot flashes within several weeks of beginning hormone replacement therapy (HRT), and many women stop having them altogether. Many women experience a decrease in blood supply to the genitals as well as decreased vaginal elasticity and bleeding, all of which lead to discomfort during sex. But HRT can reverse these effects and allow you to enjoy lovemaking once again.

Presumably due to the apparent protective effect of estrogen, women who use HRT experience fewer heart attacks or have a greater chance of surviving if they do have heart attacks. HRT prevents bone loss and reduces osteoporosis fractures. Estrogen also seems to protect your brain, possibly preventing the onset of Alzheimer's disease in older women.

Yet along with these potential benefits, HRT can cause problems for some women. Taken alone or for long periods of time, estrogen causes a buildup in the endometrial lining of the uterus, raising the risk of some cancers. Adding progestin (a synthetic form of progesterone) reduces this risk. Unfortunately, progestin can also trigger a constellation of PMS-like side effects, including headaches, spotting, and nausea, among others. (While some research suggests a small increase in the risk of breast cancer with HRT use, this has not been firmly established, as other research reports no such increase.)

You don't necessarily have to endure discomfort and inconvenience to benefit from HRT. Reducing your dose or changing the type of HRT or how you take it may help reduce side effects while still yielding long-term benefits.

"Gone are the days of one-size-fits-all hormone therapy, when all menopausal women received a standard dose of estrogen and progestin and either lived with the results or abandoned the therapy altogether," says Andrew M. Kaunitz, M.D., professor of obstetrics and gynecology at the University of Florida Health Science Center in Jacksonville and director of gynecology and menopause services at the University of Florida Medicus Diagnostic Center.

Today, hormone therapy uses various forms of estrogens (such as conjugated estrogen, estradiol, estropipate, or esterifide estrogen) and progestin (such as medroxyprogesterone acetate, norethindrone acetate, or ❯❯

micronized progesterone) in various doses. **"If you stopped taking HRT—or are worried about starting—because of side effects like headaches or spotting, don't assume it's not for you.** Unpleasant side effects can be reduced or, in most cases, eliminated," says Dr. Kaunitz.

To find the hormone mix that's best for you, talk to your doctor about tailoring therapy to your needs. Here are your options.

PILL, PATCH, OR CREAM?

The form in which you take HRT can be as important as the type and dosages that you take. The most common method of administering HRT is orally.

HRT is also available in a patch, which is ideal for women who find taking pills unpleasant, have problems absorbing the oral medication, or have high triglyceride levels.

Applied topically inside the vagina, hormone cream works especially well for women who experience sexual discomfort after menopause and tolerate neither pills or the patch. Topical treatments are so low-dose that progestin may not be necessary. But they don't treat hot flashes or protect your bones the way a pill or patch does.

Hot Flashes and Night Sweats

Sleep through a Heat Wave

It's one thing to feel a hot flash spread from your chest to your neck and your head, leaving you sweaty and flushed midday. After your first few hot flashes, you know it'll pass. Hot flashes are uncomfortable, inconvenient, and sometimes embarrassing, but like other women approaching menopause, you can deal with them.

Nocturnal flashes—night sweats—are a different story. Waking up in a pool of perspiration disrupts your sleep. So does getting up from a deep sleep to change your soaking-wet nightclothes and sheets.

"Night sweats, hot flashes, and the chills that sometimes follow are nothing to worry about and last 9 to 16 months, on the average," says Lila A. Wallis, M.D., professor of medicine at Weill Medical College at Cornell University in New York City and past president of the American Medical Women's Association. It's believed that the drop in the production of the female hormone estrogen and other hormonal changes interfere with the way the body regulates heat.

Okay, so nightly heat waves are harmless and temporary. That's no consolation if you can't get the rest you need.

Dr. Wallis, a pioneer in women's health care, offers these simple strategies to help you sleep through your next night sweat (or get back to sleep in a wink).

Sleep on all-cotton sheets and pillowcases. Cotton is a breathable fabric that wicks moisture away from the skin. Avoid flannel, satin, or cotton/polyester blends—they'll leave you feeling hot and clammy.

Continuous combined. Estrogen is taken every day along with a low dosage of progestin every day. The constant dose of progestin (which signals the uterus to shed its lining) means that you may experience erratic bleeding or spotting, with no pattern or regularity. For some women, this eventually stops.

Sequential/cyclical. Estrogen is taken every day and progestin is taken on a cyclical schedule so that bleeding occurs on a regular, predictable schedule, as if you're having a period.

Quarterly progestin. Another option is to take estrogen every day and progestin every 3 months, or quarterly throughout the year. You'll have just four periods per year.

Low-dose estrogen. Taken in a very low dose with no progestin at all, estrogen produces none of progestin's PMS-like symptoms, and the dose of estrogen is low enough that there appears to be no increased risk of endometrial cancer. However, cautions Dr. Kaunitz, "regular endometrial sampling may be appropriate for menopausal women who still have their uterus and are taking low-dose estrogen alone." ■

Keep a light cotton quilt at the foot of your bed. Pull it over you if you get the chills following a hot flash.

Buy a couple of all-cotton, short-sleeved, knee-length nightgowns. Full-length, long-sleeved gowns will be too hot and uncomfortable to sleep in.

Wear all-cotton underwear. Avoid nylon or polyester blends, which will trap rather than release heat.

Keep a dry nightie handy at the foot of your bed or on a chair next to your bed. If you have to change in the middle of the night, you won't have to get out of bed and rummage through your dresser drawers.

Keep a small cotton towel next to your bed to wipe the sweat off your chest, neck, and face.

Keep a fan next to your bed to cool those heat waves.

Take several long, deep breaths and **imagine yourself totally naked,** sliding through soft, cold snow down the gentle slope of a mountain.

Helpful Hints

Whether you experience hot flashes or night sweats, try deep belly breathing. Lie with your hands on your abdomen. Imagine that your abdomen is a balloon that you fill with air as you inhale and deflate as you exhale. Repeat six to eight times a minute. Some researchers believe that in some women, belly breathing alone can reduce hot flashes.

Sage—an ordinary kitchen herb—can help reduce or sometimes even eliminate night sweats, according to herbalists. To make a sage infusion, place 4 heaping tablespoons of dried sage in 1 cup of hot water. Cover tightly and steep for 4 hours or more. Then strain, reheat, and drink. (Used in therapeutic amounts, sage can increase sedative side effects of drugs. Do not use medicinal amounts of sage if you're hypoglycemic or undergoing anticonvulsant therapy.) ■

Hot Tubs

A Hedonist's Guide to the Warm and Bubbly

Forget clichéd images of sexy couples frolicking naked as they drink champagne in a bubbling whirlpool. As baby boomers' bones and muscles begin to show signs of wear and tear, 88 percent of hot-tub owners use them for therapy or relaxation, not parties.

The combination of heat and moving water soothes body and mind, relaxing tense, sore muscles and taking stress out of aching joints.

"No one disputes the therapeutic value of hot tubs," says Ralph LaForge, managing director of the Duke Lipid Clinic Preceptorship Program at Duke University Medical Center. "They're great—if used wisely."

Experts offers this etiquette guide—part courtesy tips, part safety advice—to help you enjoy the therapeutic and social benefits of hot tubs.

DON'T MAKE THIS MISTAKE

Women (and men) who have heart disease, seizure disorders, or high blood pressure shouldn't get into a hot tub without their doctor's okay. Hot water can lower blood pressure quickly and dramatically, which for them can be dangerous.

Do's

Shower before entering the tub. It's not a bathtub. Showering first is also easier on the filter system and keeps down the need for cleaning materials.

Wear shoes or sandals with good tread to and from the tub. They'll give you more traction than bare feet, so you won't slip near the tub. (As for a swimsuit, use good judgment, considering your company.)

Check the temperature. It should be between 90° and 100°F, 104°F at the very highest. Anything hotter can stress the heart.

Make sure the tub is clean and well-chlorinated. Warm water breeds bacteria that can lead to rashes and infections. If you're in a public hot tub, ask the person who supervises the hot tubs how often the chlorine levels are checked. The National Spa and Pool Institute recommends a chlorine level of 3 to 5 parts per million.

Drink plenty of water before getting in and after getting out. Hot tubs can dehydrate you. (Alcohol, on the other hand, is a diuretic and speeds up fluid loss.) Use plastic glasses only.

Get out of the tub if you feel nauseated, dizzy, faint, headachy, or develop an irregular heartbeat or chills.

When you leave the tub, cover it. That conserves heat and prevents others from accidentally falling in.

Don'ts

Don't go wild with the power jets. Others may prefer a gentle massage, so start out slowly and increase the force as needed.

Don't stay in the hot tub longer than 20 minutes.

Don't eat a big meal before using a hot tub. Digestion disrupts bloodflow to the heart and brain. Digesting your food while hot tubbing places undue stress on the heart, especially if you're at risk for heart disease.

Don't get in if you are taking medicine—either prescribed or over-the-counter—that makes you drowsy.

Don't roll in the snow or jump into a cold pool after being in a hot tub (or vice versa). Changing temperature quickly can lead to changes in blood pressure that stress the heart.

If you're overheated—after jogging or playing tennis—wait until you cool down to enter the tub. Your blood pressure generally drops after vigorous exercise because most of your blood vessels are dilated. Getting into a hot tub may lower your blood pressure too far. ■

Housework

Crafty Ways to Get Help—Without Nagging

Paula Jhung knows of a simple activity that can add time to your day and strengthen your family. It can make your husband more attractive and help turn your kids into upstanding members of society.

It's called housework.

Since everyone in the family benefits from a tidy house, everyone under the roof should share in its upkeep, says Jhung, an "anti-cleaning" expert in San Diego and author of How to Avoid Housework *and* Guests without Grief.

Here are some ways to inspire the whole family to take part.

Tips for the Big Guy in the House

Men's magazines are fond of asking, "What do women really want?" The answer is simple—we want help around the house, Jhung says. When a couple shares the necessary chores of daily life, they work as a team and strengthen their relationship in the process. "A guy doing his share shows compassion and care that roses can never convey," she says.

To get your guy to pitch in:

Focus on his strengths. Once you figure out what he's good at—whether it's organizing the garage or whipping up omelets—encourage his talent and give him full responsibility in that area.

Take turns doing different tasks each month. That way, neither of you is stuck doing a chore you find unpleasant for too long. ››

Acknowledge his help when he's finished. And try not to interrupt his cleaning attempts too often with suggestions on how to do it better.

Hold off criticism. If you're displeased with his contributions—or lack thereof—wait until you're both relaxed and in good spirits to voice your concerns, not when you're already in a hurry or arguing, she says.

Helpful Hint

Remind him that a clean household may cost less money. Carpets and clothes last longer when they're kept clean, and you may have less need for an exterminator when the garbage is taken out regularly.

Recruiting the Kids

Even young kids should learn to do simple tasks around the house, Jhung says. Not only will it teach them the responsibilities of being a family

Humor

It's No Joke—The Right Kind of Laughter Is Like a Spiritual Vitamin

Inside a crowded supermarket, a little girl throws a queen-size temper tantrum. She's screaming, crying, and pounding the air with her tiny fists.

But her mother seems cool and collected.

"Be calm, Jennifer," she says softly. "Don't worry, Jennifer. Be okay, Jennifer."

After the temper tantrum subsides, a stranger approaches the mother and praises her forbearance.

"It's amazing how well you deal with Jennifer," he says.

The mother pauses, smiles, and says, "I *am* Jennifer."

The story, a favorite of Joel Goodman, Ed.D., shows how humor can lighten an otherwise loathsome situation.

"This woman was talking to herself to relieve her own tension," says Dr. Goodman, founder and director of the Humor Project, Inc., in Saratoga Springs, New York, and author of *Laffirmations: 1,001 Ways to Add Humor to Your Life and Work.*

A growing body of research shows that Jennifer was on the right laugh-track. **Humor is healthy. It improves blood circulation, boosts the immune system, and suppresses stress hormones.** Many researchers believe that it also releases endorphins, the body's feel-good chemicals.

If you haven't enjoyed a good belly-laugh since Dan Quayle was vice president, here are some stress-busting tips from Dr. Goodman and one of his Humor Project colleagues: Sister Anne Bryan Smollin, Ph.D., president of Clowns on Rounds in member but the habits they pick up may also make them more self-sufficient later in life.

Instead of telling your child to do a specific task, let her choose from a few options. She may not be thrilled about emptying the wastebaskets or loading the dishwasher, but being able to pick from a number of chores will give her some sense of power.

Give the kids fun titles linked to their assignments. Jhung suggests: "Whoever keeps the hallways free of clutter is the 'Highway Patrol.' 'Spiderman' destroys competing cobwebs and 'Wonder Woman' cleans toilets in no time." ■

REWARDS WORK BEST

Instead of scolding children when they don't get the job right, reward them when they do a good job.

Albany, New York, and author of *Jiggle Your Heart and Tickle Your Soul.*

Look at stressful situations from a childlike perspective. Kids laugh 400 times a day, while adults laugh 15 times a day, so children must know something we don't. During a vacation, Dr. Goodman's wife, Margie Ingram, lost her purse with all the couple's cash and credit cards. Their 8-year-old daughter Alyssa broke the ice by saying, "Hey, Mom—now that you've lost your wallet, you'll have to get a new driver's license and maybe the new picture will look better than the old one did."

Surround yourself with cutups and cutouts. Find what Dr. Smollin calls a "laughing buddy," a good-humored friend with whom you can share the belief that the whole world's crazy except for the two of you. If you find more than one such buddy, start an informal "laughing club." Start a "joy journal" with jokes, cartoons, and wacky news stories clipped from newspapers and magazines. Keep this journal by the telephone so that you can thumb through it when you're on hold.

Laugh at yourself. "We have to learn not to take ourselves so seriously," Dr. Smollin says. "Every day, make three mistakes on purpose so you'll learn to laugh at yourself."

"That's the bottom line of humor," adds Dr. Goodman. "If we can celebrate and laugh at our imperfections as human beings, it relieves the pressure to be perfect and helps us embrace our humanity." ■

DON'T MAKE THIS MISTAKE

Use humor as a tool to build people up instead of as a weapon to tear them down. So avoid mean-spirited humor. Instead, capitalize on your natural tendency to nourish and support others. "I try not to generalize, but I think women are ahead of men on this one," Dr. Goodman says. "There's enough pain and challenge in the world. Humor is best when it helps relieve the pain."

Hysterectomy

10 Alternatives That Spare Your Uterus (and That Your Doctor May Not Mention Unless You Ask)

If you're one of the 500,000 women a year who are told by their doctors, "You need a hysterectomy," don't panic. Maybe you need surgery, and maybe you don't.

Each year, more than half a million women undergo hysterectomies (removal of the uterus) for fibroids, endometriosis, and abnormal bleeding. It's the second most common surgery in America among women in their reproductive years. (After menopause, it's far less frequent.)

But here's the real kicker: About 90 percent of women who have the surgery could have been offered uterus-sparing treatments instead, says Brian Walsh, M.D., chief of surgical gynecology at Brigham and Women's Hospital in Boston. That's important if you still want to have children, or if you want to avoid an early, surgically induced menopause.

So why aren't we told about other options? "Doctors are either unaware of the alternatives or just not comfortable with performing the procedures that require higher levels of skill," says Mitchell Rein, M.D., an obstetrician/gynecologist, reproductive endocrinologist, and associate professor at Harvard Medical School.

Hysterectomy should be necessary only if a woman's condition doesn't improve after she has explored all other possibilities, or if she has invasive uterine cancer, says Dr. Rein. The exception would be if she has very early cervical cancer and is determined to keep her uterus.

Cancer accounts for fewer than 5 percent of all hysterectomies, says Dr. Walsh. Non-life-threatening conditions make up the rest.

Following are three of the most common causes of hysterectomy and the ways to treat them that don't involve removing your uterus. If your doctor doesn't mention any of these options, ask, especially if you still want to have children.

Fibroids

As many as 4 out of 10 hysterectomies are done to remove fibroids, or uterine leiomyomas, bundles of muscle and connective tissue that can grow inside or outside the uterus. Uterus-saving treatments include:

1. Nonsteroidal anti-inflammatories (NSAIDs). Over-the-counter pain relievers like ibuprofen (such as Motrin and Advil) can sometimes help ease the pain and heavy bleeding from fibroids. For mild symptoms, they should be your doctor's first line of treatment, says Dr. Rein.

2. Uterine artery embolization. This nonsurgical procedure cuts off the blood supply to the fibroid, causing it to shrink, says Linda D. Bradley, M.D., director of hysteroscopic services in the department of obstetrics and gynecology at the Cleveland Clinic Foundation in Ohio.

Recovery is quick and side effects are few, but the impact

on fertility is questionable. "After a woman has this procedure, we don't know if her uterus is strong enough to sustain a pregnancy," says Dr. Bradley.

3. Myomectomy. This surgical technique removes fibroids but leaves the uterus intact. The size of the fibroids and where they occur determine what type of myomectomy your doctor performs. With a hysteroscopic myomectomy, fibroids are removed vaginally. Laparoscopic surgery extracts fibroids through an incision made in the abdomen. The more complex procedures for multiple and large-size fibroids are done through larger abdominal incisions, says Dr. Rein.

Endometriosis

About one out of five hysterectomies is done for endometriosis, where fragments of the uterine lining grow outside the uterus in the abdomen and on the ovaries. Fueled by estrogen, the tissue then grows and bleeds on a monthly cycle, causing chronic pain, inflammation, scar tissue, and other problems. Other ways to control endometriosis include:

4. Oral contraceptives (birth control pills). Most effective for milder cases of endometriosis, oral contraceptives alter the balance of estrogen and progesterone, slowing the progression of the disease, says Dr. Walsh.

5. Hormonal drugs. GnRH agonists, like Synarel and Lupron, are powerful hormonal drugs that reduce estrogen production and shrink endometrial tissue. They send you into early—but reversible—menopause. And they can cause premature bone loss if used long term, says Dr. Rein.

6. Laparoscopic surgery. Sometimes performed when endometriosis is diagnosed, stray endometrial tissue is destroyed with an electrical device or a laser, says Dr. Walsh. Endometriosis has a tendency to recur, but birth control pills can help keep it in check.

7. Laparotomy. More invasive than laparoscopic surgery but less so than hysterectomy, this procedure destroys the endometriosis tissue and/or associated scar tissue.

Abnormal Bleeding

Persistent or heavy bleeding that doesn't seem to let up accounts for another 20 percent of hysterectomies performed. Other options to consider:

8. Ibuprofen. In mild cases, NSAIDs such as Motrin or Advil can sometimes help slow down the bleeding, says Dr. Walsh.

9. Hormone treatment. Contraceptives like birth control pills or Depo-Provera, administered by injection, says Dr. Walsh, are often ideal for women who are not ovulating regularly and bleeding throughout the month.

10. Endometrial ablation. This destroys the lining of the uterus and the layer under it, and can be done vaginally. Ablation will usually leave you infertile. And while one-third of all patients will have no more bleeding, one-third will have spotting or a light flow. Twenty-five percent will have average periods. A few—5 to 10 percent—will be no better off than before.

Helpful Hint

It's best to seek a physician experienced in the procedure offered. ■

I

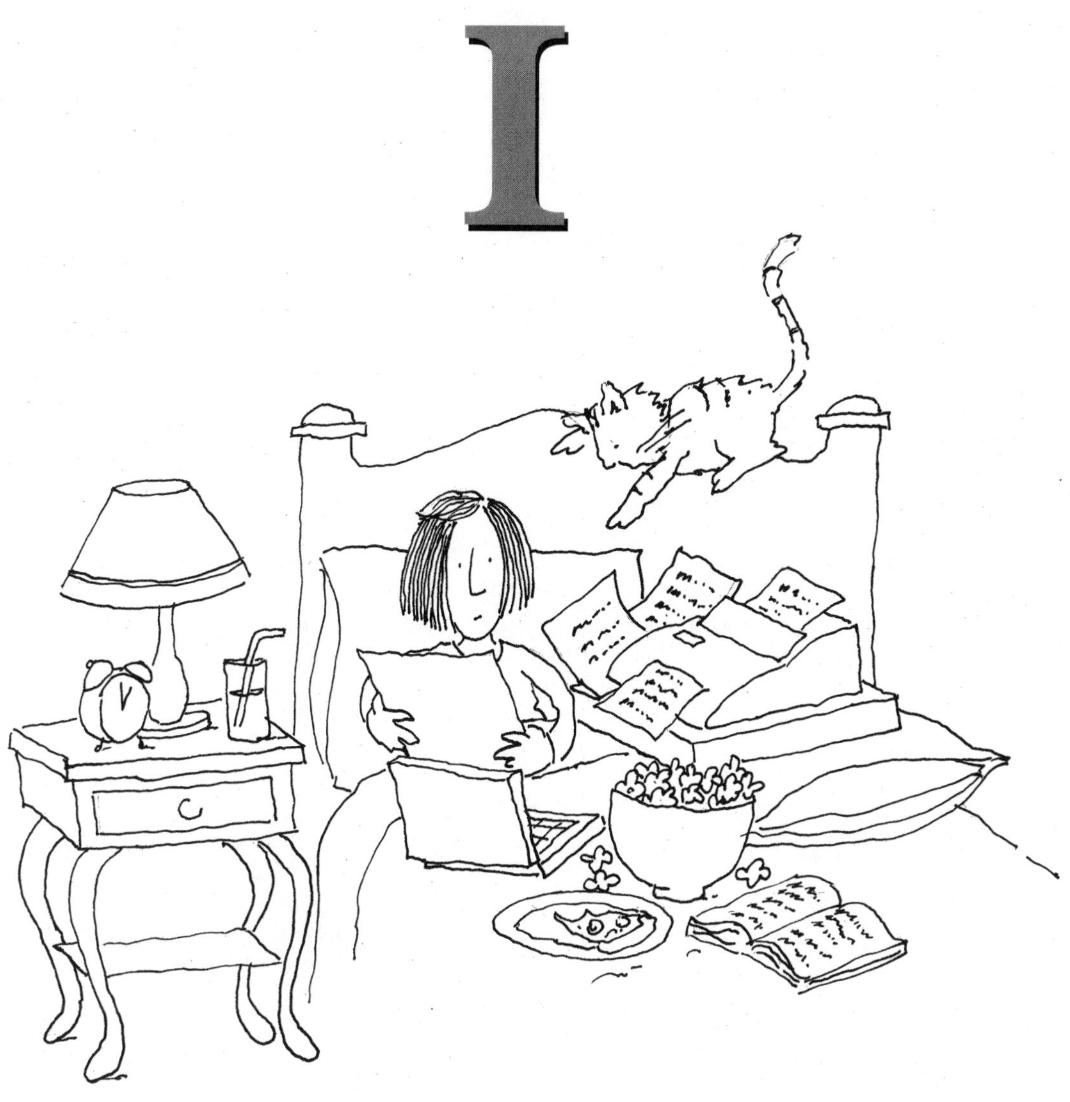

Wide awake when you should be getting your rest?
Turn to page 230.

Indecisiveness

How to Stop Agonizing and Make Faster, Smarter Decisions

Buy a van, or a sport utility vehicle? Cook Thanksgiving Dinner for your parents, or take them to a restaurant? Buy a bigger house, or remodel the one you have?

Everyone has trouble making decisions once in a while. But women tend to find decision making particularly difficult at times, says Carol Goldberg, Ph.D., clinical psychologist and president of Getting Ahead Programs, a New York–based corporation that conducts workshops on stress management, health, and wellness. "Women tend to think about others, take social relationships into consideration, and base their decisions on feelings more than men do. All of these factors make decisions even more difficult."

So how can you avoid hemming and hawing? "First of all, realize that by not making a decision, you are making a decision," says Dr. Goldberg. "In making that decision, you are giving up control of the situation."

Sooner or later, though, you're forced to choose. Here are Dr. Goldberg's tips for coming to a conclusion more readily.

If you need more information, get it. You'll feel more powerful, and you'll be more confident with your decision by going into it well-informed, says Dr. Goldberg.

When possible, make large decisions in small stages, suggests Dr. Goldberg. For instance, if you're deciding to move, consider renting in the new area for a while before buying.

List the pros and cons. Writing down the pros and cons and seeing them in black and white takes a problem from the abstract to the concrete and can help resolve a dilemma, says Dr. Goldberg. Assign point values to each item on the list, according to how important each is to you. Then add up the points on each side to see which has more value.

At work, consult a few others. One study showed that when it comes to making decisions, small groups function more efficiently than large groups, since stalemates are more likely to occur when more people are involved in a decision.

When working in a group, says Dr. Goldberg, break into small sections and select a representative for each group, then have the representatives make the final decision.

Once you've made a decision, move on. Another study showed that thinking too much about a decision makes it more difficult to actually come to a solution.

"The more you dwell on a decision, the larger and more looming it becomes," says Dr. Goldberg. Rather than letting decisions become monstrous, realize that almost everything is reversible, she advises. And don't dwell on your decision—just do it. ■

Inflammatory Bowel Disease

Tame Your Colon with Herbs, Vitamins, and Relaxation

If you have inflammatory bowel disease (IBD), you know why one doctor described it as "Montezuma's revenge that never stops." If left untreated, some women experience the diarrhea, bleeding, and abdominal cramps associated with the condition year in and year out.

There are two types of IBD: Crohn's disease, which affects the entire digestive tract, and ulcerative colitis, which affects only the lining of the colon. In both, the affected area is sore and inflamed.

Of the two, there may be a link between the use of oral contraceptives and the development of IBD, although this is inconclusive, says Melissa Palmer, M.D., a gastroenterologist in Long Island, New York. Another risk factor for IBD is heredity, since North American and West European Jews (Ashkenazi Jews) have the highest incidence.

Conventional IBD treatments include anti-inflammatory agents such as corticosteroids, immunosuppressive drugs, diets, and surgery. If you're diagnosed with IBD, you should be under the care of a gastroenterologist, since uncontrolled disease increases the risk of colon cancer.

Here are some dietary, nutritional, and lifestyle changes you can make to keep IBD under control.

Try slippery elm bark. For people with IBD who have diarrhea or constipation, slippery elm bark is often used to promote regularity and soothe irritated mucous membranes. Place a heaping teaspoon of dried slippery elm bark in a cup and gradually add enough warm water to make a paste. Continue to add water until you have a very diluted tea. Drink this once a day.

Start a food diary. Since no IBD case is exactly the same, there's no one-size-fits-all diet. So keep track of the foods that disagree with you and place them on the verboten list. Frequent offenders include milk and other dairy products, caffeine, alcohol, and laxative fruits such as prunes, figs, and cherries.

During remissions, take it easy on the fiber. Eating any kind of fiber—soluble or insoluble—is like rubbing sandpaper on an open wound. But fiber is still extremely important in a healthy, well-balanced diet. So unless it aggravates your diarrhea, it's okay to reinstate fiber into your diet once a flare-up is over, says Dr. Palmer.

DON'T MAKE THIS MISTAKE

Since IBD can cause anemia, patients are often told to take iron supplements. Try to avoid ferrous sulfate if possible. "It's very irritating to the colonic mucusa," Dr. Donovan says. Instead, take organic forms such as ferritin or ferrous fumerate. If, however, ferrous sulfate is the only form available, take it. It's very important to treat the anemia. Before taking any iron supplements, consult with your health care provider for proper dosage.

Take your vits. IBD causes malabsorption, so you should be taking a good multiple vitamin-mineral supplement that supplies 100 percent of the Daily Value for antioxidants such as vitamins E and C, beta-carotene, and selenium, plus trace minerals copper, manganese, and zinc.

Consider additional supplements. IBD medications also cause malabsorption. So if you're on sulfasalazine, you might need extra folic acid, a B vitamin. If you're on corticosteroids, you might need extra potassium, calcium, and vitamin D. To determine the correct dose, ask your doctor to test you for deficiencies. If you're low on vitamin B_{12} and have IBD, only an injection or nasal spray can correct the deficiency.

Try cod-liver oil or fish oil. Patrick Donovan, N.D., a naturopathic physician and former gastroenterology professor at Bastyr University of Natural Health Sciences in Seattle, recommends taking 1 to 3 teaspoons of cod-liver oil a day. Cod-liver oil is high in vitamin A and omega-3 fatty acids. Or you may take 2,000 to 3,000 milligrams of fish oil a day, which is high in docosahexaenoic acid (DHA) and eicosapentaenoic acid (EPA).

Take extra vitamin E. Dr. Donovan instructs women with IBD to take 400 IU of E three times a day. "I prefer vitamin E succinate, the dry form of vitamin E, because it has more aggressive anti-cancer activity," he says. If you are considering taking amounts at this level, talk with your doctor first.

Exercise, but go easy on your joints. For some people, excessive bouncing can result in cramping, pain, and an urgent need to run for the nearest restroom. It is still important for women to do some sort of weight-bearing exercise to help in the fight against osteoporosis. Low-impact exercise such as swimming or walking is preferable to high-impact exercise.

Learn to relax. "Anything that decreases your stress level is definitely rec-

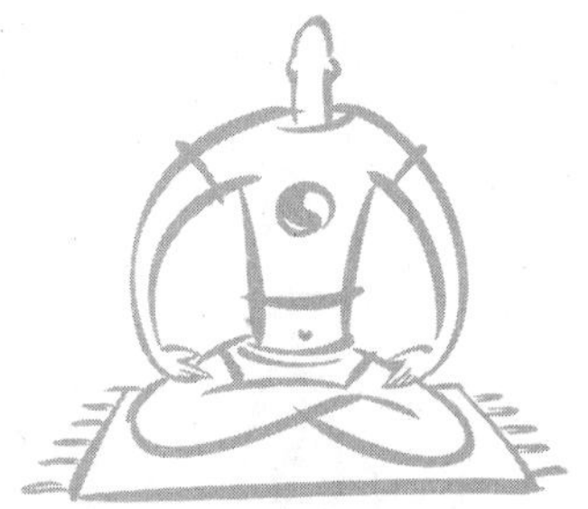

ommended," Dr. Palmer says. Among the therapies that have been found useful in treating IBD: progressive muscle relaxation, hypnosis, yoga, meditation, visualization exercises, and autogenic training, which teaches women to unwind by repeating such words as *warm* and *heavy*.

Also, know that you did not do anything to bring on this condition. Blaming yourself will only add to your stress.

Helpful Hint

Doctors sometimes diagnosis IBD when the real culprit is gluten intolerance. Dr. Donovan has treated several women suspected of having Crohn's disease who actually had celiac disease, an entirely different condition caused by a reaction to gluten, a protein found primarily in wheat. If conventional treatments are ineffective, get tested. ■

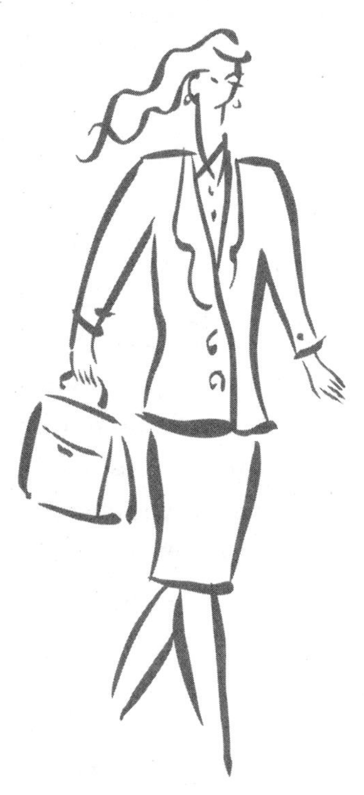

Ingrown Toenails

The Toothpick Cure

In one year, the average woman walks the equivalent of the distance between Chicago and New Orleans—often in very fashionable shoes. If you have an ingrown toenail, every step can be torturous, especially if it gets infected.

These little buggers occur when the side of a nail cuts into the surrounding skin. (It's almost always the one on the big toe.) Clipping your nails too short and picking or digging at them are common causes. So is wearing shoes that may look fabulous but are too tight.

"If you wait it out, the ingrown nail will eventually grow out," says Wilma Bergfeld, M.D., head of the clinical research department at the Cleveland Clinic and associate clinical professor of dermatology at Case Western University in Ohio. "But if you create a barrier between the sharp edge of the nail and the sensitive skin of your toe, you'll feel a lot better." Here's how.

Insect Repellent

The Bug-Free Solution

If you never, ever want to get bitten by a mosquito again, move to Antarctica. It's one place in the world where mosquitoes don't exist.

If you intend to stick closer to home, consider mosquitoes, ticks, gnats, and other pests all a part of the great outdoors. But you don't have to be their feed station.

"Preventing bites and stings is far better than having to treat them," says Edward Otten, M.D., president of the Wilderness Medical Society, an organization of physicians skilled in dealing with medical problems that arise in the great outdoors.

Possibly no one knows bite and sting control better than these doctors, who have been in the thick of the worst of it, including Alaska in June, when mosquitoes are at their meanest. So if your future plans include a trek into the wild, take this advice from Dr. Otten and his fellow doctors who have spent years of trial and error perfecting it.

• Treat clothing with permethrin spray (available at outdoor specialty stores). It works for weeks, even after washing, to repel bugs.

THE PERFECT PEDICURE

In the future, cut toenails straight across, not rounded like manicured fingernails. And never cut your toenails super-short. You'll only risk having the corners of your nails poke into your skin. Instead, leave nails long enough to not press into the surrounding skin.

• Wash your feet, then soak them in warm water for 5 to 10 minutes to soften the nail and the skin.

• Dab a pea-size amount of antibacterial ointment onto a dime-size piece of sterile cotton or gauze.

• After sterilizing it with an alcohol wipe, use a smooth toothpick or sterile cuticle pusher to gently lift the edge of the nail away from the skin. Be careful not to dig into the skin.

• Gently lift and slide the piece of sterile cotton or gauze underneath the nail. Just the edge of it will do. Make sure that the ointment is touching the skin. This will reduce the risk of infection.

• Cover the toe with a protective wrapping of gauze or an extra-thick bandage.

• Secure the dressing with tape. Be sure to wear a shoe that doesn't put pressure on the toe that's bandaged.

• Change the dressing daily until the nail grows out.

If the toe is hot, red, and painful, and you can't get your foot into a shoe, it could be infected. See a dermatologist, an orthopedic surgeon, or a podiatrist, says Dr. Bergfeld. ■

• Wear a long-sleeved shirt and pants in a fabric that is lightweight but has a tight weave.

• Spray exposed skin with an extended-duration DEET repellent, such as Sawyer Controlled Release DEET Formula or Cutter Outdoorsman. Do not apply it around your eyes, nose, or mouth because it can irritate them.

• If you're traveling with children, use a DEET repellent containing less than 5 percent of this mildly toxic ingredient. They are safer to use.

FORGET BUG ZAPPERS

Electric bug zappers may sound like they're doing a killer job, but they're really not all that effective. First, many of the insects that get electrocuted are innocent victims, like moths and butterflies. Second, with each zap, bacteria that have collected on the surface of the insect get blasted as far as 6 feet into the air.

Helpful Hint

If chemical-based repellents irritate your skin, try using a head net that protects the head and neck from biting bugs, suggests Dr. Otten. You'll find head nets at sporting goods shops and in some catalogs. ■

Insomnia

No More Restless Nights—Ever

You won't find Meg Kampen in The Guinness Book of World Records, *but she just might qualify as the longest-running case of insomnia: For 14 years, this 40-year-old resident of Lacey, Washington, survived on less than 4 hours of sleep a night. Sometimes she'd sleep only 2 to 3 hours—or not at all. And during one particularly bad stretch, she didn't sleep at all for 3 nights in a row.*

Before long, Kampen was so tense and irritable that she was unable to keep a job, and her relationships with family and friends were in shambles. "Insomnia was ruining my life," Kampen recalls.

After trying virtually every insomnia cure that medicine could offer—including prescription drugs—Kampen finally found ways to ease her insomnia: getting at least an hour a day of outdoor exercise in the sunshine and climbing out of bed the same time every day. If you're like Kampen, you've probably tried all the standard treatments for sleeplessness—pills, warm milk, white noise, melatonin supplements, maybe even a sleep clinic—without success. Perhaps you've even spent hours—often at 3:00 A.M.—searching the Internet for solutions from other sleep-deprived souls.

John Wiedman, a former chronic insomniac, collected various innovative—yet safe—insomnia cures in his book *Desperately Seeking Snoozin'*. After trial and error, here are some remedies that other world-class insomniacs recommend.

- Inhale and exhale deeply each time your mate takes a breath while he sleeps, mimicking his breathing pattern. Before long, you'll be so relaxed that you'll be on your way to La La Land. (This may not work if your guy snores.)
- Expose yourself to daylight for 30 to 60 minutes first thing in the morning. The bright light tells your brain it's time to wake up.
- Push yourself to wake up at the same time every day, whether or not you slept well the night before or even if it's the weekend. You'll keep your circadian rhythm (internal body clock) on track, so when it's time to go to bed the following evening, you will rest.

DON'T MAKE THIS MISTAKE

Don't read, work, and watch television in your bedroom, says Rafael Pelayo, M.D., at the Stanford Sleep Disorders Clinic in Palo Alto, California. Associating your bedroom with activities other than sleep isn't restful. Instead, reserve your bedroom strictly for sleeping and sex. And don't try to make up for lost sleep with a mid-afternoon nap. If you have insomnia, a daytime snooze will make it difficult to fall asleep at your normal bedtime.

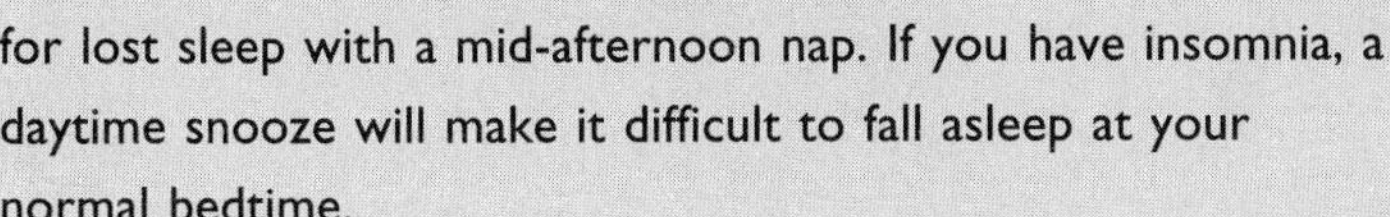

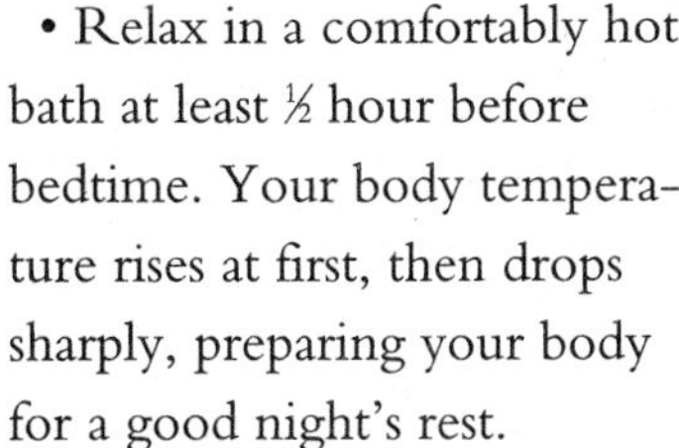

• Relax in a comfortably hot bath at least ½ hour before bedtime. Your body temperature rises at first, then drops sharply, preparing your body for a good night's rest.

• As part of your bedtime ritual, stretch your leg and back muscles in a room other than your bedroom. Taking some time to wind down in this way also lowers your body temperature, causing drowsiness.

• If you can't sleep because your mind is racing with restless thoughts, get up and write down whatever it is that's bugging you, along with some possible solutions. You'll bring closure to the problem and will be more than likely to get some Zzzs.

If those solutions don't work, consider these.

Ease into sleep with herbs. Herbalists say that kava-kava and valerian supplements, extracts, or teas (available in health food stores and pharmacies) can put you to sleep fairly quickly if anxiety and muscle tension are keeping you awake. Unlike prescription drugs, kava and valerian root aren't habit-forming and won't lose their effectiveness over time. Follow package directions for correct dosage.

While using valerian and kava-kava, do *not* do the following: drink alcohol, combine them with any sleep-inducing or mood-regulating medication, drive or operate machinery, or exceed the recommended dosage. Valerian may cause heart palpitations or nervousness in sensitive individuals. If this happens, discontinue using valerian.

Mind your minerals. Take 500 milligrams of magnesium and 1,000 milligrams of calcium ½ hour before bedtime. Together, magnesium and calcium act as mild muscle relaxers and help release sleep-related brain chemicals called neurotransmitters so you can get some sleep, says Andrew Weil, M.D., director of the program in integrative medicine and clinical professor of internal medicine at the University of Arizona College of Medicine in Tucson. (People with heart or kidney problems should check with their doctors before taking supplemental magnesium. Also, in some people, supplemental magnesium may cause diarrhea.) ■

Iron and Iron Supplements

Smart Cooking Strategies for Vegetarians

The earth's core is composed largely of molten iron. But you don't need to travel that far to get the teaspoon or so of this mineral that you need for rich, oxygenated blood. Beef, chicken, and other meats will deliver all you need. That's because animal is the richest source of heme iron, a special form of iron that's readily absorbed by your body. Vegetables, fruits, and grains also carry iron but in smaller amounts and in a less useful form, called nonheme.

Iron is a chief component of hemoglobin, a protein in your blood that transports oxygen to your brain and cells throughout your body. Women who run short of iron feel run-down, look pale, and have trouble fighting off infections.

The main reason: They eat little or no meat.

Women need a daily intake of 18 milligrams of iron a day. And if you don't eat meat, it's hard to get the heme iron that's sufficiently absorbed. And if you're menstruating, you lose iron on a regular basis through monthly bloodflow, which can contribute to the problem.

"If you're menstruating and you're vegetarian, your risk of running low on iron increases," says Helen Brittin, R.D., Ph.D., professor of food and nutrition at Texas Tech University in Lubbock, who has studied iron for nearly 20 years. Dr. Brittin urges women who don't eat meat to follow this advice.

Eat as many iron-rich plant foods as possible. These include whole grains, enriched breads and cereals, kale, spinach, chard, kelp, cooked beans, and dried apricots.

Cook in cast-iron or stainless steel pots and pans. Cooking food in iron skillets and pots increases the amount of iron in food, including nonheme iron from vegetables and grains. Studies by Dr. Brittin show that foods cooked in cast-iron pots and pans contain an average of twice as much iron as foods cooked in glassware or cookware like Corningware. Acidic foods like tomatoes and long-cooking foods like applesauce absorbed the most iron.

Stainless steel is 50 to 88 percent iron (plus chromium and nickel), and Dr. Brittin also found that some of the iron gets into the food while cooking. "Not as much as with cast-iron utensils, but it's still significant," she says.

DON'T MAKE THIS MISTAKE

Excessive or unnecessary use of iron supplements may be related to heart disease. So don't take iron supplements unless recommended by your doctor, based on a blood test.

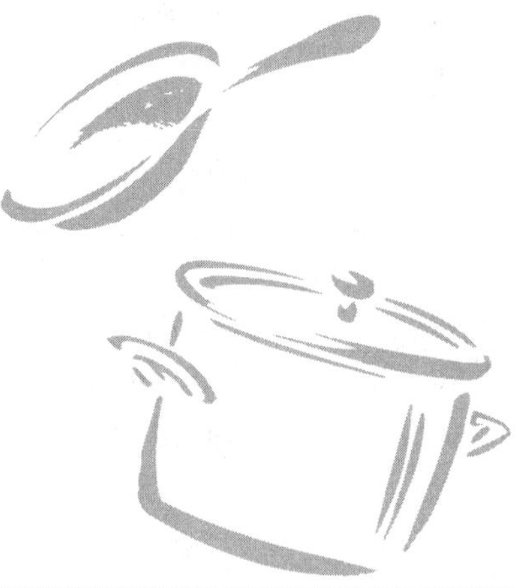

Drink orange juice with iron-enriched cereal. Vitamin C increases the absorption of nonheme iron, especially that from plant sources. At lunch, order a glass of tomato juice and a spinach salad. At dinner, follow a plate of iron-enriched spaghetti with orange wedges for dessert.

Helpful Hint

Don't drink coffee, tea, or soy milk or eat eggs, tofu, or other unfermented soy foods at the same time you eat an iron-rich meal. Substances in those foods interfere with iron absorption. However, fermented soy foods (such as miso, a soy paste used as a base for soups) will enhance iron absorption. ■

Irritability

Four Guaranteed Ways to Take the Edge Off Your Nerves

Irritability raises your blood pressure. What's more, it's contagious: One study of schoolteachers—men and women included—showed that irritability raised their blood pressures. A second study, of married men and women, found that when women are irritable, their husbands get angry, raising their blood pressures, too.

So for your loved ones' sake as well as your own, try the following quick tips for instant calm.

1. Aromatherapy. Many fragrant essential oils can help soothe your mood, says Mindy Green, director of education at the Herb Research Foundation in Boulder, Colorado. Among them: lavender, clary sage, neroli, sweet orange blossom, sandalwood, chamomile, and marjoram. If you're irritable at the end of the day, place 8 to 10 drops of one of these essential oils into your bathwater for a soothing soak. Or, mix the oils into massage lotion and ask your mate for a relaxing rubdown. The oils can also be mixed with each other in any combination that you find pleasant.

2. Kava. Taken from the root of a Polynesian plant, this herb has been used for centuries in ceremonies to help dissolve disputes. Today, it has been shown effective for relieving stress, anxiety, and irritability. Because of its bitter taste, you probably won't want to drink it as a tea. Green suggests taking kava tablets or mixing 15 to 30 drops of the extract into a glass of water. Just be sure to read the label, and don't ingest more than the recommended dose of kava, warns Green. Large amounts can leave you feeling uncoordinated or intoxicated. And don't take it with alcohol or barbiturates.

3. Exercise. "Exercise improves moods both psychologically and physiologically," says Maria Newton, Ph.D., associate professor in the department of human performance and health promotion at the University of New Orleans. ❯❯

Psychologically, it's a distraction from life's problems, it gives you a sense of achievement and power, and it helps you build confidence. Physiologically, there is a feel-good phenomenon associated with exercise: When you work out, endorphins are released in your body, which make you feel good and block out stress.

4. Sunlight. "Plenty of evidence shows that the amount of sunlight we get affects our moods," says Dan Oren, M.D., associate professor at Yale University School of Medicine. "Decreased amounts of sunlight in the fall and winter can certainly make lots of people irritable, and many others feel down in the dumps on dreary days."

Next time you're feeling under the weather, make an effort to get out in the sun, advises Dr. Oren.

- Take a walk on a sunny winter afternoon instead of staying inside and eating a heavy lunch.
- Open the curtains and blinds as much as possible and lobby for a desk near a window.
- If possible, take a trip to a warm locale. ■

Irritable Bowel Syndrome

Calm Your "Gut Reactions"

In some ways, Nancy Norton is typical of women with irritable bowel syndrome (IBS). Beginning in her twenties, Norton endured 15 years of diarrhea, abdominal pain, gas, and bloating before being diagnosed, often blaming her discomfort on her period or something she ate.

With IBS, the bowel goes into spasm, releasing stool willy-nilly. Sometimes you have constipation. Sometimes you have uncontrollable diarrhea. And it's painful. Other symptoms that can accompany IBS include cramping, heartburn, and indigestion.

"I couldn't leave the house or live a normal life," says Norton. She had to quit her job.

Like many women who have IBS but don't know it, Norton tried over-the-counter remedies for her various symptoms, with only temporary success. Once she finally realized that her symptoms were not normal and got help, she managed to get her bowel problems under control. Taking antidiarrheal medications helps. And she occasionally takes antispasmodics, often prescribed for IBS.

Treatments for IBS vary from person to person. For those whose main complaint is constipation, doctors often prescribe stool softeners to give stool consistency from day to day. Some prescribe very low doses of antidepressant drugs to treat the intestinal response, which is aggravated by stress.

"Your intestines contain the same mood-regulating neurotransmitters you have in your brain, like serotonin," explains Marvin Schuster, M.D., professor of medicine and psychiatry at Johns Hopkins University School of Medicine and director of the Schuster Center for Digestive and Motility Disorders at Johns Hopkins Bayview Medical Center in Baltimore. "The same things that make you anxious and stimulate the release of neurotransmitters in the brain also release them in the bowel," says Dr. Schuster.

Norton also used nondrug

DON'T MAKE THIS MISTAKE

Don't ignore IBS symptoms out of embarrassment, or hope they'll go away on their own. Ask your doctor for help—the sooner the better. Otherwise, IBS may get worse, not better.

treatments to calm her irritable bowel, combining antidiarrheal medications with relaxation techniques. She also uses visualization and imagery, meditation, and anal-rectal biofeedback, which monitors the activity in the rectum.

If she had known about IBS earlier, Norton would have saved herself 15 years of misery. So she founded the International Foundation for Functional Gastrointestinal Disorders, to help others help themselves. Norton travels frequently and speaks publicly, which she couldn't do unless she was able to manage her symptoms.

If you have IBS, the following strategies can help, according to Dr. Schuster.

- Eat a high-fiber diet with plenty of bran cereals, unprocessed grains, salad, vegetables, and fruits.
- Try to avoid fat and lactose (in milk and dairy products), which seem to aggravate symptoms for 40 percent of those with IBS.
- Eat regular meals. Don't go hours without eating and then gorge.
- Use relaxation tapes to relieve stress. (And avoid stress when possible.)
- Exercise regularly.

Helpful Hint

For more information, you can contact the International Foundation for Functional Gastrointestinal Disorders at P.O. Box 17864, Milwaukee, WI 53217. ■

J-K-L

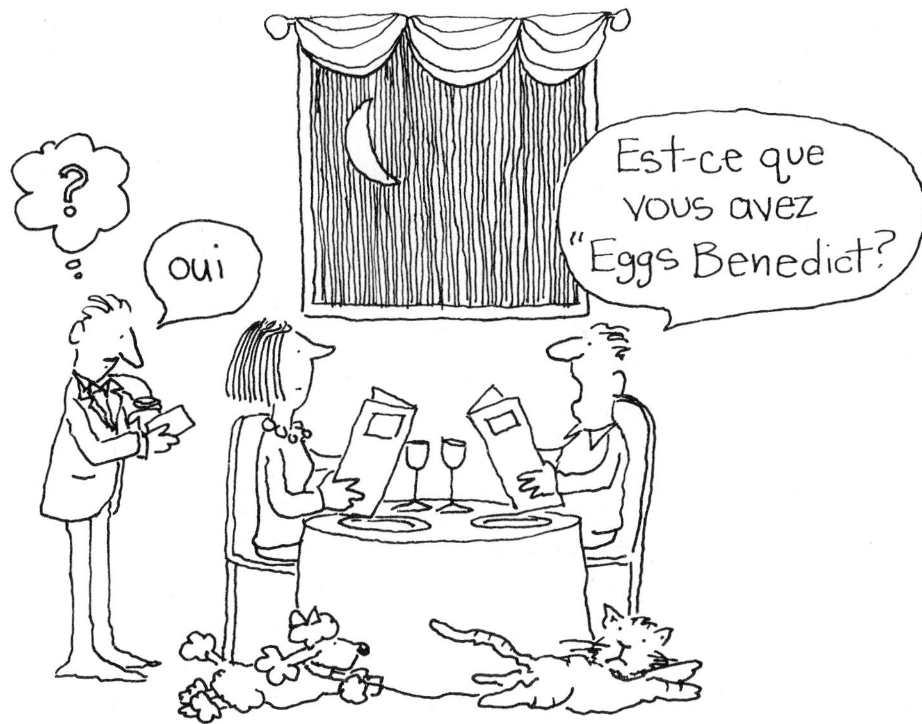

Jet lag can leave you dramatically out of sync at your destination. To adapt more quickly, see page 240.

Jealousy

Put Your Fear, Anger, and Suspicions to Rest

You know that nobody's perfect, especially your husband's ex-wife. But it infuriates you that they're still friends. It bothers you to even see them talking together. You can just picture them running away, hopping on a jet, and writing you a "Dear Joan" letter from a nude beach in Jamaica.

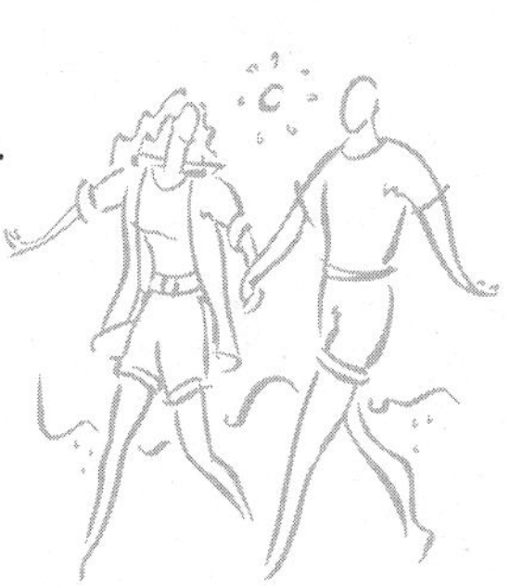

That's jealousy, a complex mix of anger, sadness, and fear that can cause irrational, uncontrollable behavior. Spying on his whereabouts. Calling him a half-dozen times a day at work, demanding to know his every move. You may believe it's a sign of devotion.

But unless you have good reason to believe your husband is fooling around, you're dead wrong. Jealousy is as corrosive as battery acid. When you turn into an inquisitor, it eats away at the core of your marriage.

Monogamous men resent being mistrusted, so they withdraw and become more protective of their privacy. This sets in motion a vicious circle in which their wives become even more panicky, paradoxically increasing the likelihood that their worst fears will come true.

"Jealous women are hard to live with. In their jealousy, they drive their husbands away," says psychologist Paul Hauck, Ph.D., of Rock Island, Illinois, author of Overcoming Jealousy and Possessiveness. *To help control your jealous tendencies, try the following:*

Turn the tables. If you've gotten into the habit of frequently calling your husband at work, stop and make him play the role of jealous spouse. Have him call you a half-dozen times a day to ask what you're wearing, who've you been with, and whether you still love him. "The men love it because they've been on the receiving end for so long," says Ayala Malach Pines, Ph.D., a psychology professor in Herzelia, Israel, and author of *Romantic Jealousy*. "The wives also like it because their husbands are making the effort to call. For them, jealousy is a show of love."

Try aversion therapy. "A jealous response is a learned response, and you can unlearn it," Dr. Pines says. "So whenever jealousy rears its head, take a whiff of smelling salts." Available at pharmacies, smelling salts are a com- »

DON'T MAKE THIS MISTAKE

Don't fall into the trap of believing that your partner "makes" you jealous. You make yourself jealous, so it's up to you to do something about it. "A wife will say, 'If you want me to stop being jealous, stop talking to other women,'" Dr. Hauck says. "That's like saying, 'I've got a headache. I want you to take the aspirin.'"

bination of alcohol and ammonia sold in little glass ampules. Popped open, they release a noxious smell to revive someone who has fainted. Sniff some whenever you feel jealous, and eventually, your brain will so strongly associate jealousy with the smell that it'll erase jealous thoughts before they can come into your conscious awareness. Just be careful not to inhale too deeply because it could bring on a coughing fit. ■

Jet Lag

How to Reset Your Internal Clock from a Travelin' Doc

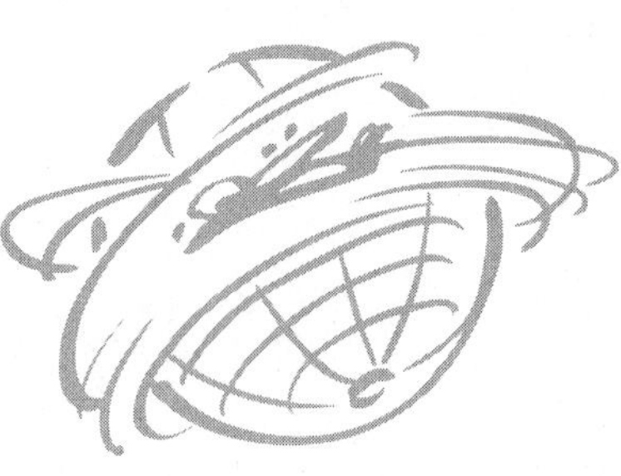

From flight attendants working international routes to secretaries making their first trip to France, frequent flyers and first-time travelers alike can encounter jet lag.

Medical experts call it circadian dischronation. But to the rest of us, jet lag simply means that our body clocks get out of sync when crossing time zones, leaving us exhausted, irritable, nauseated, and achy, with headaches and insomnia thrown in for good measure.

"The only good thing about jet lag is that it's temporary," says Dale Anderson, M.D., an emergency physician from St. Paul, Minnesota, who has traveled the four corners of the world and knows all too well how debilitating jet lag can be. Through trial and error, this globe-circling physician has found the formula for traveling with the fewest side effects.

Prep your body with extra shut-eye. Starting about 2 weeks before departure, go to bed 15 minutes earlier than usual. The extra 15 minutes of sleep help you arrive at your destination rested without feeling tired or bushed. (Beginning a trip in a state of exhaustion makes jet lag worse.)

Time your flights right. Arriving during daylight hours and spending some time outdoors is the most effective way to reset your body clock to the new time zone. Here's how.

DON'T MAKE THESE MISTAKES

If you need a morning cup of coffee to get you out of bed and to the airport in time for your flight, that's okay. Otherwise, says Dr. Anderson, you should avoid caffeine as well as alcohol and salty snacks during long flights—all contribute to dehydration.

Also, never take sleeping pills or melatonin pills (a synthetic form of the hormone produced by your brain when it is time to sleep sold over the counter) when flying unless you're under the supervision of your physician. The melatonin sold over the counter may be too strong and may actually extend jet lag by making you drowsy during the day.

When traveling east to west: Book mid-morning flights if possible. Once you reach your destination, spend some time outdoors if possible. Sunlight prompts the pituitary gland in your brain to release melatonin, a hormone that regulates your sleep-wake cycles. Plan a restful evening, but don't go to bed too early, so you get in sync with your new location.

When traveling west to east: Try to book so called "red-eye" flights that take off late at night and arrive in the morning so that you can sleep during the flight. To ensure in-flight sleep, consider packing an eyeshade to block out light, earplugs to shut out sound, and a small, comfortable pillow from home.

Stretch in the lavatory. For flights longer than 3 hours, take a few minutes to stretch to fight off muscle cramping and keep your blood circulating, especially in your legs. Lift both arms above your head. Move your head toward your right shoulder and then slowly move your head to your left shoulder. Then bend down from the waist and touch your fingertips on your shoe tops. Lift and bend your left knee with both hands. Then repeat this stretch with your right knee. Count slowly to 10 with each stretch.

Carry on some water. Bring a liter of water on board and drink 8 ounces for every hour you fly." ■

NASA ASTRONAUT BEATS JET LAG: "JUST DO IT"

If you think flying 3,000 miles and crossing two or three time zones is rough, consider what NASA astronaut Susan Kilrain experiences on a typical space shuttle flight. On one mission, Kilrain traveled 6.3 million miles, orbiting the earth 251 times in just over 2 weeks. The sun rose and set every 45 minutes, round the clock.

To prepare, the astronauts sat in rooms with very bright lights after midnight to fool their bodies into thinking it was morning every day for a week before liftoff. In the afternoons, they wore dark goggles to simulate night. Yet despite careful preparation, Kilrain still reacted to the abbreviated days and nights.

"As the sun comes up, you perk up," she says. "Forty-five minutes later when the sun goes down, you get tired." The work schedule and shared sleeping quarters on the shuttle didn't allow for naps. Shift work adds to the problem.

"You don't really adjust," says Kilrain. "You just do it."

Back on Earth, Kilrain lives in Houston and still works alternating shifts. And when she has time off, she flies to Germany to visit her husband for weeks at a time. Kilrain rarely tries to reset her body clock to the new time zone, 6 hours ahead. Instead, she sleeps while her husband is at work during the day, wakes up when he gets home, and stays up all night while he sleeps. "That way, we see each other the same hours, as if we were on the same schedule."

Job Change

Mixed Feelings? Navigate New Waters with Ease

Like marriage, a new job is cause for celebration. Someone likes you. Someone needs you. You can't wait to get started. Break out the champagne!

So why are you feeling so stressed out?

"Even under the best of circumstances, a job change is a major life stress, especially if you're uprooting a family and moving across the country," says management consultant Lynne McClure, Ph.D., in Phoenix. And now that one in five working women earn more than their husbands, it's increasingly women who are prompting the move.

"A job change can be very stressful for dual-career families," says Dr. McClure. "But sometimes it's the healthiest thing you can do." Low pay, lack of recognition, and a boss you don't get along with are all good reasons to make a change for the better.

The downside: You're leaving behind friends, familiar surroundings, and an established routine for an uncertain future. To ease the transition, follow this expert advice.

Grieve for what you're leaving behind. In one sense, a job change is not unlike a divorce or loss of a loved one. "Even if you hated your old job, there's a grieving process involved," Dr. McClure says. "Part of you has to grieve for the parts of the job you miss. If you don't, it will eventually catch up with you like all unfinished grieving."

Give yourself permission to worry. When starting a new job, many workers worry that they won't make a good impression if they can't waltz in and do the job perfectly. "It's natural to have misgivings about changing jobs," says Barbara Reinhold, Ed.D., director of the career development office at Smith College in Northampton, Massachusetts.

DON'T MAKE THESE MISTAKES

"The worst thing you can do is come in and say, 'We didn't do it that way where I used to work,'" says Dr. Manning. "The second worst mistake is badmouthing your former employer—people will tend to think you're the one who's difficult."

Ask for clear direction. Even if the job is the same as your old one, you'll still have to learn new procedures in byte-size chunks. So be clear about which tasks you're supposed to tackle first. "Don't expect to accomplish it all in a day," she adds. "It's going to take some time."

Scope out the social scene. As you settle into a new routine, remember what your mother told you in grade school: Pick your friends carefully. You're known by your associates.

"You don't know the politics, so tread lightly," says Marilyn Manning, Ph.D., management consultant in Mountain View, California.

"You could be befriended by the 'difficult' person, so don't identify yourself with any group too soon."

As a newcomer, try to associate with a variety of people: Eat lunch in different areas of the cafeteria, for example, or volunteer for such extra-curricular activities as the United Way committee, suggests Dr. Manning. ■

Jogging

Go from Walking to Running in 10 Weeks Even If You've Never Exercised Before

It happens every day. Women who want to lose weight or get in shape decide to take up jogging. So they lace up their sneakers, head out the door, and try a quick mile or two.

Half an hour later, they return home breathless and exhausted. The next day, their leg muscles scream in agony. Their career in running is over before it begins.

And that's a shame. Because if you go about it correctly, jogging can be an excellent way to shed unwanted pounds, strengthen your leg muscles, and give your heart and lungs the aerobic exercise that they need to serve you well for years, says Mona Shangold, M.D., director of the Center for Women's Health and Sports Gynecology in Philadelphia, who has run three marathons and jogs just about every day.

"If you want to take up running and haven't exercised before, the best way to start is with walking," says Budd Coates, an exercise physiologist and four-time Olympic Marathon Trials qualifier who trains beginning runners in Emmaus, Pennsylvania. "Continuous walking will slowly prepare your legs for running, prevent muscle soreness and injuries, and help you develop a consistent daily routine."

PLAY IT SAFE

Never run in remote areas, especially if you're running alone. If you don't have a buddy, run with a dog, or carry a self-defense spray. Don't approach a car if asked for directions, and never assume all runners are harmless.

Begin by walking 20 minutes a day for the first 4 days, then increase to 30 minutes a day for the following 4 days, says Coates. Then you'll be ready to run.

The following program, tailor-made for beginning runners, will turn a nonexerciser into a full-fledged jogger (without pain) in just 10 weeks. Coates suggests you do your run/walk workouts on Monday, Wednesday, Friday, and Saturday, and take Tuesday, Thursday, and Sunday off.

Week 1: Run 2 minutes, walk 4 minutes. Repeat four times. ››

Week 2: Run 3 minutes, walk 3 minutes. Repeat four times.

Week 3: Run 5 minutes, walk 2½ minutes. Repeat three times.

Week 4: Run 7 minutes, walk 3 minutes. Repeat two times.

Week 5: Run 8 minutes, walk 2 minutes. Repeat two times.

Week 6: Run 9 minutes, walk 2 minutes. Repeat, then run 8 minutes.

Week 7: Run 9 minutes, walk 1 minute. Repeat twice.

Week 8: Run 13 minutes, walk 2 minutes. Repeat.

Week 9: Run 14 minutes, walk 1 minute. Repeat.

Week 10: Run 30 minutes.

If you feel tired after completing a particular week, repeat that round of training before moving on to the following week.

Helpful Hint

Think of running in terms of minutes, not miles, until you're able to run a full 30 minutes. As a goal, time is less intimidating than distance. ■

Joint Pain and Stiffness

24 Ways to Stay Active Even If You Have Arthritis

Melanie J. Harrison, M.D., has spent nearly her entire life helping herself and others cope with arthritis. Diagnosed with juvenile rheumatoid arthritis as a toddler, Dr. Harrison, now 33, serves as an attending rheumatologist at the Hospital for Special Surgery in New York City, where she shares her expertise and empathy with men and women dealing with the kind of joint pain and swelling that she has experienced firsthand.

"With a few simple adaptations, you can do almost everything," says Dr. Harrison, who has developed some innovative strategies on her own. Even on the stickiest of summer days, she wears panty hose, for example. "My knees feel better with hose," she says.

Often used loosely to refer to pain and stiffness in the joints, arthritis actually includes more than 100 conditions affecting the body's joints, muscles, and connective tissues. Rheumatoid arthritis—an inflammatory type similar to that experienced by Dr. Harrison—isn't nearly as common as osteoarthritis, which generally strikes both women and men in their forties and older.

In normal joints, cartilage protects and cushions the ends of bones. With osteoarthritis, though, the cartilage breaks down, causing pain in the hips, knees, hands, and even the neck. Stiffness and pain can make it difficult for women with osteoarthritis to do what they need to do most: exercise the joint and surrounding muscles. "The less you move a joint, the more likely it is to become fixed," Dr. Harrison cautions. "Within a very short amount of time, you develop a limited range of motion."

If arthritis is making it harder for you to get out and do what you love—be it gardening, golf, or just getting going in the morning—consider these helpful tips from Dr. Harrison, the Arthritis Foundation, and other experts.

Keep Moving

1. Walk when you can. But avoid walking downhill, which puts more strain on the knees than walking on flat terrain. Devote some time to warmup and cooldown exercises, which provide even more protection against aches and pains.

2. Can't jog? **Try water aerobics or swimming.** Exercising in a warm (between 83° and 88°F) pool supports your joints and soothes arthritis stiffness.

3. Bring your sport indoors. Stationary cycles and rowing and skiing machines can be easier on your body than the original sports.

4. Mix up your exercise routine with dancing, low-impact aerobics and other gentle exercise. Varying your activities prevents not only boredom but also overuse of any one joint, reducing your risk of injury.

5. Build up your thigh muscles. "By building up the muscles around a joint, you strengthen the joint itself," says Dr. Harrison. She suggests this simple exercise for women with knee problems: Sit in a chair with both feet on the floor. Then raise one foot until

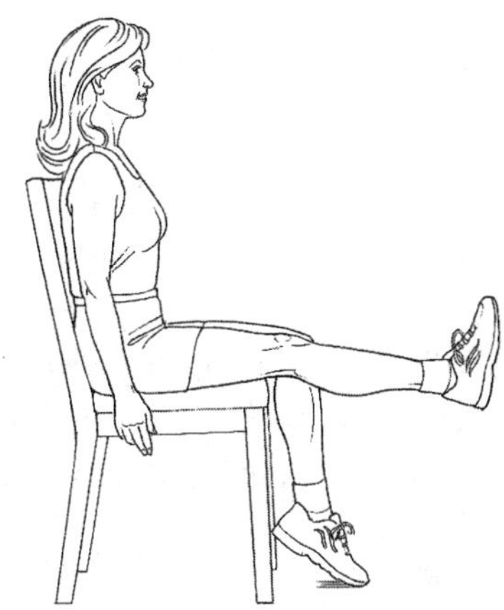

your leg is straight. Hold for 5 seconds. Lower your foot. Repeat with your other leg, doing 10 with each leg.

Stay in the Tennis Game

6. Play doubles tennis instead of singles—you don't have to work as hard to make a shot or chase down the ball.

7. Play with a shorter court. "Ping-pong tennis" uses just the service courts, widened to include the doubles alley. Use a bounce serve and always let the ball bounce before you hit it.

Golf to Your Heart's Content

8. Choose clubs with lightweight graphite shafts. They absorb shock better.

9. Switch to lower-compression balls (say, a 90 instead of a 100). They have more "give" when hit.

10. Use tees whenever you hit the ball, even when you're at the driving range. Hitting the ground can jar your joints.

11. Stabilize your wrist joints by wearing gloves or braces on both hands. Any golf glove will help your fingers grip the club, but finding the right wrist brace is trickier. Inline skating wrist protectors are too bulky for golfers. Instead, look for Neoprene wrist wraps or "resting splints" similar to what people with carpal tunnel syndrome use—shorter, more flexible plastic braces that won't interfere with your grip. Look for them in pharmacies or medical supply stores.

Garden Until You're 100 (or More)

12. Plant container gardens. Pots of peppers, tomatoes, herbs, and other plants can be more manageable than a full-size vegetable garden.

13. Buy or build raised garden boxes or terraces. You won't have to bend down to the ground to weed and plant.

14. Buy young plants instead of seeds. They're **››**

less labor-intensive than seeds, which require lots of hands-on TLC, from sowing to thinning, to survive and thrive.

15. Use long-handled garden tools so that you can stand instead of kneel when caring for your plants.

16. Instead of large, elaborate, high-maintenance shrubs, **grow dwarf trees or miniature fruit trees in pots** so that you don't have to do a lot of pruning.

Cook Up a Storm

17. Slide heat-resistant foam-rubber grips, sold in medical supply stores, over handles of saucepans and kitchen utensils, making them easier to grab and hold.

18. Use gadgets such as food processors, electric can openers, and other labor-saving electric appliances that cut down on troublesome culinary prep work and cleanup.

19. Reorganize your kitchen so your most-used utensils, pots, pans, and staples are stored at arm level to eye level, within an arm's reach, instead of tucked away in bottom cabinets where you

Kava

A Natural Sedative from Pacific Islanders

When English explorers and missionaries first visited the South Pacific islands in the 1700s, they noticed that the inhabitants were unusually calm and relaxed. The secret to their laid-back state? A native pepper plant known as kava-kava (or simply "kava"), used for centuries to make a ceremonial drink. Thus, kava earned its botanical name, *Piper methysticum,* or "intoxicating pepper."

In truth, kava relieves anxiety, relaxes muscles, and calms while promoting alertness. On islands like Tahiti and Fiji, it's a social beverage. Kava bars outnumber alcohol bars, and residents stay content and clearheaded.

"Pacific Islanders typically meet over kava after work to talk about their problems, unload them, and then go home feeling a bit euphoric and relaxed and ready to relate well with their families," says Hyla Cass, M.D., assistant clinical professor of psychiatry at the University of California, Los Angeles, UCLA School of Medicine and author of *Kava: Nature's Answer to Stress, Anxiety, and Insomnia.* "It's an excellent, natural sedative."

Dr. Cass sipped her first cup of kava in Samoa several years ago. Within seconds, her tongue was slightly numbed by the tea's pungent, muddy taste. Within minutes, she felt her entire body relax, her mind clear, and her mood elevate.

Curious, Dr. Cass decided to study this herb in detail. Among other noble qualities, she discovered that kava is nature's safe solution to stress-induced anxiety and insomnia. That's due in large part to its active ingredients, known as kavalachave to kneel to get them or above your head where you need to extend your reach.

No-Fuss Clothing Tips

20. Buy a button hook to help you fasten pesky buttons. Look for them in "independent living" or "adaptive aids" catalogs.

21. Wash and hang your shirts, blouses, and cardigans partially buttoned, with the top three buttons undone so you can pull them over your head each time you wear them.

22. Have Velcro fasteners sewn onto your bras instead of tiny hooks and snap-in-back design, which are frustrating for women with arthritis.

23. Buy walking shoes (or any shoes) with Velcro closures instead of shoelaces.

Bonus Tip

24. Doors equipped with levers are easier to open if you have arthritis in your hands. To convert knob handles into easier-to-use levers, look for doorknob adapters in specialty catalogs for people with special needs. ■

tones. Studies suggest that these constituents act on the limbic system, the brain's emotion headquarters, and directly relax your muscles. The real beauty of kava is that unlike prescription sedatives, it is nonaddictive and keeps users clearheaded.

If a pending airplane trip, a job change, marriage, divorce, or any other stressful event is leaving you anxious or unable to sleep, Dr. Cass says kava can help.

Ease anxiety. Keep yourself calm—but alert—by taking a standardized kava extract in capsule form two or three times a day. Since dosage is based on kavalactones, the extract should contain 40 to 70 milligrams of kavalactones per capsule. Do not exceed 70 milligrams per dose or 210 milligrams of kavalactones per day—it can be intoxicating in high doses. Alternately, you can take 40 drops of tincture three or four times a day.

Get a good night's sleep. If you have trouble sleeping, take a total of 135 to 250 milligrams 1 hour before you're ready to sleep or 1 to 2 dropperfuls of tincture. Kava does not interfere with the deepest sleep known as REM (rapid eye movement), so you'll be sure to get a good night's rest.

DON'T MAKE THIS MISTAKE

Do not take kava along with alcohol, barbiturates, or medications that depress the central nervous system, and do not take if you are pregnant or nursing. Also, don't take it for prolonged periods of time, or a temporary yellow rash may appear on your skin, hair, and nails. And don't use this herb before driving or operating equipment.

Helpful Hint

When buying kava, read labels and select standardized extract products containing 30 percent kavalactones. ■

Kegels

Recondition Your Leaky Bladder—With Biofeedback, Not Surgery

Lolly Morrison, a former operating room nurse from Brightwaters, New York, battled urinary incontinence for 38 years. Her bladder leaked urine at unpredictable times. At first, her doctors prescribed Kegel exercises—standard procedure for women with incontinence. To perform Kegels, you repeatedly contract and relax the pubococcygeal (PC) muscles, which hug your urinary tubes and stop and start the flow of urine. Doctors usually recommend practicing them four times a day—during meetings, at your desk, driving in your car, and so forth.

Kegels didn't work for Lolly (not her real name). In fact, her condition got worse. "I didn't know whether I was doing them right or whether I was capable of doing them," she remembers. "So I stopped."

Desperate for a cure, Lolly endured three surgeries and a lot of pain and frustration. And still, there was no change. Her doctor tried a collagen injection, which helped a little, but not for long. Then she was referred to Howard I. Glazer, Ph.D., clinical associate professor of psychology in obstetrics and gynecology and PC-muscles specialist at Cornell University Medical College in New York City, and she finally found relief.

Dr. Glazer used surface electromyography biofeedback (EMG), a computerized treatment method that measures the strength of the PC muscles (which run from the pubic bone to the tailbone). EMG gives you immediate feedback on whether or not you're doing your Kegel exercises properly.

After being treated for one month, Lolly no longer needed to wear incontinence pads—a daily accessory for the previous 10 years. **You can do standard Kegels until you're blue in the face, but unless you're doing them correctly, you're wasting your time.**

"Telling women to do them at a traffic light or by squeezing off the flow of urine is at the least ineffective and at the worst potentially harmful," says Dr. Glazer. The purpose of the PC muscles is to keep the uterus, bladder, and bowel in place. Weaknesses in these muscles can cause different types of incontinence, bowel problems, uterine prolapse (the uterus descends into the vagina), and inability to achieve orgasm or other sexual problems. And each condition affects different areas of the muscles that require their own unique set of exercises. And the only way to do Kegels correctly is with EMG."

EMG-assisted Kegels are taught in a doctor's office. A tamponlike sensor is inserted into your vagina. A wire connects the sensor plugs into a

WHERE TO FIND A PERSONAL KEGEL TRAINER

To find a doctor familiar with EMG (called biofeedback pelvic floor muscles specialists and urogynecologists), contact the following organizations. (If your doctor says that surgery is the only option you have to repair damaged pelvic floor muscles, get a second—or even third—opinion from a board-certified PC-muscles specialist familiar with EMG first. You may not need surgery after all.)

- **The Biofeedback Certification Institute of America**, 10200 West 44th Avenue, Suite 310, Wheat Ridge, CO 80033. Send a self-addressed, stamped, business-size envelope for free information and a national listing of board-certified practitioners. Or, visit their Web site to locate a doctor in your area at www.bcia.org.
- **American Association of Electrodiagnostic Medicine**, 421 First Avenue SW, Suite 300 East, Rochester, MN 55902. Check their Web site for a listing of member doctors at www.aaem.net.
- **American Urogynecologic Society**, 1200 19th Street, NW, Suite 300, Washington, DC 20036. You'll receive information on incontinence and other pelvic floor muscle conditions. Check their Web site for a listing of urogynecologists in your area at www.augs.org.
- **National Kidney and Urologic Diseases Information Clearinghouse**, 3 Information Way, Bethesda, MD 20892-3580. Write for free information on electromyography biofeedback and pelvic floor muscle disorders. No physician referrals are provided. Browse their Web site at www.niddk.nih.gov.

computer. First you do a number of Kegel exercises to test the muscles' strength. The computer analyzes what's going on, identifying weak spots that are causing your symptoms. "Using EMG, I can prescribe the right type of Kegel exercises to rehabilitate those muscles," says Dr. Glazer.

To perform the Kegel exercises on their own, women need to rent or buy a portable EMG trainer device. Before using this device, see a specialist to rule out other causes of incontinence, including infections, neurological disease, or hormonal problems. Also, see a biofeedback expert with special training in pelvic floor muscle rehab first so you can have the equipment properly demonstrated before using it at home," says Dr. Glazer.

EMG trainer devices are distributed primarily through hospitals, and though the cost varies, they may be covered by insurance depending on your policy.

Typically, you'd start doing 20 minutes of Kegels a day twice a day, then gradually cut back to 15 minutes three times a week, says Dr. Glazer. ■

Keloids

A Head-to-Toe Guide to Scar Prevention

For many women, especially African Americans, a cut, surgical incision, or other injury to the skin can lead to smooth, thick, elevated scar known as keloid.

These unsightly and sometimes painful protrusions can appear almost anywhere, but often form on the earlobes (if your ears are pierced) or on the shoulders or chest (if you have acne). Keloids can also form on your lower abdomen if you give birth by cesarean section.

"Keloids tend to run in families, so some women are more disposed to these scars than others," says Susan C. Taylor, M.D., a dermatologist at Society Hill Dermatology in Philadelphia.

Doctors don't know why African Americans and other women of color are more prone to keloids than Caucasians. "But you can make keloids smaller, eliminate the scars, or prevent them altogether," says Mary Ruth Buchness, M.D., associate professor of dermatology and medicine at New York Medical College in Valhalla and chief of dermatology at St. Vincent's Hospital and Medical Center in New York City. If keloids run in your family, here's what experts advise.

Pierced Ears, Navels, and Other Body Parts

You should never pierce any part of your body if you are prone to keloids. Foreign bodies in the skin, such as earrings, are a chronic irritation, says Dr. Buchness. If you are already pierced, wear 14- or 18-karat gold jewelry. An allergic reaction to nickel alloys found in costume jewelry can cause a rash, inflammation, a secondary infection, and—finally—a keloid, says Dr. Buchness.

Ask your doctor about wearing pressurized earrings after getting your ears pierced. They'll compress the area surrounding the hole and either prevent a keloid from forming or keep a small scar from getting bigger.

Never get a second or third hole in either ear if you have a keloid. (And don't even think of piercing any other part of your body.)

Everyday Cuts and Scrapes

• Before shaving your legs or underarms, lather generously with shaving cream or gel, and shave slowly. Replace the blade every 3 or 4 shaves to prevent cuts and skin irritations. And select a razor specifically designed for women.

• Wear elbow and knee pads and wrist and shin guards if you cycle or skate, to protect against accidental scrapes or abrasions.

Acne

• See a dermatologist if you're prone to acne on your chest and upper back. Your doctor can prescribe medication to clear up your blemishes and inject the pimples with a steroid to speed healing and prevent acne-related scars and keloids.

• Resist the urge to pop pimples. You can injure your skin and trigger a keloid.

Cesarean Section or Surgery

• If your doctor suggests a cesarean section, tell her if you're susceptible to keloids or if they run in your family.

• Ask your doctor about steroid injections, silicone patches, and scar-reducing creams to minimize the risk after a C-section or other surgery.

• Avoid any unnecessary surgery.

Helpful Hint

If you need surgery for any reason, your doctor can inject a steroid at the incision site 2 to 3 weeks after the procedure to prevent a keloid from forming.

If you want to have a keloid removed, find a dermatologist or plastic surgeon experienced in treating keloids of all types who can find the right solution for you. ■

Knee Pain

Three Ways to Get Back in Motion

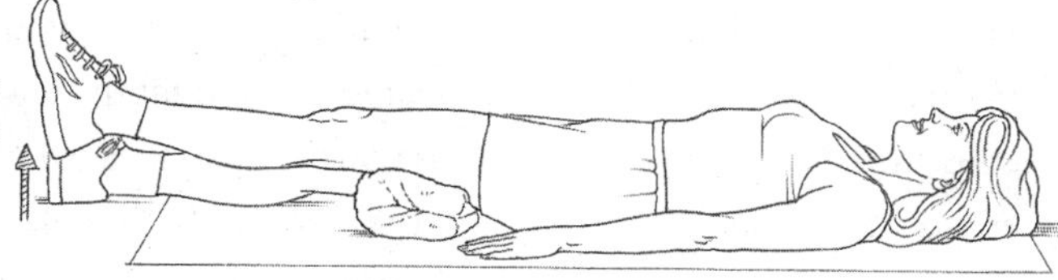

What do being a women and high-impact exercise have in common?

Patellofemeral stress syndrome, what we more commonly know as knee pain.

"Kneecap pain is one of the most common problems among women who exercise," says Paul Raether, M.D., physical medicine and rehabilitation specialist at Kaiser Permanente Medical Center in Portland, Oregon, and a former 2:16 marathon runner. "That's because women have wider hips than men, which causes their kneecaps to slide out of alignment during exercise. Normally, the kneecap slides up and down its track on the thighbone while exercising. When it goes off track, nerve endings are aggravated, and pain often results," he says.

You can alleviate (and prevent) knee pain by strengthening your quadriceps, the muscles in the front of your thighs. Strong quads will keep knees in place and can pull an errant kneecap back into alignment.

If you have problems with your knee or knees, the following three exercises will help strengthen your quads and quell the pain. Use them mainly to help prevent future flare-ups, but they are also effective to lessen pain while you are experiencing it. If you have any hip, back, or other musculoskeletal problems, check with your doctor first.

1. Short-arc leg extensions *(above).* Lie on your back on the floor with your legs outstretched in front of you. Place a rolled towel or cushion (about 6 inches thick) under the thigh of the affected leg. ››

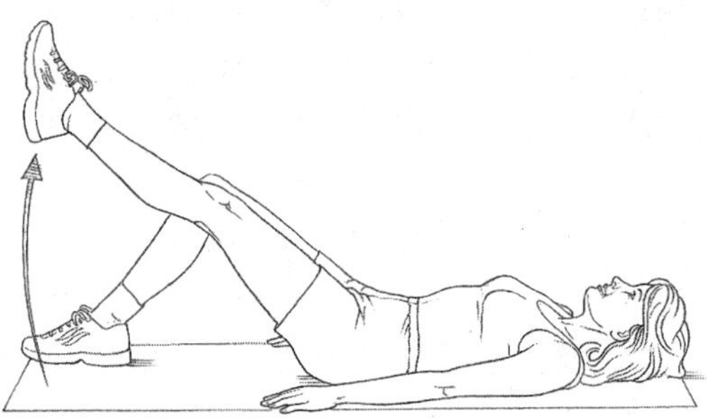

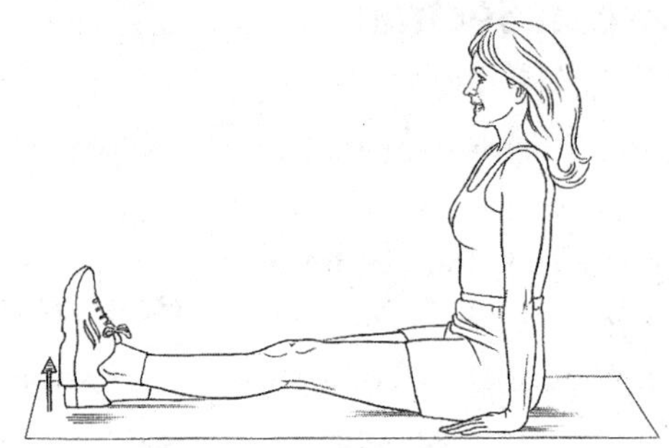

Tighten your thigh muscle as you raise your heel as high as possible while keeping your leg on the towel or cushion. Hold 5 seconds, then slowly lower your heel until your knee is straight, but avoid overextending your joint. Do three sets of 10 repetitions twice a day.

2. Straight-leg lifts *(top left).* Lie on your back on the floor and bend the knee of your unaffected leg. Tighten the quadriceps muscle of your affected leg, and lift the leg as high as your bent knee, as shown. Hold 5 seconds, then slowly lower your leg. Do three sets of 10 repetitions twice a day.

3. Quadriceps clenching *(top right).* Sit on the floor with your legs stretched out straight in front of you. Flex your foot and tighten the quadriceps muscle of your affected leg so that your heel rises slightly off the floor. Hold 5 seconds. Do three sets of 10 repetitions twice a day. ■

Labor Pain

A Gentle Way to Ease into Childbirth

It all began in the Garden of Eden. After Eve ate the forbidden fruit, God said he would greatly increase her pain in childbirth. And that's a reality to which all women who've borne children can relate.

When Cain and Abel came along, Eve didn't have Lamaze and prenatal exercise classes to see her through childbirth. She also didn't have the Alexander Technique, a unique process that can prepare you mentally, physically, and emotionally for the challenges of labor and delivery.

Luckily, you do.

How does it work? An instructor studies how you sit, stand, walk, and bend in order to teach you to correct your postural and tension-related habits and help you increase your awareness of how you might move more naturally. As a result, you'll minimize the common aches and pains of pregnancy, and you'll learn how to manage the pain and stay in control while delivering your baby, says Judith Stern, a physical therapist and Alexander Technique teacher in Rye, New York.

"We teach women how to free their breathing to remain calm during the birth," says Stern. "You learn how to relax between contractions, become aware of your body in preparation for the contractions to come, and stay focused on what your body is doing while paying attention to the labor process. And that takes skill," says Stern. What you learn from the Alexander Technique can be used alone or with other childbirth preparation techniques such as the Bradley and Lamaze methods.

The technique also helps you deal with the fear of giving birth and associated reactions to pain. "Fear is a major factor in how much pain you experience," says Stern. "So the less afraid you are, the less pain you'll have."

It takes anywhere from 10 to 30 sessions to learn the Alexander Technique. Sessions last 30 to 45 minutes and cost $45 to $100 each. The best time to start is the moment you learn that you're pregnant.

Here's a sampling of the type of exercises you'd be doing to prepare yourself for that big day, courtesy of Hope Gillerman, a board-certified Alexander Technique instructor in New York City and spokesperson for the American Society for the Alexander Technique.

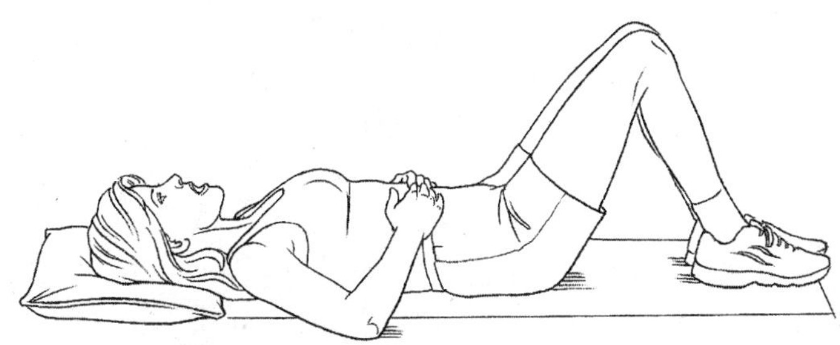

Breath control (*top*). Lie down on your back with your knees bent and your feet flat on the floor. Use an exercise mat or a blanket. Don't try this pose on a bed, as it is not firm enough. Support your head with a pillow. Start by exhaling through your mouth while whispering an "ah" sound (as in "father") until you run out of breath. Close your mouth and inhale through your nose. As you inhale, notice how easily your chest springs up as you fill your lungs with air. Repeat 10 times, or until you feel completely relaxed. Practice this exercise when you're feeling short of breath, tired, or irritable, says Gillerman. This is best performed in the early months of your pregnancy. If you are no longer comfortable lying on your back, try it on your side with pillows supporting your head, neck, back, and knees.

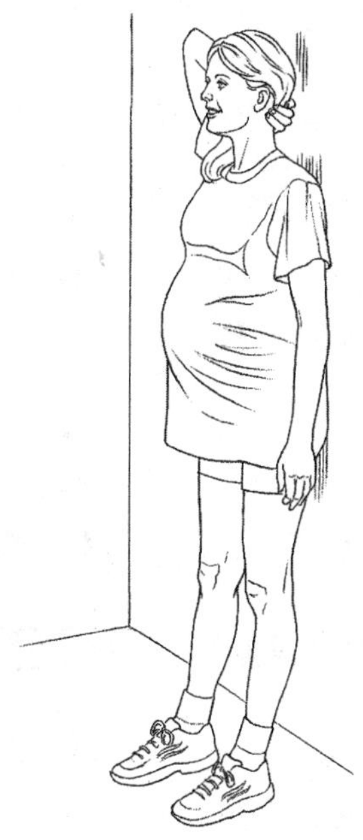

Muscle relaxation (*above*). Stand with your heels 6 inches from the wall, hip-width apart, with your back up leaning against the wall. (Your head should not be touching the »

wall.) Wrap one hand with your fingers together around the back of your neck. Tighten your neck muscles by jutting your chin forward. Hold for 2 seconds. Return your head and chin to their normal position while focusing on those muscles you've just tightened, and let the back of your head lift up off your shoulders. Repeat four times.

Back stretch (*right*). Facing the edge of an open door, with your arms straight but not locked, grasp both doorknobs with your hands. Your feet should be shoulder-width apart. As you hold the doorknobs, lean your whole body

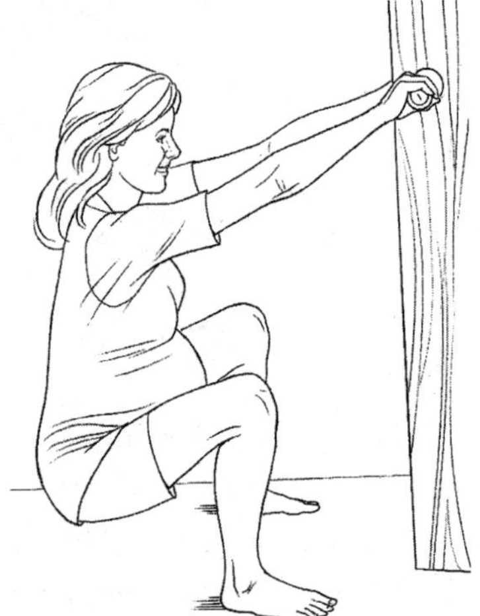

backward. Bend your legs as if you were going to sit in a chair, then continue into a squatting position until your hips are slightly below knee level. Make sure that your knees are aligned with your ankles and pointing straight forward, not out to the sides or in toward each other. Holding your head above your shoulders, not slumped forward, relax your neck muscles and drop your shoulders. Hold for 5 seconds and return to the starting position. Repeat four times.

Helpful Hint

Board-certified Alexander Technique instructors are qualified to prepare women for childbirth. To locate a teacher in your area, write to the American Society for the Alexander Technique, 401 East Market Street, Charlottesville, VA 22902. ■

Lactose Intolerance

More Calcium—Without Bloating

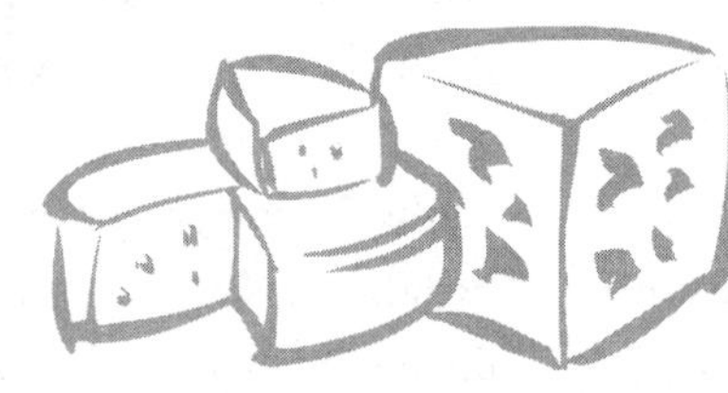

Once girls grow into women, some produce less lactase—the enzyme that digests lactose, the sugar naturally present in milk. If you have lactose intolerance, the undigested sugars in milk, ice cream, and other dairy products travel to the large intestine undigested. There, they ferment, producing hydrogen, carbon dioxide and other gases, causing bloating, cramping, gas, or diarrhea.

Not all women develop lactose intolerance. It seems to be inherited. If you're a Black American or of Asian heritage, you're more apt to develop lactose intolerance than White Americans with northern European backgrounds.

Problem is, you never outgrow your need for calcium, an essential bone-building mineral generously supplied by milk and milk products (like cheese). Avoiding dairy products puts you at risk for osteoporosis, marked by thin bones that break easily and tiny, painful fractures in your spine. After menopause, when production of the female hormone estrogens wanes, bones weaken even faster.

DON'T MAKE THIS MISTAKE

Don't automatically avoid all lactose-containing foods. Lactose tolerance varies, and some women may be able to digest small amounts of lactose, says Dr. Altman. Experiment to find your personal level of tolerance.

Women who switch to fat-free or reduced-fat milk may find it harder to digest than whole milk, because the fat in whole milk helps make lactose easier to digest.

But you have plenty of other options.

"Women who are lactose-intolerant should go out of their way to make sure they are getting enough calcium," says Daryl Altman, M.D., director of Allergy Information Services in Baldwin, New York. "Make it your goal to get calcium any way you can, even if you can't digest milk or dairy products." Here are some of her suggestions:

• Take a supplement that contains 1,200 milligrams of calcium every day.

• Buy lactose-reduced or lactose-free milk and cheese.

CALCIUM-RICH, LACTOSE-LIGHT

These foods supply a fair amount of calcium, but they're short on lactose. In comparison, an 8-ounce glass of milk has about 300 milligrams of calcium and about 13 grams of lactose.

Food	Calcium (mg)	Lactose (g)
Sardines, 3 oz	371	0
Soy milk	300	0
Molasses, 2 Tbsp	274	0
Oysters (raw), 1 cup	226	0
Tofu (processed with calcium salts), 3 oz	225	0
Turnip greens (cooked), 1 cup	194–249	0
Ice cream/ice milk, 8 oz	176	6–7
Salmon with bones (canned), 3 oz	167	0
Processed cheese, 1 oz	159–219	2–3
Chinese cabbage (bok choy; cooked), 1 cup	158	0
Collard greens (cooked), 1 cup	148–357	0
Milk (whole, low-fat, fat-free, buttermilk), 4 oz	146–158	6–7
Yogurt (plain), 4 oz	137–208	6–7
Sour cream, 4 oz	134	4–5
Kale (cooked), 1 cup	94–179	0
Broccoli (cooked), 1 cup	94–177	0

• Take lactase tablets to help you digest the lactose. (You can buy them at most pharmacies and supermarkets. Follow package directions.)

• Eat foods that are low in lactose but high in calcium. You'll get a host of other nutrients along with the calcium.

Helpful Hint

If you're lactose-intolerant, look for foods marked "parve" or "pareve." They don't contain milk, to conform to kosher food laws. For example, regular frankfurters may contain milk fillers, but kosher franks do not. ■

Laryngitis

Common (but Unsuspected) Causes and Cures

Sometimes, a throaty voice sounds sexy. But unless you're husky-voiced entertainer Brenda Vaccaro, laryngitis is more of a liability than an asset.

Laryngitis can be caused by any number of problems: Talking too much, straining your voice, a cold or throat infection, or excessive smoking or drinking all can leave your larynx irritated and inflamed. Take care of the cause, and your voice should return to normal. Allergies can also be a cause, says John A. Henderson, M.D., an ear, nose, and throat allergist and director of the Henderson Clinic in San Diego. Here are several ways to help get your voice back.

Soothe with steam. Turn your bathroom into a steam room by turning up the hot water and waiting for the steam to fill the air. Then inhale for 5 minutes. The moist air will soothe your vocal cords. You can use a humidifier to accomplish the same task, but be sure to clean it after every use. Otherwise, mold and mildew can build up in the device, and you'll risk exposing yourself to more voice-stealing particles.

Skip the cocktails. On its own, alcohol has a harsh effect on the delicate tissues of the voice box—it dehydrates your throat. But if you're prone to laryngitis, you'd do well to steer especially clear of dark-colored, fermented drinks such

DON'T MAKE THIS MISTAKE

Resist the tendency to whisper. Contrary to what you might think, it will strain your vocal cords and your throat more than speaking in a normal tone of voice will. And if hoarseness continues, see your doctor to rule out a tumor of any kind.

IS YOUR MATTRESS MAKING YOU HOARSE?

If you've ruled out common causes of laryngitis and still can't talk—or if you experience frequent episodes of laryngitis—your mattress may be the culprit.

"If you have recurrent laryngitis, you may have undetected allergies," says Dr. Henderson. "Molds, dust and dust mites are three of the most common culprits. And when you sit on a mattress, it kicks up a 2-foot-high cloud of particles from mold, mites and dust that you can't see, but you breathe all night long. The next morning, you wake up tired and with upper respiratory problems that can lead to laryngitis."

The solution: Buy a waterproofed mattress, or an allergy-sensitive mattress cover. These will seal out the particles that can cause allergy-induced laryngitis. Cover your water-proofed mattress with one or two mattress pads and the pillows with two or three cases. Or use your regular mattress with your allergy-sensitive cover. This, along with washing bedding twice a week in hot water, will control the mold, mites and dust you breathe.

as scotch and bourbon. Fermented liquors contain mold, a major allergen and hidden cause of laryngitis. You may not see it, but each time you imbibe the darker drinks, you're sending a load of mold straight down to your larynx, says Dr. Henderson.

Steer clear of cigarette and cigar smoke. Smoking aggravates the already dry mucous membrane lining of the larynx and covers it with polyps, or small lumps of tissue, especially in women with untreated allergies. This causes the larynx to thicken and become inflamed, which is why smokers often have raspier voices than others. ■

Lavender

A Tension Tamer That Fights Blemishes, Too

The purple-flowered lavender has worn many hats in its lifetime as a healer. In the Middle Ages, it was considered a dependable remedy for palsy, convulsions, and all manner of female "hysteria." Even in more enlightened times, aromatherapists say that the highly concentrated, or essential, oil of the lavender plant is a sure cure to help relieve skin problems, headache, insomnia, and stress.

"Aromatherapists consider lavender the universal healer. I never leave home without it," says Marilyn Johnson Kondwani, an aromatherapist in Stone Mountain, Georgia.

Here are just a few of the effective uses that Kondwani suggests.

As an acne fighter: For that ill-timed angry red pimple that pops up on your chin, cheek, or nose, chase it away by placing 1 drop of lavender oil directly on it. Repeat a drop as needed to restore smooth skin. Unlike other essentials oils that need to be diluted before they're applied, lavender is so gentle that you can apply it to the skin undiluted.

As a headache healer: For those temple throbbers, relax tightened muscles that constrict bloodflow and trigger headaches by dabbing 2 or more drops of lavender essential oil on each temple as needed. Gently rub in the lavender with a circular motion of your index fingers. The soothing scent of the oil can help melt tension fast.

As a neck pain pacifier: For muscle tightness in the neck area from hours of driving or a full day of stress, wet a washcloth with warm water and then wring it out. Put 3 to 5 drops of lavender essential oil on the cloth. Lay the warm, herbal-scented cloth across the back of your neck for a few minutes to relieve tension.

As a stress soother: When everyday hassles get you revved, restore tranquillity almost immediately. Find a quiet spot. Place 3 to 5 drops of lavender essential oil on a moist, cool washcloth (wring out the excess water), and place the cloth over your closed eyes. Clear your head of the day's clutter, then slowly and deeply inhale and exhale.

Or simply place an opened bottle of lavender essential oil about 6 inches from your nose and gently wave your hand over the top, breathing in lavender's calming aroma. ■

Leg Cramps

Stretch Away Middle-of-the-Night Pain

If you've ever had a nighttime muscle cramp, you've most likely heard of the common cure: Get out of bed and put your heel on the floor to get rid of a leg cramp.

"Getting out of bed with a leg cramp may be easier said than done, and putting your heel on the floor at that time is virtually impossible for some people," says Alison Lee, M.D., medical director of Barefoot Doctors in Ann Arbor, Michigan.

If you have a leg cramp and can't get out of bed, then:

Consciously relax and breath deeply. (Tensing up with pain only makes the cramp worse.)

Gently stretch the calf muscle, says Jessica Seaton, D.C., a Los Angeles chiropractic orthopedist. Lie on your back with the cramping leg in the air and pull your toes down, flexing the foot, until you feel a gentle calf stretch. (If you can't reach your toes, loop a towel or bathrobe belt around your foot.) Pull gently until the pain subsides, probably about 60 seconds. Don't force.

Massage the entire calf lightly, paying special attention to where it hurts the most. "Avoid deep massage—you may further injure the muscle," cautions Dr. Seaton.

To prevent leg cramps from recurring:

Quit smoking and get some exercise. "Two very common causes of night cramps in leg muscles are tobacco and inactivity," says Andrew T. Weil, M.D., director of the program in integrative medicine and clinical professor of internal medicine at the University of Arizona College of Medicine in Tucson.

If you have been exercising harder than usual, cut back. You may be exercising too vigor-

Light Therapy

Blast Your Way Out of Dead-of-Winter Depression

Joyce Fitzstephens spent her winter in a lethargic haze. Some days, she couldn't even get out of bed to get to her job as secretary at Western Michigan University in Kalamazoo. Her doctor dismissed her symptoms as depression. But Fitzstephens knew what depression felt like, and this was different. Her condition continued through the winter. "I kept trying to figure out what was wrong with me. I tried to exercise, and it felt like walking up a stone wall," recalls Fitzstephens.

Then came spring, and she sprang back to life—until the next November, when her winter doldrums hit again. Her doctor put her on antidepressants, which just made her apathetic. Then she read about seasonal affective disorder (SAD) and how to treat it. Her problem was solved.

SAD feels a lot like depression—you may feel blue, lethargic, irritable, indecisive, ously or too soon for your fitness level.

Drink plenty of water before, during, and after exercise and throughout the day. Dehydration is a common cause of muscle cramps, says Dr. Seaton. For tips on working eight 8-ounce glasses into your daily routine, see page 461.

Limber up and stretch your calf muscles before exercise.

Stretch a few times during the day, even on days you don't exercise.

Take a warm bath and stretch your calves before bedtime.

Quit caffeine, which may contribute to muscle tension and fluid loss. This should improve overall sleep quality as well.

If You Still Have Occasional Cramps . . .

Here's what else experts suggest.

- Magnesium supplements (500 to 1,000 milligrams per day). If you have kidney problems, check with your doctor before taking this supplement. If high doses give you diarrhea, cut back.
- Calcium supplements (1,000 to 1,500 milligrams per day)
- Foods that supply potassium (one banana daily, plus plenty of spinach, oranges, and other fresh fruits and vegetables)
- Tonic water (contains quinine, which may help prevent cramps). If you're prone to anemia, check with your doctor first.
- Quinine sulfate tablets, with a doctor's prescription

If leg cramps persist despite your efforts, see your doctor to rule out a vascular problem or other underlying condition that needs treatment.

Helpful Hint

Acupuncture sometimes succeeds when other methods fail. ■

uninterested in activity, and generally worthless. While depression has many possible causes, SAD is specifically linked to a decrease in natural light. Some experts theorize that a lack of light can affect hormones and brain chemicals related to our moods or energy levels. Whatever the cause, the result is the same: The darker the days, the darker your mood. As the days get brighter, so do you.

During the darker months of fall and winter, the best way to deal with SAD is to get some light therapy, explains Norman Rosenthal, M.D., senior researcher on biological rhythms at the National Institute of Mental Health in Bethesda, Maryland, and author of *Winter Blues*. This involves exposure to extremely bright light—25 to 100 times brighter than typical indoor lighting. To make sure you're getting that level of light, most doctors recommend renting or buying a light box, which is specially ›› designed to give you the dose of light you need. This can be expensive, however. Prices range from $250 to $500. Some health insurance plans may pay for part of the cost. Light boxes may be purchased through Apollo Light Systems, 352 West 1060 South, Orem, UT 84058, or The SunBox Company, 19217 Orbit Drive, Gaithersburg, MD 20879, among others.

If You Can't Afford a Light Box

Simply trying to get more light into your life may help. Dr. Rosenthal recommends these methods.

Get outdoors while it's daylight. In the winter, days are short, so it's best to try and get out during the brightest part of the day. So take a stroll in the late morning or during a lunch break. Always wear a sunscreen to protect your skin from the sun's ultraviolet rays.

Paint rooms a light color. This will help amplify whatever natural light may be coming through the windows.

Increase indoor light with lamps and skylights. Add mirrors, too, which reflect light and make a room even brighter.

Longevity

A Life-Extension Program That Pays Dividends Now

Ever wonder why your neighbor looks as though she's in her early forties, but is really 55? Or, why your 90-year-old grandmother has as much spunk and mental sharpness as women half her age?

"Some people don't just look young for their age, they are *young for their age," says Michael F. Roizen, M.D., a preventive gerontologist and professor of medicine, anesthesia, and critical care at the University of Chicago and author of* RealAge. *"They are physiologically and mentally as active and vibrant as those who are much younger. As a result, they live longer, healthier lives." And luck has little to do with it.*

"Genes do play part of the role," says Dr. Roizen. "But lifestyle choices and behaviors have far more impact on longevity and health than heredity." In fact, research conducted by Dr. Roizen shows that daily aerobic exercise; strength training; a low-fat, nutrient-rich diet; and lots of social interaction can make you feel up to 26 years *younger.*

Feasting on antiaging foods is one way to add years to your life and life to your years (see page 8). Here's what else Dr. Roizen recommends.

Pop a "life insurance" supplement. Taking a multivitamin each day will help ensure that you're getting all the nutrients you need even when you're not eating right. The best kind: One without added iron and with less than 8,000 IU of vitamin A. High iron intake may be linked to heart disease. Too much vitamin A can cause many problems, ranging from headaches and nausea to bone problems and liver damage.

You'll also want to supple-

DON'T MAKE THIS MISTAKE

Steer clear of tanning booths—they won't help SAD symptoms. Besides the fact that your eyes are covered during tanning sessions, the ultraviolet light given off by tanning beds doesn't work as well as other types of light. What's more, the UV light can damage your skin.

Eliminate anything that might block natural light. That includes hedges or branches in front of your windows. It also means washing windows regularly—you'd be surprised how much brighter a room looks with clean windows.

Plan a winter vacation in a sunny place.

Helpful Hint

Designate one room in your home as a "bright room." Ideally, it should have the biggest windows that let in the most light. Give it a bright coat of paint. Clear out all dark rugs and furniture, and fill it up with lamps and mirrors or other light-reflective surfaces. ■

ment with 600 milligrams or more (up to 2,000 milligrams) of vitamin C, 400 IU of vitamin E, and 1,200 milligrams of calcium daily, says Dr. Roizen. **Vitamin C and E are powerful antioxidants that mop up free radicals, those menacing molecules that damage cells, age arteries, and weaken your immune system.** Without them, you're at a greater risk for heart disease, cancer, and other forms of aging. Calcium preserves bone density, keeping your bones strong no matter how many candles you have on your birthday cake. Excess vitamin C may cause diarrhea in some people. If that happens, cut back.

Break a sweat. Daily aerobic exercise such as brisk walking, swimming, jogging, cycling, or dance aerobics slows down your body's aging process. How? "Any physical activity that gets your heart and lungs pumping will lower your risk of heart disease, heart attack, stroke, colon cancer, breast cancer, arthritis, and diabetes—debilitating diseases that prematurely age you," says Dr. Roizen. For example, in the Nurses' Health Study, an ongoing study of 80,000 women, researchers found that women who walked at least 3 hours per week had a 40 percent lower risk of heart attack and stroke than women who got little or no exercise.

Pump some iron. Unlike aerobic exercise, strength training—with dumbbells or weight machines—builds muscle. By building muscle, you'll get stronger. And that means that daily activities ››

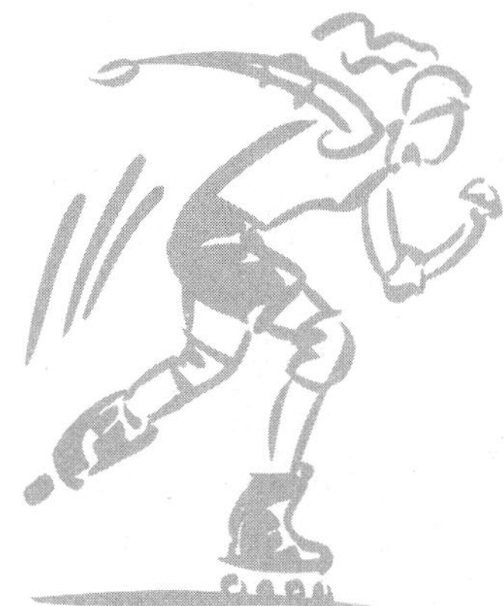

such as carrying groceries and walking up and down stairs won't be a chore, even as you age.

You'll also prevent osteoporosis (the loss of bone density) and the bone fractures that often follow, because strength training preserves and builds bone, says Dr. Roizen. Shoot for three weight-training workouts a week and make sure you exercise all your major muscle groups such as your chest, back, shoulders, arms, legs, and abdominals. **You can work out in a gym, but all you really need is a pair of 2- to 5-pound dumbbells or whatever is right for you.** Begin with a weight that you can comfortably do one set of 8 to 12 reps for each exercise. Then try to work up to two and finally three sets. (See the whole-body workout beginning on page 467.)

Brush and floss your teeth daily. Preliminary studies show that gingivitis and periodontal disease lead to the release of inflammatory or toxic substances and certain bacteria into the bloodstream. That, in turn, sets up an immune reaction that enables plaque to form in arteries, leading to heart disease and possibly stroke.

Eat breakfast. One study found that people who ate breakfast each day were less depressed and stressed than those who did not. Breakfast eaters were also less likely to smoke, plus they drank less alcohol and ate healthier diets, all factors that lead to longevity.

Get 7 hours of sleep a night. Sleep deprivation makes you more prone to accidents and other life-threatening situations.

Laugh more often. Laughter is a whole-body stress reducer that relieves anxiety and tension.

Get some sun—but not too much. Ten to 20 minutes of sun each day helps your body produce active vitamin D, which aids calcium absorption.

Own a dog—and walk it. Dog owners stay young longer, presumably because they get exercise caring for their dogs, and they benefit from the canine companionship. ■

STRENGTHEN YOUR FAITH

Lots of research shows that people who attend worship services regularly and practice their faith are far less likely to get sick and suffer from stress than people who don't.

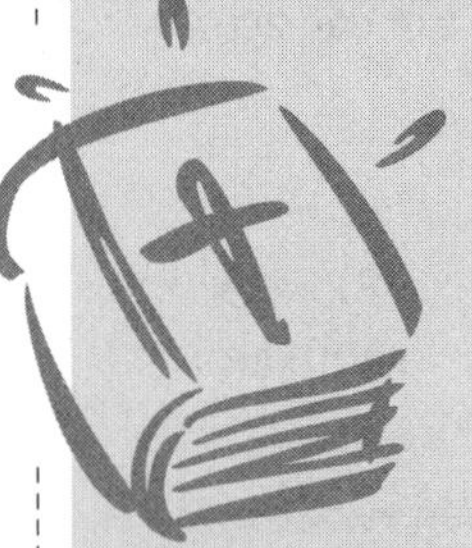

What's more, one study showed that women who attend church once a week or more are one-third less likely to die prematurely than those who don't. And that's after taking into account smoking, drinking, exercise, and weight status. Part of the reason: increased social interaction with fellow believers. As a result, they have lower blood pressure, lower incidences of heart disease, emphysema, suicide, and often recover faster from physical and mental illness. So you if don't already pray, meditate, or attend religious services regularly, now is a good time to start.

Lukewarm Sex

From So-So to Sizzling

If things have been a little, well, bland in the bedroom lately, you're not alone. Half of women over the age of 40 experience some decrease in sexual desire at this point in their lives. Or they're just not connecting as often as they'd like to.

There's no reason you and your husband shouldn't enjoy an exciting and fulfilling sex life for years ahead, says Patricia Love, Ed.D., sex educator and coauthor of Hot Monogamy. *The strategies that follow can create more sexual electricity between the sheets.*

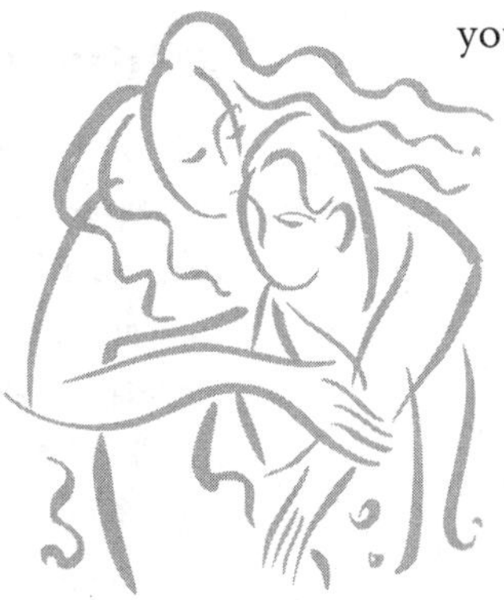

Try something new. "When women lose interest in sex, it's often because they're bored with the routine," says Dr. Love. "It's very common for lovemaking to become somewhat ho-hum if you do it the same way for 20 years." So try something different—you never know what will turn you on. A new position, new lingerie, or acting out fantasies with which you are both comfortable can breathe new life into your libido.

Try stop-and-go lovemaking. During foreplay, back off just as you get to the brink of orgasm. When your arousal decreases, start building toward climax again. "This type of 'teasing' builds momentum so that when you finally do climax, it will be more powerful," says Dr. Love. Performed properly, Kegel exercises can also strengthen your genital muscles, making orgasms stronger, says Dr. Love. (To learn more about Kegels, turn to page 248.)

Tune in to what you need. "Many women don't even know exactly what gets them in the mood, and often when they do know, they're afraid to ask their husbands for it," says Dr. Love. Think about what catches your eye in movies or books. Or, you may need more help with the kids, more time alone, or more time with your girlfriends. "For some women, the most powerful aphrodisiac is having her husband take the kids to the park for the morning so that she can sleep in." In any case, make sure your husband knows what you need.

Allow yourself to feel sexy. You probably already know that when your body image is low, you don't particularly feel like taking off your clothes and jumping into bed. "Do something to help yourself feel good about yourself—get a pedicure or a facial," says Dr. Love.

Help yourself to the aerobic aphrodisiac. "Exercise is one of the best things you can do to feel better about your body. And when you have an improved body image, an improved sex life almost invariably follows," says Dr. Love. Better yet, work out together as a couple.

Pretend you're on vacation. Ever wonder why sex seems to be better when you're on vacation? "When you're ›› away from home, you're removed from the stress of everyday life, and you have plenty of time on your hands," says Dr. Love. "And stress and lack of time are both deadly for the sex life." Early in a relationship, couples make plenty of time for each other, but as time passes, spending time together becomes less of a priority. But time is the very

VIAGRA FOR WOMEN?

Sold under the brand name Viagra, sildenafil is designed to be used to help boost sexual performance in men. But evidence indicates that the little blue pill helps women, too, says Bonnie Saks, M.D., clinical associate professor of psychiatry at the University of South Florida in Tampa. Among postmenopausal women she counsels, nearly 80 percent experienced higher sexual arousal after taking Viagra. The drug sustains vaginal lubrication and arousal, but it's not a magic pill—so communication, touching, listening, and other forms of intimacy are still key in having a healthy, satisfying sex life, says Dr. Saks.

Lyme Disease

How to Find and Remove a Tick

Standard advice for anyone who ventures outside in tick-infested areas, be it your backyard or the backwoods, is to check yourself for ticks, head to toe. And for good reason: Ticks may carry bacteria that cause Lyme disease and other infections. If untreated, Lyme disease may cause joint, nerve, and heart problems and occasionally, a serious, lingering illness that may resemble rheumatoid arthritis.

Doctors often overlook the symptoms of Lyme disease in women, assuming that they don't spend a lot of time in the woods and aren't at risk (an erroneous assumption). So you have to look out for yourself.

If you find a tick on yourself, don't panic. It takes 48 to 72 hours for a tick to infect your bloodstream. Don't delay, however—remove the tick immediately, says Laura Tenner, M.D., a dermatologist with Kaiser Permanente Medical Center in Hayward, California, who specializes in wilderness medicine.

Ticks can be really tough to pull off for two reasons, says Leonard Sigal, M.D., medical director of the American Lyme Disease Foundation, director of the Lyme Disease Center, and chief of the division of Rheumatology at the University of Medicine and Dentistry of New Jersey–Robert Wood Johnson Medical School in New Brunswick. "First, their mouthparts have reverse barbs, which make the upward tugging less effective in removal. Additionally, **ticks secrete cementum, which will literally cement their mouths to anyone they bite.**"

To remove a tick you'll need tweezers, sold in department stores, pharmacies, and best investment you can make in a relationship, says Dr. Love.

Helpful Hints

"Some women simply have less of the sex hormone testosterone and, therefore, a lower sex drive than others," says Dr. Love. "That's perfectly okay. You just need to make an extra effort to get in the mood." Make sure you communicate and tell your partner what you need to get turned on, says Love. You might need to set a weekly or monthly lovemaking date with your husband. It'll give you both something exciting to look forward to. Doing things to prepare for the date—like taking a bath, putting on perfume, or lighting candles—can help you to get in the mood.

Hormonal changes that occur after childbirth, as a result of taking birth control pills, or during menopause can cause a decline in libido, says Dr. Love. Hormone replacement therapy can help adjust these imbalances, or talk to your doctor about switching to a different type of birth control pill. ■

sports shops. Look for thin, sturdy, pointed tweezers that allow you to grasp the tick's mouthparts as close to your skin as possible, says Dr. Sigal. Pull in the opposite direction in a smooth, steady motion.

After removal, treat the skin with a first-aid antiseptic. If feasible, put the tick in a jar, to help your physician identify it.

Don't try to dig out any mouthparts that remain in your skin after removal. They're difficult to remove thoroughly, and you may do further damage. Leave them alone—they'll work their way out eventually, says Dr. Sigal.

If you spend a lot of time outdoors in areas where Lyme disease is prevalent (the Northeast, northern Midwest, and the northern Pacific states, for example), be sure to thoroughly check your entire body for ticks at the end of the day.

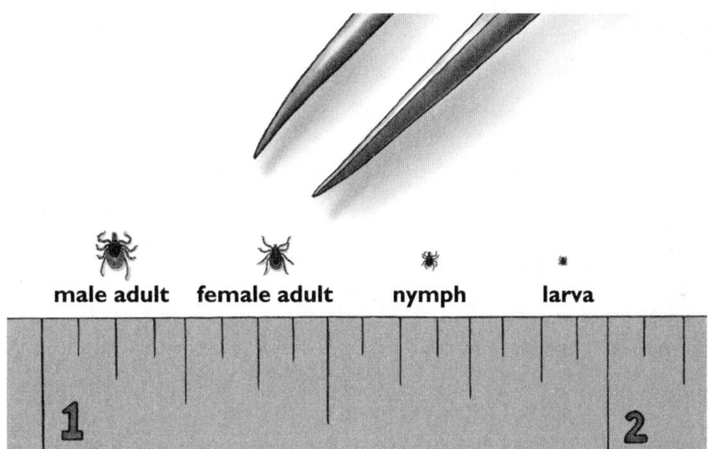

The deer tick that carries Lyme disease is orange-brown with a black spot near the head. It's tiny—the size of a poppy seed—when it is in the nymphal stage, and grows to $^1/_{16}$ of an inch as a female adult (shown here). The disease is most often spread by the female, usually (but not always) in the nymphal stage. To remove a tick, use thin, sturdy tweezers with pointed tips, as shown.

"You can get Lyme ››

disease right in your own backyard," explains Dr. Sigal, "but a tick does not survive for more than a few days on an open lawn in the bright sunshine." The possibility of coming across a tick is far greater in the leaf clutter, brush, or shrubs found at the edge of a forest, he says.

DON'T MAKE THIS MISTAKE

Don't put a lit match or hot pin on a tick to remove it. This rarely works, and it may cause ticks to regurgitate infectious secretions into your skin, says Dr. Tenner. And if you notice a ringlike rash on your skin and suspect a tick bite, see a doctor without delay. It's a symptom of Lyme disease.

Helpful Hint

If you spent a lot of time outdoors, your doctor may suggest a Lyme disease vaccine. Keep in mind that the vaccine takes 1 year to take effect, is not 100 percent effective, and doesn't protect against other infections carried by ticks. So even if you get the Lyme vaccine, it's still important to check yourself thoroughly for ticks and remove any you find. You should still wear insect repellent and long sleeves and pants when outdoors, says Dr. Tenner. ■

M

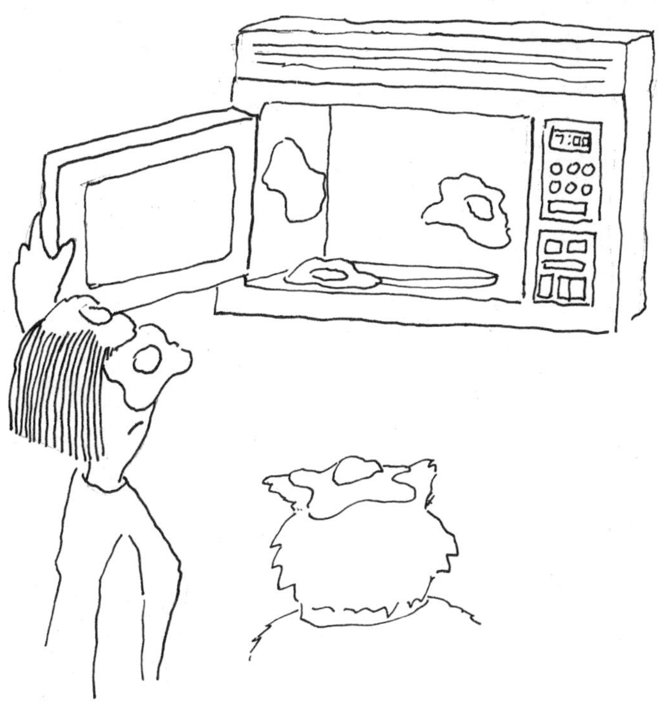

Eight foods you should never cook in the microwave (or you'll end up with egg on your face—literally).

See page 284.

Magnesium

Asthma? Breathe Easier with This Mineral

Your body contains no more than an ounce of magnesium. Yet that tiny amount of the mineral plays an active role in more than 300 bodily functions, helping muscles to contract, nerves to travel far and wide, bone to grow strong, and more.

Magnesium in the form of magnesium sulfate is the active ingredient in Epsom salts, sold in drugstores. A cup of Epsom salts poured into a warm bath relieves achy muscles.

For women with asthma, magnesium offers an extra-special blessing: Scientists are not sure why, but consuming magnesium seems to help reduce wheezing and other asthma symptoms, often aggravated by spasms in the smooth muscles that help your airways expand and contract as you breathe.

"Magnesium seems to have an antispasmodic effect on the smooth muscles of the upper respiratory tract," says John G. Gums, Pharm.D., professor of pharmacy and medicine at the University of Florida in Gainesville and a member of the National Magnesium Board.

A study conducted at the University of Nottingham City Hospital in the United Kingdom, for example, showed that **men and women diagnosed with asthma who took 400 milligrams of magnesium supplements daily experienced less airway obstruction than when they did not take these supplements.**

Though magnesium is available in a wide range of foods, experts say it's hard to get your Daily Value of 400 milligrams a day in your diet. **For maximum benefit, it is important to balance magnesium with your calcium intake,** says Judith Turnlund, R.D., Ph.D., a research nutrition scientist with the USDA Western Human Nutrition Research Center in Davis, California. The two minerals complement one another: Magnesium helps muscles relax, while calcium helps them contract. So if you're taking 1,200 milligrams of calcium, through food or supplements, you need 300 milligrams of magnesium.

12 HANDY WAYS TO GET MAGNESIUM

Experts encourage women to get as much magnesium as they can through food. Here are some top sources.

Food	Magnesium (mg)
Cashews (⅓ cup)	110
Sliced almonds (⅓ cup)	98
Halibut, baked (3 ounces)	90
Mackerel, baked (3 ounces)	82
Swiss chard, boiled (½ cup)	75
Artichoke (1)	72
Tofu (soybean curd), ½ cup	58
Potato, baked with skin	54
Navy beans (½ cup)	53
Peanut butter (2 tablespoons)	50
Watermelon (1 slice)	50
Spinach spaghetti (½ cup)	43

Helpful Hint

Supplements of magnesium oxide may cause diarrhea. If that's a problem for you, switch to magnesium gluconate. ■

Mammograms

Visualize a Pain-Free Exam

Elaine Filose, 52, had a severe case of mammogram phobia. The night before a mammogram, she worried herself sick. Her chest tightened and her heart raced with fear and anxiety, followed by stomach cramps and diarrhea. She couldn't eat, sleep, or stop herself from shaking.

Fears of breast cancer terrified Filose, and the discomfort of the exam didn't help. Her mammograms never showed any sign of cancer. Nevertheless, "I was a total wreck," says Filose.

After years of this annual ordeal, a good friend introduced Filose to Laurie Nadel, Ph.D., a doctor of clinical hypnotherapy in New York City who has coached many women in calming mammogram jitters.

After four sessions of relaxation and visualization exercises, Filose overcame her phobia.

"Just about every woman experiences a certain degree of apprehension when getting a mammogram," says Dr. Nadel, whose first mammogram was so painful that she put off scheduling another one for years. "I used mental imagery to pick up the phone and make another appointment."

The trick is to give yourself a boost by remembering a positive experience, says Dr. Nadel.

If your mammogram appointment is just

Marital Conflict

His and Hers Fighting Styles: Follow These Ground Rules

Many women have been taught to believe that the only functional marriage is an argument-free marriage.

"That's a myth," says Michele Weiner-Davis, couples counselor in Woodstock, Illinois, and author of Divorce Busting *and* Getting Through to the Man You Love. *"In any relationship, conflict is inevitable. Women need to know that. Happy couples simply find ways to deal with these differences."*

Money is the number one issue couples fight about, followed by children, chores, communication, in-laws, and careers.

Since women are the ones who typically bring up the subjects that men would rather not discuss, they need to know the ground rules.

Timing is everything. Ask your guy if now is a good time to talk. If not, ask if some other time within the next 24 hours would be better.

Start on a positive note. "The outcome of a chess game can be dictated by the first move. So, too, in conversation," Weiner-Davis says. Suppose you're upset that your husband hasn't been spending enough time with you lately. "Many women will say, 'I feel like you just don't care about my feelings.'" Weiner-Davis says. "At that point, he'll start to defend himself." Instead, around the corner, practice this exercise three times a day, then again just before you step up to the mammography plate.

Ball up your hands into fists. Close your eyes and think about a wonderful place where you once felt calm, relaxed, and safe. Remember the sights, sounds, and smells as you relive every moment.

To enhance your sense of peace, add more color to that picture-perfect place in your mind. Make the images larger or sharper, or increase the tightness of your fists until your calmness reaches its peak like a chord or music.

As your anxiety slowly fades, release your hands, shake them out, and open your eyes. To recapture that warm, fuzzy feeling, make those fists again and say to yourself, "Take me back."

The more you practice this exercise, the faster your brain will make the connection between your fists and total calm, says Dr. Nadel. "The painful part takes 3 seconds, then it's over. If you learn to quickly flood your body with feelings of happiness, you'll reduce the perception of anticipated pain."

Helpful Hint

Schedule your mammogram about 1 week after the last day of your menstrual period, when breast swelling and tenderness is minimal. Also, a few weeks before your appointment, cut down on caffeine and start taking 200 to 400 IU of vitamin E daily to further reduce discomfort. ■

turn your complaint into a compliment. Say, "I've really been missing you lately. I wonder if we could spend more time together."

Stick to the point. "A woman should list two or three points she wants to make, state them in a positive way, and stop talking," Weiner-Davis says. "If she's not succinct, she'll lose his attention."

Carefully scan his response. Although two-thirds of what he does say might be critical ("You're so invested with the kids that you wouldn't notice if I was around. You don't even notice what I do around the house."), the other third might be positive ("But I do agree it would be great if we could spend some time together"). "Filter out the stuff that won't lead anywhere and listen for those gems," Weiner-Davis says. "That's what you should respond to."

Fight fair. Take turns talking without interruption. Strive for clarity. Suggest compromises. If you don't reach an understanding immediately, give him a few days to come around.

If the temperature's rising, call a time out. ››

DON'T MAKE THIS MISTAKE

Resist the temptation to bring up every offense your spouse has ever committed. Stay focused on the here and now. "I've seen so many women go on and on about their feelings, giving example after example, and raising points from the past," Weiner-Davis says. "When they do that, they lose their partners."

You may enjoy a "lively" conversation, but he doesn't. "Women always complain that men shut down and don't want to talk," Weiner-Davis says. "But research shows that men tend to get more physiologically agitated than women do during heated debate." Clamming up is his way of calming down.

Find your make-up style. How you make up after a fight is as important as how you conduct it. Study what softens your man. "I used to think you shouldn't ever go to bed angry, but if I approach him in the evening when he's still angry, it'll make it worse. But if I approach him in the morning, he'll be Mr. Friendly."

Helpful Hints

With men, actions often speak louder than words. "A man once told me his wife had been nagging him for years to fix a leaky sink," Weiner-Davis says. "One day, while he was taking a shower, she stuck the necessary tools in the bathroom sink. When he got out, he immediately fixed the leak." ■

Marital Romance

Recreate Intimacy without Looking Silly

Over the years, women have been offered some incredibly silly advice about romancing a stone-cold marriage.

They've been told to wrap their naked bodies with cellophane and greet their husbands at the door with a dry martini. They've been instructed to lower their voices so they sound as seductive as Lauren Bacall. One women's magazine even advised its readers to drape themselves with Christmas-tree lights, a strategy that could be literally electrifying if a martini spilled in the wrong place.

"All that stuff is ridiculous," says Polly Young-Eisendrath, Ph.D., a psychologist in Burlington, Vermont, and author of You're Not What I Expected: Love after the Romance Has Ended *and* Women and Desire. *"Women need to find out what gives them pleasure."*

"Women spend all their time trying to fulfill some perfect image," Dr. Young-Eisendrath says. "Then they feel empty because they haven't explored their wants and pleasures."

"Women in marriages that have lasted a long time are especially likely to go on automatic pilot," adds Michele Weiner-Davis, a couples counselor in Woodstock, Illinois, and author of Divorce Busting.

START YOUR ENGINES

Don't wait until you feel romantic to take romantic action. If you grab the old bull by his horns, it might seem a bit awkward at first, but eventually, you'll experience more tender emotions. "Even the most inhibited woman can find the wild woman within," Weiner-Davis says.

Here's what you can do to find your pleasure points in a marriage that seemingly has lost its spark.

Discover what turns you on. "For some women, it's candlelight and romantic music," Dr. Young-Eisendrath says. "For others, it's just deep breathing." Experiment with touch, atmosphere, and context to find the combination that's right for you.

Remember your courting daze. "Every couple has a litany of actions they engaged in during more romantic times of their lives," Weiner-Davis says. "If you recall what those were, you have a blueprint for change, like giving each other cards, flowers, and gifts for no reason."

Get a babysitter and go steppin'. "Going out with your husband isn't the icing on the cake," Weiner-Davis says. "It *is* the cake. You can't afford to put your marriage on a back burner, even for your children. The best thing you can do for your children is to put your marriage first."

Surprise your guy. Men like surprises, too, including ones that don't cost any money. If your husband looks particularly sharp one morning on his way to work, pay him a compliment. If you see that his exercise program is working, playfully squeeze his bicep. A gesture like that can put him in a lovey-dovey mood for weeks. ■

Massage

How to Give Yourself the Perfect Neck Rub

Why does massage feel so good? Because it's good for *you.*

"Massage puts you in a relaxed state," says Tiffany Field, Ph.D., director of the Touch Research Institutes at the University of Miami School of Medicine and Nova Southeastern University, which study the effects of massage in five research centers around the world. Not simply a luxurious form of relaxation, the pressure of massage slows heart rate and blood pressure and reduces stress hormones. The reduction in stress hormones leads to increased immune function.

"Regular massages should be right up there with diet and exercise, because people are basically touch-deprived," says Dr. Field.

If you have the time or money for weekly trips to a professional massage therapist, great. If you don't, you can at least give yourself a tension-relieving neck rub (shown on page 274), says Laura Favin, a licensed massage therapist practicing in New York City. (Consult a doctor first if you've had a serious neck injury such as whiplash.)

1. Pre-massage stretch: Drop your chin toward your chest. Breathe. Drop your right ear toward your right shoulder, lowering the shoulder. Put your right hand on your ››

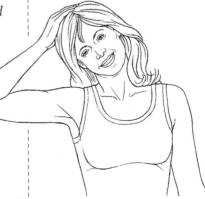

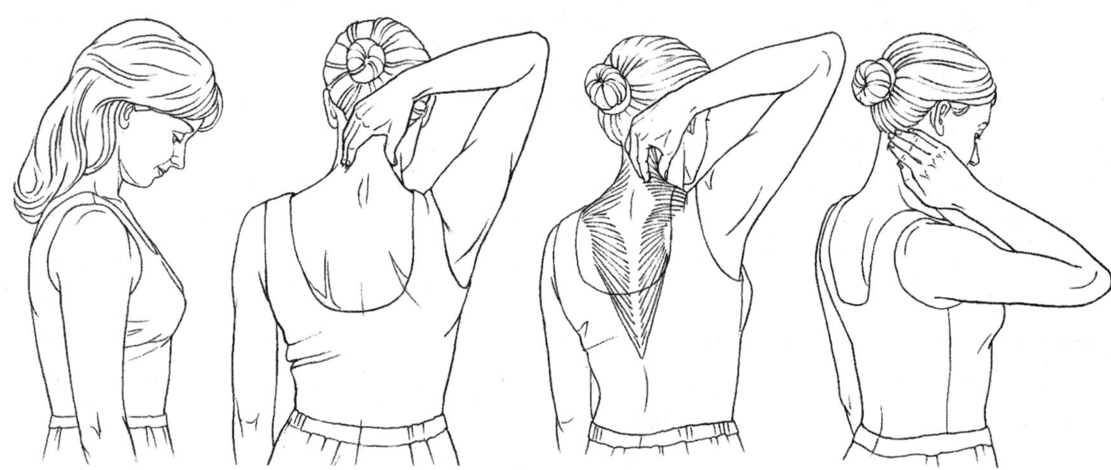

head and gently coax it down toward your shoulder. Repeat on the other side.

Helpful Hint

To find a certified massage therapist in your area, contact the national locator service of the American Massage Therapy Association at 820 Davis Street, Suite 100, Evanston, IL 60201-4444, or check their Web site at www.amtamassage.org.

2. Center your neck, letting the weight of your head gently pull your head forward.

3. Squeeze the back of your neck with your right hand, fingers on one side and thumb on the other. Start at the base and work your way up, squeezing and lifting the muscle away from either side of the vertebra. Knead upward as if you were kneading bread dough. Move your head up or down to reach different parts of the muscle.

4. With your right hand, pinch the muscle that goes from your neck to your right shoulder. Follow it down around the shoulder blades and rub with your fingertips, applying as much pressure as is comfortable.

5. Follow that muscle along the sides of the spine back up to the base of the skull and rub the ridge at the base of the skull.

6. Repeat steps 3 to 5 with the left hand on the left side. ■

Mastectomy

Tips for a Natural-Looking New Breast

Years ago, women had little choice but to stuff their bras with cloth or paper to simulate a breast removed due to cancer. Today, they can choose either breast reconstructive surgery or a prosthesis, an artifical breast that resembles a natural breast.

"A prosthesis is a nice choice for many women who can't bear the thought of or aren't physically able to have additional surgery," says Dixie Mills, M.D., a general surgeon specializing in breast surgery at Maine Medical Center in Portland. "The correctly fitted prosthesis can help you feel as comfortable and confident as you did before surgery."

Finding the right prosthesis has benefits beyond good looks (although that's important). When a breast is removed, one side of your chest weighs more than the other, which can cause poor posture and strain the muscles in your shoulders, neck, and back. "Because prostheses come in different weight measures, this won't be a problem," says Dr. Mills. "And you can wear one while you exercise and swim, which is important for your overall health and a full emotional recovery."

Ask your surgeon to refer you to a professional prosthesis fitter, and follow these tips.

Consider the type of breast surgery you've had. Specific shapes and sizes are required for women who've had, say, a radical versus a modified mastectomy, or a lumpectomy. Your fitter should match the texture and shape of the prosthesis to your healthy breast so that it looks natural, says Josephine Murphy, a prosthesis consultant at Evelyn H. Lauder Breast Center Memorial Sloan Kettering Cancer Center in New York City.

Buy a surgical bra with a built-in pocket to hold the prosthesis. Your fitter (often an employee of a shop that sells lingerie or undergarments for women who've had mastectomies) can find the right one for you—they're specially trained. Or, ask your fitter to sew pockets into the bras you already own, including exercise bras. If you want to wear a strapless dress, a prosthesis that adheres directly to your body is another option. Many insurance companies, including Medicare and Medicaid, will cover the cost of surgical bras and prostheses.

If you swim, ask for a prosthesis that's made for the water. Your fitter can sew a pocket into a swimsuit's bra. Or, she can provide you one with pockets to accommodate the prosthesis.

Helpful Hint

Ask yourself: Does the prosthesis match the size, shape, skin tone, and texture of your healthy breast? Do you like the bras you've chosen? Does the prosthesis fit well inside your bras? When you wear the prosthesis directly on your chest, does it feel comfortable? Does it look natural in your clothes? "If you answer yes to all of these questions, then you've chosen the right prosthesis," says Murphy. ■

Meditation

A Speed Bump against Stress

Every workday morning, Linda Ferris rushes out of her home in Ventura, California, at 6:30 A.M. and—on a good day—returns home at 7:00 P.M. As a sales director for a large electronics company, a typical work week includes meetings with branch managers and salespeople, several presentations, and two or three plane trips.

As if her schedule weren't stressful enough, Ferris sustained a head injury in an automobile accident caused by a drunk driver. The headaches were intolerable, aggravated by her job stress.

Ferris didn't try to slow her work pace, though. She didn't know how. She just kept on going, despite the pain.

Then Ferris learned meditation for stress and pain management, and turned her life around. "I learned to stop and take care of myself. Sometimes, between sales calls, I pull my car over and meditate at the side of the road. My headaches have gotten much better. When I do get one, I know how to handle it, and they no longer take over my life."

"There's a cost to extending yourself," says Margaret Caudill, M.D., Ph.D., codirector of the Department of Pain Medicine at Dartmouth Hitchcock in Manchester, New Hampshire, and author of *Managing Pain Before It Manages You*. "You can't use your debit unless you put money in the account. We have to give back to the body, particularly as we age," says Dr. Caudill, who taught Ferris how to meditate.

Meditation—repetition of a thought, word, or focus over an extended period of time—is one effective way to give back to the body. "When the mind wanders, you direct it back to the focus," explains Dr. Caudill. **The repetitive focus of meditation, similar to repetitive prayer, elicits the relaxation response, which quiets the body.**

Mediterranean Diet

Eat More Garbanzos, Less Pepperoni

You've probably heard that the Mediterranean diet promotes health by protecting against cancer and heart disease. And it does. But that doesn't necessarily mean you can feast on baklava and pepperoni pizza.

Even experts are sometimes confused about what constitutes a Mediterranean diet. Women in Athens don't cook the same foods that women in Naples do, for example. Even within Italy and Greece, people eat different foods from region to region. And the working classes eat differently from the rich.

In fact, experts say the ideal Mediterranean diet is typical to what the working class in Crete, Greece, and southern Italy ate in the 1950s and early 1960s: Vegetables, fruits, whole grains, peas, beans, olive oil, and fish were mainstays.

Some types of meditation (like prayer) are defined by a certain belief system, others simply by a specific focus. "You can focus on a candle flame, a rippling brook, the rain on the roof," says Dr. Caudill.

Breathing is an important part of meditation. "Many women aren't aware of how much the breath is altered with anxiety and negative moods," says Dr. Caudill. You can prove this by making a fist. What happens to your breathing? "It's automatic to hold your breath when you create tension," she says. **Meditation teaches you to relax through attention to breathing.**

To put the brakes on tension and stress, learn this basic breathing meditation and practice it whenever you feel like you're on a runaway train.

1. Sit up straight, either in a chair or on a pillow on the floor with your legs crossed.

2. Breathe in and out slowly, for a count of 10, without thinking of anything—just being aware of your breathing. Continue for 5 to 10 minutes.

Helpful Hint

If you think you don't have time to meditate, combine it with exercise, suggests Dr. Caudill. Match your breathing rhythm with the movement of your legs as you use a treadmill or stationary bike or walk in a quiet place. Take a passive approach by again letting go of your thoughts, letting them float away, no matter what your focus point is.

3. If your mind gets distracted, start counting again at 1.

4. When thoughts float into your mind, picture them as fish in an aquarium. Label them "thoughts" and let them swim away as you go back to focusing on your breathing.

"After a while, your breathing will start to slow down and get deeper," says Laurie Nadel, Ph.D., a psychotherapist in New York City who specializes in mind/body therapies for stress-related conditions. "Your focus and sense of calm improves." ■

Dessert was fresh fruit, not sweets, and red meat was eaten rarely.

Many studies support the health benefits of the Mediterranean diet. Best known is the Lyon Diet Heart Study, which followed 605 men and women from Lyon—the gourmet capital of France known for its rich cuisine—who'd had heart attacks. Half went on the Mediterranean diet described earlier. The others ate less fat but also ate fewer plant foods (vegetables, fruit, grains, legumes) and more animal foods (meat and dairy products). After 4 years, fewer of the men and women on the Mediterranean diet died of heart disease, cancer, or other causes. **And they found the Mediterranean diet easy to stick to.**

The Mediterranean diet contains more fat—about 40 percent of calories—than the 30 percent or less amount that doctors usually recommend. But the primary source of fat is olive oil, which is very low in saturated fat, so it's less apt to raise cholesterol.

"Mediterraneans also consume enormous quantities of vegetables and legumes," says Dimitrios Trichopoulos, M.D., professor of cancer preven- ››

tion and epidemiology at Harvard School of Public Health. Growing up in the 1950s in Greece, he recalls that most people were poor and ate very little meat. "And in the 1960s, Greece had the lowest mortality among adults in Europe, even though they had poor medical care—and smoked."

In addition to diet, Dr. Trichopoulos credits the Mediterranean tradition of a daily siesta and plenty of exercise (Mediterraneans had to do a lot of walking to get around.) **He offers these simple guidelines for adopting the best traits of the Mediterranean diet and lifestyle.**

- Use olive oil instead of butter or other vegetable oils.

DON'T MAKE THIS MISTAKE

If you're trying to lose weight, go easy on fat, even if it's olive oil. It's still 100 percent fat and a plentiful source of calories, about 120 per tablespoon.

- Eat generous portions of vegetables, fruits, legumes, and salads.
- Eat moderate amounts of fish and seafood.
- Eat minimal amounts of red meat, margarine, saturated fat, and animal fat.
- Choose whole grains rather than white bread.
- Eat lots of tomatoes. (Cooked may be healthier than raw). They contain lycopene, which is a red pigment that seems to protect against some cancers.
- Use garlic freely. It's been shown to lower cholesterol and may thin the blood, which might help prevent heart disease and stroke.
- Get more physical activity.

The Mediterranean diet also includes a glass or two of wine with dinner.

If you're at risk for breast cancer, you may want to omit the wine, because alcohol in any form may increase that risk, says Dr. Trichopoulos. (Same goes if you need to avoid alcohol for other reasons.) ■

Menopause

Herbs That Work with, Not against, Hormones

At around age 40, production of female hormones like estrogen and progesterone begins to dwindle. Your body is easing out of its reproductive responsibilities. As you reach your fifties, they drop sharply,and you've officially reached menopause.

"Menopause is a powerful and profound rite of passage," says Susun S. Weed, an herbalist and herbal educator from Woodstock, New York, and author of the Wise Woman *series of herbal health books, including* Menopausal Years: The Wise Woman Way. *"It gives a woman the opportunity to realize her full potential and strength as a human being. And it's a time to take extra special care of her bones and her heart."*

Menopause has system-wide effects. Increased hormones trigger hot flashes and other annoyances and may precipitate changes in your heart and bones unless you get lots of minerals and high-quality fats, explains Weed. Minerals protect your heart, and fats provide raw materials to make estrogen. Estrogen reduces total cholesterol and raises HDL cholesterol. And it helps your body pump calcium to your bones. When estrogen dwindles, you lose those protective effects.

Luckily, nature provides women with a number of herbs that can protect and nourish heart and bones. Some contain high levels of calcium, which keeps bones strong, and magnesium, which helps bones absorb calcium.

Black cohosh. Used for centuries by Native American women—long before the Pilgrims settled in North America—black cohosh has been approved by Germany's Commission E (similar to our FDA) for the relief of hot flashes and other menopausal symptoms.

Researchers deem black cohosh a good alternative to hormone replacement therapy, which can increase a woman's risk for high blood pressure, vaginal bleeding, and endometrial and breast cancer. In fact, evidence suggests that black cohosh may boost the ability of the drug tamoxifen to slow the growth of breast cancer cells.

In rare cases, women report mild stomach upset, headache, dizziness, weight gain, nausea, vomiting, and uterine contractions when taking black cohosh. If you experience any of these symptoms, stop using it. Black cohosh should not be used for more than 6 months.

Hawthorn. This herb relaxes and widens coronary arteries, rebuilds blood vessels, and strengthens the heart muscle, helping to counteract any tendency among women to develop heart disease. You can drink a potent tea (or infusion) of hawthorn daily, but take a week off every 8 weeks, advises Lisa Alschuler, N.D., a naturopathic physician and chair of the department of botanical medicine at Bastyr University in Bothell, Washington. If you've already been diagnosed with a heart condition, talk to your doctor before trying hawthorn.

Red clover. Red clover tastes like black tea and has 10 times more plant estrogens (phytoestrogens) than soy, says Weed. It's known for strengthening your heart and lungs, and keeping your breasts healthy. The herb is also loaded with calcium, chromium, magnesium, niacin, potassium, selenium, phosphorus, and vitamins A and C. According to Weed, an 8-ounce cup of infusion yields 375 milligrams of calcium and 88 milligrams of magnesium. (An 8-ounce glass of milk contains 300 milligrams of calcium.)

Stinging nettle. "Nettle is a wonderful menopause ally," says Weed. "It keeps your heart healthy, your bones strong, and your menopausal journey on a smooth road." This herb brims with calcium, magnesium, iron, phosphorus, selenium, and other minerals that build bone. And it contains vitamin D to keep bones flexible, says Weed. An 8-ounce cup of the infusion provides 250 milligrams of calcium and 215 milligrams of magnesium, according to Weed.

Oatstraw. Nicknamed "herbal Viagra" because it nourishes the sex drive, oatstraw also contains calcium, magnesium, chromium, silicon, and other potent minerals to strengthen your heart, bones, and nerves, says Weed. An 8-ounce cup of infusion contains 375 milligrams of calcium and 300 milligrams of ❯❯

magnesium. Do not use if you have celiac disease (gluten intolerance), as it contains gluten, a grain protein.

Helpful Hint

The beneficial minerals in the herbs mentioned here aren't available in tinctures or capsules. To get the health benefits of these mineral-rich herbs, advises Weed, you need to make an infusion—a lot of dried herb brewed for a long time. Place 1 ounce of the dried herb in a quart jar. Fill it with boiling water. Seal it tightly and allow it to sit for 4 to 8 hours. Drink at least 1 cup of the strained liquid and up to a quart a day. The infusion will last up to 2 days in the refrigerator. For best results, take one herb for a day or two, then switch to another one. Mint can be added to give the herbs a lift. ■

Menstrual Cramps

A Nutritional Prescription for Periodic Pain

As a young woman, Jeanne Wallace, Ph.D., suffered from severe menstrual cramps that made her miserable. "I would throw up. I'd miss 2 days of school," she recalls. "I'd lie on the bathroom floor wishing I was dead." Even massive quantities of ibuprofen—24 capsules in a 24-hour period, she admits—failed to bring her relief.

Today, the certified nutrition consultant is cramp-free, thanks to a nutritional regimen that she devised and tested based on scientific research. "I finally gave up on the drugs," Dr. Wallace says.

Menstrual cramps—and the gastrointestinal discomfort that may accompany them—stem from chemicals known as prostaglandins, which are released in abundance during menstruation and cause your uterus to contract. Over-the-counter menstrual painkillers such as ibuprofen (in Midol IB, for example) block the formation of these inflammatory prostaglandins, preventing the contractions. But these drugs don't always work. Your body can also make isoprostanes, which cause cramps, too, but don't respond to ibuprofen or similar drugs (such as Pamprin, which contains acetaminophen.)

Give your body the right nutrients, though, and you can stop cramps before they start.

Eat more fish, dark leafy greens, and flaxseed oil. These are high in omega-3 fatty acids, which create anti-inflammatory prostaglandins—not agonizing cramps.

DON'T MAKE THIS MISTAKE

Herbalists often recommend evening primrose oil for PMS, but it shouldn't be used to relieve menstrual cramps, since it contains omega-6 fatty acids that can stimulate inflammatory prostaglandins, Dr. Wallace says.

Cut down on meat. Meat contains omega-6 fatty acids, which stimulate cramp-producing prostaglandins. Omega-6's are also found in corn, safflower, soybean, and sunflower oils.

"You should have about a 1-to-1 ratio of omega-3's to omega-6's in your diet if you're trying to get rid of cramps," Dr. Wallace says. "Most women's ratios are more like 1 to 20 or 1 to 40."

WHEN TO SEE THE DOCTOR

If you experience severe abdominal pain associated with missed or delayed periods, see your gynecologist, says Dr. Rao. You may need medical treatment. Same goes if you experience any of the following:

- Menstrual cycles shorter than 21 days or more than 45 days long
- Skipping two cycles
- Periods lasting longer than 10 days
- Heavy soaking of tampons or pads, especially when accompanied by dizziness and fatigue (a possible indication of iron-deficiency anemia)
- Bleeding between periods
- Severe cramps or pain unrelieved by over-the-counter medications

Consider Supplements

Omega-3's. Two tablespoons of flaxseed oil daily will boost the levels of omega-3's in your body—the "good" fatty acids you want. Use it to replace other oils in salad dressings. Because flaxseed oil is sensitive to heat, don't use it for cooking. You can take a fish oil supplement with at least 1.8 grams of omega-3 fatty acids twice daily. Or, eat three servings weekly of fish that contain omega-3's, such as salmon, lake trout, bluefish, mackerel, herring, sardines, or tuna.

Vitamin E. Taking 400 IU of vitamin E daily will support the cramp-reducing properties of omega-3 fatty acids and prevent unstable compounds known as free radicals from creating inflammatory prostaglandins, Dr. Wallace explains.

Magnesium. A muscle relaxant, magnesium will also inhibit the production of inflammatory prostaglandins. Take a total of 400 milligrams daily, splitting that between two doses, advises Dr. Wallace. Women with heart or kidney problems should check with their doctors before taking supplemental magnesium. Supplemental magnesium may cause diarrhea in some people.

Vitamin B_6. This vitamin works with magnesium to create anti-inflammatory prostaglandins, but women generally don't get enough B_6. Dr. Wallace recommends taking 100 milligrams daily during cramping, 25 to 50 milligrams daily otherwise.

Niacin. This B vitamin can help convert omega-6 fatty acids into the anti-inflammatory prostaglandins you want. Dr. Wallace recommends taking 25 to 50 milligrams of niacin daily (look for supplements labeled "flush-free" or "nonflush"), and during your period, upping that dose to 100 milligrams twice daily. ››

Doses above 35 milligrams must be taken under medical supervision. And if you have diabetes, check with your doctor before supplementing with niacin. Women with liver disease, gout, or peptic ulcers should also stay away from niacin supplements.

Other antioxidants. To prevent free radicals from creating isoprostanes—and cramps—in your body, Dr. Wallace suggests taking 500 to 1,000 milligrams of vitamin C and 10,000 IU of natural beta-carotene with mixed carotenoids daily.

Helpful Hint

If you're feeling crampish, indulge in Indian food. As little as one-quarter teaspoon of turmeric can give you the anticramp and antioxidant power you need. Other culinary cramp fighters include garlic (one clove daily) and ginger (steep ½ inch gingerroot in 1 cup of water for 10 minutes for an anticramp ginger tea). ■

Menstrual Irregularities

Get Back on Track with This Herb

You're not pregnant. You're not approaching menopause. And your doctor has ruled out fibroids, endometriosis, and polycystic ovary disease. But for some reason, your periods have become erratic: They may come every 22, 35, or 45 days or at completely irregular intervals. What's going on?

"Probably nothing. You're perfectly normal," says Meena Rao, M.D., assistant professor of obstetrics and gynecology at Emory University School of Medicine in Atlanta. "Anytime you have a period that's 22 to 45 days apart, and there are no underlying reproductive health problems, there's really no cause for alarm. Your period is just late."

That's a relief. But if you're one of those women who hates having no idea when her period might start, you may want to try the herb chasteberry.

"It's the best herb you can use to regulate your period," says Tori Hudson, N.D., a naturopathic physician, professor at the National College of Naturopathic Medicine, and medical director of A Woman's Time, a women's natural health clinic in Portland, Oregon. Chasteberry stabilizes your reproductive hormones so you'll ovulate consistently—and on schedule.

Take one pill of the standardized extract or 40 drops of the tincture every day for 3 to 4 months. Just be patient. Your cycle will likely return to its old predictable self. If you're taking birth control pills and want to try chasteberry for health problems of any sort, be forewarned: Chasteberry can interfere with the effectiveness of birth control pills. ■

Metabolism

The Only *Real* Way to Burn More Calories

A lot of women are frustrated to find themselves gaining 10 pounds at midlife for no obvious reason. They aren't eating any more than usual. Or they're eating less, but can't seem to drop an ounce.

The problem? Slow metabolism.

Aging per se doesn't slow your metabolism (the rate at which your body processes food, stores energy, and burns calories). What does slow metabolism are hormone changes associated with menopause combined with a drop in your activity levels.

"Ovarian hormones, such as estrogen and progesterone, are not just reproductive hormones," says Elizabeth Lee Vliet, M.D., medical director of HER Place women's health centers in Tucson and Dallas. "They play a metabolic role in your body and help build muscle and bone. So when these hormones decline, so does muscle and bone mass, and the body stores more fat."

A pound of muscle burns about 35 to 50 calories a day, while a pound of fat burns much less—about 2 calories a day. Your body stores those extra calories as fat.

"Here's where things can spiral downward," says Susan Bowerman, R.D, executive assistant to the director of the UCLA Center for Human Nutrition in Los Angeles. "The body fat you gain not only burns significantly fewer calories but it also adds extra weight. Carrying around those extra pounds makes you feel tired, draining your desire to exercise. That can lead to greater fat gain and muscle loss."

DON'T MAKE THIS MISTAKE

Many women erroneously blame weight gain and slow metabolism on a faulty thyroid. While it's true that this tiny gland is the warehouse manager of calories—overseeing storage and usage—problems are not common. A blood test can tell you if, indeed, a thyroid problem is to blame for weight gain. If it is, medication can help.

In fact, it's not unusual for women to lose 5 pounds of muscle in a decade, which, in the average woman, is replaced with 10 pounds of metabolically sluggish fat.

Starving yourself (and depriving yourself of the nutrients that foods provide) won't do anything to boost your metabolism. Neither will loading up on caffeine, capsaicin (an ingredient in hot peppers), or ephedra (a dangerous amphetamine-like herb). They stimulate calorie burning only slightly, and their effect is temporary. "After 4 to 5 weeks, your body adapts, and you no longer benefit," says Bowerman.

A better solution: **››**

Strength training—that is, restoring lost muscle mass by working out with some kinds of weights or resistance bands.

"While aerobic exercises are great for burning calories and building cardiovascular health, you won't build significant amounts of muscle unless you do some kind of strength or resistance training, like lifting weights," says Bowerman. When muscles regularly encounter resistance—whether from hoisting dumbbells, pressing a barbell, or lifting bags of kitty litter into your car—they grow to meet the extra demand. Hence, you restore the metabolically active muscle mass you need to avoid unwanted weight gain.

You don't have to spend several hours a day in a gym to restore lost muscle. Spending 20 minutes, 3 days a week will do it. All you need is a set of dumbbells. Use a weight that is light enough for you to lift at least 8 times but heavy enough that you cannot possibly lift it more than 15 times. Work all the major muscle groups: legs, arms, shoulders, and back. For a whole-body workout, turn to page 467. As a bonus, you'll also strengthen your bones. ■

Microwave Cooking

What You Can Nuke (and What You Can't)

In 1957, home-economics student Carolyn Dodson was selected to demonstrate a new cooking appliance on a nationwide promotional tour. It stood nearly as tall as she did and cost $2,000, but could bake a potato in just 4 minutes.

Dodson saw then that the microwave oven would someday play a key role in a society that was moving faster, and her career was decided. She went on to write several microwaving cookbooks, conduct seminars, and star in a microwave cooking series on cable television.

Over the years, microwave ovens have become much smaller, cheaper, and easier to use. But you still can't heat just anything in them. Like most women, you probably already know that it's dangerous to put anything metal in the microwave unless it's labeled as microwave-safe. A spark can leap between the metal and the inside wall of the microwave, starting a fire or damaging the appliance. But did you know that cups and plates embossed with a gold or metallic finish can also cause a fire? Same with leaded crystal, silverware, or even twist ties with a metal wire.

Here are several other items—and some foods—you should never microwave, says Dodson.

Nonmicrowavable containers. When superheated, margarine tubs, refrigerator storage dishes, plastic wraps, and plastic trays may melt and possibly leach chemicals into your food. Instead, use plastic dishes and other cookware labeled safe for the microwave. (You can use plastic wrap to cover a container to hold in steam, so long as it's not touching the food.)

Brown paper bags. Never use brown paper bags, paper towels, and newspaper. They may contain tiny particles of metal, which can create sparks. Instead, use waxed paper.

Oil and oil-soaked foods. Don't try to "deep-fry" any

DON'T MAKE THIS MISTAKE

No matter how quickly you need to dry off damp shoes, socks, towels, clothing, or other nonfood items, don't put them in the microwave. They could catch on fire.

food in the microwave. Hot oil can easily overheat and catch fire. Also, cook greasy foods like bacon in small amounts (no more than 3 or 4 strips at a time).

Breast milk or baby formula. If you're breastfeeding an infant and freeze expressed breast milk for later use, don't defrost it or heat it in the microwave. It can destroy nutrients in the milk. Plus, heating milk of any kind creates hot spots that can burn the baby.

Bones. Debone large pieces of meat, such as pork chops, chicken, or other meat before microwaving. Bones block microwaves, leaving undercooked spots in meat.

Eggs in their shell. If you try to hard-cook an egg in the microwave, it will blow up. Honest. Same goes for clams or oysters in the shell. ■

Migraine Headaches

New Options for Women Who Have Tried Everything

If you're one of millions of women who get migraines, you've no doubt made the round of doctors in search of relief. You've cut out suspected migraine triggers like caffeine, aspartame (an artificial sweetener), alcohol, chocolate, aged cheeses, and MSG.

And still, your head throbs. Nightmarish symptoms are part of your life, putting you out of commission for hours—or days. The only thing that helps is lying down in a dark, quiet room—if you're lucky.

You might think you've tried everything—pain pills, herbs, relaxation therapy, you name it. Yet the secret to eventual relief may be a different drug, another form of alternative therapy, or a combination of treatments.

Are You Taking the Wrong Drug?

"Don't give up on medication because you think you've 'been there, done that,' " says Lisa K. Mannix, M.D., neurologist at the Headache Wellness Center in Greensboro, North Carolina, who sees only headache patients all day, every day. "Perhaps you weren't taking enough. If you were taking a daily medication designed to prevent migraines or make them less severe, maybe you haven't given it enough time. They take at least 4 weeks to kick in. And sometimes, a combination of drugs works better than any one drug alone."

Sit down with your doctor and review your treatment. Include the doses and duration of medications, side effects, and benefits.

If you've tried a triptan without success, try another one. Taken when a headache attack occurs, triptans bring relief to many people with migraines. They include sumatriptan (Imitrex), zolmitriptan (Zomig), rizatriptan (Maxalt), and naratriptan (Amerge), which provide fast relief for most, says Dr. Mannix.

"The triptans have revolutionized migraine treatment," says Dr. Mannix. They all work somewhat differently ››

GIVE FEVERFEW A SECOND TRY

If you get migraines, daily doses of feverfew, a popular herb found in pharmacies and health food stores, may prevent future attacks—but only if used correctly, says Fred Sheftell, M.D., headache specialist and director of the New England Center for Headache in Stamford, Connecticut.

Because feverfew isn't regulated by the FDA, how much you get varies from product to product. Feverfew tea won't give you a consistent, reliable dose. Dr. Sheftell suggests feverfew in tablet form, such as Migrafew (available in health food stores), which has a standardized amount of parthenolide, the active ingredient. Take one tablet every day and give it time to work—4 to 6 weeks. If you have no side effects, continue taking it for 6 months.

Feverfew is not recommended for pregnant women or lactating mothers, women with ulcers or gastrointestinal disease, or anyone taking aspirin or nonsteroidal painkillers like ibuprofen, warns Dr. Sheftell.

If you get mouth sores or gastrointestinal discomfort from feverfew, Dr. Sheftell suggests these other natural remedies.

Ginger. Take a 300- to 400-milligram capsule three or four times a day. "Ginger has some anti-inflammatory qualities, and it eases nausea without the side effects that feverfew may trigger," says Dr. Sheftell.

Riboflavin. Start at 200 milligrams for a week, then go to 400 milligrams. Take it with a B complex or multivitamin, not alone. It may take several months before showing a decrease in migraine frequency.

Magnesium. Take 400 milligrams a day in supplement form as a muscle relaxant. If you're the one out of two women who are magnesium deficient, you'll see a response in 2 to 3 months. Women with heart or kidney problems should check with their doctors before taking supplemental magnesium. Supplemental magnesium may cause diarrhea in some people.

for different individuals. If one doesn't work, talk to your doctor about trying another.

And keep checking with your doctor. "New classes of drugs will likely be developed as we learn more about the physiology of migraine," says Dr. Mannix.

Consider a preventive medication. If you have to take pain relief medications more than 2 days a week, discuss other options, such as a preventive medication. Your doctor may prescribe an antidepressant used for migraine (such as amitriptyline, or Elavil), an antihypertensive (such as propranolol, or Inderal), or an anticonvulsant (such as divalproex sodium, or Depakote).

The Alternative Route

When the pain is sudden and severe, you may instinctively try applying ice to your head and neck. "Like rest, sleep, or massaging your head, these techniques provide symptomatic relief only," says Dr. Mannix. "They feel good, and they help distract you from the pain." You may still need to take medications to fully stop the headache. In fact, for stubborn headaches like migraine, alternative treatments may work best when used in conjunction with medications, says Dr. Mannix. Here's what else to try.

Biofeedback. This technique provides body-change feedback—so you can see how much your forehead muscle is contracting, for example. Under the direction of a qualified biofeedback therapist, you view this feedback on a computer at first, then later learn skills to observe and control it.

Guided imagery. A method for creating sensory-rich images in your mind that help you relax, this, too, is best learned from a health care professional qualified in imagery and visualization.

Acupuncture. Fine needles are inserted in specific body areas that correspond with pain relief in other areas. Look for someone who is certified by the National Certification Commission for Acupuncture and Oriental Medicine (NCCAOM).

Physical therapy. This helps stretch and strengthen muscles in the upper back, neck, jaw, and head, where tight muscles make headaches worse. Ask your doctor to refer you to a physical therapist in your area. ■

Moisturizers

Has Your Face Cream Stopped Working?

If you're like most women, you've probably been using a moisturizing lotion or cream for years. Maybe even the same type or brand. So far, so good: Your skin needs some kind of barrier to seal in water and natural oils while shielding it against the drying effects of sun, wind, cold, or dry indoor air. Skip your moisturizer, and chances are you'll notice the difference: Your skin will feel tight or look flaky. Foundation makeup won't go on smoothly—it drags across your face.

You may be using moisturizer faithfully, every day and night. But are you using the right moisturizer? With age, your skin gets drier and more sensitive to cold. And depending on your job or your exercise habits, you may be spending more (or less) time outdoors. The moisturizer that you've relied on until now may no longer meet your needs.

Your moisturizer must be able to repair the barrier layer of the skin, says Edward M. Jackson, Ph.D., president and CEO of Jackson Research Associates in Sumner, Washington. Dr. Jackson has worked to help produce skin care products for companies such as Neutrogena, Jergens, and Noxzema.

Emollients, such as petrolatum, prevent moisture from leaving your skin too quickly. But if all you needed to moisturize your face was an emollient, plain old vegetable oil would do. But that would be silly—a moisturizer also needs to be light and greaseless and able to meet your skin's changing needs.

To find a moisturizer that meets *all* your skin's needs, says Dr. Jackson, look for these ingredients.

Humectants, such as glycerin. This is vital: Humectants help repair the skin, which then can do its job of holding in moisture. Other humectants include propylene glycol and urea. **››**

An SPF of at least 15. "Sun exposure can damage skin all year," says Dr. Jackson. "And damaged skin is dry skin." So if you haven't yet scouted out a moisturizer with sunscreen, now is the time to start.

Alpha hydroxy acids (AHAs). Compounds that occur naturally in grapes, apples, citrus fruits, sour milk, and sugar cane, AHAs help lessen wrinkles and improve dry skin, acne, and age spots. They speed up turnover of "old" skin cells, helping your skin look younger. But by thinning out dead surface cells, AHAs also help moisturizers do a better job. (So do beta hydroxy acids, which also are found in some moisturizers.)

DON'T MAKE THIS MISTAKE

Just because a moisturizer is the most expensive lotion on the shelf doesn't mean it's the best for you. Buy what you need based on content and comfort, not price and packaging, says Dr. Jackson.

Tint. If foundation makeup clogs your pores or streaks when you exercise, but you feel pale wearing moisturizer alone, try tinted moisturizer in a shade for your complexion.

Once you've selected the right moisturizer, make sure you use enough. "Don't be afraid you'll use too much," says Dr. Jackson. "You'll automatically stop applying it before it gets too thick."

Helpful Hint

Switch moisturizers when the weather turns nasty. "I recommend a light moisturizer like Oil of Olay or Purpose moisturizing lotion for milder days and a heavier cream, such as Eucerin, with an SPF of 25 for really bitter, windy weather," says Jonith Breadon, M.D., dermatologist and codirector of the dermatology surgery clinic at Cook County Hospital in cold, windy Chicago. ■

Monday Mornings

Launch Your Day with Verve

Unless you happen to have a recording contract, singing the Monday morning blues won't make your life any better.

Instead of griping about Mondays, try some of these tactics to get your week off to a high-energy start.

Forget about cleaning your desk. When you head home on Friday, leave all your work supplies and information out on your desk, says Lee Silber, a motivational speaker and author of *Time Management for the Creative Person.* Then on Monday morning, you won't have to drag out everything you need to start working, which can lead to procrastination.

Write a memo to yourself. Purposely leave a project unfinished, then attach a note to it that will remind you on Monday how you planned to continue the task, Silber says.

Spend your weekend productively. Many of us have jobs in which the work we complete tends to be abstract. So on the weekend, make a project with your hands or work on a chore that you can look at when you're finished—like mowing the lawn or vegetable gardening.

Hit the ground running. Set your coffeemaker to start brewing before you get up on Monday morning, suggests Robert Epstein, Ph.D., a university research professor of psychology at the United States International University in San Diego and editor in chief of *Psychology Today.* Set out your toast, bagel, muffin, or other breakfast food. Assemble your clothes the night before. Then, when the alarm sounds, everything you need to start your day will be ready for you to get going. ■

Monosodium Glutamate

The Real Culprit behind Chinese Restaurant Syndrome

More than 30 years ago, a physician wrote a letter to the New England Journal of Medicine *reporting that his wife experienced strange symptoms—headaches, dizziness, and heart palpitations—when she ate Chinese food.*

The editors slapped the headline "Chinese Restaurant Syndrome" on the letter, and—voilà!—a new malady was born.

Some Americans believe they've experienced Chinese Restaurant Syndrome, blaming monosodium glutamate (MSG), a flavor enhancer sometimes used in Asian food, as well as canned soups, lunchmeats, and other processed foods.

MSG is a synthetic form of glutamic acid, a nonessential amino acid otherwise found in tomatoes, Parmesan cheese, and other foods. MSG is used to enhance the flavor of hundreds of processed and prepared foods, including restaurant pizza, and is sold on supermarket shelves under such brand names as Accent.

Whether MSG in Chinese food—or any food—causes problems is debatable. Proponents say it's chemically identical to natural glutamic acid and therefore safe. MSG opponents say it's chemically different and therefore toxic.

"I've had an MSG headache, and I think it's terrible," says Nancy Lonsdorf, M.D., director of the Maharishi Ayurveda Medical Center in Rockville, Maryland. "I think it should be outlawed."

Dr. Lonsdorf's sentiments are shared by such consumer groups as the Chicago- ››

based Truth in Labeling Campaign, which claims that MSG causes potentially life-threatening cardiac, neurological, and respiratory reactions.

But the FDA and the Institute of Food Technologists scoff at such claims. The FDA considers MSG "a safe food ingredient for most people when eaten at customary levels."

In an effort to settle the issue once and for all, the Federation of American Societies for Experimental Biology, an independent body of scientists, released a 350-page report on MSG. Although the report was mostly favorable to MSG, it identified two groups who might be MSG-sensitive: people who consume 3 or more grams on an empty stomach (a typical serving is less than 0.5 gram) and people with severe, poorly controlled asthma. Since then, double-blind studies have disproved the MSG-asthma link. Australian researchers gave as much as 5 grams of MSG to 12 men and women with asthma who perceived themselves to be MSG-sensitive. It had no effect.

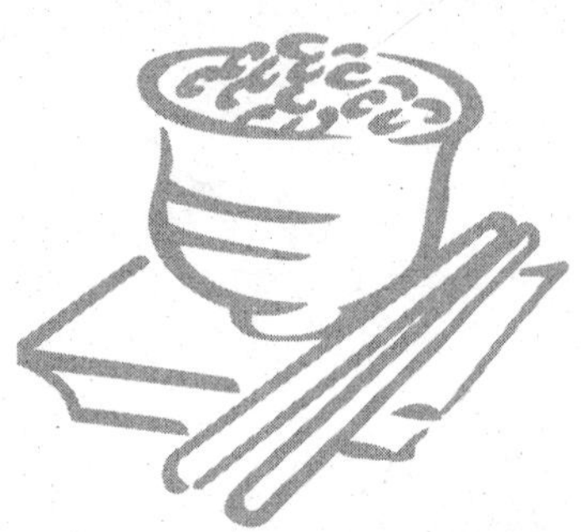

Other double-blind studies also have concluded that MSG is essentially harmless.

"MSG has gotten a bad rap," says Susan Hefle, Ph.D., a food toxicologist at the University of Nebraska in Lincoln. After reviewing 30 years' worth of MSG research, Dr. Hefle believes the real culprit behind Chinese Restaurant Syndrome is histamine, not MSG.

Plum, teriyaki, and other sauces used in Oriental cooking contain high amounts of histamine, which is the same sniffle-inducing substance released by the body when it overreacts to such allergens as ragweed pollen. "If you eat histamine in enough quantity, it can cause some of the reactions people are seeing when they say they have a reaction to MSG," Dr. Hefle says. If you think you are sensitive to histamines, avoid ingredients common to Chinese cooking, such as soy sauce, black beans, and shrimp paste, which can form histamines as they are fermented.

As for MSG, not even its most avid defenders rule out the possibility that some men and women may be sensitive to it. If you think you're one, here's what you can do to minimize potential reactions.

Check food labels. Federal regulations require manufacturers to include MSG on the ingredient statement as "monosodium glutamate."

Try a food-elimination diet. Exclude all processed foods from your diet for 3 weeks, then slowly reintroduce them one at a time to see if there are any reactions. Keep a detailed food diary you can show to your doctor.

See an allergy specialist. She can give you MSG orally, restrict your contact with other potential reaction triggers, and observe your reactions for up to 48 hours to see if you have a true sensitivity.

Helpful Hint

A board-certified allergist is best qualified to administer a test for MSG sensitivity. ■

Mood Swings

Self-Rescue for When You Feel Sad and Crabby

Mood swings are like sudden shifts in the weather. Nobody expects them. Nobody likes them. But a sudden change in your emotional weather is a force to be reckoned with.

"This isn't bipolar disorder," says Leah J. Dickstein, M.D., director of attitudinal and behavioral medicine at the University of Louisville School of Medicine. "Mood swings are common, everyday occurrences."

Still, mood swings aren't entirely benign. If you frequently veer off into sadness, guilt, irritability, and regret for no apparent reason, it can impair your ability to get along with yourself, your family, and your coworkers.

It also can become overwhelming.

The next time you feel yourself floating off into a bad mood, take a time-out. Consider what is going on around you. Are you or someone close to you going through some kind of crisis, large or small? You may or may not be able to do anything to resolve it on the spot, but at least you'll know why you feel the way you do. Then, to help even out your mood, try the following relaxation techniques.

Try the "navel release." This is a simple exercise from qigong, an Eastern belief system in which the navel is the center of existence. "Qigong can refresh the body in a short period of time," says Dr. Dickstein. Sit with your palms cupped, the heels of your hands together at your navel. Open them very slowly. "Think of pulling energy into your body," Dr. Dickstein ››

DON'T MAKE THIS MISTAKE

If you're feeling really rotten, don't isolate yourself at home or at work. "The worst thing you can do is hide in your house, contact nobody, and try to go it alone," Dr. Dickstein says. "If you feel or believe you will be like this forever, you set yourself into a pattern of unhappiness or hopelessness. Make a plan to do something positive."

ADD THESE MOOD-FRIENDLY OILS TO YOUR DIET

Omega-3 fatty acids, substances found in fish known for keeping hearts healthy, may also help mood disorders.

"The brain is essentially made of fat," explains Joseph Hibbeln, M.D., researcher at the National Institutes of Health. "Some fats necessary for brain functioning, such as polyunsaturated fatty acids found in fish, cannot be manufactured by the body. You have to get them from your diet."

His suggestions include canola oil, flaxseed oil, and fish oil supplements—all available in health food stores.

says. "Feel softness moving into the center of your body, replacing bad feelings." Repeat the entire process, beginning with the time-out as often as you feel a need to.

Helpful Hint

If self-help techniques fail to control your mood swings—or you're experiencing mood swings on a daily basis—seek professional help. And don't be embarrassed to ask for medical or psychiatric advice; you may have an underlying condition that, once treated, eliminates mood swings. ■

Morning Sickness

Five Ways to Hold On to Hold Down Breakfast (and Lunch)

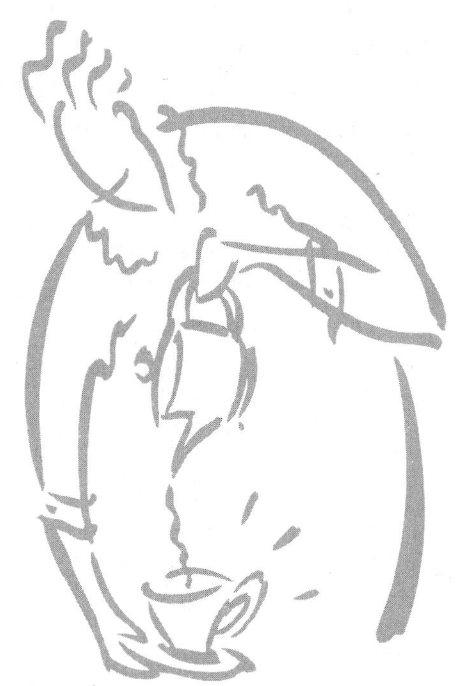

For many pregnant women, that healthy glow and eager anticipation of bringing a new life into the world is sometimes put on hold by episodes of nausea and vomiting.

Starting between the 4th and 6th weeks of pregnancy, as many as 9 out of 10 women feel queasy in the morning—anywhere between 6:00 A.M. and noon. "But you can experience it at any given time during the day," says Brian Fenmore, M.D., chairman of the department of obstetrics and gynecology at Encino/Tarzana Regional Medical Center in California. It usually disappears around week 14.

What's making you queasy? A surge in estrogen and progesterone combined with a slowdown in gastrointestinal activity. Exactly how or why they make your stomach churn is a matter of speculation.

A lucky few don't experience morning sickness during pregnancy. But for women who do, here are some tips for much-needed relief.

1. Have breakfast in bed. Keep a box of your favorite dry cereal or crackers at your bedside and eat some before you get out of bed, says Dr. Fenmore. Putting food in your stomach first thing in the morning will prevent the nausea before it starts.

2. Sip on ginger. Wash down your breakfast with some flat ginger ale (regular, not diet) or ginger tea. "Ginger is great for settling the stomach," says Teresa

Hoffman, M.D., an obstetrician-gynecologist at Mercy Medical Center in Baltimore. Let the open can or bottle sit out overnight to disperse the carbonation.

You can buy the tea at health food stores or make your own with fresh ginger from the supermarket. Chop about ¼ inch of fresh ginger into small cubes. Place them in a nonaluminum pot, and add 1 cup of water. Cover the pot and let it simmer for 15 to 20 minutes. You can drink up to 3 cups a day. Ginger beer, a nonalcoholic soda, is also a big help.

3. Munch on watermelon. If eating or drinking liquids turns you off, sink your teeth into some juicy watermelon. It's a solid liquid, so you'll fill your stomach and get your fluids at the same time, says Miriam Erick, R.D., senior perinatal nutritionist at Brigham and Women's Hospital in Boston, where she works with women hospitalized for severe morning sickness, and author of *Take Two Crackers and Call Me in the Morning!* and *No More Morning Sickness*.

DON'T MAKE THIS MISTAKE

See your doctor immediately if you are pregnant (or think you might be) and you haven't eaten or been able to drink liquids for 24 hours, you're vomiting every 2 hours, you're not gaining weight, or you're losing weight. Severe morning sickness can lead to dehydration, which requires hospitalization.

4. Eat five or six small meals a day instead of three large ones. It's easier for your stomach to digest a little bit of food at a time. And you'll avoid going for long periods without eating, which leads to an upset stomach.

5. Ask your doctor about B_6. Taking 25 milligrams of vitamin B_6 three times a day relieves nausea for many women, says Dr. Hoffman. Vitamin B_6 is available in supermarkets and drugstores. You can buy 50-milligram tablets and break the pills in half. Use caution, though: The Daily Value for vitamin B_6 is 2 milligrams a day, and very high doses—more than 100 milligrams a day—can be toxic. So check with your doctor before taking it during pregnancy.

Helpful Hints

Fatigue worsens nausea. So make sure you get enough sleep, and take naps during the day when you're feeling tired. "For some reason, women who have other child-care responsibilities while they're pregnant are more likely to have morning sickness," says Dr. Fenmore. So ask your spouse or another family member to help out with the other kids until you're feeling better.

Ask your doctor about the ReliefBand, the only FDA-approved wrist-band device that prevents nausea and vomiting by stimulating nerves on the inside of your wrist with a gentle electrical current. ■

Motion Sickness

Stop the Queasiness and Enjoy the Ride

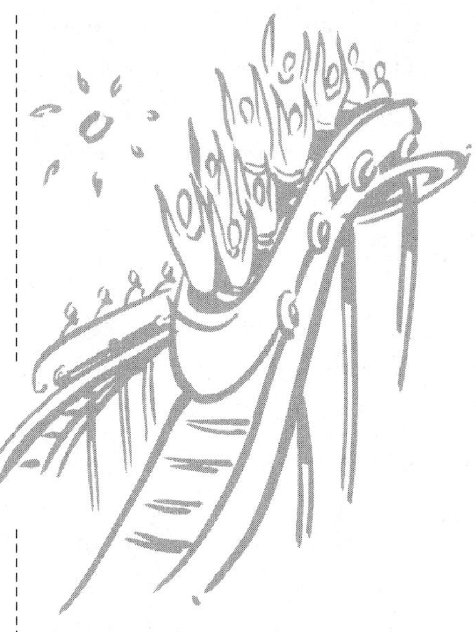

Even roller-coaster enthusiasts sometimes get motion sickness. "It seems like the body will let you go upside down twice, but after that, you're asking for trouble," says Carole Sanderson, vice president of the 6,000-member association of American Coaster Enthusiasts.

No riding the looping, hanging-upside-down roller-coasters after dark for her. "Not being able to focus on anything can be disorienting, making me more susceptible to motion sickness," says Sanderson, who's ridden more than 400 different roller-coasters around the world. Riding on a full stomach is also risky.

Motion sickness occurs when the signals from your brain, inner ear, and body conflict about how your body is moving. Aside from amusement-park rides, typical triggers include boats, trains, cars, or airplanes, or even an elevator or swing. When you're on an airplane, for example, your inner ear senses the turbulence as the plane bounces up and down, but your eyes see a stable cabin—not the roller-coaster ride your stomach is experiencing. As a result, you start to feel nauseated, dizzy, faint. You may break out into a cold sweat or even throw up.

Women are particularly susceptible to motion sickness, especially if you're on birth control pills or your period is about to start, because of a fluctuation in the female hormone progesterone, says Glenda Lindseth, R.N., R.D., Ph.D., professor of nursing at the University of North Dakota who has studied airsickness in pilots of both genders.

Whether you're determined to conquer coasters or just quell your car sickness, here's what motion sickness experts recommend to keep your stomach calm on the water, road, or in the air.

Get some rest. "If you're tired, you tend to get more motion-sick," says Dr. Lindseth, perhaps because your body can't tolerate added stress. Don't stay up late to pack your bags the night before a trip. Plan ahead and get a good night's sleep instead.

Stay away from salt. "Sodium tends to make people sicker," Dr. Lindseth says.

Choose small, light meals—and plan ahead. The best time for soft ice cream or a chili dog is *after* your ride, not before. "You want something in your stomach, but it needs to be easy to digest," Dr. Lindseth advises. Avoid dairy products and high-fat foods. Instead, snack on fruits, vegetables, and carbohydrates (such as low-salt pretzels). Eat your last meal no later than 2 to 3 hours before your trip.

Think calm. "Some women get so anxious about air travel that by the time they get on the flight, you can almost predict they're going to get sick," says Dr. Lindseth. Take deep breaths. Or meditate.

Cool yourself. Warm airplane cabins and cars may exacerbate motion sickness. If you're flying, dress in layers so you can cool yourself off by shedding a sweater; if you're in a car, open the window or turn up the AC.

Take control. If you start to feel ill in a car, ask if you can take the wheel, suggests Thomas Stoffregen, Ph.D., associate psychology professor at the University of Cincinnati. You'll feel better because you can prepare for the road's ups and downs, rather than being caught off guard in the backseat.

Focus on a fixed point. "If you can see the horizon, keep your eyes open and focus on it," Dr. Stoffregen advises. Doing this will stabilize your system.

Minimize your activity. Closing your eyes and lying down (or even just resting your head on a traveling pillow) will slow down the conflicting body signals that are making you feel sick, Dr. Stoffregen says.

Try herbs. Soothe your stomach with ginger. One hour before your trip, take a teaspoon of grated fresh ginger, two ginger capsules, or 60 drops of ginger extract (also known as a tincture). Don't use ginger of you have gallstones, because it may increase bile secretion. A cup of peppermint tea might work in a pinch.

Apply pressure. Sold in pharmacies, special elastic bands (such as Sea-Bands) designed to apply gentle pressure to certain points on your wrist that correspond to motion control centers in your brain may help relieve your nausea. Or, you can try ReliefBands, a battery-operated device prescribed by doctors for motion sickness and other forms of nausea.

Helpful Hint

If nondrug remedies don't work, talk to your doctor. She may prescribe a scopolamine patch that you can apply to your arm or neck. ■

N

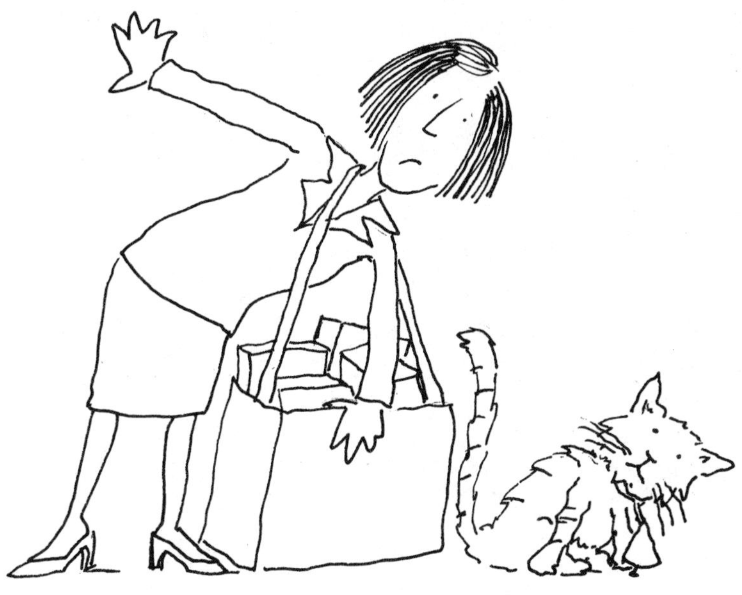

If your purse qualifies as carry-on luggage,
you could end up with neck pain.
To lighten the load, see page 302.

Nail Biting

Breathe Your Way to Prettier Nails

Women have tried just about everything to quit biting their nails. Hypnosis. Regular manicures. Foul-tasting polish. But if those methods don't work for you, relaxation techniques just might, says Allen Elkin, Ph.D., director of the Stress Management Counseling Center in New York City.

His favorite nail biting remedy is a yoga breathing technique called rapid relaxation that has worked for many women.

Sit quietly with your right hand resting on your lap. Inhale deeply through your nose. Hold the breath as you squeeze your thumb and index or middle finger of your right hand. Hold this position for 4 to 6 seconds, then exhale through parted lips. Let your hand relax and allow the tension to leave your body. Repeat any time you feel the urge to bite your nails. ■

Natural Childbirth

Ease Labor and Delivery with Personal Pregnancy Trainers

Athletes have trainers and opera singers have voice coaches. Why not enlist a trainer or a coach to help you ace childbirth?

You can do both—by enlisting a certified nurse-midwife (CNM) and a doula, health care professionals who work together to ease childbirth in different ways.

CNMs are registered nurses who specialize in delivering babies. They graduate from advanced education programs accredited by the American College of Nurse-Midwives (ACNM). And they must pass a national certification exam and meet strict requirements set by state health agencies.

"We're able to give women more personalized care than obstetrical doctors are able to offer, and we go the extra mile to give the mother-to-be the birth experience she wants," says Kathy Slone, a certified nurse-midwife in Baltimore.

Nurse-midwives have a proven track record. Experience shows that if a CNM performs your delivery:

- You're less likely to need an epidural injection or other pain-relieving drug.
- You may be less likely to need an episiotomy (an incision to widen the vaginal opening).
- You're less likely to need a cesarean section.

A doula (a Greek word meaning "woman's servant") is trained and experienced in maternity care, labor, and childbirth and is equipped to deal with the emotional and physical needs of women during childbirth and the immediate postpartum period. Certification is offered by local, national, and international organizations. ››

A doula teaches you breathing and relaxation techniques and coaches you on positioning to make labor and delivery as comfortable as possible. She also provides psychological reassurance and information to you and your family during the birth, says Sandy Szalay, a doula in Seattle and president of Doulas of North America (DONA), a non-profit organization that offers training and certification. Most doulas are women.

Doulas even make house calls. "She can comfort you during early labor right in your own home," says Szalay. "Doulas specialize in non-medical tasks—we leave that to the CNM." The two work together as a team.

According to the Doulas of North America, when a doula provides assistance:

- Your labor may be shorter.
- You're less likely to experience difficulty and complications.
- You're less likely to need oxytocin, a drug given to in-

Natural Hormones

What Are the Alternatives? And Do They Work?

Women who choose to avoid synthetic hormone replacement therapy (HRT) because of fear of increased risk of breast cancer or other medical concerns will find various "natural" hormone products on the market.

What are natural hormones, anyway? And do they work as well as HRT?

Good questions.

"Everybody defines 'natural' differently," says Kurt Barnhart, M.D, reproductive endocrinologist and epidemiologist at the University of Pennsylvania Medical Center in Philadelphia. Certainly, any hormones that occur in the female body—such as estrogen and progesterone—are natural to your body. But if you swallowed a dose of natural progesterone, your body would quickly digest it, break it down in your liver, and excrete it before it could get to your reproductive organs and have any positive effect. So traditional HRT uses progestin (a synthetic version of progesterone), which is not excreted as quickly.

Hormones derived from plants, like certain compounds in yams or soy, or animals, like estrogens from pregnant mares, are natural to those plants and animals. But they may or may not be natural to the human body.

Of these, plant products, like progesterone derived from wild yams, are most often marketed as natural.

"Just because it comes from a plant doesn't mean it's natural to people," says Dr. Barnhart. In fact, wild yams do not contain progesterone at all. They contain diosgenin, a chemical that labs convert into a replica of the body's progesterone.

Another distinction: Prescription hormones are drugs, and therefore subject to rigorous testing and require FDA approval for use. So-called natural duce labor, or forceps to pull the baby out of the birth canal.

• Your baby may be able to leave the hospital sooner.

To find a certified nurse-midwife in your area, write to the American College of Nurse-Midwives, 818 Connecticut Avenue NW, Suite 900, Washington, DC 20006. Or, visit their Web site at www.midwife.org. To find a doula, write to Doulas of North America, 1100 23rd Avenue East, Seattle, WA 98112. You can also check local birth centers and hospitals for referrals.

Helpful Hint

Insurance coverage will vary from state to state, provider by provider, for many doula and CNM services. Sometimes home and hospital deliveries will be considered differently. Check with your provider as early in your pregnancy as possible for details. ■

hormones (such as progesterone cream made from wild yams) are classified as supplements and require no testing. There are no national standards for purity, safety, or effectiveness. **Some brands may contain more progesterone than others, and some may not contain any, despite their claims.** It's difficult to get enough of the hormone and impossible to know (without lab tests) if you are. For example, one popular brand of natural progesterone cream claims to contain 930 milligrams of progesterone in one 2-ounce jar. An independent test found just 200 milligrams of the hormone present.

That's not to say natural hormones aren't without merit. There's some evidence that natural estrogen can be beneficial if you're also taking estrogen postmenopausally. For example, natural progesterone may be better than synthetic at preserving more of estrogen's beneficial effects on the heart. However, it's a more recent form of treatment, and a "correct dosage" is still subject to some debate, says Dr. Barnhart.

All things considered, your best bets may be the following two forms of natural hormone therapy, both available by prescription only.

Micronized progesterone (Prometrium). This natural progesterone in pill form was tested in a major study, the Postmenopausal Estrogen/Progestin Intervention Trial (PEPI), and found to provide the same benefit as progesterone (that is, protecting your uterus against estrogen) without progesterone's uncomfortable side effects, which are commonly associated with HRT therapy. It's formulated by breaking down progesterone into very tiny particles that are absorbed before they're metabolized by the liver.

Taking micronized progesterone before bedtime minimizes drowsiness, the only real side effect of this therapy.

Crinone. Applied to the vagina, this natural progesterone-containing gel delivers progesterone directly to your uterus. Unlike vaginal creams and suppositories, the gel doesn't cause a messy discharge. In a series of studies, it effectively protected women taking estrogen from endometrial cancer, and was found to have a calming effect. ■

Nausea and Vomiting

How to Stop Throwing Up—Fast!

Let's face it: If you're sick to your stomach, you're not all that concerned about the cause, be it a stomach bug, questionable food, or a little too much liquid cheer the night before. You just want that horrible feeling to stop—the sooner, the better.

But rushing in with the wrong remedy may make matters worse. Here's what to do.

Try liquids first. When your stomach stops heaving, sip some flat soda, plain (not carbonated) water, Gatorade-type fluid-replacement drink, or chicken broth (canned broth is fine) once or twice every 5 minutes. Chamomile or ginger tea may also help. (If you're allergic to ragweed, skip the chamomile—they're related.)

"It a good idea to stay hydrated so that vomiting is easier when it does come," says Amy Rothenberg, N.D, a naturopathic physician in Enfield, Connecticut.

If you're sick for more than 3 days or you frequently feel nauseous for no apparent reason, see a doctor, particularly if you're also experiencing abdominal pain or losing weight unintentionally.

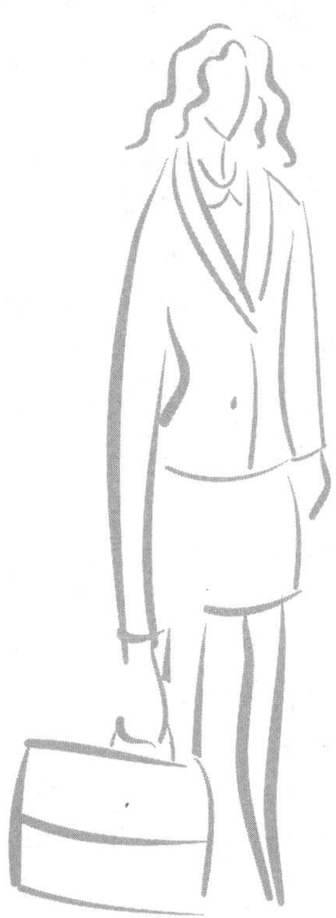

Neck Pain

Put Your Purse on a Diet

For years, Rachel Lyn Honig kept shoving more and more into her purse: Car phone. Makeup bag. Monthly organizer. Apple. Paperback novel. Brush. Handful of coins.

"Like a lot of women, I think I must be prepared for everything, so it got to the point where my purse was like a small suitcase weighing heavy on my shoulder," says Honig, a New York City public relations executive. Hauling all that stuff around was turning out to be a real pain in the neck. Literally.

Honig and other women are common victims of "purse creep," the inclination to pack more and more into a purse, including items for husbands and children, says Susan Isernhagen, physical therapist and director of Isernhagen Work Systems in Duluth, Minnesota. Eventually, this pack-mule behavior exacts a physical price.

"By wearing a heavy purse on one shoulder, the neck muscles on that side contract and give you pain. The heavy strap puts pressure on the blood vessels and nerves in that area," says Isernhagen.

Helpful Hint

Peppermint is one of the oldest known remedies for nausea, says James S. Sensenig, N.D., distinguished visiting professor at the University of Bridgeport College of Naturopathic Medicine in Connecticut and founding president of the American Association of Naturopathic Physicians. It's so enduring because it usually works. "Mint has a very relaxing effect on the intestinal muscles," Dr. Sensenig says.

To be ready for your next bout of nausea, pick up some peppermint tea at a health food store or supermarket. Check the label to be sure that it's made from peppermint and not just regular tea with peppermint flavoring. ■

SICK TO YOUR STOMACH? PRESS HERE

This simple do-it-yourself acupressure technique sometimes works to relieve nausea. Massage the acupressure point at the weblike area between your thumb and pointer finger of either hand, using firm, deep pressure for several minutes, says Dr. Rothenberg.

Isernhagen offers these tips to lighten your load and still feel fashionable.

Think diagonally. Place the purse strap over your head and diagonally across your body so that it distributes the weight of the contents more across your body and not just a single shoulder.

Select thick straps. They shoulder the weight of the purse better than spaghetti-thin straps.

Switch to backpacks and fanny packs. Both help keep your hands free, and both provide a better weight distribution than a purse.

Pluck out coins. They can

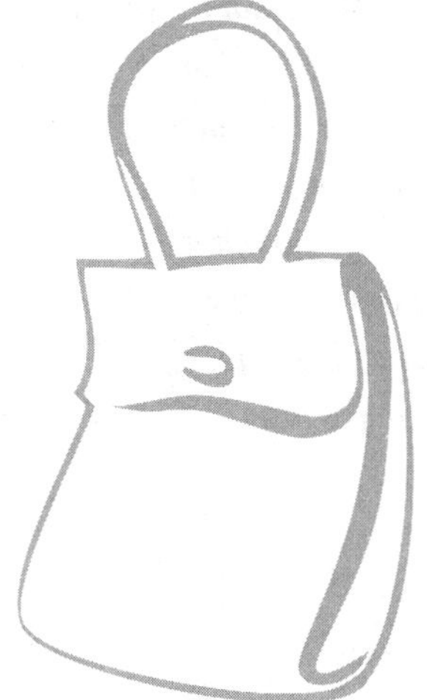

really add weight to your purse. Store some change inside the car or your office desk drawer. Save a few coins to drop in a jacket or pants pocket. Store the rest in a jar at home. "We put all our coins in a glass jar. The last time we went on vacation, we had $250 to spend on souvenirs just from those coins," says Isernhagen.

Leave makeup at home or the office. Only pack lipstick. It can redden your lips and double as blush for your cheeks.

Let your car do the carrying. Cell phones are major weight items. Try keeping your cell phone in your vehicle. Same goes for your sunglasses and stash of supermarket coupons.

Ditch the day planner. Go digital. Lightweight, com- ❯❯

puterized planners and address books take up less room and offer greater storage capacity.

Buy small. Your husband or children are less apt to ask you to carry their books, toys, keys, and other items when you pack an itty-bitty purse. On family trips, make sure each of you has his own backpack or fanny pack to distribute the cameras, guidebooks, and other trip items.

Consolidate your cards. Take a major credit card, driver's license, cash card, and paper money and leave all those cards for department stores, video stores, and other places at home. You'll have the major forms of identification, and there will be fewer cards to report in case your purse is lost or stolen.

Helpful Hint

Once a week, take inventory of your purse contents and remove unnecessary items. "I prevent my purse from getting overloaded by cleaning it out the same day I do my laundry," says Isernhagen. ■

Negative People

Deflective Strategies for Naysayers

"It won't work. It never did. It never will. If you think it might, you're kidding yourself."

What makes some people so negative?

"Life. Biochemistry. Childhood problems. Unresolved issues. Constantly being defeated. Not having a lot of success. Not being acknowledged or respected. Not being appreciated. Not feeling they have what they want in life or in a relationship," says Lillian Glass, Ph.D., communications consultant in New York City and author of nine books, including Toxic People.

Sometimes it's easy to deal with negative people—you just ignore them. But what do you do about friends, relatives, or coworkers who have a tendency to see the proverbial glass as half empty?

For starters, don't try to change them.

"You always hope the person will change. You hope you can do something to make her not act that way," says Dr. Glass. The problem is, you can't change another person. (Didn't you try that with a boyfriend or two?) But you can change your own behavior and attitude and the interaction between the two of you.

The next time you encounter a negative friend, try these tactics.

• Every time she says something negative, say, "Smile," "Say something nice," or "Let's not go there." Don't scold—that only adds fuel to the fire.

• Cut her off kindly, letting her know you don't want to deal with it. Say, "Let's not talk about this. It upsets both of us."

• Agree with her. Say, "You're right. It won't work. Not even you could find a way to make it work." Continue with these kind of responses to every negative comment until the only way she can contradict you is to switch to a positive position and argue that yes, she can make it work, says Rick Kirschner, N.D., a naturopathic physician in Ashland, Oregon, and coauthor of *Dealing with People You Can't Stand*.

• Really listen to her. "When someone is discouraged, they don't need others to tell them exactly what they think they should do. That only makes them uncomfortable and may make them dig deeper into the hole," says Michele Novotni, Ph.D., assistant professor of counseling at Eastern College in St. Davids, Pennsylvania. Instead, simply let the negative person express what she is feeling. **By encouraging a person to identify the problem area causing the discouragement, we help them keep it in perspective.** It's one problem, not her whole life.

• Suggest that at the end of each day, the person make a list of positive things that happened, little or big. This will help her look for goodness in her life.

• Insist on respect in a positive way. Say, "When you put me down, it doesn't do good things for our relationship. I'm on your side." You may find this technique valuable when your friend misdirects her frustrations and anger at you. Be assertive to keep the direction of the conversation positive. Respond with, "I really want to be helpful, but you're making it hard for me. Let's refocus on your situation and see if there's something we can come up with that would help," says Robert D. Kerns, Ph.D., chief of psychology service at VA Connecticut Healthcare System in West Haven, Connecticut, and associate professor of psychiatry, neurology, and psychology at Yale University.

• Focus on your own attitude instead of your friend's. Instead of trying to change her mind and ultimately feeling negative yourself, maintain your own sense of well-being by taking whatever she says and telling yourself the opposite. "If she says, 'You'll never get it to work,' tell yourself, 'I'll find a way to make it work.'" If this isn't enough, "take a deep breath and think of something relaxing, peaceful, and distracting," says Dr. Kerns. Your goal should be to relax and respond to her in a rational and reasonable manner instead of becoming unnecessarily angry.

Chronic negativity can be a sign of deep disappointment—perhaps she wants to protect you from the same thing. If she feels the need to keep warning you of things, simply say, "I don't want anything to go wrong either." This should help relieve some negative people of the responsibility they feel to announce disaster or constantly point out harmful things to you, says Dr. Kirschner. However, it can also be a sign of serious depression. If her attitude is seriously interfering with her life in any way, encourage her to get help.

Helpful Hint

Realize that the problem is not you, and don't take her attitude personally. ■

Negative Thinking

Find the Optimist Within

Are you convinced that your health will suffer unless you become an incurable optimist who goes around with a smile on your face and a song in your heart?

That's what such apostles of positivism as Norman Vincent Peale, author of The Power of Positive Thinking, *would have you believe. For decades, they've been preaching that positive thinking will save you from disease, disability, and an early grave.*

Not necessarily so, says Susan Robinson-Whelen, Ph.D., a researcher at the Center of Excellence on Healthy Aging with Disabilities at the Houston VA Medical Center.

Dr. Robinson-Whelen is coauthor of a study that examined how optimism and pessimism affected the health of 224 middle-aged and older adults—mostly women—over a period of several years. She found that embracing optimism isn't as strongly associated as you might think with high levels of self-reported health and low levels of stress and anxiety.

What's more important, the study suggests, is avoiding pessimism. In other words, you don't have to always expect the best. Just don't always expect the worst.

If you're locked into a negative mind-set, you'll enjoy better health and more peace of mind if you at least allow for the possibility that every endeavor won't turn into a disaster. Optimism and pessimism are traits that don't fluctuate much through life, however. So you'll have to work at changing your world view.

Here are some strategies you can use to neutralize negative thinking, says Ayala Malach Pines, Ph.D., clinical and social psychologist and professor at the School of Management at Ben Gurion University in Beersheva, Israel.

Identify the source of your negativity. "You need to figure out where it's coming from. For example: Is there a particularly negative sentence you frequently heard as a child? And does it serve a function in your life? For example: Do you use it as an excuse to avoid doing certain things?" Dr. Pines says. If you can't answer these questions on your own, a therapist may be able to help.

Give yourself a reality check. Intimate relationships are at the center of women's sense of self, and they can cause negative thinking. "We worry about being abandoned, losing love, or that something will happen to our loved one," Dr. Pines says. Realistically consider how likely it is that such worst-case scenarios will come true. After careful reflection, you may well conclude that it's not very likely.

Get support. Find friends who identify with you. "Seek out others who see the world the way you do," Dr. Pines says. "They will give you emotional support. They will challenge you. They will tell you if they think there's something wrong about a situation and also if they think you're crazy to think a certain way."

Rant to the music. Suppose you're worried that you'll get a bad review at work, that your husband will be laid off from his job, or that your daughter's wedding will turn into a soccer brawl. "Summarize the worst of your fears in one sentence. (For example: 'If this happens, I'm going to die.') Put on music with a very powerful beat," Dr. Pines says. "Then repeat that sentence over and over and over again to the beat of the music. Somehow, the repetition takes the sting out of the worry." ■

Neighborhood Disputes

Make Peace, Not War

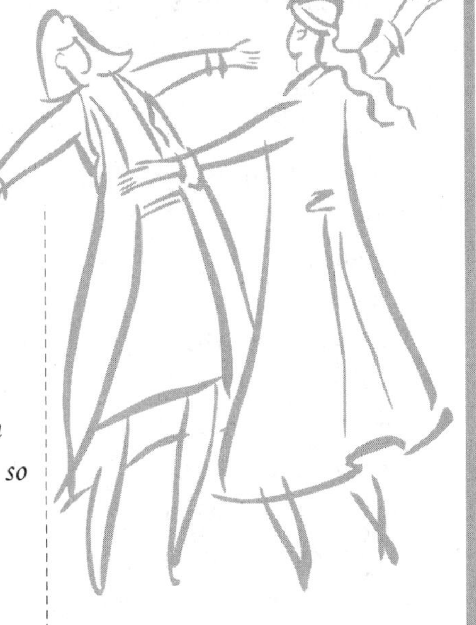

When a Philadelphia family installed a new swimming pool, they left their old kiddie pool in the next-door neighbor's yard.

Although it was supposed to be a gift, the neighbors considered it trash. But instead of voicing their complaint, they silently simmered.

Then the kids from both families began arguing, and one of them turned to vandalism. As the situation escalated, the mothers became so enraged that they hurled raw eggs at each other.

Fortunately, the case reached the Good Shepherd Mediation Center in Philadelphia before these modern-day Hatfields and McCoys got out their shooting irons. In just a few hours, a mediator got to the bottom of the 6-month-long feud.

"Even though it was ostensibly about the kids, it all went back to the swimming pool," says Cheryl Cutrona, the center's executive director. "What started the conflict was a simple misperception."

Neighborhood disputes typically start with a real issue such as a rowdy kid, barking dog, noisy stereo, or overhanging tree. They can turn surreal as the warring parties draw imaginary lines in their sandboxes.

Cutrona recalls a Philadelphia man who shoveled a curbside parking place during a snowstorm and reserved the spot with a lawn chair. After a neighbor removed the chair, the man shot him.

If you have a beef with your neighbor, follow this 6-step process for resolving interpersonal conflicts.

1. Set the stage for peacemaking. Call your neighbor, tell her you have an issue to discuss, and ask when and where it would be convenient to meet. "You may not want to use either house, because ›› that's turf," Cutrona says. When you meet, decide who will speak first. Usually, it's the person who arranged the meeting since she may be the only one who knows what the issue is about.

2. Express your concerns without blame and accusations. Use lots of "I" statements, calmly state your concerns, then yield the floor. Agree to take turns speaking without interruption until each of you understands the other's perception of the situation.

3. Share ideas that might resolve the conflict. Brainstorm as many solutions as you can without rejecting any of them out of hand. Don't be afraid to offer humorous suggestions ("Maybe you could replace your outdoor stereo system with a nice, relaxing fish pond.") to help break the ice.

4. Evaluate the options. "Ask yourselves what the consequences would be if you did this or if you did that," Cutrona says. "Feel free to reject, modify, or combine options or add new ones as the discussion progresses."

DON'T MAKE THIS MISTAKE

When neighbors get out of line, women often refuse to challenge them because it wouldn't be "nice." In serious disputes, nice women finish last, Cutrona says. "If you're always an avoider or an accommodator, you're never going to have your needs met. Eventually, you're going to explode."

5. Collaborate until you reach a win-win agreement. After finding a solution you both can live with, be specific about how it will be implemented. Spell out who will do what, where they'll do it, when they'll do it, and how it will be accomplished.

6. Put your agreement in writing. Not only will it help everyone remember what they agreed to do but it'll also give you both something to take to court if someone violates the agreement.

What should you do if it turns out the agreement isn't worth the paper it's written on? Should you go to court?

Not right away, advises Cutrona.

Since the 1970s, nearly 600 community mediation centers have opened nationwide. Their mission is to offer individuals and families a free or inexpensive alternative to the legal-justice system. The center will provide a trained mediator to facilitate the discussion without taking sides.

Although mediation isn't legally binding, Cutrona says that 85 percent of cases result in a written agreement that's acceptable to both parties.

Helpful Hint

Even if you have a laundry list of grievances against your neighbor, resist the urge to air them all. If you bring up the time your neighbor accidentally blew some leaves onto your lawn, it'll weaken your complaint about the graffiti that her kids spray-painted on your garage. "If there's something you can take care of yourself, why make a big deal of it?" Cutrona says. ■

Nutritional Supplements

What Do You Really Need?

Ever felt overwhelmed walking down the vitamin aisle of a drugstore, supermarket, or health food store? Bottles of individual vitamin and mineral supplements sit on the shelves like puppies at the pound longing to be taken home.

If you have special needs, your doctor or other health care practitioners may very well recommend individual supplements geared to your needs. But if you're basically healthy—and want to stay that way—you may need to consider no more than a handful of individual supplements, says Richard J. Wood, Ph.D., associate professor at the School of Nutrition at Tufts University in Medford, Massachusetts, and Laboratory Chief of the Mineral Bioavailability Laboratory, as well as Scientist I, both at the Jean Mayer USDA Human Nutrition Research Center on Aging at Tufts.

Folic acid. This B vitamin has been proven to prevent birth defects and seems to protect against heart disease in women. Although leafy green vegetables are excellent sources of this B-vitamin, heat and poor storage can destroy as much as half of their folic acid. Plus, drinking alcohol or coffee or taking birth control pills or steroidal anti-inflammatory drugs (such as Prednisone) can deplete your folic acid reserves. So meeting your Daily Value (DV)—400 micrograms per day—is challenging through diet alone.

Recommended amount: 400 to 800 micrograms a day for pre- and postmenopausal women, and 800 micrograms per day for pregnant women

Best form: Folate or folic acid

Vitamin C. This vitamin builds collagen, a basic building block of bone and skin, and speeds wound healing. It also boosts immunity and works as an antioxidant to prevent heart disease, cancer, and other degenerative health problems. The DV is 60 milligrams per day.

Recommended amount: 60 milligrams a day for nonsmokers and 100 milligrams a day for women who smoke. Women who have diabetes may need 200 milligrams per day.

Vitamin E. Also an antioxidant, convincing evidence indicates that vitamin E goes a long way to preventing heart disease. Best sources are vegetable oils, nuts, and seeds—all of which are high in fat. So it can be difficult to get enough of this vitamin if you're trying to lose weight.

Recommended amount: 200 to 400 IU per day

Best form: Natural forms of E, typically labeled as "vitamin E mixed tocopherols," include d-alpha, d-beta, d-gamma, and d-delta tocopherols. Synthetic forms that start with "dl," like dl-alpha tocopherol, are not absorbed as well.

Vitamin D. Blocking ultraviolet rays with sunscreen not only prevents wrinkles and skin cancer but it also prevents the formation of vitamin D in your skin, needed to protect your bones. But instead of giving up your sun protection, just make sure you're getting D in supplement form. ››

Recommended amount: 400 IU per day

Calcium. Unless you've been locked away for years in a news-deprivation chamber, you know that calcium is vital for strong bones. But did you know that eating excessive amounts of protein can deplete your body of calcium, increasing your need for it? Plus, women in menopause who don't take hormones need even more of this mineral.

Recommended amount: 1,000 milligrams for women who are premenopausal or taking hormones; 1,500 milligrams per day for women in or past menopause

Best form: Calcium citrate and calcium carbonate. Calcium carbonate has the highest amount of calcium by weight and is best absorbed with food. Calcium citrate, however, is better absorbed on an empty stomach.

Magnesium. Without this mineral, your muscles couldn't contract and your lungs couldn't function. You'd also lose the calcium in your bones and teeth. The richest food sources of magnesium are beans, nuts, and green vegetables. Unfortunately, like calcium, women don't get enough of this artery-protecting mineral from their diets—increasing their risk for high blood pressure and heart attacks.

Recommended amount: 300 to 400 milligrams per day (Anyone with a heart or kidney problem should check with her doctor before taking supplemental magnesium.) Supplemental magnesium may cause diarrhea in some people.

Best form: Magnesium oxide has the most magnesium per weight of a pill and it's fairly well absorbed.

Helpful Hint: If constipated, try magnesium citrate. It has a slight laxative effect

DON'T MAKE THESE MISTAKES

More isn't always better—especially when it comes to folic acid. Too much of this nutrient can mask a vitamin B_{12} deficiency. To avoid this problem, do not exceed 800 micrograms a day.

Large amounts of vitamin E can thin blood, interfering with blood clotting and may even lead to a hemorrhage. To prevent these problems, do not exceed 400 IU per day.

Steroidal anti-inflammatory drugs, like Prednisone and Decadron, can deplete your vitamin D. If you're taking one of these medications, consult your pharmacist. You may need more of this bone-strengthening, cancer-preventing nutrient.

Calcium decreases the effectiveness of a number of antibiotics. If you are prescribed an antibiotic, check with your pharmacist to see if it interacts with calcium.

Helpful Hint

When buying a mineral supplement, you'll find two values listed: One is the total amount of mineral salt in the tablet. The other—the elemental value—is more useful. It tells you the maximum amount that your body can absorb from the product. That's the number you want. "If the label doesn't list the elemental values, don't buy it," says Dr. Wood. ■

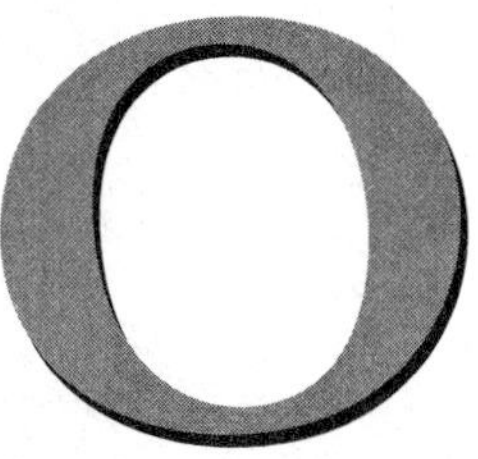

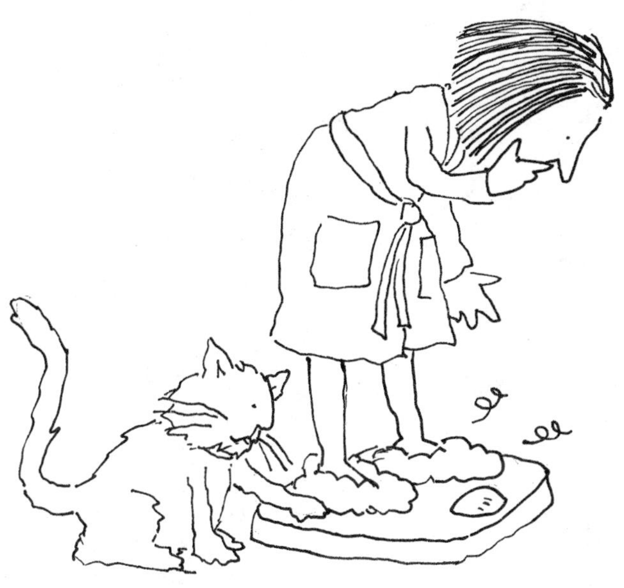

Can't seem to lose weight?
Maybe you're trying too hard.
See page 326.

Oatmeal

Jazz Up This Heart-Saver Cereal

Loaded with fiber, oatmeal was the first food to break the FDA's health claim barrier. Oatmeal fit the bill by having enough soluble fiber to meet the government's guideline for claims linking specific health benefits to specific foods.

"About 1½ cups of cooked oatmeal, or a cup of oat bran, or 3 cups of an oat-based cereal a day will reduce your cholesterol by 5 to 6 percent, which reduces your risk for heart disease by 10 to 12 percent," says Constance Geiger, R.D., Ph.D., research assistant professor in the division of food and nutrition at the University of Utah in Salt Lake City. "It helps control blood cholesterol levels by binding bile acids made from cholesterol in your digestive tract. Think of oatmeal as a sponge that soaks up cholesterol and carries it out of your body."

"As a bonus, oatmeal leaves you feeling full, so you don't get hungry quickly and you eat less at your next meal," says Dr. Geiger. Because oatmeal is bland, it accommodates other flavors nicely. To jazz it up, add your favorite fruits, nuts, sweeteners, or spices, says Jill Nussinow, R.D., president of the Vegetarian Connection in Santa Rosa, California. She and Dr.Geiger suggest these exciting new ways to prepare heart-healthy oatmeal.

- Cook oatmeal with half apple juice and half water, adding raisins and cinnamon while cooking. After cooking, add maple syrup and sprinkle with a tablespoon of chopped walnuts.
- In a blender, combine your favorite fruit juice and a banana, then pour on cooked oatmeal instead of milk. Top with sliced almonds and your favorite berries or seasonal fruit.
- Add apple slices during the last few minutes of cooking, or mix in chunky applesauce afterward. Top with low-fat granola.
- Top with toasted nuts, dried cranberries (or any kind of dried fruit), freshly ground flaxseed, and brown sugar.
- Add ½ teaspoon of real vanilla per serving of cooked oatmeal. Grate a sprinkling of nutmeg over the top and add fruit in season. Top it off with fat-free apricot yogurt. ■

DON'T MAKE THIS MISTAKE

To keep your oatmeal heart-healthy, don't pile on the butter, warns Dr. Geiger.

Graham Kerr's Gourmet Oatmeal

When his wife, Treena, suffered a heart attack some years ago, renowned cookbook author and celebrity chef Graham Kerr changed his culinary focus. Gone were the copious quantities of cream, butter, egg yolks, and deep-fried foods he relished as television's Galloping Gourmet. Oatmeal—among other heart-healthy foods—became a staple.

"Treena and I love to eat oatmeal all year round," says Kerr. Here are two of Kerr's favorite oatmeal recipes. Both recipes serve two people.

Winter Oatmeal with Cranberries and Raisins

- ½ cup rolled oats
- ¼ cup dark raisins and dried cranberries, mixed
- 2⅔ cups fat-free milk
- ¼ cup Graham's Seed Mix (recipe follows)
- 2 teaspoons brown sugar

In a small saucepan, combine the oats, raisins, and milk. Cover and simmer over low heat until warmed through and the fruit is plump. Raise the heat to medium and stir vigorously until creamy-thick in texture, less than 1 minute. Add the seed mix and brown sugar.

Summer Muesli with Fresh Apple

- ½ cup rolled oats
- ¼ cup dark raisins
- 1 Granny Smith apple, grated
- 2 tablespoons lemon juice
- 2 tablespoons fat-free evaporated milk
- ¼ cup Graham's Seed Mix (recipe follows)

Soak the oats and raisins in a bowl of water overnight. In the morning, drain and stir in the grated apple and lemon juice. Stir in the milk.

Sprinkle with the seed mix and serve.

Graham's Seed Mix

- 1 cup raw sunflower seeds
- 1 cup unhulled sesame seeds
- 1 cup green pumpkin seeds
- 1 cup sliced almonds
- ½ cup flaxseeds

In a large bowl, combine the sunflower seeds, sesame seeds, pumpkin seeds, almonds, and flaxseeds. Store in an airtight jar in the refrigerator, ready for use on your cereal each morning.

Oily Hair

Go Botanical

It's not fair, but even the most fastidious shampooers can develop oily hair. Some women have especially active oil glands, so their hair starts to develop an oily sheen within hours after shampooing. But other factors play a role, too.

"Did you ever go out in a convertible and come back and feel your hair? Or play with your hair for an hour because your were anxious?" asks Carlo Cantavero, owner of Carlo and Company Salon in Greenwich, Connecticut. "It will feel soiled and oily because the stimulation makes the blood circulate in your scalp, and that causes the secretion of oil," he explains.

Wearing a hat does the same thing.

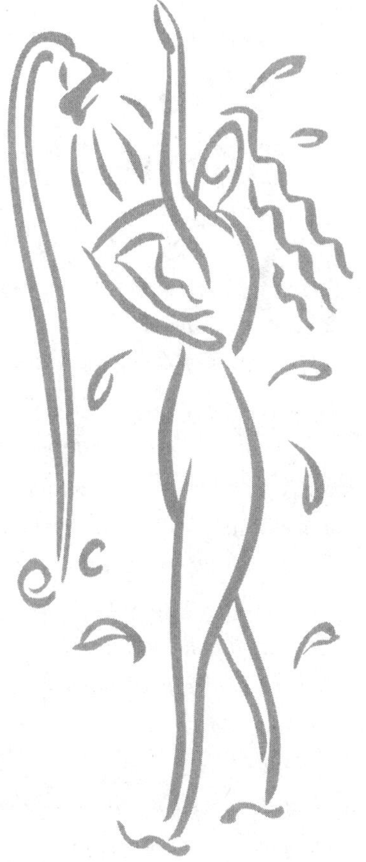

Short of shampooing your hair every hour on the hour, what can you do to keep your hair clean throughout the day? Try these tactics.

Use a shampoo advertised as a "balancing" or "botanical" formula. These are gentler on the scalp and more likely to clean your hair without overstimulating the oil glands, as more alkaline shampoos do, says Cantavero.

Avoid conditioning shampoos and two-in-one products. If your hair is naturally oily, adding a conditioner or shampoo-with-conditioner will only make things worse, says Diana Bihova, M.D., a dermatologist in New York City and author of *Beauty from the Inside Out.*

Wear a silk scarf instead of a polyester hat. Synthetic fabrics cause the scalp to sweat, which can make your hair appear oily. Natural fabrics, in contrast, allow your scalp to breathe, which helps keep your hair dry. Also, don't wear anything too tight on your head; this will also make your scalp sweat.

Helpful Hint

If your hair looks oily but you're too rushed to shampoo, lightly dust some talcum or baby powder on your brush, then run it through the part of your hair that looks oily. Or put a little talcum on your fingers, shake off the excess and run your fingers through your hair. The talcum will help separate the hairs that hang together and eliminate the oily look. If any talcum remains visible, just fluff it out with your fingers. ■

Oily Skin

Two Ways to Cut the Shine

Depending on how you look at it, oily skin can be a woman's best friend or her worst enemy.

Nestled just beneath your skin are tiny glands that pump out an oily, waxy liquid—called sebum—onto your face. The oil keeps your skin soft, supple, and well-hydrated. You'll look years younger than all your girlfriends who have dry skin because they'll begin to wrinkle prematurely as they age and you won't.

Too much of this skin-protecting oil, though, and you're likely to experience a makeup meltdown just 2 to 3 hours after you've applied it. Plus, it's the number one contributor to adult acne, says Leslie S. Baumann, M.D., director of cosmetic dermatology at the University of Miami.

But there are ways to enjoy the benefits of oily skin—without drowning in a sea of sebum.

1. Vinegar and water. Place ¼ cup of tap water and ¼ cup of white vinegar in a small container. Douse a cotton ball in the solution and wipe it all over your face. The vinegar will remove oil and debris deep within your pores. It will strengthen your skin and leave it less susceptible to environmental irritants, which can crank up oil production, says Zein E. Obagi, M.D., director of Obagi Dermatology, Plastic Surgery, and Laser Center of Beverly Hills.

If the vinegar stings your face, dilute the solution with more water. You may have to build up a tolerance. So try using it once or twice a week. Once your skin gets used to it, you can use it as often as twice a day, every day, says Dr. Obagi.

2. Retin-A (tretinoin). Revered as a wrinkle remover, Retin-A cream puts the squeeze on sebaceous glands, reducing oil production so that your skin won't be as slick. It also speeds the removal of the top layer of skin cells, keeping your pores free of dirt and debris. Retin-A is a derivative of vitamin A and is available in different concentrations by prescription only.

DON'T MAKE THIS MISTAKE

Using alcohol pads or other harsh astringents to wipe off oil is a big facial no-no. You'll leave your skin dry, which will trick your oil glands into thinking that they need to crank out more oil.

Helpful Hint

If your oily skin isn't responding to good skin care, and you're seeing more than your share of blackheads and whiteheads, you may want to see a dermatologist. She'll suggest a topical cleanser or astringent that's right for you. ■

Omega-3 Fatty Acids

Help Yourself to These "Good Fats" (Even If You Don't Like Fish)

What do flaxseed, walnuts, and a common California garden weed have in common? They are all great sources of omega-3 fatty acids, normally found in cold-water fish such as tuna and salmon.

Like an all-natural antifreeze, omega-3's help keep the tissues in fish functioning in icy waters. But in you, omega-3's lower your risk of several diseases.

Heart disease. Despite having more body fat and consuming a high-fat diet, Eskimos rarely have heart disease. Researchers suspect that their fish-laden diet should get the credit. In fact, studies have shown that eating these heart-friendly fats regularly can lower cholesterol and may even reverse atherosclerosis.

Cancer. Men and women who cook up two or more servings of omega-3-rich fish a week are 30 to 50 percent less likely to develop cancer of the esophagus, stomach, colon, and pancreas. Some studies suggest that omega-3's may boost your number of detoxifying enzymes—our first line of defense against environmental cancer causers. "You need these enzymes to break down carcinogens found in secondary smoke, car or bus fumes, pesticides, and environmental PCBs (polychlorinated biphenyl)," says Mitchell L. Gaynor, M.D., director of medical oncology at Strang Cancer Prevention Center at Cornell University and author of *Dr. Gaynor's Cancer Prevention Diet.* He advises everyone to take daily omega-3 supplements.

Cataracts and other eye problems. Without omega-3's, your brain and eyes couldn't develop normally. And as we age, diets rich in these fats as well as antioxidants lower our risk of degenerative eye diseases, like macular degeneration and cataracts.

HEMP OIL SKEWS TEST RESULTS

While hemp seed oil is a great source of omega-3's—about as high as flaxseed oil—there's one potential drawback: cannabinoids. These are the active ingredients in cannabis that cause positive drug tests.

Inflammation. While inflammation does fight microscopic invaders and disposes of damaged cells, overzealous immune activity can cause psoriasis, rheumatoid arthritis, ulcerative colitis, allergies, and even asthma. Like volume control for immunity, omega-3's turn down inflammation to a kinder level. But fortunately, they don't turn it off—like many over-the-counter medications.

Mental ills. People with schizophrenia, bipolar dis-❯❯

order, and depression may all benefit from fish or omega-3 supplements—especially those containing fish oil. Most fish oil supplements contain two omega-3 fatty acids, eicosapentaenoic acid (EPA) and docosahexaenoic acid (DHA). Studies show that EPA may reduce symptoms of schizophrenia, while depressive patients may benefit from DHA. Another study found that fish oil supplementation could help alleviate the symptoms of bipolar disorder.

Omega-3's for Women Who Don't Care for Fish

Since omega-3's help keep fish tissues working even in cold water, the colder their watery home, the more omega-3's fish contain. Some superior deep-sea sources: salmon, white albacore tuna, mackerel, herring, and sardines. But if you're a total vegetarian or simply don't like strong-tasting fish, you can also get a useful version of these fats in flaxseed or other plant foods. Once consumed, your body converts the omega 3's in plant foods into a version similar to what's supplied by fish.

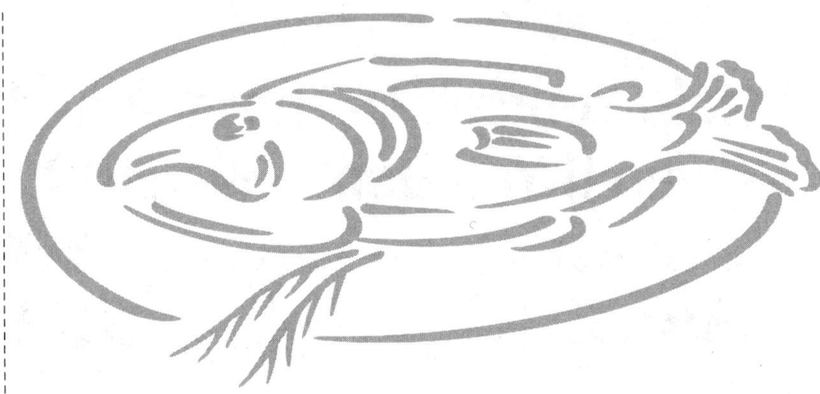

If you'd rather hold the anchovies, try a few of these nonfish sources. While there is no RDA for omega-3's, some studies have found that a minimum of 1 gram per day is beneficial. To get this amount, eat a serving of any of these foods every day. (You'll find them in most health food stores and some supermarkets.)

Flaxseed or flaxmeal

Serving size: 1 tablespoon of flaxmeal or ½ tablespoon of flaxseed

Mix flaxmeal in oatmeal or yogurt. Toss flaxseed on salad or in a plastic bag with dried fruit for an afternoon snack.

Flaxseed oil

Serving size: 1 to 3 teaspoons

"You can add flax oil to just about any cold dish, like salad, cereal, or yogurt," says Dr. Gaynor. "Just don't cook with it. It'll go rancid."

Canola oil or soybean oil

Serving size: 1 tablespoon

Good for salads and cooking—alternate use with olive oil. Since processing removes some omega-3's from the oils, look for unrefined varieties in your supermarket or health food store. These have a higher omega-3 content. And keep these oils refrigerated; they spoil quickly at room temperature.

Butternuts (white walnuts) and English walnuts

Serving size: about 2 tablespoons of each

Toss on salad or in cereal.

Walnut oil

Serving size: 1 tablespoon

Mix with red or white wine

SHOPPING TIPS FOR FISH OIL SUPPLEMENTS

If you don't eat fish twice a week, chances are you get only about one-fifth the omega-3's you need. If you don't like fish—or if eating it several times a week gets boring—getting up to 1 gram of omega-3 fatty acids from fish oil capsules is a safe option, say experts. Most capsules have about 0.3 gram of EPA (eicosapentaenoic acid) and DHA (docosahexaenoic acid).

Take a 1,000-milligram gel capsule three times a day with low-fat foods, like chicken, 1 percent milk, or low-fat yogurt, recommends Dr. Gaynor.

These supplements go rancid within 3 months, so it's important to buy fresh products.

• If a strong fishy odor wafts from the container after you open it, take it back. It's rancid.

• To protect your fish oil from heat and prevent spoiling, refrigerate it after you open the container.

• Throw away an open bottle after 3 months or when it develops a fishy stench.

Fish oil capsules can cause indigestion in some people. If this happens to you, switch to flaxseed oil. Also, fish oil supplements can cause nosebleeds and easy bruising, so don't take them if you have a bleeding disorder or uncontrolled high blood pressure or if you take anticoagulants (blood thinners) or use aspirin regularly. You should also avoid them if you have diabetes or are allergic to any kind of fish. Make sure you take fish oil, not fish-liver oil, which is high in vitamins A and D, which are toxic in high amounts.

vinegar for a salad dressing. The unrefined type has more omega-3 fatty acids.

Wheat germ oil

Serving size: 1 tablespoon

Mix into a fruit smoothie.

Purslane

Serving size: 2 cups

Toss with romaine lettuce for a salad. If you can't find purslane, try dandelion, another common weed that contains a small amount of omega-3's. It's available in early spring in many farmer's markets and supermarkets. Other green leafy vegetables, like spinach and collards and even broccoli, offer some omega-3's.

Chicken eggs from hens fed flaxmeal and fishmeal

Serving size: two eggs

Substitute these for regular eggs. Look for them in health food stores.

Helpful Hint

Eating too many trans-fatty acids or hydrogenated fats—found in processed foods like margarine, white bread, pastries, french fries, potato chips, and some salad dressings—can deplete omega-3 fatty acids. So read labels and cut back on foods that contain hydrogenated fats. ■

Osteoporosis

The Do's and Don'ts of Healthy Bones

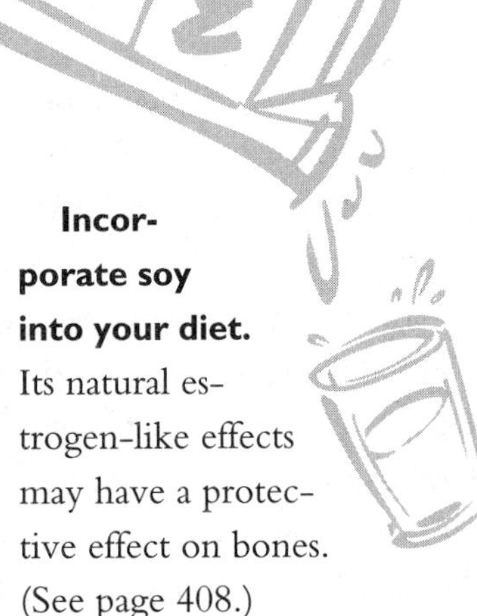

Forget the notion that your bones automatically grow weak and brittle with age. True, at menopause, the drop in production of the female hormone estrogen interferes with your body's natural ability to maintain sturdy, fracture-resistant bones. But there are several simple strategies you can use to help maintain strong bones well into your seventies, eighties, or nineties.

"Just because you're getting older, you don't have to end up bent over or out of commission with a hip or wrist fracture," says Karl Insogna, M.D., director of the Yale Bone Center at the Yale School of Medicine. "The good news about osteoporosis is that there is lots you can do to protect your skeleton."

Once you reach menopause—at about 51, for most women—you should have a bone density test, especially if you have a family history of osteoporosis or if you've had a bone fracture, advises Dr. Insogna. If you have low bone density, your doctor may suggest estrogen therapy, which has been shown to have a protective effect on bone.

Maintaining bone health naturally will also help. Starting today, maximize your bone density with these bone-saving strategies.

Get milk—and other calcium-rich foods. Since calcium is the brick and mortar of bones, consuming plenty of calcium helps you build and keep bone mass and prevent fractures. Make sure you get 1,000 milligrams every day (1,300 to 1,500 milligrams if you're over 50 and not on estrogen replacement therapy). (To find out how, see page 74.)

Remember your vitamin D. It's important for calcium absorption, yet many women have vitamin D deficiencies and don't even know it. You need 400 to 600 IU daily, from vitamin D–fortified milk, a multivitamin supplement, or from 20 minutes or so of sunlight every day.

Incorporate soy into your diet. Its natural estrogen-like effects may have a protective effect on bones. (See page 408.)

Get ½ hour of exercise at least five times a week. Incorporate weight-bearing aerobic exercise and resistance training, such as weight lifting, into your routine. The gentle push-and-pull on your bones stimulates bone growth and helps reduce your risk of falling.

Sidestep These Calcium Thieves

To truly safeguard your skeleton, you also need to avoid certain bone robbers.

Watch your salt intake. Consuming more salt than the recommended daily amount of 2,400 milligrams—about a teaspoon's worth, from processed foods or seasoned food—interferes with calcium absorption.

Don't crash diet. Women who limit their calorie consumption long term are shown to have lower bone density, increasing their chances of developing osteoporosis. Make sure you get at least 1,200 calories every day.

If you smoke, quit ASAP. Women who smoke tend to have earlier menopause, triggering osteoporosis and doubling their risk of fracture. Cigarette smoke is also thought to damage bone cells and prevent new bone growth, and it may reduce your body's ability to absorb calcium.

Minimize your need for steroids. Though effective in treating medical problems such as rheumatoid arthritis, asthma, or lung disease, when steroids are taken for more than 2 months, they can cause rapid bone loss and lead to osteoporosis. Talk to your doctor about nonsteroid approaches to control these conditions. ■

Overactive Bladder

A Workout That Holds Water

As a former model and busy sales representative, Bettye Roussos of Ormond Beach, Florida, takes pride in her appearance. When an overactive bladder left her with the repeated need to find a bathroom at a moment's notice, she was determined to master the problem, even though it meant some inconvenient changes.

"I carried extra underwear, panty hose, and incontinence pads with me," Roussos recalls. "And I changed my wardrobe from suits to long, full skirts, where I could hide them if I had a problem."

And as problems go, an overactive bladder can be one of the most frustrating, and one of the most confusing. It's not stress incontinence, a more common problem among women, where urine leaks out of the bladder during a sudden physical action, such as a sneeze or a laugh. With overactive bladder, the urge to urinate comes on more frequently—as much as a dozen times a day—and more suddenly. Unless you're close to a bathroom, the urge can lead to a sudden emptying of the entire bladder. What's more, the cause of overactive bladder isn't entirely clear. It may come on after a urinary tract infection, or it may be linked to certain neurological disorders, including Parkinson's disease or multiple sclerosis. On the other hand, it can often occur for no apparent reason.

In Roussos' case, medication eventually proved helpful in moderating the problem. But there are several things women can do to control an overactive bladder without medication, says Mary Jane Minkin, M.D., clinical professor of obstetrics and gynecology at Yale University School of Medicine.

She and others recommend these tactics.

Kick it with Kegels. Also known as pelvic floor exercises, kegels involve nothing more than contracting your pelvic muscles as described on page 248.

Turn off the faucet. When you feel the urge to uri- ››

nate, try to relax and contract your pelvic muscles as forcefully as you can. "That will set up a reflex that will shut off the urination reflex," says Alan Wein, M.D., chief of the urology department at the University of Pennsylvania School of Medicine in Philadelphia. The longer you've been doing

DON'T MAKE THIS MISTAKE

Generally, when people have problems with their bladders, they tend to drink a lot of fluids to clear it out, says Dr. Wein. That might be fine advice for an infection, but it can only make an overactive bladder worse. So, while fluids play an important role and shouldn't be decreased or eliminated, don't make a special effort to increase the amount of fluids you drink each day.

Overeating

Hide the Cookies in the Garage (and Other Ways to Show Your Appetite Who's Boss)

Things you never hear women say:

"I ate so much spinach last night, I felt like I was going to burst."

"I'd love a third helping of steamed carrots, but I'm watching my waistline."

"If I let myself go, I could easily eat a quart basket of strawberries, but then I'd hate myself afterward."

If you're like most women, you're more likely to overindulge in spinach dip, carrot cake, and strawberry cheesecake than their namesake foods.

An occasional indulgence is no big deal. "It's when you slip up again and again that it starts to be a problem," says Allan Geliebter, Ph.D., research psychologist at the Obesity Research Center at St. Luke's Hospital in New York City. "Chronic overeating can lead to weight gain and feelings of discomfort or guilt—especially since people tend to overeat high-calorie foods, not healthy things like fruits and vegetables."

Here are some tips to help put the brakes on overeating.

Eat only at the dining table, with a proper place setting—never in front of the TV, standing at the sink, or while talking on the phone. These activities distract you from your food, and before you know it, you might gobble down a whole bag of chips or cookies.

Hang a mirror near your dining table. Two studies have shown that watching yourself in a mirror while eating reduces consumption of high-fat foods by 22 to 32 percent. "When people see themselves in a mirror, they become more your kegels, the more effective this method will be.

Train your bladder. It may be possible to condition your bladder to hold urine for longer periods of time. Start by urinating every hour on the hour, whether you feel the need to or not, and keep it up for 3 to 4 days. Then extend it to every 90 minutes. Then extend it again to every 2 hours, 2½ hours, and so on until you reach your maximum capacity (about 4 hours).

Identify irritants. Alcohol, fruit juices, spicy foods, garlic, or chocolate can make some women urinate more often because they can irritate the bladder. If you consume a lot of these or other foods, try going without them for a few days and gauge how it affects your control, or the urgency to urinate, says Dr. Wein. "It's important to try to keep track of what bothers you and avoid anything that falls into that category." ■

aware of themselves and their goals," says Brad Bushman, Ph.D., lead researcher and associate professor of psychology at Iowa State University in Ames. "This prompts them to think twice about what they're eating, which prompts them to choose less-fattening foods."

Stop and think before you eat. "Simply taking a second or two to think about what you're about to eat and why you're eating it can have a big impact on your food choices," says Dr. Geliebter.

Place tempting foods in the garage, in a high cabinet, or other inaccessible spot. This will make it more difficult to absentmindedly grab them and eat, says Dr. Geliebter.

Look to nonfood sources of comfort. "Many women eat because they are upset or stressed and needcalming," says Dr. Geliebter. Instead, take a walk, listen to music, or take a bath. You'll find these activities even more soothing than eating cheesecake because you won't feel guilty afterward.

List what you plan to order before leaving for a restaurant. If you plan to have the grilled chicken or fish, rice pilaf, and a salad, but no more, write it down. Then stick to your list. Don't be seduced into add-ons like hot buttered rolls, appetizers, cream soup, or the special of the day.

Take the lead when ordering (or not ordering) dessert. The ritual is all too familiar: You're dining out with friends. The bread basket, salad plates, and dinner platters have been cleared away. Everyone at the table is stuffed to the gills. Yet when the server offers dessert, everyone is game. Unless you're truly famished (not very likely), take the lead and pass. "Most of ››

BANKING CALORIES BACKFIRES

Don't "save" an entire day's worth of calories for the big night out. "If you're ravenous when you go out to dinner, you're more likely to overeat," says Dr. Geliebter. Instead, eat a small, healthy snack like fruit or yogurt an hour before going to the restaurant, to help control your appetite.

the time, if one person orders dessert, others will too," says Dr. Geliebter. "To beat the temptation of getting chocolate cake after everyone else orders, speak up first. Try to choose something low-calorie like fruit or coffee, or have nothing at all—just say, 'No dessert for me, thanks.' The others may follow suit."

Helpful Hint

Most often, we overeat because we're feeling a certain way, and what we're feeling isn't hunger. "There is a link between emotions and eating," says Dr. Geliebter. "Don't confuse hunger with boredom for example. Before long, you may start to think you're hungry every time you're actually bored."

To break this habit, keep a food diary. "Write down everything you eat, and note your emotional state beside it. Before long, you may start to see a pattern emerge that tells why you're overeating," he says. Then deal with it: Irate? Confront the source. Angry? Address the issue head on. Frustrated? Voice your feelings. ■

Overexertion

Are You Exercising Too Much?

Overtraining is no better than not getting any exercise at all. Take Hannah Rothlin, for instance. As an exercise physiologist and personal trainer in Sebastopol, California, Rothlin knew better than to try to do a triathlon in 110-degree heat. Rothlin always told others to test but not push their limits. But this time, she ignored her own advice.

"I'd trained for a year, and dropping out was not an option I considered," says Rothlin. She completed the first two of the three events—the 2½-mile swim and the 112-mile bike ride. She dragged herself through most of the 26.2-mile run/walk.

Then, with only 3.2 miles to go, Rothlin's body and mind turned to mush. "I couldn't think straight—I couldn't focus," she recalls. "My legs were wobbly. My heart was beating too fast." She had to quit.

You don't have to do a triathlon in 110-degree heat to overexert yourself. Pushing yourself beyond your fitness level can leave you hurting and exhausted.

"You can overexert yourself in two ways—by doing too much too quickly or by ignoring discomfort or pain thinking that you can push through it," says James Garrick, M.D., director of the Center for Sports Medicine at St. Francis Hospital in San Francisco.

Not sure if you're working too hard? Take this quick quiz.

1. Are you fatigued most of the time, not just right after exercising?

2. Even though you're tired, do you have trouble sleeping?

3. Are you irritable (or do other people tell you that you are)?

4. Do you frequently get colds or other illnesses, and does recovery take longer?

5. Are you less motivated

GO EASY ON THE POST-WORKOUT PAINKILLERS

Don't rely on handfuls of ibuprofen or other over-the-counter painkillers to get you through exercise-induced aches and pains, especially if you work out in the heat. Combined with the stress of prolonged exercise and dehydration, taking too much ibuprofen or other nonsteroidal anti-inflammatory drugs, such as naproxen sodium and ketoprofen, can tax your kidneys and cause permanent damage, say researchers at the Noll Physiological Research Center at Pennsylvania State University in University Park. (Acetaminophen seemed to have less potential for damage.)

And skip the post-workout beer—alcohol only makes matters worse.

and less interested in your exercise program?

6. Is your resting heart rate getting higher?

7. Do you have a muscle or joint pain that is getting worse or doesn't go away after you stop exercising?

If you answered yes to any one of these questions, you may be overtraining. If you answered yes to more than one, you're definitely overtraining.

Unless you're injured, you don't have to stop exercising. Instead, "Back down and see if the symptoms go away," says Dr. Garrick.

Exercise less often. If you usually work out 6 days a week, do 4. If you're still tired, cut back to 3.

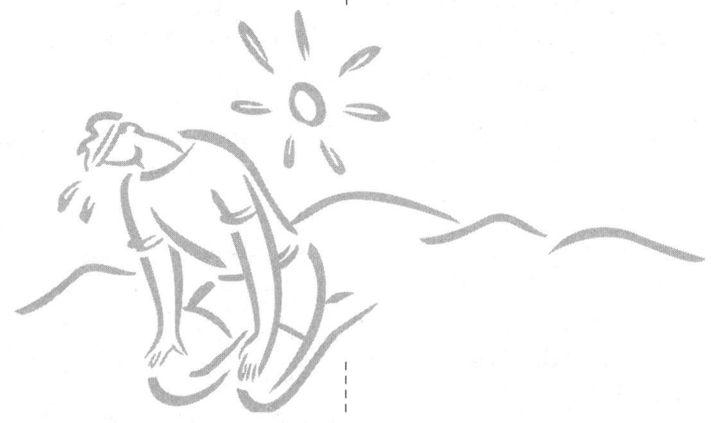

Don't work so hard. If you usually run, walk. If you cycle hills, stick to flat terrain. If you do step aerobics, lower your risers. If you strength train, lift less weight. Substitute a gentler exercise like yoga or tai chi for one of your workouts.

Cut your workouts short. If you're used to an hour of aerobics, do ½ hour. If you're used to a 2-hour bike ride, do 1 hour.

If exercising less often, less intensely, or for shorter periods of time helps, stay at your new level for a week to 10 days, then start increasing slowly, says Dr. Garrick. In the future, know your limits.

Helpful Hint

Treat any pulled muscles or sprains with R.I.C.E. (You'll read about how on page 379.) If you've simply overexerted yourself working or playing too hard and hurt all over, soak in a warm bath with Epsom salts. Heat brings damage-repairing white blood cells to the area; the salts open pores to allow heat access to your muscles. ■

Overweight

10 Simple Ways to Lose Weight

More protein. No carbohydrates. More cardio boxing. No pasta.

Try to lose weight, and you'll get dizzy trying to listen to the latest "official" advice.

Getting rid of unwanted pounds—and keeping them off—doesn't have to be confusing. Just follow these 10 commandments of weight loss from Prevention *magazine.*

1. Take a few minutes to think about the reasons you've decided to shape up.

Write them down. Keep the list someplace where you'll look at it often. Think about how much better you'll feel—and how great you'll look—as you move toward your weight-loss goals. Know that you can do it.

2. Set daily or weekly goals to change some bit of behavior that's been standing between you and your weight loss.

Working within a series of small, achievable goals has proven again and again to keep dieters more motivated and generate far better results than one big goal. It's good to increase your goals, but make sure they remain doable.

3. Heap your plate with juicy, sweet, wonderful-tasting fruits; filling, satisfying grains; and colorful, crunchy vegetables.

Losing weight and slimming down doesn't mean you'll have to be hungry, skip meals, or live on iceberg lettuce and celery sticks. Also, eating five or six mini-meals a day, rather than two or three large, heavy meals, keeps your body revved up and burning off calories.

4. Learn to distinguish false hunger from real hunger.

Record what, how much, and when you eat. Weigh and measure your food until you know what the recommended portions look like.

5. Find something that you like to do, and get moving.

Studies have shown time and time again that women who exercise are generally healthier, happier, and feel better about themselves than those who never get off the couch.

6. Work with weights, at home or in a gym.

When combined with aerobic exercise, some easy weight training will build muscle and keep your metabolism moving the way it should. Thirty minutes, 2 or 3 days a week, is all it takes to build up your muscles and get a sleeker, firmer, more toned look.

7. Figure out what makes you binge and recognize binge triggers.

The more you're aware of what you're doing, the easier it will be to control. Then steer yourself away from food and toward another source of comfort.

DON'T MAKE THIS MISTAKE

However you decide to reward yourself, it shouldn't be with food. As tempting as it might be to celebrate your 20-pound weight loss with a chocolate brownie sundae, it's not a good idea. Putting too much emphasis on "forbidden" food sets you up for a binge.

If you find yourself about to start on a binge or, worse still, in the middle of one, walk away.

8. Find the right weight-loss buddy.

Buddy up with your husband, your sister, your son or daughter, your best friend, or a neighbor. As long as it's someone you can count on to be there for you, a buddy can be more valuable than gold to your weight-loss plan.

9. When the weight-loss program blahs set in, jump-start your motivation.

Review your goals, and see how much you weighed and how much you've lost. Think about the reasons you started working out and watching your food intake in the first place. Congratulate yourself on the job you've done so far and adjust your goals to get you where you want to be. Don't throw it all away by giving up now!

10. Reward yourself.

Compliments from others tend to reinforce our efforts, and they can be great motivators. Even more important than the rewards you'll get from others are those that you'll give yourself. Do something that you really love but don't normally take the time for. ■

Overwork

Say No without Getting Fired

Remember those predictions that robots would be doing most of our work in the 21st century and that our biggest problem would be too much leisure time?

Hah! Since 1973, the average American workweek has actually increased 15 percent, and leisure time has decreased 37 percent.

For women workers, this time squeeze can be suffocating.

"Not only are women feeling the same workload and pressures that men have always felt but they're still responsible for worrying about the kids, groceries, and dinner," says Lynne McClure, Ph.D., management consultant in Mesa, Arizona.

Overwork takes a toll, mentally and physically. One study shows that women who juggle heavy work and family responsibilities are more likely than men to experience high blood pressure on the job that persists through the night. The landmark Framingham Heart Study cautions that stressful work may nearly triple a woman's risk of developing heart disease. Overwork is even associated with shorter menstrual cycles. The length of a woman's menstrual cycle may affect fertility, osteoporosis, and breast cancer.

Dr. McClure says the archetypal overworked woman is a mid-level manager with several subordinates, or a worker with a 12-hour shift schedule, either of whom may have a husband who won't help out at home. At her kids' soccer games, she's the mom who has one eye on the ball and the other on a pager.

"Women need to set boundaries," says Dr. McClure. "No matter how much glory they think they'll get, they need to set limits on how much responsibility they take from other people. Ironically, the more they overdo it, the lower the quality of what they do."

Beg off graciously. Whether it's tactfully telling your boss you can't work late or gracefully informing family members that you no longer can stage a four-star Christmas all by yourself, saying no ›› more often can be a strong first step toward avoiding overwork. "Women have to speak up for themselves and be assertive to management about what they need," whether it's flex time, better resources, or more realistic deadlines, Dr. McClure says.

Set off-duty hours. With only 24 hours in a day, you need to have some time you can call your own. If your boss is in the habit of loading you up with take-home work or calling after hours with perceived emergencies, explain why you can't accommodate these requests. At home, give yourself daily downtime when it's your mate's responsibility to clean up, run errands, and handle children's temper tantrums. "Women need to say when they'll be available and when they won't be," Dr. McClure says.

Create your own co-op. Are you tired of being a chauffeur/baby-sitter during your so-called free time? If you're a busy, disciplined worker during the day, use your hard-earned organizational skills to create a neighborhood car pool or baby-sitting co-op. Finding alternatives to these daily challenges can really lighten your load, Dr. McClure says.

Divvy up the chores. Is your "second shift" more of a grind than your first? If you find yourself fixing dinner, doing the laundry, checking the kids homework, getting them ready for bed, and paying all the bills, it's time to negotiate a more equitable arrangement with your spouse, Dr. McClure says. "Choose words that show you are not blaming anyone, but that you're simply taking care of your own needs. For example, don't say "You never help me." Instead say, "I need a break. Can we take turns fixing dinner?" Practice saying "I need."

DON'T MAKE THIS MISTAKE

You say you thrive under pressure? Forget it. Health risks are especially high for I-can-do-it-all women. "In many cases, women love their work," Dr. McClure says. "They can get so caught up in the excitement of it that they don't realize what's happening to them physically and emotionally. Eventually, they fall apart." Early warning signs that you are falling apart include: feeling angry or upset most of the time, sleeping too much or too little, having no energy, feeling depressed, acting differently than you usually do, eating too much or having no appetite, frequent illnesses, or wanting to "run away" from your job or family. Any of these symptoms could mean that you need a change in how you operate. When your life is balanced, you feel good.

Helpful Hints

If you want time for yourself, you have to book it. "It's not going to happen spontaneously," Dr. McClure says. "You aren't going to open up your calendar one day and say, 'Wow, Thursday's free!' "

Also, if you use a pager in your line of work, turn it off when you're off duty. Perhaps you and a coworker can arrange to be on call during alternate weeks. ■

P–Q

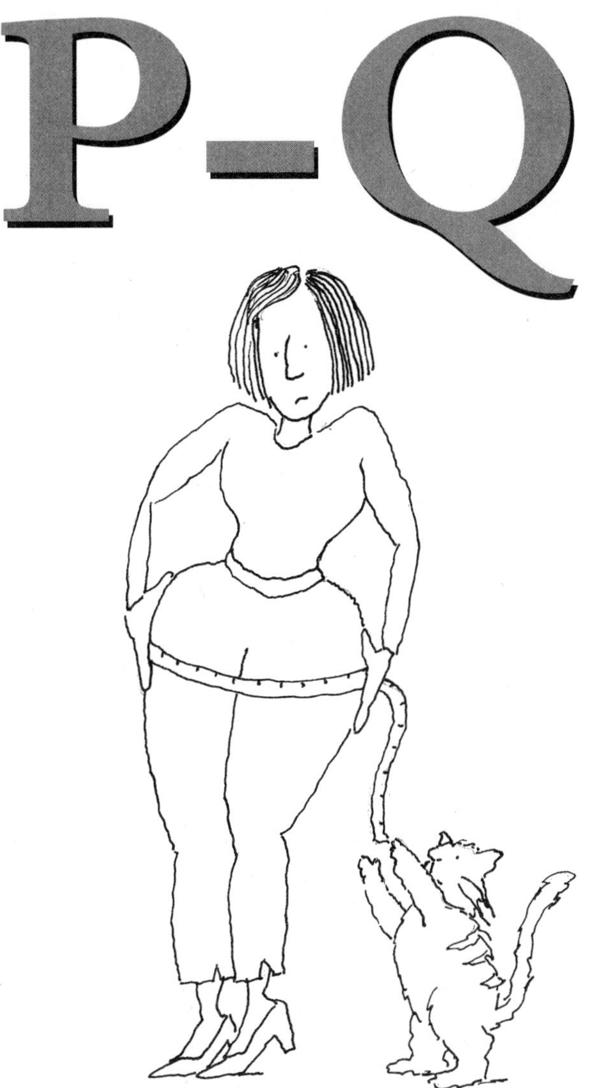

Are your periods getting lighter
while your hips are getting heavier?
Find out why on page 338.

Painful Intercourse

Why Suffer in Silence?

At one time or another, every sexually active woman experiences pain during intercourse. But if it becomes frequent, unbearable—or both—you have a problem.

"Sex is not supposed to hurt," says Sujatha Reddy, M.D., an obstetrician-gynecologist and assistant professor at Emory University School of Medicine in Atlanta.

Yet there are a lot of women out there who grit their teeth and bear the pain to accommodate the men in their lives. And they shouldn't. Sex should be fun, not painful, says Tori Hudson, N.D., a naturopathic physician and professor at the National College of Naturopathic Medicine in Portland, Oregon.

You may be experiencing painful intercourse for many reasons. In menopausal women, it's often vaginal dryness. (Read more about that on page 440.) Other possible causes range from a simple yeast infection to uterine fibroids.

Until your problem is diagnosed, there's not much you can do on your own. So speak up. You can expect your doctor to ask the following questions to pinpoint what's causing the problem and begin treatment. ››

WHEN YOUR MAN IS TOO BIG

If your husband's penis is large, don't worry—you can still make love comfortably.

"The vagina is a very stretchable tissue. If a baby can pass through it during childbirth, a woman should be able to accommodate a large penis—with room to spare," says Barbara Bartlik, M.D., clinical assistant professor of psychiatry in the departments of psychiatry, obstetrics, and gynecology at Weill College of Medicine at Cornell University in New York City.

If size is a problem, in most cases, the man isn't too big. Rather, the woman may be too small, says Dr. Bartlik. Here's what you can do to put the pleasure back into your sex life.

Spend a little extra time on foreplay. Focus on kissing and caressing each other from head to toe. Ask your husband to stimulate your clitoris with his fingers or mouth, bringing you to orgasm. "After you've experienced pleasure, and you're fully aroused—and relaxed—then let your husband slowly and gently proceed with intercourse," says Dr. Bartlik.

Minimize deep thrusting. Get on top or assume the missionary position with your legs somewhat straight. Don't make love doggie-style, on your hands and knees while your hubby enters you from behind, says Dr. Bartlik.

Ask your doctor for a vaginal dilator. It's a phallic-shaped probe that you insert into your vagina. You move it around from side to side and front to back to stretch the vaginal walls. If you use the dilator 20 minutes a day, your lovemaking will feel more comfortable in a week or two, says Dr. Bartlik.

• Is the pain deep within or at the opening of the vagina?

• How long have you had the pain?

• At what times during the month do you feel the pain? (At midcycle? During menstruation?)

• Does it hurt to insert a tampon?

• Is there pain with any type of urogenital contact, such as wiping yourself after using the toilet or receiving oral sex?

To learn about remedies for common causes of painful intercourse, turn to Yeast Infections. ■

Panic Attacks

Float Your Way Out of Flood-Stage Anxiety

They're not called panic attacks for nothing. A racing heart, chest discomfort, shortness of breath, hyperventilation, dizziness, nausea, and feeling out of control are scary, especially if you have no good reason for panic.

A panic attack lasts anywhere from 10 to 30 minutes, but it feels like forever.

Panic attacks can begin at any age and don't discriminate according to sex. But according to Pepi Granat, M.D., professor of family medicine and community health at the University of Miami, for some women, the emotional upheavals of menopause may cause greater anxiety, which can lead to panic attacks.

"First, understand what's happening and realize that you will be okay," says John Vanin, M.D., professor of psychiatry and family and community medicine at West Virginia University School of Medicine in Morgantown. Otherwise, the attacks become a self-fulfilling prophecy. "Most men and women who have had panic attacks become so fearful of another one that they become even more anxious, which makes the problem worse."

Unfortunately, when you're in the middle of a panic attack, there's little you can do to stop it, says Dr. Granat. In fact, fighting the attack as it is happening makes it worse because your anxiety becomes heightened. Instead, Dr. Granat suggests the F-A-F-L method, developed by Australian researcher Claire Weeks, D.Sc.

Face it. Don't fight the attack, but face the fact that it is happening.

Accept it. Accept the fact that there is nothing you can do to stop the attack from happening.

Float through it. Try to detach yourself from the feelings of anxiety and float through them by thinking calming, relaxing thoughts. You may want to rely on your belief system during this phase and pray or meditate to relax. Or, suggests Dr. Granat, imagine that you actually are floating on a raft in a calm pool of water.

Let time pass. Remain in the floating state and allow

time to pass. You will eventually see that nothing actually happens, and you'll be all right.

To prevent future attacks:

Pay attention to what seems to set you up for an attack, and learn how to handle the triggers. Anything that increases your heart rate and makes you anxious or not able to sleep well can trigger an attack, says Dr. Granat. This includes caffeine, alcohol, certain over-the-counter drugs (especially those that warn people with high blood pressure against taking them), stress, and even scary movies or stressful television dramas.

Take steps to buffer stress in your life. "Anything that helps you stay relaxed will help prevent panic attacks from occurring," says Dr. Vanin. Adopt relaxing hobbies, do yoga or meditate, practice your faith, take a leisurely walk, or work out.

If you have recurrent attacks, attacks that are disrupting your life, symptoms of depression or anxiety, suicidal thoughts, or you are avoiding places (agoraphobia), it's time to see your doctor to discuss treatment options. ■

Paper Cuts

First-Aid for Fumbling Fingers

Anyone who has ever sliced her finger opening the mail is painfully aware of just how sharp paper can be. And a manila folder? It's the Ginsu steak knife of paper cutlery.

From gift wrap to food wrap, Americans handle about 187 billion pounds of paper and paper goods a year. Sooner or later, you're bound to get cut. "We're always in a hurry," says Mary Ruth Buchness, M.D., chief of dermatology at St. Vincent's Hospital and Medical Center in New York City. "I know I'm always rushing when I get a paper cut."

Don't take paper cuts lightly, says Dr. Buchness. "Any opening in the skin, even a microscopic cut, can let bacteria through. Keep it clean and protected from environmental dirt and germs." Here's how.

Rinse the cut with warm water. Then clean it with a little peroxide to prevent infection. Next, apply an antibacterial ointment, such as bacitracin. Finally, cover it with a bandage. "In general, wounds heal better if they're covered," says Dr. Buchness.

Close the cut with Krazy Glue. "I've done it myself," says Dr. Buchness. "It is sterile and seals the skin, so it prevents dirt and germs from getting into the wound." Simply rinse the cut with warm water, dry, then dab a little Krazy Glue (or Super Glue) on a ››

DON'T MAKE THIS MISTAKE

If you have a paper cut, keep it clean and covered. "One woman I treated was hospitalized for 3 days because she got a splinter in her hand, then gardened and picked up bacteria," says Dr. Buchness. The same thing can happen with a paper cut. If you have redness, swelling, or pus, see a doctor within 12 hours. "Those are signs of infection," she says. "Any infection on your hand calls for immediate treatment."

cotton swab and apply it to the cut. The glue will immediately seal the cut and relieve any pain.

(If you are allergic to nail cosmetics, avoid using Krazy Glue. "It contains some of the same ingredients found in nail glue," says Dr. Buchness. Stick with old-fashioned peroxide and antibacterial ointment instead.) ■

Pap Tests

Tips for a More Comfortable Pelvic Exam

If you shudder at the thought of lying on an examination table with your feet propped up on stirrups, join the crowd.

"No wonder so many women dread Pap tests—they tend to be uncomfortable and embarrassing," says Lila A. Wallis, M.D., clinical professor of medicine at Cornell University Medical College in New York City, leading advocate for quality women's health care, and author of The Whole Woman. *"All too often, bad experiences cause many women to postpone this exam. Some don't go at all."*

Your doctor needs to see you at least once a year to detect problems in your reproductive organs and elsewhere in the pelvic area. If you're anxious about going to the gynecologist, here's what Dr. Wallis says you can do to make your exam as painless and as comfortable as possible.

Tell your doctor how you feel about the procedure. If she knows you've experienced pain or discomfort in the past, she can put you at ease by telling you what to expect and what not to expect during the procedure, and take extra care to reduce your fears of the unexpected.

Empty your bladder. Going to the bathroom just before the exam makes the Pap test a lot more comfortable. Besides, a full bladder prevents your doctor from examining your uterus properly.

Move your bowels. You'll also feel less discomfort with an empty colon, says Dr. Wallis. And you'll make it easier for your doctor to check your ovaries as well as the front and back of your uterus for any abnormalities during a rectal-vaginal exam.

Relax your abs. Tense abdominal muscles will prevent your doctor from manually examining your uterus, fallopian tubes, and ovaries effectively. Ease the tension by breathing in and breathing out deeply, focusing on relaxing your tummy.

Helpful Hints

That funny-looking metal clamp your doctor places inside your vagina to peek at your cervix during a gyn exam is called a speculum. If it's cold, especially in the

A BETTER TEST FOR DETECTING CERVICAL CANCER

Next time you make an appointment for your annual Pap test, ask your doctor if she can perform a PapSure exam when she takes the usual cervical tissue sample. This screening procedure—also called speculoscopy—allows doctors to immediately see precancerous or cancerous cells on the cervix during a pelvic exam that the Pap test doesn't generally detect.

Studies show that speculoscopy can raise the accuracy rate of the Pap test from 40 percent, when used alone, to 90 percent for the tandem procedure.

winter time, it will send chills up your spine. So ask your doctor to warm it up for you in a water basin before inserting it into your vagina, says Dr. Wallis.

Most doctors use a one-size-fits-all speculum, which tends to be large. So if your cervical exam hurts, ask your doctor to use a smaller speculum, says Dr. Wallis. ■

Passive Smoking

Kindly Ways to Clear the Air without Alienating Your Friends

In the not-so-distant past, American society and government turned its focus toward urging people not to engage in an offensive, potentially disease-spreading habit in public.

Health-conscious people posted signs and carried placards prohibiting this habit except in very specific places. Scofflaws who did it anyway risked a fine, or at least a stern scolding.

The time was the early 1900s. The health scare was tuberculosis. And the social no-no was spitting in public.

A century later finds us in a similar situation as we try to eliminate breathing secondhand smoke. This time, though, the turf isn't a messy sidewalk. It's our workplaces, public places (especially restaurants), homes, and cars.

When nonsmokers breathe someone else's cigarette smoke, they dramatically increase their chances of lung cancer and heart disease, as well as a wheezing attack if they have asthma. Secondhand smoke can be lethal, so even nonsmokers need to avoid tobacco smoke, says Michele Bloch, M.D., Ph.D., chair of the tobacco control and prevention subcommittee of the American Medical Women's Association. So, until we're all protected by legislation, she offers these suggestions to clear the air around you.

Protect your home with love. Most smokers know where their habit won't be welcome. But if you have to ask a friend or relative not to light up in your home, be sure they know it's the smoke you dislike—not the smoker. Give them the option to smoke in a comfortable outdoor place with good ventilation, such as a porch. Or take a walk with them. Sometimes smoke is ›› less bothersome if you're outdoors or in a well-ventilated area. Permit indoor smoking only as a last resort.

Use the sign of the times. Place a small, simply worded sign, like "Welcome to a smoke-free home," near your front door to head off awkward confrontations.

Give smokers a break on car trips. Because cars are so enclosed—and rolling down the windows doesn't give enough ventilation—secondhand smoke is even more intense on road trips than in a building, Dr. Bloch says. If you're sharing a car with a smoker, make an agreement that you'll stop periodically to stretch and give them a chance to light up.

Vote with your dollars. Patronize smoke-free restaurants. If you do dine at a restaurant with a smoking section and are bothered by the smoke, politely tell the manager or owner that the setup isn't working and you won't be able to return until it's fixed.

"Restaurant owners aren't foolish. If people complained about the food, they'd do something about it," Dr. Bloch says. "They need to hear from nonsmokers that they're not pleasing them. And by putting the smokers off in a room with the same air is like having a nonchlorinated section of the swimming pool."

Let your voice be heard. Ask your elected officials to support measures to eliminate secondhand smoke in work places and public places. ■

Peanut Allergy

Be Your Own Detective

Avoiding an allergy to peanuts might seem simple: Don't eat any peanuts. But peanuts can show up in the most unlikely foods—like spaghetti sauce.

"Trying to avoid peanuts in every way, shape or form can be time-consuming—and frustrating," says Daryl Altman, M.D, director of Allergy Information Services in Baldwin, New York. "You have to be supremely aware of everything that goes in your mouth." Her advice:

Make as much food as possible from scratch. Eating in restaurants can be especially chancy.

When you must buy packaged food, read every food label, every time you buy it. Manufacturers change ingredients, so even a product that is safe to buy today may not be so tomorrow.

DON'T MAKE THIS MISTAKE

A few women are so sensitive to peanuts that they can become extremely sick, even die, if they eat food cooked with utensils that were used to prepare peanut-containing foods. If you have a serious peanut allergy, make sure you're never without an emergency Epi-Pen or Ana-Kit, so you can inject yourself with epinephrine at the first signs of a reaction.

Helpful Hint

To help identify technical terms for peanuts and other common food allergens, contact the

Pectin

Not Just for Grape Jelly

Remember that magical powder your mom—or grandma—used to make homemade jelly when you were a kid? Experts say it has three unexpected health benefits: It lowers cholesterol, blood sugar, and your risk of cancer.

Added to liquids like grape juice, pectin turns liquids into solids. Inside you, this water-soluble fiber becomes a gelatinous cleaning lady, removing cholesterol components, cancer-causing compounds, and glucose as it works its way through your intestines. That lowers your risk for coronary artery disease, cancer, and diabetes. This colonic "Hazel" does its best work when you get 20 to 35 grams of total dietary fiber a day. If you include fruits, vegetables, and legumes in your daily diet to meet this recommendation, you can get plenty of pectin from foods along with other beneficial fibers.

JELLY DOESN'T COUNT

Although jellies and jams are made with pectin, they aren't great sources of fiber. You'd have to eat seven of those restaurant jelly packets to get just 1 gram of fiber and 27 packets to get as much as in one medium apple.

Studies have found that using 15 grams of pectin supplements can lower cholesterol. No need to rush out ››

Food Allergy Network and ask for "How to Read the Label," available for a small fee. For additional, free information about food allergies, send a self-addressed stamped envelope to the Food Allergy Network at 10400 Eaton Place, Suite 107, Fairfax, VA 22030-2208. They track ingredients for hundreds of food products, including fast foods. And they publish a newsletter that details the peanut content of new foods on the market and notifies consumers of product recalls due to incorrect food labeling. ■

SURPRISING SOURCES OF PEANUTS

Avoiding peanut brittle and peanut butter is a cinch. Avoiding other sources of peanuts isn't so easy. Chefs may add peanut butter to certain kinds of sauce, so always ask questions before eating food prepared by someone else. Here are some likely (and some highly unlikely) foods that may contain peanuts, according to the Food Allergy Network.

- Chili
- Chinese, Vietnamese, Indonesian, and Thai foods (including egg rolls)
- Chocolate candy, such as plain M&Ms
- Desserts such as cookies and other baked goods
- Fried foods
- Garnishes for almost every meal
- Gravies
- Ice creams
- Nougat
- Pastries
- Spaghetti sauce

and buy some pectin supplements, sold in health food stores, though.

"Just eat an apple," says Jerry Hickey, R.Ph., a pharmacist specializing in nutritional supplements and drug-food interactions and coauthor of *Dr. Gaynor's Cancer Prevention Program.* Pectin is the most commonly found soluble fiber in produce. It's what makes ripe fruit feel firm. **Other great fruit sources include bananas, grapefruit, oranges, nectarines, peaches and pears with their peels, tangerines, dried figs, dates, prunes, and blackberries.** Pineapple, melons, blueberries, cherries, raspberries, and strawberries are lower in pectin (although they have other nutritional attributes).

Vegetables and legumes, like beans and peas, also contain pectin. In fact, just five servings of fruits or vegetables a day can supply some of those all-important 15 grams. One way to get them: Eat half a grapefruit for breakfast, a small mixed garden salad sprinkled with dried cranberries for lunch, and ½ cup of steamed peas and a baked potato with dinner.

Perimenopause

Herbs That Restore Your Menstrual Rhythm

You might call the decade before menopause "period pause." Your period used to arrive like clockwork, every 28 days. Now it's early one month and late the next. Sometimes it doesn't show up for months. And when it does, it may last 2 weeks or more. Your periods may be very heavy, or very light.

Meanwhile, you're starting to have an occasional hot flash and bouts of insomnia. What's going on here?

If you're in your forties but not yet menopausal, your hormones may be on the blink. Levels of the female hormones estrogen and progesterone—which used to fluctuate on cue—may surge one month or be released at odd times the next. Also common are hot flashes and night sweats as well as insomnia, irritability, anxiety, forgetfulness, and fatigue.

"Menopause is like puberty," says Susun S. Weed, an herbalist and herbal educator in Woodstock, New York, and author of the *Wise Woman* series of herbal health books, including *Menopausal Years: The Wise Woman Way.* "You may have symptoms you haven't had since you were a teenager: cramps, PMS, fatigue, headaches. It's a complex change in the symphony of hormones that are being played inside a woman's body. But it's a normal passage that every woman goes through."

Even so, that doesn't mean you have to put up with problem periods. Two female-friendly herbs can help you navigate the transition from super tampons to none.

Motherwort. Available at health food stores, this herb "will make erratic periods less erratic," says Weed. It also cools hot flashes and relieves anxiety, insomnia, PMS, and menstrual cramps. A dose is 15 to 25 drops of Motherwort

Here are some other ways to ensure that you harness the power of that disease-fighting custodian.

Can the juice. If it's pectin you want, pick up a piece of fruit, not a carton of juice. Extracting juice from fruit leaves most pectin behind. If you want to have juice, choose one that has pulp or is not clear—that means it has some of the fiber left in.

Sweeten your selection. If you're a card-carrying member of the vegetable-haters club, munch on a bunch of grapes and any other fruits you enjoy. Five servings daily of these light delights still provide plenty of pectin, as well as its partners in disease prevention: antioxidants and phytochemicals.

Helpful Hint

The less rain that crops get, the smaller fruits and vegetables will be and the more concentrated the pectins will be. So if your region experiences a midsummer drought, purchase fruits and vegetables locally. You'll not only help your neighborhood farmer but you'll also boost your pectin. ■

tincture (available at health food stores and made from the fresh flowering plant) in a small amount of water. Take as needed up to four times a day. Motherwort can be used regularly for many years.

Shepherd's purse. If your periods are heavy, use motherwort sparingly. To stop flooding, use shepherd's purse instead. This is one of the best herbs to stop heavy uterine bleeding. A dose is 1 full dropperful in some water or juice. Repeat this dose every 15 minutes, or until bleeding slows down. You may bleed more heavily after the first dose since shepherd's purse contracts the uterus. If flooding is severe—if you're going through a super tampon every hour or having frequent accidents—place the tincture under your tongue instead, says Weed. You can continue with two or three doses a day until the bleeding is completely controlled. And if your bleeding seems too severe, you should see your doctor to make sure that you're not anemic.

If you can't find shepherd's purse at your health food store, try lady's-mantle and follow the same dosage for shepherd's purse. Lady's-mantle also works as a preventive .

DON'T MAKE THIS MISTAKE

If your periods are very heavy, you should also avoid taking red clover tincture, alfalfa sprouts, cleavers tincture, pennyroyal tincture, willow bark tincture (although the infusions are okay for these), or wintergreen in any form. These herbs can make matters worse.

Do not take shepherd's purse if you have a history of kidney stones.

Helpful Hint

Snack on flaxseed. Flaxseed contains lignans, substances that your body turns into weak estrogens. Added to your changing supply of estrogen, flaxseed may help balance your shifting hormones. Try 1 tablespoon of freshly ground flaxseed on your cereal or salad. Grind the seeds right before eating. ■

Perm Problems

Reactivate Tired Waves

Hairstylists don't use the term *permanent wave* anymore.

"Now we say that we 'restructure or alter the texture of the hair for style support,'" says Leslie Correa, owner of Capelli D'oro, a full-service day spa in New York City.

Call it what you will, using chemicals to make straight hair wavy presents the same problems that women and their hairstylists have always faced: The perm looks fine at first but goes flat in a few weeks.

You can't reperm too soon, though. Perming hair that already has some perm left in it can seriously dry the hair. Wait at least 6 weeks for a root perm and 3 to 4 months to reperm the entire head, says Leslie.

Meanwhile, here's what you can do to perk up a pooped-out perm.

Get it trimmed. Cutting the hair can help re-

Pesticides

The Right Way to Wash Fruits and Vegetables

"Eat five fruits and vegetables a day." The message is everywhere—it's even printed on the plastic bags dispensed in the produce section of your supermarket. And for good reason: Loads of evidence says that eating plenty of fruits and vegetables decreases your risk of a number of health problems, from high blood pressure to cancer.

But what about all the pesticides that growers spray on fruits and vegetables to kill insects, fungus, and weeds? After all, pesticides are by nature toxic. At least to pests. In repeated doses. But how do they affect you?

Experts at the National Institute for Environmental Health Sciences claim that pesticide residues on fruits and vegetables are so small that they are unlikely to be unhealthy. **Your risk of illness is much greater, they say, if you avoid eating fruits and vegetables.**

"The benefits of eating fruits and vegetables, which provide essential vitamins, minerals, and phytonutrients, far outweigh the dangers of pesticides," says Martha Smith Patnoad, cooperative extension food safety education specialist in the department of food science and nutrition at the University of Rhode Island in Kingston. For peace of mind—and to get rid of dirt—

DON'T MAKE THIS MISTAKE

Avoid washing your fruits and vegetables with soap or even with the fruit washes that are now available, Patnoad says. These products can soak into food and are difficult to wash off. You're just trading one chemical for another.

store movement and curl by taking off unnecessary weight.

Apply gel at the roots and distribute to the ends of your hair. Then grab a small handful of hair, gently scrunch it, and let it air-dry. Or, hold it up and direct medium-temperature air from a blow-dryer with a diffuser starting at the ends and pushing up to the roots. This will help restore body.

Try a curl rejuvenator. Available at most salons and stores, these products make the most of any natural curl you have by bumping up the hair texture and giving you beautiful curl, says Correa.

Pin it back or tie it up. If your hair is shoulder-length or longer, try pulling it up and pinning it to the top of your head. This will make the most of the curls you have left while the bottom layer grows out.

Helpful Hint

If you have the opposite problem—your perm is too curly, too kinky, and you hate it—apply a creamy leave-in conditioner or styling gel after shampooing, says Correa. "They will weigh the curl down and make the hair manageable." ■

clean them correctly. Here's how.

• Peel fruits and vegetables whenever possible, and throw away or compost the outer leaves of leafy vegetables. This gets rid of their surface pesticides.

• Thoroughly wash all fruits and vegetables under cool running water, even if you plan to peel them. Then drain them in a colander. "When you're peeling them, you could transfer some of the pesticides from the peel to the part you eat," says Patnoad. "Rinsing first washes pesticide residue, dirt, and other possible contaminants right down the drain."

• Rinse foods that have nooks and crannies with special care. Fruits like raspberries and vegetables like lettuce tend to collect pesticides and dirt easily.

• Scrub fruits and vegetables that have lots of surface dirt, like potatoes, with a firm brush or washcloth. ■

BUY LOCAL, BUY ORGANIC

The easiest way to avoid eating pesticides on your fruits and vegetables is to buy organic fruits and vegetables, grown without chemical fertilizers, stimulants, antibiotics, or pesticides, says Nell Newman, daughter of actor Paul Newman and founder of Newman's Own Organics, an Aptos, California, company that sells all-organic products like pretzels and tortilla chips. (As a coincidence, they go well with Newman's Own Salsa, distributed by her dad's nationwide food company.)

"I was introduced to organic foods by my parents at an early age, so I've always been concerned about the potential health effects of pesticides," says Newman.

"Support your local farmers," urges Newman. Produce that has to travel long distances must be treated with more chemicals to control fungus and rot as the fruits and vegetables travel and sit in storage and on grocery store shelves. Since their produce doesn't travel as far as food distributed by commercial growers, local farmers can use fewer pesticides.

Pet Allergies

Live in Peace with Furry Friends

A few years ago, Joanne Howl noticed that her eyes were constantly itchy and watery, her nose was either stuffy or runny, and her whole body felt like a battery in need of recharging. A doctor confirmed that she had developed allergies to dogs and cats. But she wasn't about to surrender her pets nor her career—as a veterinarian.

Dr. Howl, who practices in West River, Maryland, told her allergist that getting rid of her two dogs and three cats wasn't an option. Neither was quitting her job and embarking on a new career. Luckily, she didn't have to.

As it turns out, people with pet allergies can still mingle with their furry friends and keep the wheezing and the sneezing to a minimum. Dr. Howl, along with Mary Ann Michelis, M.D., chief of the division of allergy and immunology at Hackensack University Medical Center in New Jersey, offer ways to lessen, if not avoid, allergy flare-ups for pet owners.

Make your bedroom a no-pets zone. Otherwise, you'll end up breathing in their dander all night as they sleep with you. Keep the door shut when you're gone during the day. Wash the sheets weekly in hot water to keep dust mites or other allergens to a minimum.

Invest in a filter. Many allergy specialists recommend HEPA (high-efficiency particle arresting) room air filters to clear the rooms of allergens. HEPA filters come in various sizes and are available at most home supply stores.

If you can afford it, Dr. Howl suggests asking your heating and/or air conditioning service to add an electrostatic or hypoallergenic filter to your furnace. They're more expensive, but more effective.

Lather up your pet weekly. Washing dogs—and if possible, cats—once a week with a gentle shampoo made for pets can diminish dander production, prevent dry skin, and nourish the skin and fur. They also get rid of pollens and grass allergens the pet may have collected on its coat from being outside. "With practice, you can do a complete routine allergy bath in 5 minutes," says Dr. Howl. Ask your vet to recommend a brand of shampoo.

Wipe your pet's coat in the morning and in the evening. Use a damp cloth (or damp oven mitt used only for pets) to get rid of dander or other allergens that accumulate between baths.

Buy dust-free litter for your cats. This limits dust that is known to collect pet dander.

When you vacuum, use double-filtration or microfiltration vacuum bags. They trap airborne allergens and can be purchased where vacuum-cleaner supplies are sold. ■

Pierced Ears

First-Aid for Telephonitis and Other Rips, Redness, and Rashes

Compared to body piercing—rings adorning the belly buttons, eyebrows, and tongues of young people—plain old pierced ears may seem a bit quaint and harmless.

Yet even pierced ears can cause problems, including redness, swelling, blisters, itchiness, and pain, says Rebecca L. Euwer, M.D., a dermatologist in Dallas.

If you're going to have a problem, most likely it will occur shortly after the piercing is done, and stem from an infection or allergy. Infection from piercing usually starts within 1 week of piercing, but allergic reactions can occur anytime—even years after piercing.

Here's what you can do to help prevent trouble right from the outset—and treat a problem if something goes wrong.

Make sure the piercing device is sterile. One surefire clue: "The earring that will be used should come in a wrapped plastic or cellophane package that the person doing the piercing has to pull open and out. If they just pull it out of a box, something's wrong," says Euwer. The ears should be cleansed with rubbing alcohol, and the person doing the piercing should wear gloves.

Avoid wearing costume jewelry. Use only earrings with 100 percent stainless-steel posts. This will prevent exposure to nickel, a metal commonly used in jewelry, which many women are allergic to. Usually, 14-karat gold is okay, but not always.

DON'T MAKE THIS MISTAKE

Many women clean their earrings with alcohol, to prevent infections. Not a good idea, says Dr. Euwer. "Alcohol can start to erode the coating, which may cause the nickel to leech out," she says, "and potentially cause an allergic rash and subsequent infection. Instead, clean your earrings only when they look cruddy along the post."

Don't tighten earring backs. Loosely-adjusted backs will allow air to get to the hole and keep it free of unnecessary pressure.

After putting on your earrings, try not to touch your ears during the day. If your hands aren't clean, you could cause an infection.

Take off your earrings before lengthy phone calls. Prolonged pressure against your ear can prevent air from getting to the hole and cause the hole to elongate, which may eventually make it impossible to wear earrings at all. Do not take them out right after the piercing is done. Wait until they've healed. ››

Avoid "chandeliers" and hula hoops. Heavy earrings, too, can tear the hole, especially if you're on the phone a lot or the earring gets pulled.

Always remove your earrings before going to bed. This will also allow air to get to the hole and help prevent tearing.

Helpful Hints

If you develop an allergic reaction to your earrings—itching, redness, swelling, or tiny oozing blisters—apply a cortisone cream daily until it clears up.

If you have an infection—characterized by slight to moderate pain—stay away from neomycin, a topical antibiotic ointment that may cause allergies. Instead, apply bacitracin, an antibiotic cream or ointment, or rubbing alcohol, daily. If your ear is infected and doesn't get better within 48 hours of cleaning and ointment, remove the earrings. If the infection hurts badly or if redness has spread beyond the earlobe to the surrounding skin, consult a doctor. You may need a prescription antibiotic. ■

Pizza Burns

Quick Relief for a Hot Singed Roof

When searing-hot cheese meets tender tissue on the roof of your mouth, the result is predictable: You get a pizza burn. Within hours, the scalded skin begins to shed. As new cells replace the old, your mouth may be supersensitive to hot food.

"As irritating as pizza burns are, wounds in the mouth heal more quickly than they do elsewhere on the body," says Irwin Ziment, M.D., hot-food lover and professor and chief of medicine at Olive View–UCLA Medical Center in Sylmar, California. "That's because the surface cells of the mouth and tongue grow rapidly and seem to heal more easily than skin cells."

The next time a pizza slice singes your mouth, don't just cry, "Mamma mia!" Hasten the healing by following Dr. Ziment's advice.

Suck on an ice cube, pronto. For the first 5 to 10 minutes after being burned, rely on ice cubes. Your mouth contains pain receptors and heat receptors, which transmit messages to the brain. Ice cubes seem to slow down these pain signals, thereby reducing the pain sensation. Ice water also helps.

Chew on a clove. After the ice cube, fight the pain and burn by chewing and sucking on a whole clove. If whole cloves aren't available, you can substitute powdered clove or a drop of oil of clove. The chewing and sucking action releases eugenol from the cloves. This substance acts as a natural anesthetic. Dr. Ziment recommends chewing on one clove every hour for the first few hours of a pizza-burn attack.

Consume dairy products. For the first day or so after a pizza burn, soothe the site by eating frozen yogurt or ice cream or drinking milk. The ingredients in cold dairy products help turn off the heat and pain receptors in the mouth as well as coat the tissues with a light, protective film while they mend.

Helpful Hint

Even though you may be able to hold a slice of pizza in your hand, the cheese may still be hot. (This is less apt to be a problem with most home-delivered pizza.) Wait a couple of minutes before biting into pizza that has just come out of the oven. ■

Pneumonia Shots

The Vaccination That Fights Super Germs

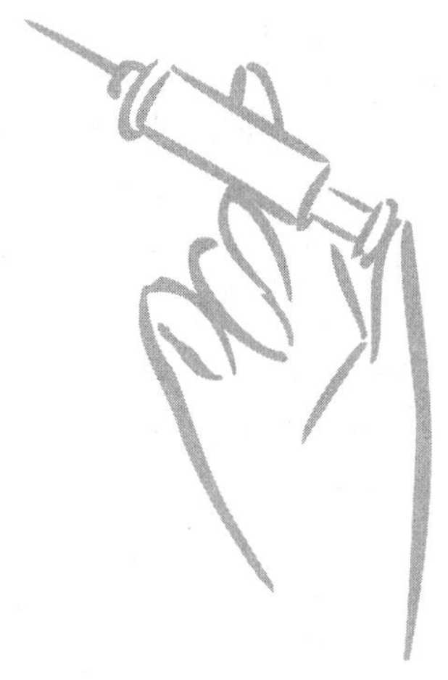

Many health-savvy women line up every autumn to get flu shots. Getting a pneumonia shot may be just as important, yet few women (or men) are even aware of it.

In this country, pneumonia and other diseases caused by the pneumococcus bacteria kill thousands of people a year. A simple vaccine can prevent half of those deaths. The elderly have the greatest risk of dying from pneumonia or its consequences, such as respiratory failure, says Andrew Fishmann, M.D., pulmonary disease specialist at Good Samaritan Hospital in Los Angeles.

At one time, doctors could count on antibiotics like penicillin to cure pneumonia. No more: newer strains of pneumococcus (Streptococcus pneumoniae) are drug-resistant. Your best bet may be to take preventive action by getting the pneumonia shot, which kills 23 different strains of pneumonia. (It doesn't contain live bacteria.)

There's no question that everyone age 65 or older should get the vaccine, though only 45 percent actually do, says Raymond Strikes, M.D., medical epidemiologist at the National Immunization Program at the Centers for Disease Control and Prevention. And anyone with certain chronic diseases—namely, heart disease, diabetes, lung disease, cancer, sickle cell disease, alcoholism, HIV or other immunosuppressant disorder, or kidney failure or transplant. Anyone who has no spleen, and therefore has lowered immunity to infection, should get a pneumonia shot.

What about the rest of us? Given that antibiotics are less effective in treating bacterial pneumonia than they used to be, some experts believe that anyone over the age of 60, or possibly even 50, should have the shot, even if they're relatively healthy. If you have reason to suspect you may be at increased risk from pneumonia due to asthma, your line of work, or other health or lifestyle factors, your doctor can help you determine if a pneumonia shot would be a prudent safeguard. ››

The shot costs more than a flu shot—about $40—and leaves you with a sore arm for a couple of days. It's a small price to pay for protection. You can get it when you receive your annual flu shot, but not in the same arm. Women under age 65 may have to shoulder the cost themselves—it's covered by Medicare, but private insurance may or may not cover it, depending on your plan. Protection wanes over time, so you'll need to be revaccinated every 6 years. ■

DON'T MAKE THIS MISTAKE

If you develop symptoms of pneumonia—sudden onset of fever, shaking chills, chest pain, shortness of breath, and rapid breathing and heartbeat—get medical help immediately, whether or not you've had a pneumonia shot. The pneumonia shot protects against only one form of bacterial pneumonia, and it doesn't protect against viral pneumonia.

Poison Ivy, Oak, and Sumac

Try the Water-Bottle Rescue

Good thing the Coasters weren't dermatologists: It turns out you don't need an "ocean of calamine lotion" if you develop a rash from poison ivy (or related plants). All you need to do is wash your skin with soap and water to get rid of urushiol, the sticky oil causing the itchy, weeping rash typical of poison ivy.

Doctors agree, it's best to wash off the urushiol within 10 minutes of contact before it binds to the skin and triggers a rash. It's also a good idea to change clothes that have urushiol on them—standard advice—and apply some over-the-counter hydrocortisone cream if a rash develops. Then wash your clothes, following standard washing directions. It's safe to mix them with other clothes. And be sure to wash your hands thoroughly after loading the clothes into the washer.

That's fine if you're at home working in your backyard when you encounter the wicked weed. But what if you're hiking or picnicking when you break out?

"If you don't have soap, plain old water will do," says Laura Tenner, M.D., a dermatologist with Kaiser Permanente Medical Center in Hayward, California, and a member of the Wilderness Medical Society. Water inactivates the urushiol, she says. In fact, any sort of liquid will do. To preempt poison ivy in a pinch, here's what Dr. Tenner suggests, depending on what you have on hand.

- Rinse the contact area with water from a stream or lake (and rinse any infected items).
- Wet a handkerchief or item of clothing with liquid from your water bottle—even if it's Gatorade or juice—and wipe skin that's affected.
- Rub the affected area with ice from your cooler, if you have one.
- Use a premoistened towelette, such as a baby wipe, if you have any with you.

Helpful Hint

Creams formulated to shield the skin from urushiol work

well. But remember to apply them *before* exposure. Available in pharmacies and sporting goods stores under brand names such as IvyBlock and Works Outdoors, they work by preventing the urushiol from binding to your skin on contact. Showering removes the cream and the urushiol, preventing a rash. ■

OATMEAL SOUP FOR POISON IVY

If you come in contact with poison ivy or poison oak and don't have any way to wash off the oil afterward, you can treat the rash with oatmeal, says David Pomeroy, M.D., clinical instructor in the department of family medicine at the University of Washington School of Medicine in Seattle. For soothing relief, make some soupy oatmeal. Let it cool. Then, spoon the mixture into an old sock, strain out the liquid, and apply to the rash as a compress for 10 minutes every 2 hours (except overnight).

Or, you can strain the oatmeal mixture and just smear the liquid over your rash five times a day, or as often as needed, says Dr. Pomeroy. Do this until the symptoms subside.

Pollution

Show Indoor Toxins the Door

You don't have to stand downwind from a factory smokestack or drive along a traffic-clogged highway to breathe air pollution. In fact, you don't even have to leave your house.

Pollutants can waft through the air in your house from a variety of sources, ranging from the ground beneath the home to the products you use to clean it, chemicals in pressed wood cabinets, or a poorly maintained furnace. Potential reactions to indoor air pollution can range from mild wheezing or flulike symptoms (from some pollutants) to life-threatening symptoms (from exposure to elevated carbon monoxide levels), says Elissa Feldman, associate director of the indoor environment division of the Environmental Protection Agency.

Here are some ways to make your home-sweet-home a safer place to live and breathe.

Check for carbon monoxide. Have all the gas-burning appliances in your home—including your stove, heater, and water heater—checked by a trained professional at the start of each heating season, Feldman advises. Hundreds of people die accidentally every year from carbon monoxide poisoning caused by malfunctioning or improperly used fuel-burning appliances.

Install a carbon-monoxide detector. This lifesaver, which works much like a household smoke detector, will alert you if the odorless gas is leaking into your home. To make sure it works, test it following ›› the manufacturer's instructions. Carbon monoxide hampers your body's ability to use oxygen, which could be fatal.

Turn on your radon radar. Radon is an invisible, radioactive gas produced by naturally decaying uranium in the soil that can enter into your home. It's known to cause lung cancer, even at very low levels. Radon is the second leading cause of lung cancer in the United States.

Pick a radon test kit at hardware and retail stores, or consult the Environmental Protection Agency's (EPA) Web site at www.epa.gov to find the name and phone number for your state's radon program. Set the kit in the lowest level of your home for the specified time, then return it to the indicated laboratory for analysis. You can use a short-term test (which you set out for 2 to 90 days) or a long-term test (more than 90 days), though the long-term test is more likely to reflect your annual average. **If your radon level is 4 picocuries per liter of air or higher, the EPA recommends hiring a certified contractor to deal with the radon.** Your state radon program can provide lists of such contractors.

SKIP THE "AIR FRESHENERS"

Hanging strongly scented faux fresheners around your house may do more harm than good. Same goes for aerosol sprays.

"Rather than removing odors, they just make it impossible to smell them," says Lance Wallace, Ph.D., environmental scientist at the Environmental Protection Agency office of research and development. Many fresheners have chemicals that have been found to cause cancer in animals.

"And it's not just aerosols that are dangerous. In tests, the solid air fresheners were found to have high concentrations of some of the nastier chemicals."

Keep household cleaners to a minimum. Especially try to avoid aerosols, scented products, and chlorine bleach. (Use an oxygen bleach such as Clorox 2 instead.) If a product doesn't smell good, don't use it. "The molecules get into your bloodstream, and your body doesn't know if you ate it or breathed it," says Alfred Zamm, M.D., a Kingston, New York, dermatologist and environmental medicine physician and author of *Why Your House May Endanger Your Health*. Good substitutes include: baking soda, vinegar, and other biocompatible products that are nontoxic to humans and won't harm the environment.

Let your car air out. If your garage is attached to your house, leave your vehicle outside for 2 hours when you arrive home to allow the engine to cool down and release fumes outdoors.

Put a lid on pesticides. Don't stockpile household pesticides, fertilizers, and weed killers, and use only biocompatible forms. When not in use, store them in a garbage can with a tight-fitting lid in a storage shed or garage.

Knock on (real) wood. Cabinets and furniture made of pressed wood can release formaldehyde fumes, Feldman says. Consider choices made of solid wood, but if you buy pressed-wood items, make sure they're laminated and that the laminate covers all the surfaces. Avoid sealants that contain formaldehyde. ■

Poor Night Vision

Turn On the Night Light

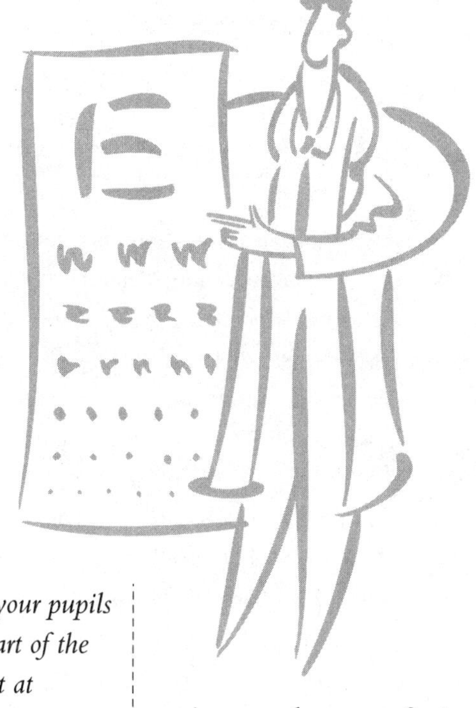

Do you find yourself leaning forward over your steering wheel as you drive at night, straining to see what's ahead? Do you ever come close to missing a highway exit at night because you can barely read it in time? Is navigating in a new area of town impossible after dark because you can't read the street signs?

If your vision is blurrier at night, you're not alone. You and a significant portion of the population are experiencing night myopia—night nearsightedness.

Your eyesight or your corrective lenses may work just fine in the clear light of day, yet you can't read the license plate of the car right in front of you at night. "It's because your pupils dilate in the dark, and the image goes through a different part of the lens, so some women (and men) can become nearsighted just at night," says Anne Sumers, M.D., an ophthalmologist in Ridgewood, New Jersey.

Night vision gets worse with age. "You need more light to see, the older you get," says Dr. Sumers. You've seen kids reading by a lamp across the room, while if you're over 45, you struggle with a menu in a restaurant with mood lighting. "Women who are 40 need twice as much light as women in their twenties," says Dr. Sumers. "When you hit 55, you start changing all the lightbulbs from 65 to 100 watts."

As you get older, you're also bothered more by glare from bright lights. When you're in your sixties and seventies, the glare from oncoming headlights can be startling.

The solution: night glasses, designed specifically to correct night vision.

"It makes a huge difference," says Dr. Sumers. If you wear contact lenses, you'll wear your night glasses over your contact lenses.

To be fitted for night glasses, you'll need an eye exam from an ophthalmologist or optometrist. But first, try getting your lenses professionally cleaned or polished. Often, vision impaired by scratched lenses can make you think that your prescription is wrong. If your glasses have a tint or reflection-free coating, they can wear off, like peeling paint, affecting your vision.

Helpful Hint

If you're over 40, get your eyes checked every 2 years, says Dr. Sumers. If you have glaucoma, diabetes, or a family history of these, get checked every year. If you're over 65, get your eyes checked annually. ■

Poor Resistance

Boost Your Immunity with Jazz, Vitamins, and a Smile

No one can avoid an occasional bout of the sniffles. But if you're forever coming down with repeated colds, sore throats, or bouts of the flu, there's a whole lot you can do to improve your resistance to infections.

"By keeping your immune system functioning at an optimal level, you can decrease your susceptibility to colds and the flu as well as the likelihood of developing autoimmune diseases like type 1 diabetes, and possibly influence the course of some forms of cancers," says Bruce Rabin, M.D., Ph.D., professor of pathology and psychiatry and director of the Brain, Behavior, and Immunity Center at the University of Pittsburgh.

Here are 14 proven ways to boost your immunity, from eating more potatoes to listening to Miles Davis.

Nutrients You Need

1. Get your fair share of vitamin E. Found in nuts, fish, whole grains, dark leafy greens, and vegetable oil, vitamin E has been shown to enhance the immune system and resistance to infectious diseases, including viral infections and respiratory diseases, according to research done by Simin Nibkin Meydani, Ph.D., chief of the nutritional immunology laboratory at the USDA. For optimum protection against germs, aim for 100 to 400 IU of vitamin E per day. (You'll need to take supplements to get this amount.)

2. Focus on vitamin C. Found in peppers, potatoes, tomatoes, and orange juice, vitamin C is linked to a protein that activates the immune system, beefing up T-cells and increased natural killer cell activity, two key markers of strong resistance. You should aim for about 200 to 500 milligrams daily for optimum protection, according to Marianne Frieri, M.D., Ph.D., associate professor of medicine and pathology at State University of New York at Stony Brook. If large doses of vitamin C give you diarrhea, cut back.

3. Sneak in a little extra selenium. When you feel the sniffles coming on, reach for this trace mineral. Research has shown that taking up to 800 micrograms daily for 3 days can help your body resist a cold. Doses above 200 micrograms, however, must be taken with a doctor's supervision.

4. Eat foods rich in beta-carotene. Found in broccoli, spinach, and sweet potatoes, beta-carotene fights infection and protects the mucous membranes, the slippery defensive tissues that line your mouth, throat, and digestive tract and act as your body's shield against germs.

5. Look to vitamin B_6. Found in beans, cabbage, walnuts, and potatoes, vitamin B_6 has been shown to strengthen immunity.

Enlist an Herb or Two

6. Pop some echinacea. It won't relieve your symptoms if you're already sick, but taken as a tincture, tablet, or capsule, it will stimulate your immune system and increase your body's ability to fight in-

DON'T MAKE THESE MISTAKES

Using antibacterial products may actually increase our chances of getting sick, because they kill off the beneficial bacteria that protect us from the undesirable bacteria. Experts at the Center for Adaptation Genetics and Drug Resistance at the Tufts University School of Medicine who have studied this effect say that your best bet is to **save antibacterial soaps and disinfecting gels for occasions where you really might encounter unusual bacteria, like when camping.**

The same theory applies to antibiotics. Overuse of antibiotics can suppress your immune system, allowing other (more harmful) bacteria into your body. **Don't coerce your doctor into prescribing antibiotics for every sniffle**—it just may make you worse.

fections. According to Andrew T. Weil, M.D, director of the program of integrative medicine at the University of Arizona College of Medicine in Tucson, if you take it at the first hint of a sniffle, it can jump-start your immunity so that the infection can't take hold. Follow recommended dosages on the package for tablets and capsules. For the tincture, use 1 dropperful (about ½ teaspoon) in a little warm water four times a day until symptoms go away. But if you have tuberculosis or an autoimmune condition such as lupus or multiple sclerosis, don't use echinacea. Same goes if you're allergic to closely related plants such as ragweed, asters, or chrysanthemums.

7. Have a cup of yarrow or elderflower tea. These herbs are antiviral and stimulate the immune system. Herbalists suggest adding 1 to 2 teaspoons of dry leaves to 1 cup of boiling water. Steep for 10 to 20 minutes, strain, then drink. Continue drinking 2 to 3 cups a day until symptoms disappear.

Around the House

8. Get enough sleep. Your immunity is compromised when you're fatigued, so take your sleep seriously. If you have trouble dozing off, try taking valerian, an herbal sleep promoter, after dinner according to label instructions. You can also take ½ teaspoon of the tincture form. Don't use valerian with other sleep-enhancing or mood-regulating medicines. Also, avoid eating or exercising right before bedtime—it tends to interfere with sleep.

9. Listen to music. Listening to music (particularly smooth-jazz style, or mellow, elevator-style background music) boosts the body's production of protective antibodies, which helps defend against all diseases.

Out and About

10. Make friends. Who would have thought that shmoozing works like a vitamin? A study conducted at Carnegie Mellon University in Pittsburgh found that men and women who had a variety of social relationships had 20 percent better immune function than more introverted people. Researchers speculate that social ties may help us cope better with stress.

11. Attend worship. One study revealed that men and women who attend religious ›› services at least once a week have lower levels of interleukin-6, an immune system protein linked to some autoimmune diseases, such as cancer and heart disease. Researchers speculate that this may be related to increased social contact, or increased relaxation.

Attitude Adjustments

12. Laugh. Research has shown that the positive emotions associated with laughter actually decrease stress hormones while increasing and activating immune cells.

13. Don't let stress get the better of you. When you're stressed, your body produces stress hormones. These hormones bind to immune system cells and decreases those cells' ability to function. When those cells don't function, you get sick—and we're not just talking about colds. You become more susceptible to autoimmune diseases like rheumatoid arthritis and diabetes, and even cancer, according to Dr. Rabin.

14. Work out. Exercise activates the same areas of the brain that are activated by stress. Once those areas are activated by exercise, it become more difficult for them to be activated by psychological stress—which means that the stress has less of an effect on altering the concentration of hormones in the blood that influence the function of the immune system. According to Dr. Rabin, moderate amounts of exercise (done at an intensity that permits you to carry on a conversation) daily or every other day are the most beneficial. ■

Pore Strips

Strip Away Blackheads in Minutes

Under a microscope, the pores on your face may look like dimples on a golf ball. But they serve a purpose: Skin pores distribute sebum—oil produced by tiny sebaceous glands underneath the surface. In just 1 year, your face can produce more than a quart of sebum, which protects and moistens your skin. But if sebum backs up, you end up with acne cysts. Pores can also collect dirt, bacteria, and dead skin, leaving you with unsightly blackheads.

Enter pore strips, special tapes designed to neatly coax accumulated oil and debris out of your pores.

"When used correctly, pore strips temporarily unload clogged pores," says Deborah Sarnoff, M.D., a dermatologist in Manhattan and assistant clinical professor at New York University Medical Center. Simply lay the strip over different parts of your face, especially the nose, cheek, and chin areas. After a few minutes, gently lift off the strip.

"Women find it satisfying to remove the tape and see all the oil extracted from their pores," says Dr. Sarnoff. And pore strips are safer than trying to squeeze pimples or blackheads with your fingers, which can rupture blood vessels and infect the skin with dirt from underneath the fingernails.

Portion Control

Cut Your Calories in Half

Some days, it seems that we're all either turning into the Incredible Shrinking Woman, or the foods that surround us are growing larger.

Actually, the food portions we encounter are swelling in size, says Lisa Young, R.D., Ph.D, adjunct faculty member at New York University in New York City who has studied portion sizes. And we're getting bigger right along with them.

"In many cases, we often bite off or gulp down more than we should because we don't want to pass up a bargain," says Dr. Young. At fast-food restaurants, super-size servings of french fries and soda cost just a few cents more than regular, for example. The 20-ounce bottle of soda at the convenience store looks tempting because it offers more for our money than the 12-ounce can. Yet ordering the jumbo size can double the amount of calories you consume from that food.

"If you have a big portion every now and then, you won't necessarily get fat," says Young. "But if all your meals are big portions and you have no idea how much you're eating, then you have a problem."

Here's how to keep from being lured into the "bigger is better" trap.

Just say no to supersizing. If you must give in occasionally to a fast-food craving, keep it simple and stick with a small burger, small fries, and small drink. ››

DON'T MAKE THIS MISTAKE

If you've been diagnosed with rosacea, have extremely sensitive skin or inflamed acne, or use vitamin A topically, consult your dermatologist before using pore strips. The slight friction created by pulling the adhesive strip off your face can cause reddening and swelling.

As a bonus, pore strips help prevent future blemishes: When your pores are open and operational, your protective glands can work better against bacteria and other foreign invaders.

Pore strips may indirectly help shrink enlarged pores. Technically, you can't actually shrink or expand your pores. Pore size is predetermined by heredity and influenced by weather (hot, humid weather makes your pores appear to expand, and cold, dry days make them appear to contract). But built-up sediment can stretch pores' openings and make them appear larger. Regular cleaning returns them to normal size.

Pore strips have their limits. If y ou have tiny pores, you may not get great results. If the bottom of the plug is larger than the tip, there isn't enough adhesion to pull out the plug. Pore strips do not work on impacted blackheads, which need attention from a dermatologist.

Helpful Hint

You don't need to apply pore strips more than once or twice a week. If you use them daily, you risk irritating your skin and depleting it of adequate oil. ■

Think twice about eating a whole bagel. The average bagel has grown to a hefty 4 ounces—the equivalent of about four large slices of white bread. You get a whopping 310 calories, compared with 79 calories for a slice of toast. If you're still going to eat that bagel, cut back on a similar food later—for example, don't eat pasta that night, says Dr. Young.

Buy snacks in small packages. To keep from eating a few too many handfuls of potato chips, buy them in single-serving bags.

ENTREES IN DISGUISE

Never automatically assume that appetizers are diminutive. A plate of chicken wings supplies 583 calories, and an order of nachos supreme provides 770 calories. Order one plate for the whole table and set aside a fraction of the total for yourself.

Divide and conquer. Some restaurant platters are up to 18 inches across and hold the equivalent of two or three entrées—per person. Ask for a child-size portion, or have the excess wrapped before you dig in. You'll cut calories by one-half to a third.

Helpful Hints

Use these comparisons to limit portions of other foods.

Cheese = four dice

Meat = deck of cards

Baked potato = computer mouse

Pasta = baseball

Wine = half a can of soda

Slice of bread = CD case

Pat of butter = teaspoon ■

Postnasal Drip

Why Moister Is Better

Call it a nose that runs in reverse. Postnasal drip feels like something is draining down the back of your throat. You might think something's wrong with your nose. But the fact is, your body is doing exactly what it's supposed to.

Postnasal drip is actually your body's healthy attempt to clean and humidify the nose, says Michael Benninger, M.D., former chairman of the speech, voice, and swallowing committee of the American Academy of Otolaryngology–Head and Neck Surgery, and chairman of the department of otolaryngology–head and neck surgery at Henry Ford Hospital in Detroit. When irritants get into those olfactory openings, the glands around your nose and throat secrete greater or thicker amounts of mucus to keep your passages moist, or to flush out the offending matter. Unfortunately, those extra secretions have to go someplace, and often as not, they follow gravity and slide down the back of your throat. Yuck.

The best solution is to avoid the irritants—allergens, dust, dry air—that trigger the drip. But if you already have postnasal problems, your best course of action is to keep nasal passages moist to avoid triggering more mucus, or to thin the mucus so it won't tickle your throat as much. Here's how.

Tame it with tea. Herbal tea is a great home remedy for a variety of reasons, says Dr. Benninger. First, a steaming cup of tea can help moisturize the nasal passages and avoid the dryness that often triggers

CONSIDERING SURGERY? NOT SO FAST!

"I've seen many people undergo surgery for postnasal discharge, and they still have the problem," says Mark Loury, M.D., an otolaryngologist/head and neck surgeon at Pudore Valley Hospital in Fort Collins, Colorado. Gastroesophageal reflux may push saliva into your throat, causing a drip sensation. But it's not postnasal drip, and surgery won't do any good.

postnasal drip. Second, herbal teas contain no caffeine, which actually make the secretions thicker. Add a little lemon—which stimulates saliva flow, so you can swallow easier—to any herbal tea of your choice, and you've got yourself a tasty and soothing tonic. Drink as needed.

Steam the flow. Running a vaporizer in the wintertime or simply taking a hot shower seems to alleviate postnasal drip, says Jack Anon, M.D., chairman of the nasal and sinus committee of the American Academy of Otolaryngology–Head and Neck Surgery. Or, heat up water in a bowl, place a towel over your head, lower your face to the captured moisture, and inhale through your nose for a stimulating steam treatment, adds Dr. Anon. Keep your face about 18 inches away from the water.

Use a saltwater spray. A simple saline spray can keep your nasal passages moist and help flush away irritants that might cause postnasal drip. Most pharmacies sell them, or you can make your own. Mix a teaspoon of salt with a pint of clean, warm water, put the solution in an atomizer, and spritz it into your nose a few times a day, advises Dr. Benninger.

Avoid clearing your throat in an attempt to clear away the phlegm. It does nothing to alleviate postnasal drip. In fact, it sets up a cycle of irritation that strains the throat and actually causes the mucus to stay put, says Dr. Benninger. ■

Postpartum Depression

You Don't Have to Go It Alone

For many new mothers, a mild bout of the baby blues is as common as smelly diapers, round-the-clock feedings, and sponge baths. Three out of four new mothers find themselves crying for no reason or experiencing mood swings, insomnia, and irritability. In most, feelings of unhappiness fade within days and should be gone completely within a couple of weeks.

If your sadness deepens, however, or you develop anxiety, a fear of losing control, a lack of interest in your baby, and/or thoughts of harming yourself and your little one, you may have postpartum depression (PPD), a serious psychiatric disorder that occurs in one out of five women who've given birth, says Anne Stoline, M.D., director of women's mental health at Mercy Medical Center in Baltimore. ››

No one knows exactly what causes it. "But doctors believe it's a result of the major shifts in estrogen and progesterone levels that occur immediately after delivery. After all, the brain is affected by hormones,"says Dr. Stoline. Women with histories of depression face a higher risk of developing PPD, as do women with family histories of the illness. But there are mothers who don't have any prior history of depression and still end up with PPD, which means that there are other factors involved.

"You also have to take into account the woman's circumstances at the time of delivery. Is she a single parent? Is her family supportive? Did she have a traumatic delivery? Does she have an ill baby? These types of negative events will increase her vulnerability to PPD."

Once diagnosed, postpartum depression can be treated. So if you think you have postpartum depression, don't feel ashamed—seek help without delay. Here's how.

Call a support group. Depression after Delivery, a national organization that specializes in PPD referral services, can put you in touch with qualified psychologists or psychiatrists in your area. They also supply a list of telephone contact volunteers—women

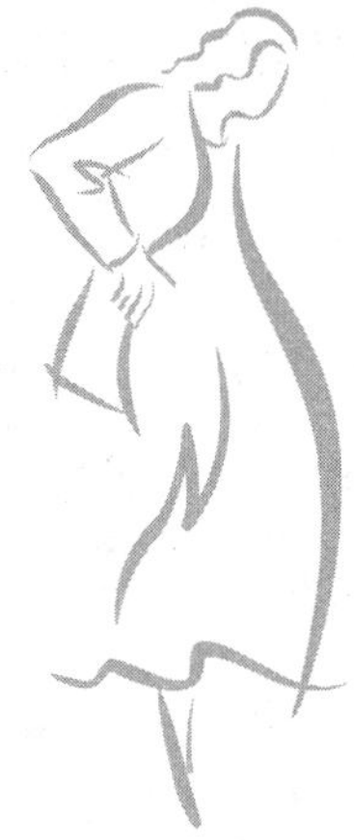

who themselves have gone through PPD and are willing to speak about it to others. You can write to them at 91 East Somerset Street, Raritan, New Jersey 08869 to request the free referrals and information on PPD. Or, visit their Web site at www.behavenet.com/dadinc.

Prayer

Take This High-Spirited Path to Super Health

"Walking with God" takes on special meaning for Larry Dossey, M.D., author of *Healing Words* and one of the leading authorities on healing and prayer. Dr. Dossey believes that when you combine prayer with brisk walking, the health benefits become twofold.

"There's a ton of evidence supporting the positive effects that prayer has on health," he says. "When people pray, their blood pressure comes down, heart rate falls, stress is relieved, adrenaline levels drop, and the body simply becomes healthier."

Studies have shown that women who live spiritual lives and who attend church once a week or more are one-third less likely to die prematurely than those who do not. They have lower incidences of heart disease, emphysema, and suicide and often recover faster from physical and mental illness, surgery, and addiction.

"This is a result of putting your trust in a higher power beyond yourself," Dr. Dossey explains. "It's believing that you don't have to rely on yourself to do everything. This is immensely comforting to people.

Work with your doctor. "Many women are reluctant to seek help for this little-known complication of childbirth, but those who do generally are very relieved to find experts who understand their condition and can provide the appropriate support for it," says Dr. Stoline.

Helpful Hint

If you've ever had postpartum depression and plan to have another child, ask your doctor about supplemental estrogen therapy. She can place a patch on your hip after delivery that will give you a steady dose of the hormone throughout the postpartum period. ■

Pregnancy Discomfort

Round-the-Clock Strategies for Your Tummy Troubles, Back Pain, and More

Unless you're a kangaroo, carrying your progeny around your middle for 9 months can put a lot of stress on your body.

"As the uterus grows during pregnancy, it alters a woman's sense of gravity and balance," says Teresa Hoffman, M.D., an obstetrician-gynecologist at Mercy Medical Center in Baltimore. And the extra weight a woman normally gains during pregnancy can put quite a strain on your hips, knees, ankles, feet, and back.

Here are some handy ways to relieve discomforts most commonly associated with pregnancy.

Heartburn

As your baby grows, the esophageal sphincter muscle located at the top of your stomach may weaken and no longer be able to prevent ››

"Add to that the health benefits of brisk walking such as improved muscle tone, weight loss, endurance, elevated mood, reduced stress, and stronger cardiovascular and immune systems," he continues, "and you have the perfect recipe for physical and spiritual fitness."

Eager to get started? Here is a step-by-step guide to prayer walking for a healthier body, mind, and spirit, courtesy of Linus Mundy, author of *The Complete Guide to Prayer Walking: A Simple Path to Body-and-Soul Fitness.*

Lace up a good pair of walking shoes, step on your treadmill, or head out the door. As you begin walking, concentrate on each breath and the number of steps you take as you inhale and exhale. Take three or four steps when inhaling and three or four steps when exhaling, silently saying "one, two, three"—one word with each step. Then substitute a three- or four-word prayer or mantra for the counting. You could say, for example, "Praise be to God" or "God give me strength." Repeat the phrase throughout your walk.

Keep your mind in the present. When past anxieties or future worries enter your head, don't hold on to them. Say something like, "Cast your cares on the Lord and he will sustain you," or "He is my refuge and my fortress, my God, in whom I trust." And feel the stress melt away. ■

stomach acids from creeping up your throat, says Charles Moniak, M.D., an obstetrician-gynecologist at Fountain Valley Regional Hospital and Medical Center in California.

Don't eat and lie down right away. In fact, avoid eating anything 3 hours or less before you go to bed. That's when your stomach acids are the most active. Eat small, frequent meals throughout the day. And choose low-fat, healthy foods instead of hot, spicy, and high-fat fare. What's more, stay away from tomato-based sauces, grapefruit juice, chocolate, coffee, tea, and colas.

Lower-Back Pain

Usually around the second and third trimesters, your back starts to ache as the muscles in your back and spine respond to changes in the center of gravity.

The solution: Wear a pregnancy girdle designed to support your lower back. They're available in maternity shops. You also can place a heating pad on your lower back, soak in a warm bath, or get a massage, says Dr. Hoffman.

Or, ask your doctor to give you three or four different strengthening and flexibility exercises for your back and abdominal muscles. The exercises she gives you will depend on how far along you are in the pregnancy and how fit you are to begin with, among other factors, says Kathleen Francis, M.D., medical director of women's health services at the Kessler Institute for Rehabilitation in West Orange, New Jersey.

DON'T MAKE THIS MISTAKE

If your hands and face swell, don't pass it off as edema. See your doctor immediately. You could have high blood pressure, which can be a major complication in pregnancy.

Sleep Difficulties

In the third trimester, sleeping on your back or your stomach isn't an option. And that can mean restless nights if you're not used to resting on your side. Your baby can also keep you up if he or she starts kicking at 2 o'clock in the morning.

There's no solution for a rambunctious baby-in-the-works. But since you can't sleep on your back, make sure you rest on your left side. On your right is a large blood vessel that carries blood back to your heart called the vena cava. So if you sleep on your right, you'll put pressure on the blood vessel, preventing it from doing its job.

To get comfortable, place a fluffy pillow under your left hip and one between your knees to cushion your bones. Or, buy a body pillow to help support your lower and upper back, hips, and legs.

Edema (Accumulated Fluid)

During pregnancy, your body produces extra blood and other fluids that run through your blood vessels. But when these vessels get filled to the brim, some fluid seeps out into surrounding tissues, causing your feet and ankles to swell, says Dr. Moniak.

Elevate your feet higher than your hips for 10 minutes every hour to drain the fluid. Eat a low-salt diet to prevent water retention, and drink lots of water to flush out excess sodium, says Dr. Moniak. ■

Premenstrual Syndrome

Add Minerals, Subtract Tension

Premenstrual syndrome was first identified in 1953 by two physicians—one a woman—in Britain. Dr. Katharina Dalton and Dr. Raymond Greene were the first health care experts to label the bloating, aches, irritability, and other complaints that many women have come to associate with that time of the month. They called it PMS.

Women affected by PMS may experience any combination of 17 or more different symptoms during the week or so before their monthly menstrual flow: Mood swings. Sadness. Tension. Nervousness. Short temper. Insomnia. Crying spells. Ankle swelling. Breast tenderness. Abdominal bloating or cramping (or both). Backache. Headache. Or aching all over. Increased appetite. Loss of appetite. Cravings for sweets . . . or salt. And perhaps worst of all, weight gain.

Not all women notice significant changes before their periods. But if you do, separate studies on magnesium and calcium found that these easy-to-find minerals work to relieve the worst of premenstrual symptoms (and possibly prevent PMS entirely).

In one of the largest studies of calcium for PMS, researchers found that women who take 1,200 milligrams of calcium daily for three menstrual cycles experience significantly less pain and water retention, fewer food cravings, and a more positive mood.

The researchers suspect that calcium relieves PMS by easing depression and muscle pain, but they don't know how. "Unfortunately, most women don't get enough calcium in their diets—you need 1,200 milligrams a day," says Susan Thys-Jacobs, M.D., endocrinologist at St. Luke's–Roosevelt Hospital Center at Columbia University College of Physicians and Surgeons in New York City and lead study author.

What calcium can't tackle, magnesium will. In another study, women who took 200 milligrams of the mineral daily for two menstrual cycles reported improvements in weight gain, water retention, breast soreness, and abdominal bloating versus those who received a pill that looked like magnesium but did nothing.

"Magnesium works by reducing inflammation triggered by certain hormonal changes that occur 7 to 10 days before menstruation," says Ann F. Walker, Ph.D., senior lecturer in human nutrition at the University of Reading in the United Kingdom and lead study author. What's more, women who consume too little magnesium run short of dopamine, a brain chemical that regulates mood, which may explain why some women with PMS are tense and irritable before their periods, says Dr. Walker.

For best results, Dr. Walker recommends taking calcium and magnesium supplements together, in a ratio of 2 (calcium) to 1 (magnesium). In other words, if you take 1,200 milligrams of calcium per ❯❯

day, you should take 600 milligrams of magnesium. Women with heart or kidney problems should check with their doctors before taking supplemental magnesium. Supplemental magnesium may cause diarrhea in some people.

Helpful Hint

For an easy way to feature more PMS-fighting foods in your day-to-day diet, think dairy, greens, and beans. For calcium, include low-fat or fat-free milk, cottage cheese, yogurt, and cheese, plus broccoli and calcium-fortified orange juice. For magnesium, opt for soy beans, pinto and navy beans, and leafy green vegetables, such as spinach and Swiss chard, plus halibut, oysters, brown rice, nuts, seeds, and wheat germ. ■

Prozac

A Breakthrough Drug—But Is It for You?

When the Rolling Stones wrote about "mother's little helper" back in the 1960s, Prozac hadn't been discovered. Back then, heavy-duty antianxiety agents like Milltown and Librium saved the day for harried housewives coping with the stress of everyday life.

Twenty years later, along came Prozac. Hailed as a breakthrough for depression when first introduced, Prozac and other SSRIs (selective serotonin reuptake inhibitors) such as Zoloft and Paxil have fewer side effects than tricyclic antidepessants, the most commonly used agents at that time. And they're less likely to cause dependency or overdose than Valium, Librium, or Xanax, used for anxiety and insomnia. Plus, Prozac is less likely to cause weight gain, and many women even lose weight while taking it.

Yet the popular antidepressant Prozac doesn't come without side effects. Men and women alike complain that it lowers their sex drive. Other common side effects include headache, fatigue, drowsiness, lightheadness, nausea, diarrhea, upset stomach, dry mouth, insomnia, anxiety, or nervousness—trading one problem for another. Plus, it's expensive—about $100 a month. For the cost of a years' supply, you could take a Caribbean cruise (which may be all you really need.)

Nevertheless, Prozac has experienced great popularity and tremendous sales since its introduction. Some critics say Prozac is overprescribed. Others argue that it's underprescribed. Which is it?

In fact, both claims are true, says Margaret Jensvold, M.D., former director of the Institute for Research on Women's Health, in Rockville, Maryland. "On the one hand, many physicians who don't really have the training to assess emotional problems (or aren't taking the time to do so) are sending women off with prescriptions for antidepressants like Prozac. At the same time, many women experiencing serious depression are not getting help."

If you're stressed out or depressed, you're probably wondering if you should ask your doctor about Prozac. Here's what to consider.

Ask yourself if you're really depressed or just blue. "A truly depressed woman is so low that she may not be able to get out of bed in the morning—she feels deeply sad, hopeless, helpless, without energy, inadequate, and guilt-ridden. She cannot concentrate properly. Often, her sleep and appetite are impaired. Some women even feel as if life is not worth living, or even have thoughts of suicide," says Vivien Burt, M.D., Ph.D., director of the Women's Life Center at the Neuropsychiatric Institute of UCLA. If you feel sad on an occasional basis, however, you may not need an antidepressant. Because depression can be life-threatening, if you feel hopeless or suicidal or persistently sad and fatigued, consult a doctor.

Go to the right doctor. Your family doctor or the ob-gyn you see once a year for your annual checkup may not be the best person to consult for emotional problems, says Dr. Jensvold. Instead, she says, you should consult a psychiatrist—in particular, one who will thoroughly evaluate you to determine the best treatment for you.

DON'T MAKE THIS MISTAKE

If your doctor decides that Prozac is right for you, you may not need to take it forever. But even if you feel better, don't discontinue drug treatment on your own. Consult your doctor.

Look for the right traits. "Is your doctor listening to you? Has she proposed an approach that makes sense to you? Is she following up on your symptoms?" asks Dr. Burt.

Rule out underlying medical problems. In treating women complaining of depression, Dr. Jensvold does a basic blood test to rule out hyper- or hypothyroidism (abnormalities in the thyroid gland) and anemia (a deficiency of iron in the blood), easily corrected problems that can mimic or cause depression. A more extensive exam may be needed to rule out chronic fatigue syndrome or other, more complicated causes of depression.

Consider nondrug approaches. You might not be truly depressed—maybe you've just developed a depressing way of thinking, based on depressing assumptions, says Dr. Jensvold. "Women tend to dwell on their thoughts and not take action," she says. Talk therapy can help you change how you think or do something about whatever is causing your problems, rather than just medicating them away.

Know what to expect. If you and your doctor decide that Prozac is right for you, rest assured: It won't make you "spacey" or "high." "Prozac is not a 'happy' pill," says Dr. Jensvold. Rather, it subtly helps you return to a state of "normalcy" from which you can better deal with the root of your problems. "Women say it's like a cloud gradually lifting or a curtain opening," she says.

Helpful Hint

Prozac and other SSRIs may take about 8 weeks to kick in. So don't feel discouraged if you don't start to feel better immediately. ■

Psoriasis

Clear Your Skin with Meditation and Light Therapy

You might describe psoriasis as a kind of whole-body dandruff gone amok: The outer layer of skin grows at a greatly speeded rate, causing inflammation and scaling. Itchy, red, scaly spots appear on your scalp, ears, elbows, or knees. The skin surface is red but sheds silvery white scales. If you scratch it, you bleed.

Psoriasis is often inherited, though other factors can trigger the disease or make it worse, most notably, stress.

A standard treatment for psoriasis is phototherapy, or ultraviolet light treatments. Combining light therapy with stress reduction is even better, says Thomas G. Cropley, M.D., associate professor of dermatology at the University of Massachusetts Medical School in Worcester.

In one study, Dr. Cropley and fellow researchers discovered that psoriasis cleared up more quickly in men and women who practiced mindfulness meditation, a form of stress-reduction therapy, while receiving phototherapy. "In fact, their skin cleared up twice as fast—and needed only half as many light treatments—as others who had only the light treatments," says Dr. Cropley.

The mindfulness meditation group listened to tapes that directed their breathing and taught them how to empty their minds and focus on the feeling of warmth in their skin from the light melting their psoriasis and making it go away.

Margaret Jarvis was one of the women who benefited from the combined approach. She knew that stress triggered and worsened her outbreaks. At one time, her skin was completely clear. Then she went through a stressful incident, and boom, a few days later, she was covered with itchy, scaly sores. When she practiced mindful meditation, outbreaks cleared up much faster. What's more, she felt like an active participant in her treatment—she could do something to hasten clearing. "Your mind and body work together," says Jarvis. She practices mindful meditation every day, not just when she is having an outbreak.

Mindfulness meditation is a way of staying focused on the present moment, and it takes some training. If you'd like to try it, enroll in a class at one of the 240 clinics worldwide that offer it. For best results, practice daily, not just when you're having a flareup, says Dr. Cropley. And take other steps to manage stress, such as exercise, stress-management workshops, and counseling. If these don't work, anti-anxiety medications (such as Xanax or BuSpar) may also help.

Helpful Hints

Some medications make psoriasis worse, such as Lithium (for manic depressive illness or bipolar disorder) and beta blockers (for high blood pressure). Don't stop taking your medication, however. Instead, talk with your physician about how to manage both psoriasis and your other condition most effectively.

If psoriasis affects your scalp and you're treating it with medicated shampoo, be sure to wash your hair often, preferably daily, says Dr. Cropley.

Natural ultraviolet light—sunlight—helps psoriasis to some degree. Be careful not to risk sunburn, though. "Start with 10 to 15 minutes a day, and apply sunblock or cover any areas that don't have psoriasis. Leave only the affected areas exposed," suggests D'Anne Kleinsmith, M.D., a cosmetic dermatologist at William Beaumont Hospital in Royal Oak, Michigan. ■

RELIEVE ITCHY SCALP WITH OLIVE OIL

If psoriasis is making a mess of your scalp, try this soothing treatment offered by Dr. Kleinsmith.

1. Heat olive oil until it is warm, but not hot.
2. Massage the oil into your dry scalp.
3. Leave the oil on for 20 to 30 minutes minimum or overnight. (Wear a shower cap to protect your pillowcase.)
4. Wash out the oil with a dandruff shampoo.

Apply the oil nightly until the psoriasis is gone, then continue to use it once or twice a week, as needed.

Psyllium

An Emergency Tool for Sluggish Bowels and Stubborn Cholesterol

If your daily diet contains oatmeal or oat bran, peas, beans, citrus fruits, blackberries, or apples, you're getting plenty of soluble fiber, which will keep your bowels regular and your cholesterol at a safe level. But if the closest you get to those foods are oatmeal cookies, lemon pie, and a beanbag chair, you may want to consider adding a little psyllium to your diet.

Made from seeds of the psyllium plant, this concentrated form of fiber absorbs liquid to form a gel. Added to a low-fiber diet, it softens stools, helping to relieve constipation and irritable bowel syndrome. (You'll find psyllium sold under brand names like Metamucil and Fiberall.)

Research indicates that psyllium also lowers artery-clogging cholesterol. Psyllium-fortified products containing at least 1.7 grams of this soluble fiber are permitted to claim that, when combined with a diet low in saturated fat and cholesterol, they help reduce the risk of heart disease.

But there's more to using psyllium than grabbing it off the shelf at your local pharmacy and knocking it back, says David Lineback, Ph.D., food scientist and director of the Joint Institute for Food Safety and Applied Nutrition at the University of ››

Maryland in College Park. Here's what you need to consider.

Be a dietary detective. While some psyllium products are high in sodium and sugars, others are not. If you're trying to avoid either one, read the list of ingredients. Experts recommend a 2,400-milligram sodium limit for the day. Products labeled "low-sodium" contain 140 milligrams or less per serving.

Fill 'er up. To prevent choking when taking psyllium mixed with juice or water, make sure you use the portions of liquid and powder recommended on the label. And remember to keep a beverage handy if you're eating psyllium-fortified products—they can be difficult to swallow.

Keep your powder dry. Since psyllium absorbs liquid to form a gel, sprinkling it on top of your cereal—or any other moist dish—may not be the most palatable approach. Instead, mix a little into dry foods, like bread dough, says Dr. Lineback.

Make sure you get enough. If lowering your cholesterol is your goal, you'll want to make

Puffy Eyes

Classic Kitchen Cures That Work

Poets say that eyes are the window to the soul. But doctors can tell you that puffy ones reveal a lot more than that.

When your eyes look like you stayed awake all night crying, it may be caused by an allergy to smoke, pollen, or a cat; premenstrual hormone changes; an adverse reaction to a medication, alcohol, or the sun; a thyroid problem or kidney ailment; or heredity. Or maybe you did, indeed, stay up all night crying.

"The periocular skin, around the eye, is perhaps the thinnest skin on the body and therefore more susceptible to any trauma, including lack of sleep," says Seth Matarasso, M.D., a dermatologist in San Francisco.

If you've inherited a tendency toward puffy eyes, the only permanent solution is cosmetic surgery. If it's from a medical problem, like a thyroid imbalance, treating the problem should get rid of puffiness.

THE RIGHT AND WRONG WAY TO USE CONCEALER

If you put concealer cream directly on the puffy surface of your eyes, it will reflect the light and make your eyes look even more swollen. A better approach is to apply concealer just above your cheeks, right on the line of the bottom rim of the eye sockets.

You've probably heard that wet tea bags, cucumbers, and egg whites can help get rid of temporary puffiness. The reason the same remedies surface again and again is simple:

sure you get enough psyllium from fortified products.

In the most promising study, researchers found that taking roughly 7 grams of soluble fiber from psyllium a day—4 servings from fortified products—can lower total blood cholesterol and harmful LDL cholesterol without lowering HDL cholesterol, which is beneficial. ■

DON'T MAKE THIS MISTAKE

Don't rely on psyllium to completely undo low in roughage and high in artery-clogging strategy should be a diet that's focused on high-fiber low in saturated fat. Supplement with psyllium only if dietary tactics don't work or if your cholesterol is stubbornly high. A 1-teaspoon serving of psyllium provides as much soluble fiber as a cup of cooked oat bran sprinkled with raspberries.

They work. Pick the one that suits you best.

- Make a cup of chamomile or green tea, using two tea bags. After steeping the tea, drain and chill the tea bags in the refrigerator. Then lie down and place one of the bags over each eye for 2 to 5 minutes. The combination of pressure and coldness relieves the swelling.
- Apply two cucumber slices, two cool spoons, or a cool washcloth on your eyes—or just close your eyes and relax—for 15 minutes.
- Smooth raw egg white directly under your eyes. Leave on for 3 to 5 minutes until dry. Then gently rinse off with cool tap water and blot dry. This will help tighten the skin and help wrinkles disappear for a few hours, says Dr. Matarasso.

Helpful Hint

"If you're thinking, 'I have 2.5 kids, a mortgage, and a job, and I don't have time to sit with cucumbers on my eyes,' take heart," says Dr. Matarasso. "Gravity alone—simply standing—will get rid of eye puffiness by midday." The other techniques simply speed up the process—use them if you want to look your best for a special event. ■

IS IT YOUR LAWN—OR NAIL POLISH?

If you look as though you've been partying all night but you've actually been out mowing the lawn, your puffy eyes may be caused by allergies. Ask your doctor to prescribe eye allergy drops—either an anti-inflammatory or an antihistamine. Used just before you take out the mower, they can prevent swelling.

If you have had puffy eyes for several days, it may be due to an allergy to cosmetics like eye shadow or nail polish. Switching brands—or going without—may help.

ercetin

The Allergy Fighter in Your Food

You may not know how to pronounce it (KWER-se-tin), but chances are, you eat it—in apples, onions, nuts, seeds, tea, cabbage-family vegetables, and berries. You also swallow it if you take herbs such as ginkgo biloba, elder, and St. John's wort.

Quercetin is a flavonoid, a type of antioxidant that benefits health in various ways. Evidence indicates that quercetin can protect against allergies, heart disease, stomach ulcers, cancer, viruses such as herpes simplex and HIV, inflammation associated with asthma and gout, cataracts, arthritis, and complications related to diabetes.

Quercetin is best known for its powerful effects on allergies and asthma. "Quercetin acts as an antihistamine and an anti-inflammatory," explains Kathleen Head, N.D., a naturopathic physician in Dover, Idaho, and co-editor of Alternative Medicine Review. *"Quercetin strengthens the membranes of cells that secrete histamine so they don't break open as easily to release the histamine. And as an anti-inflammatory, it inhibits enzymes that trigger inflammation."*

You can get quercetin from either food or supplements. Studies show it's absorbed better when consumed from foods, says Dr. Head. But if you're aiming for a particular dose, you can't tell how much you're getting from food sources.

"If you want to use it therapeutically—say, to help control asthma or allergies—you're better off taking a concentrated supplement in addition to foods," says Dr. Head. A typical dose is 400 to 500 milligrams twice a day, usually taken before meals.

As for which type of quercetin to buy, Dr. Head recommends quercetin chalcone, available in some pharmacies, because it's water-soluble for better absorption. Capsules are better than tablets, says Dr. Head—the binders interfere with absorption, and the powder is messy and not very water soluble.

Helpful Hints

If you're taking quercetin for allergies, be sure to take it regularly, says Andrew Weil, M.D., director of the program in integrative medicine and clinical professor of internal medicine at the University of Arizona College of Medicine in Tucson.

"It acts as an allergy preventive rather than as a symptom reliever," he explains. "Give it a full 6 to 8 weeks to show its full effect." ■

R

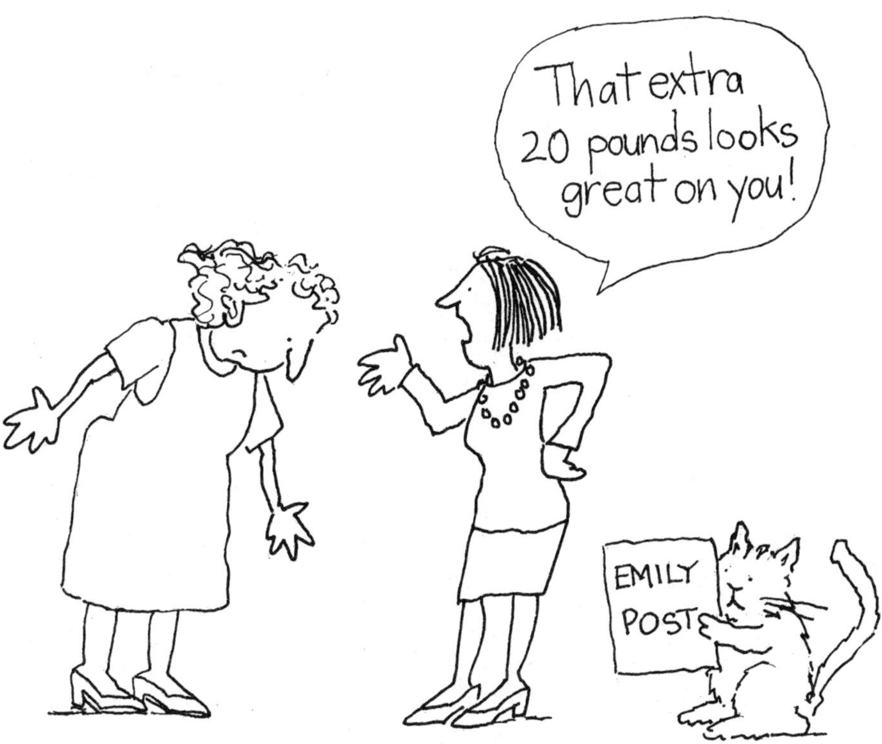
That extra 20 pounds looks great on you!
EMILY POST

Snappy comebacks are the *worst* way
to handle rude remarks.
To find out what you *should* say, see page 382.

Rashes

Stop the Itch-Scratch Cycle with These Soothing Remedies

Everything from perfumes, makeup, and body lotions to medications and stress can make you break out in itchy bumps or scaly patches, says Susan C. Taylor, M.D., a dermatologist at Society Hill Dermatology in Philadelphia and director at the Skin of Color Center in New York City. Other common, often unsuspected causes include laundry detergent, nickel jewelry, and even fake fingernails.

Assuming you avoid whatever's making you itch, a rash will probably heal within 5 to 7 days. Meanwhile, you're scratching yourself raw. That starts a vicious scratch-itch cycle. If you scratch, you'll itch more; if you itch, you'll scratch more, says Dr. Taylor. So here's how to make yourself comfortable.

• Take an antihistamine such as Benadryl before bedtime. Antihistamines not only alleviate itching but they also cause drowsiness, so you'll get a good night's sleep. Follow the label directions for proper dosage.

• Soak yourself for 5 minutes in a colloidal oatmeal bath with mineral oil two or three times a day. Available in drugstores and supermarkets nationwide, colloidal oatmeal will also soothe your skin and ease the itch. Be very careful getting out of the tub afterward—the oil will make the tub, and you, slippery.

• Smooth 100 percent petroleum jelly on your rash if it's dry and itchy. Keeping your rash lubricated will also help relieve itching.

• Dip a washcloth in milk or cool water. Place on the itchy area as a compress for 10 minutes two or three times a day. It will reduce swelling and relieve itching.

DON'T MAKE THESE MISTAKES

• Avoid antibiotic ointments that contain the ingredient neomycin. Normally, neomycin is an effective antibacterial for cuts and scrapes. But if you're allergic to neomycin, it will make matters worse.

• Avoid hot water. The heat will dry out your skin and make it even itchier.

• Never use someone else's prescription anti-itch cream. Just because it was prescribed for a similar-looking rash doesn't mean that it's right for you.

• Don't try to tough it out if things get ugly. Call a doctor if a week goes by without relief, if you don't know why you're itching, if the itching gets worse, or if you develop blisters, pus, and a fever along with the rash.

• Rub on an over-the-counter cortisone ointment. Used twice a day, this old standby will temporarily stop the itching and reduce inflammation. Follow the label directions. ■

Razor Nicks

Shave Your Legs without Bloodshed

Stone Age women relied on things like sharpened rocks and seashells to scrape off unwanted hair. American women of the late eighteenth century resorted to crude methods like burning away leg hair by applying poultices of caustic lye.

Today, women use more civilized tools to clear-cut the follicle forest of 11,000 or so hairs poking through the top layers of skin on each leg. But one errant swipe, and the cry is "ouch" instead of "timber."

"Women, unlike men, generally shave in the shower, where it's slippery, wet, and difficult to get a steady hand," says Jerome Litt, M.D., a dermatologist and assistant clinical professor of dermatology at Case Western Reserve University School of Medicine in Cleveland.

Using a razor designed for men makes shaving all the more difficult. Women have to shave over uneven terrain—over the anklebones and knees—territory for which men's straight-edged razors are ill-equipped.

For a perfect shave—close and smooth, without nicks or bloodshed—follow these tips from Dr. Litt and "shaving engineers" at the Gillette Company in New York City.

Select a razor designed for women. Putting a razor in a pink package doesn't necessarily make it a woman's razor. Look for a textured slip-proof rubber grip, single or double blades, pivoting heads for moves around ankles and kneecaps, and lubra, which are smooth strips coated with aloe and moisturizers. A number of makes and models are available.

Lather up with moisturizers. Moisturizing soaps, gels, or shaving creams like Skintimate Cream and Gillette Vitamin Enriched Shaving Gel that contain vitamin E and other moisturizing ingredients keep leg hair moist so the razor can easily glide over the skin, minimizing drag and nicks. These products won't dry the skin and clog the razor like bath soap.

Follow the 2-to-15 rule. For nick-free shaves, take your first swipe at least 2 minutes after stepping into a warm shower and finish within 15 minutes. The 2-minute soak softens and plumps up the hairs. After 15 minutes, water clogs the hairs, causing skin to wrinkle and

ONE SWIPE WILL SUFFICE

Never run your razor over a patch of skin more than once. Once the razor removes the follicles on the first swipe, repeated swipes can slice your top layer of skin, causing bleeding and possibly infection.

swell slightly so you won't get as close a shave.

Save hard-to-shave areas for last. Leave the shave gel or cream on the ankles, knees, and backs of the thighs for 2 minutes to make hair easier to cut.

Finish with a blot and lotion. Lightly towel-dry your legs. Then, while they're still damp, apply a moisturizer.

Helpful Hints

Replace your blade every four shaves. Dull blades cause cuts and skin irritations. Can't remember when you need to change the blade? If you shave twice a week, then replace the blade on the 1st and 15th of every month or every other Sunday.

Women with denser, fast-growing hair may need to replace their blades sooner than women with fine, slow-growing hair do. ■

Reflexology

Stressed Out? Rub Your Feet

Your feet are home to nearly 15,000 nerve endings. No wonder it feels so good to kick off your shoes or massage your feet.

Reflexology takes foot massage to a higher level, using finger pressure on the feet (and sometimes hands and ears) to reduce stress, thereby helping alleviate stress-related health problems such as back, shoulder, and neck pain; headaches; chronic indigestion; and anxiety.

"Reflexology is based on the principle that there are reflex areas in the feet that correspond to every organ, gland, and part of the body," explains Laura Norman, a certified reflexologist in New York City and author of Feet First: A Guide to Foot Reflexology. *She trains and certifies reflexologists internationally. "It's mainly a form of deep relaxation. Stress acts as a tourniquet. Deep relaxation, on the other hand, helps improve circulation by reducing vascular constriction, so that your blood and nerve supply can flow more freely."*

Reflexology is thought to affect the nervous system, which affects all the other systems, including the circulatory, muscular, urinary, and reproductive systems, says Norman.

DON'T MAKE THESE MISTAKES

Avoid caffeine before and after a reflexology session—it interferes with the relaxation response. Don't do reflexology on a recent injury or open sore. If you're pregnant, don't work the area on the inside of the foot from the heel to the anklebone. During pregnancy, ankle reflexology can induce labor.

"It's sort of like making a telephone call," explains Valerie Voner, certified reflexologist and instructor of reflexology at New England Institute of Reflexology in Onset, Massachusetts. Your feet are the telephone dial. You're sending a message »

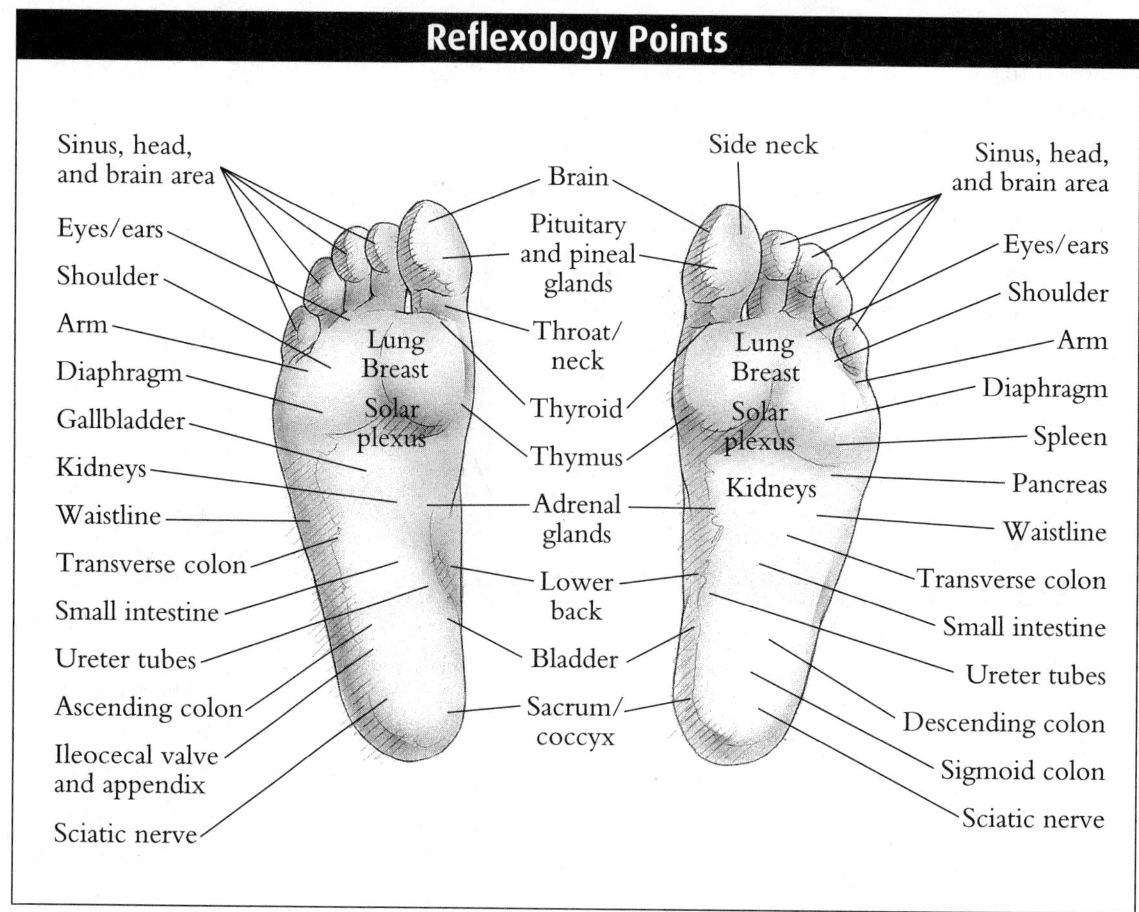

through the nerve pathways (phone line) to the brain (central switchboard). The brain answers your call and sends the correct message to your body parts (phones connected to the switchboard). "The brain is telling the entire body, mind, and spirit to work in balance with each other," says Voner.

You can learn various reflexology points and how to stimulate them at a weekend workshop or school of reflexology. "But you can try a simple reflexology technique on your own," says Voner. "If you're holding stress in your back and neck, for example, the corresponding reflex points are along the inside of the foot, from just above the heel all the way to the middle of your big toe."

"For reflexology to be truly effective, the receiver should be given a full treatment (both feet), and then the giver may go back and work the areas that need extra attention," says Voner. "Working on oneself is considered an interim approach."

First, massage both feet all over using the fingers and thumbs of both hands.

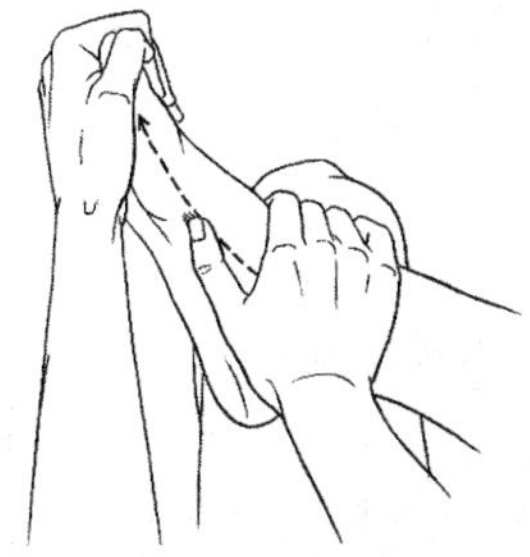

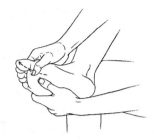

Hold the foot with your thumb along the inside ridge and your index finger at the bottom of your foot. Starting at the heel, push back and forth as your index finger and thumb walk along the foot to the big toe, pushing in a back-and-forth motion, like pressing into Play-Doh.

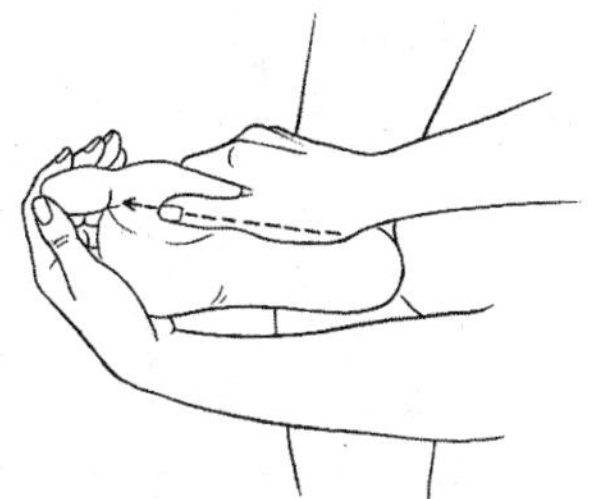

Take your thumb and walk along the whole ridge again, this time pressing like a caterpillar: Press in, and walk, press in, and walk. This releases stress in the back.

When you get to the big toe, do a small replica of the caterpillar finger-walk with thumb and index finger

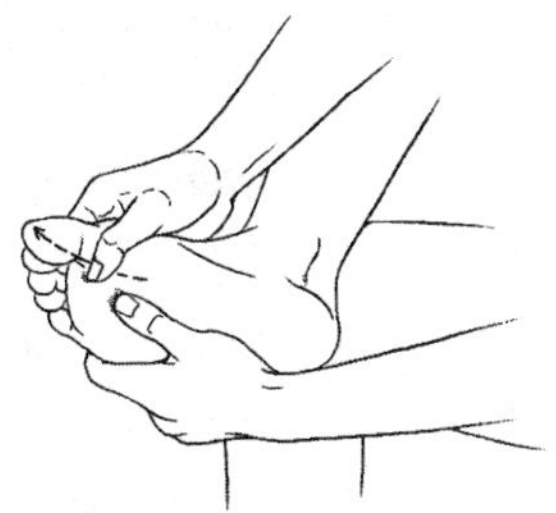

around the neck of the big toe. This releases stress in the neck.

Helpful Hint

Use a light pressure, not heavy. If the area you're working on is sensitive, work it a little, leave it, and return to it later. ■

Relaxation Tapes

More Than Just Quiet Music

When you're searching for a relaxation tape, the choices are many. Bird songs, ocean waves, or music. A soothing voice, or no voice. Images of brooks, meadows, or forests.

"Relaxation tapes are more than just soothing sounds," says Laurie Nadel, Ph.D., a Manhattan-based psychotherapist specializing in mind/body therapies for stress-related conditions. "They're combinations of sounds, words, and images specifically designed to help you get into a hypnotic state, accessing the part of the unconscious that knows how to relax completely and that can accept suggestions."

Any symptom that is made worse with stress can be improved by relaxation, says Dr. Nadel. Dr. Nadel and others have "prescribed" relaxation tapes to help women change their eating habits, control their weight, relieve insomnia and headaches, quit smoking or other bad habits, enhance their moods, relax before surgery, and even reduce the nausea associated with chemotherapy.

Most relaxation tapes start with some kind of progressive relaxation. You tense and ›› relax your muscles, starting at one end of the body and ending at the other. Or maybe a color or a wave of relaxation is described as flowing through your body. Once you're relaxed, the tape uses imagery to put you in a lovely, natural setting, where you experience the soothing sights, sounds and smells of that environment. When you're in a state of very deep relaxation, you're more receptive to suggestions for healing and well-being, says Dr. Nadel. "You can resolve an issue from your past, for example, or see yourself when you no longer smoke or you're 20 pounds thinner."

DON'T MAKE THIS MISTAKE

Never listen to a relaxation tape while driving, riding a lawn mower or operating other machinery. And don't use relaxation tapes as a substitute for getting medical help or professional therapy for depression or other serious problems.

How do they work?

"Relaxation tapes function as a pause button for our normal train of thought," says Dr. Nadel. "They slow down your breathing, which in turn slows your brain waves into the alpha state (gentle relaxation) and the theta state (deep relaxation, between sleeping and waking). In the theta state, your brain comes up with creative ideas or solves problems.

When selecting a relaxation tape, consider the following, then look for the features that

Rest

Are You Getting Your RDA of Quiet Time?

The Bible speaks about God creating the world by working for 6 days and then resting on the 7th. If we're over 50, we remember when whole towns closed down on Sundays, with no stores or businesses open. Now, our culture seems to consider rest a waste of time. But rest is essential for our health and our psychological and spiritual well-being.

"Rest is a natural and necessary part of life and of work," says Stephan Rechtschassen, M.D., cofounder of the Omega Institute for Holistic Studies in Rhinebeck, New York. He points out that the heart beats every second. "We might say that it works all the time. But in fact, it contracts for one-tenth of a second and then rests for nine-tenths of a second." It's easy to see that if the heart kept contracting without resting, it wouldn't function.

Like our hearts, we too need regular rest breaks.

"We need to step off the wheel," says Wayne Muller, ordained minister and psychotherapist in Mill Valley, California, and author of *Sabbath: Restoring the Sacred Rhythm of Rest*. "Life works in rhythm—the seas, the tides, the body, everything. If we're only on one track—producing and working, without time for reflection and regathering—we're doing harm."

If you don't make time for rest, your body will demand it—by getting sick. Researchers in the Netherlands say that excessive tiredness—a state they call vital exhaustion, typified by fatigue, irri-

appeal to you, as noted on the cover.

1. Do you prefer music or nature sounds?
2. What setting would you find most peaceful?
3. Do you want direct, vocal suggestions? A subliminal track (which means that you can't hear the voice, you just hear music or nature sounds)? Or no verbal directions at all?
4. If you prefer vocal direction, would you find a male or female voice more soothing?

Dr. Nadel recommends tapes made with the Hemi-Sync process, a patented process that produces a stereophonic pulse that stimulates both the left (analytical) and the right (creative) sides of the brain, creating both an alpha and a theta state. One brand that uses this process is Mind Food tapes, available from Interstate Industries, P.O. Box 505, Lovingston, VA 22949.

Helpful Hint

If you have a specific goal, you'll get best results with a personalized tape created for you, says Dr. Nadel. For example, if you're not sleeping because a relationship has ended, an insomnia tape won't work as well as one that helps you make peace with your loss. A hypnotherapist can make a customized tape for you, says Dr. Nadel. To find a licensed psychologist who is trained in hypnosis in your area, contact the American Society of Clinical Hypnosis, 33 West Grand Avenue, Suite 402, Chicago, IL 60610. ■

tability, and demoralization—may double your chance of heart attack, for example.

So no matter how busy you are, you can (and should) find ways to rest. Here's how.

• Start your day with yoga, meditation, or a walk.

• Take three deep, slow breaths before answering the phone, starting the car, serving the kids lunch, or any other activity.

• Take a long bath at the end of the day, with candles, music, and a good book. Let your family know that you must not be disturbed.

• Build time into your schedule for play and fun with the family. No cell phones or pagers allowed!

• Reserve some hours each week to spend with your spouse or a close friend, where you enjoy a special meal and share an activity.

• Take back the Sabbath as a day of rest for family, leisure, and worship. Don't spend the day mowing the lawn, grocery shopping, or catching up on office work.

Helpful Hint

Don't feel guilty about spending some time relaxing when you have a lot to do, because a change of pace can make you more productive. "If you leave a problem for a while and do something else, your mind will work on it in the background," says David Neubauer, M.D., associate director of Johns Hopkins Sleep Disorders Center in Baltimore. "It's like when you're doing one thing on your computer, and Windows is working in the background." ■

Restless Legs Syndrome

Counteract It with Action, Distraction

Sheila Connolly calls them her jumpy legs. Whenever she sits still, what feels like waves moving in her legs makes it impossible for her to resist moving her legs up and down to relieve the uncomfortable and irritating sensation. The only time it goes away is when she stands.

"I garden, I cook, and I read standing up," says Connolly who runs a nonprofit preschool in Massachusetts. "I stay constantly physically or mentally active all day."

Connolly has restless leg syndrome, characterized by an uncontrollable urge to move the extremities (it can affect the arms, too). No one knows what causes it. It also is a mystery why many pregnant women get it, and why it sometimes comes and goes. But anyone who has restless legs knows it: Many say that restless legs syndrome feels like bugs crawling inside your bones. It typically strikes just when you want to rest. And it can wreak havoc with your sleep, says Mark Buchfuhrer, M.D., medical director of the Southern California Restless Legs Syndrome Support Group and medical advisory board member of the Restless Legs Syndrome Foundation in Rochester, Minnesota.

Fortunately, there are many things you can do to calm your legs when you need to sit still or get some sleep.

Put your mind in gear. One of Connolly's solutions—staying mentally active—is one of the best daytime cures for restless legs, says Dr. Buchfuhrer, especially when you know you'll be sitting still for a long time. When you're in the car or on a plane, for example, play a computer game or tune your radio in to a talk-show station so you can argue with the host. Whatever engages your mind will disengage the restless legs.

Cut off the caffeine. Caffeinated drinks like coffee, tea, and cola will only stimulate your nervous system and make an irritating case of restless legs even more annoying.

Soak it out. To get an uninterrupted night's sleep, take a hot bath before bed to relax your muscles.

Rub out the restlessness. Another before-bed tip: Massage your legs, vigorously if possible, with your hands or a loofah sponge. Doing so may release endorphins, natural painkillers in the body that may counteract the jumpiness.

DON'T MAKE THIS MISTAKE

While exercise can keep restless legs at bay during the day, too much exercise—especially in the evening—can be counterproductive. You might minimize the restlessness in your legs, but your metabolism will be so revved that you won't be able to sleep anyway. Dr. Buchfuhrer recommends taking an evening walk—but do it at least 4 hours before bedtime.

Helpful Hint

Consider supplementing your diet with iron and folic acid (a B vitamin) if you're not already getting the Daily Value (DV) of both. Some researchers think that a deficiency of iron or folic acid may lead to restless leg symptoms. Be sure you're getting your DV for each—400 micrograms of folic acid and 18 milligrams for iron. ■

Rheumatoid Arthritis

What to Do When Medicines Aren't Totally Effective

Unlike osteoarthritis, which wears down pads of cartilage cushioning the bones in weight-bearing joints, rheumatoid arthritis affects more than your hips, knees, ankles, feet, or back. With rheumatoid arthritis, the body releases harmful substances that eat away at the silklike joint lining (synovial membrane). Rheumatoid arthritis also triggers inflammatory reactions elsewhere in the body. Why this happens isn't clear, but as a result, rheumatoid arthritis is a whole-body disease, capable of causing not only painful, swollen joints but other, more generalized discomforts, like fever or fatigue.

Rheumatoid arthritis is two to three times more common in women. One theory suggests that it may possibly be linked to the fact that women process proteins less effectively than men. While osteoarthritis tends to occur at age 50 or older, rheumatoid arthritis most commonly affects women between the ages of 20 and 40.

Luckily, the prognosis for rheumatoid arthritis is brighter than ever, says Teresa Brady, Ph.D., national medical advisor for the Arthritis Foundation in Atlanta.

When Dr. Brady was diagnosed with rheumatoid arthritis during the 1970s, most doctors started patients on nonsteroidal anti-inflammatory drugs (NSAIDs), then gradually added more aggressive disease-modifying drugs. They often used only one drug at a time, combined with NSAIDs.

But studies found that this go-slow approach didn't slow the disease's progression and prevent disability, so most doctors now favor a more aggressive approach. They routinely start those who are newly diagnosed with rheumatoid arthritis on a variety of potent prescription medications, such as leflunomide (Arava) and etanercept (Enbrel). **Remarkably effective, these drugs help slow the progression of rheumatoid arthritis, especially when used early.**

"They have, in effect, inverted the treatment pyramid," says Dr. Brady, who manages her condition with a combination of medications, heat, rest, and exercise.

Given that rheumatoid arthritis is controllable but not yet curable, your best bet is to augment medical treatment with self-care tips from Dr. Brady and other arthritis experts. ››

Protect your joints. Switching from a heavy purse to a backpack can save wear and tear on your fingers, wrists, and shoulders. Building up the grips on household items, such as by encasing pens and pencils in foam hair curlers, can spare you writer's cramp.

Get moving. Doctors no longer restrict all women with rheumatoid arthritis to simple range-of-motion exercises. They now recommend low-impact conditioning exercises, such as swimming, walking, stationary bicycling, road cycling, and cross-country skiing. Some even recommend strength-training programs. Ask your doctor what activities might best suit you. A lot depends on how much inflammation you're experiencing at any given time.

Helpful Hint: When you try a new activity, follow what clinicians call the 2-Hour Rule. You may experience some initial discomfort, but if your pain recedes to its normal level within 2 hours after exercise, you probably can keep on doing the activity. If the pain persists longer than 2 hours, change the way you do the activity or how long you do it.

Pass the pepper cream. Capsaicin-based creams block the transmission of pain signals. They might sting at first, and it might take 1 to 2 weeks of daily applications to see results. Follow label instructions, and be sure to wash your hands well after applying it so you don't get any in your eyes.

Take extra calcium. Since steroids inhibit calcium absorption in the stomach, women taking these drugs for rheumatoid arthritis are at increased risk of osteoporosis. To preserve bone density, take three 500-milligram calcium tablets with vitamin D every day.

Be a realistic optimist. Studies show that having an upbeat attitude is at least as important as following doctor's orders. "Rheumatoid arthritis isn't a bed of roses, so I don't think anyone can convince themselves that having it is fun," Dr. Brady says. "But they can tell themselves, 'This is hard, but I can do it.'" You can change your negative thoughts by keeping an hourly diary of your thoughts and consciously trying to replace the "I cant's" with "I can's."

QUACK CURES TO AVOID

Resist the temptation to jet off to a foreign clinic promising a miracle cure for rheumatoid arthritis. Most likely, the treatment that you receive will either be ineffective or unsafe or will use higher-than-recommended doses of substances such as corticosteroids. Also, avoid extremely restrictive "antiarthritis diets," which can send you to the hospital with malnutrition.

You can also try these less traditional but still effective approaches.

Go fishing. For fish oil, that is. More than a dozen studies show that fish oil can relieve tender, swollen joints and ease morning stiffness. But you must take it daily for at least 12 weeks to see any results. In order to get the recommended amount of omega-3 fatty acids (2.5 to 3 grams), you'll need to take 8 to 10 capsules a day. Or, you can eat 6 ounces of a fatty fish like Atlantic salmon. Since omega-3's are metabolized very rapidly, you need to take them daily. Do not take fish oil if you have diabetes, a bleeding disorder, or uncontrolled high blood pressure, take anticoagulants (blood thinners) or use aspirin regularly, or are allergic to any kind of fish. Do not take fish liver–oil supplements, which are high in vitamins A and D and are toxic in high amounts.

Consider GLA. Also known as gamma linolenic acid, GLA is an unsaturated fatty acid found in evening primrose oil. In one study, researchers found significant improvements and minimal side effects in participants who took 2.8 grams of GLA a day. If you are taking aspirin or anticoagulants (blood thinners) regularly, have a seizure disorder, or are taking epilepsy medication, use GLA only under the supervision of a doctor. GLA should be taken after meals and may cause headaches, indigestion, nausea, and soft stools.

Finding the remedy that works for you may require some trial and error—and patience. ■

R.I.C.E.

The Initials for Instant Relief

What do you get when you combine a disposable diaper, an elastic bandage, a pair of scissors, and a bag of frozen corn? Why, a recipe for instant R.I.C.E., of course. Not the kind you cook in a pot, but the kind that rescues you from the pain and swelling that follow ankle sprains, twisted knees, and myriad other sudden injuries. Here's what you need to know about this amazing acronym.

Rest. If you're luckless enough to suffer a strain or sprain, steer clear of the activity that caused the injury until the pain is completely gone. You want to rest the injured area, but that doesn't mean you have to stay in bed. You can stay active in ways that don't aggravate the injury and don't cause pain. If you got an ankle sprain from running or tennis, for example, you may be comfortable swimming—as long as this doesn't make the ankle pain flare.

Ice. Apply ice or another cold preparation immediately after the injury for 15 to 20 minutes every 4 to 6 hours for the first 24 to 36 hours to deaden pain and alter blood circulation. The best cold preparations are crushed ice or a bag of frozen corn, says James Garrick, M.D., head of the Center for Sports Medicine at St. Francis Hospital in San Francisco. Frozen vegetables work so well because you can reshape the bags to conform to the contours of the injured body part.

DON'T MAKE THIS MISTAKE

Since applying ice can slow down bloodflow, avoid it if you have health conditions that already affect bloodflow or circulation, such as diabetes or a blood supply that is less than normal due to surgery or vascular disease.

Before you ice, wet a dish towel or a length of elastic ››

bandage and lay it over the injured area to protect it from direct contact with the cold. Otherwise, the ice can cause frostbite and blisters, warns Dr. Garrick. If you want to use the bag again later, make sure it's clearly labeled before putting it back in your freezer. Never eat food that has thawed and been refrozen.

Compression. Between icings, wrap the injured area firmly (but not tightly enough to cut off circulation and cause tingling or numbness) with a padded bandage to prevent swelling and decrease pain. The trick is not to leave any recessed areas that aren't compressed, because these areas will swell, says Dr. Garrick. If this is an ankle injury, for example, he recommends cutting a horseshoe out of the center of a disposable diaper (or any padded material that is ¾ inch thick), with the sides of the horseshoe approximately 1 to 1¼ inches wide and the open spot about 1 inch wide. (Avoid diapers with gel.) Place the curved part of the horseshoe around the ankle knob, and wrap the entire ankle with an Ace bandage, as shown above.

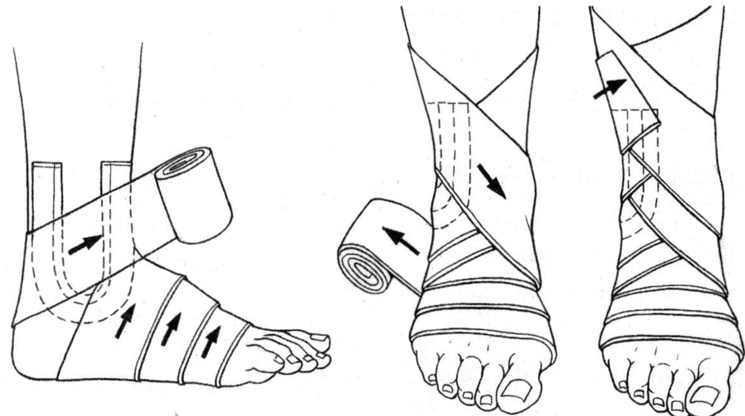

Start wrapping at the ball of the foot, continuing under the foot from inside to outside, overlapping one-half of the previous layer with each wrap. Do this two or three times, moving closer to the ankle with each turn. When the bandage is on the outside of the foot, begin a figure-eight turn by bringing the bandage over the instep and inside around the ankle.

Continue down inside of the foot, around the heel, up over the instep, down under the foot, and back up completely around the ankle.

Repeat the figure-eight rap two or three times, rising above the ankle with each turn, before you fasten the bandage with the fasten method provided.

If time is an issue, simply wrap the bandage from the ball of your foot to up above your ankle, covering the entire horseshoe. "The idea is not to have any voids under the wrap," says Dr. Garrick. "You really want the pressure where there are hollow spots."

Elevation. If the injury is in an arm or leg, keep it elevated whenever you can to minimize swelling and pain.

Helpful Hint

Heat isn't part of R.I.C.E. "Heat increases the blood supply to the area, so you get more swelling," says Dr. Garrick. Although it may seem to feel good at first, heat can make swelling and bleeding worse. Much later, when the injury is healing nicely and no longer swelling, and stiffness is your worst complaint, heat may make you more comfortable. ■

Road Rage

The Common-Scents Approach to Senseless Drivers

Rush hour. Downtown Atlanta. A rude driver whips in front of Marilyn Johnson Kondwani. Moments later, the same driver turns abruptly—without signaling, of course—and careens down another street, the proverbial accident looking for a place to happen.

Even the least confrontational of us might feel a rebuttal was in order—a retaliatory flashing of lights or honking of the horn, perhaps even some indelicate sign language. But not Kondwani. Her reaction to the road hog? She simply kept both hands on the steering wheel and continued to take deep, refreshing breaths.

"People are always going to cut you off in their hurry to get somewhere, but I've found a way to keep my cool," says Kondwani, an aromatherapist.

Anyone who takes a seat inside her navy blue Lincoln Continental quickly discovers why. The interior of the car is scented with one or more essential oils known to calm, refresh, and cool moods. Aromatherapy is the use of essential, aromatic oils for emotional and physical health. Geranium, lemongrass, peppermint, lavender, and grapefruit essential oils work best against road rage, says Kondwani. These oils are distilled from flowers, leaves, fruit, bark, and roots of plants.

DON'T MAKE THIS MISTAKE

Do not respond to aggressive acts by making obscene gestures at the offending driver, blocking the passing lane, tailgating, or flashing high beams. These acts of retaliation may intensify the situation and lead to injury or possibly a fatal crash, according to studies by the American Automobile Association Foundation for Traffic Safety in Washington, D.C.

Like Kondwani, you too can use calming scents to help you steer clear of the emotional ravages of road rage. Try any of these aromatic options.

Buy an aromatherapy diffuser for your car. These cylindrical-shaped electric diffusers plug directly into your cigarette lighter. Manufacturers such as Aeron International of Fairfield, Iowa, offer diffusers and essential oil aromas in three distinct categories: alertness, ambiance, and floral botanical. "You simply add a few drops of essential oil to the diffuser, insert the unit into your cigarette lighter, and enjoy." says Jeffrey L. ››

Smith, president of Aeron International. To purchase a diffuser, check your local health food store or visit the company's Web site. To contact the company directly, write to them at 406 West Depot Avenue, Fairfield, IA 52556.

Make your own road rage–fighting diffuser. Take a 4-ounce plastic spray mister, fill nearly to the top with distilled water, and add 20 to 50 drops of your favorite calming essential oil. Secure the cap, shake a few times, and then spray 6 to 8 times. Pump a few sprays every 20 minutes when you've stopped driving.

Keep a bottle of Rescue Remedy handy. Rescue Remedy is a water-based homeopathic blend of five flower essences (star of Bethlehem, rockrose, impatiens, cherry plum, and clematis) that can restore calm, says Mark Stengler, N.D., a naturopathic physician in Oceanside, California. "Place a few drops directly on your tongue and within 10 to 15 seconds, you'll feel stress and anxiety disappearing." To purchase Rescue Remedy, check your local health food store. ■

Rudeness

Deflective Tactics for Thoughtless Remarks

No matter what social circles you travel in, sooner or later you're bound to be blindsided by a rude remark. Anything, it seems, is fair game: your weight, your marital status, or even your children's parentage.

If you're like most women, you'll probably react in one of three ways: (1) You'll counterattack with a snappy comeback, (2) you'll plead that you don't have time for such nonsense, or (3) you'll explain why such remarks are hurtful. "All those responses are wrong," says Suzette Haden Elgin, Ph.D., a psycholinguist in Huntsville, Arkansas, and author of How to Disagree without Being Disagreeable. *"They give the attacker your full, undivided attention—which is exactly what she is after. Rudeness is a form of hostility, and hostile people are like little kids who'd rather be spanked than ignored. They know they'll be rewarded if they say something mean."*

Dr. Elgin recommends countering rude remarks with what she calls the Boring Baroque Response. It goes something like this.

DON'T MAKE THIS MISTAKE

If you encounter a rude waitress or waiter, responding in kind increases the odds that you'll get a burnt offering for dinner. "A lot of times, they're only snapping at you because things have been going wrong for them," Horn says. "If you treat the person kindly and ask sympathetically, 'Has it been one of those days?' oftentimes they'll just melt."

Hostile person: "Your children look foreign. Is their father Chinese?"

You: "You know, hearing you say that reminds me of a story I read the other day in the *Wall Street Journal* about mixed-race children. Or maybe it wasn't the *Wall Street Journal.* Maybe it was the . . ."

"Usually, they're long gone before you can name the second newspaper because they're thinking, 'Uh-oh, here comes this long, boring explanation I don't want to hear,'" Dr. Elgin says. "It tells them you're not going to take the bait, but in a way that doesn't make them lose face or make you lose your dignity."

Just be sure to deliver your response with a straight face and a neutral voice. "If you say it sarcastically," Dr. Elgin says, "it's like picking a fight."

But what if the rudeness isn't intentional, just gauche? Either ignore it or have fun with it, says Sam Horn, professional speaker, president of Action Seminars in Maui, Hawaii, and author of *Tongue Fu!: How to Deflect, Disarm, and Defuse Any Verbal Conflict* and *Conzentrate.*

Here are some of her favorite comebacks to thoughtless remarks.

"Why aren't you married?" I think, therefore I'm single.

"When are you going to have children?" We thought having kids was a spectator sport.

"Where did you go to college?" (If you didn't.) U.H.K. (the University of Hard Knocks).

"I didn't know you were pregnant!" (When you're not.) "Rosie O'Donnell has a great comeback for that one," says Horn. "She says, 'I'm having twins. They're called Ben and Jerry.'"

Helpful Hint

Learn to recognize the difference between intentional and unintentional rudeness. "Women waste a lot of time reacting to people who are just socially inept," Dr. Elgin says. "In English, hostile language is usually marked by not only your choice of words but also emphasis on words or parts of words, as in '*WHY* do you *EAT* so much?' as opposed to 'Why do you eat so much?'" ■

S

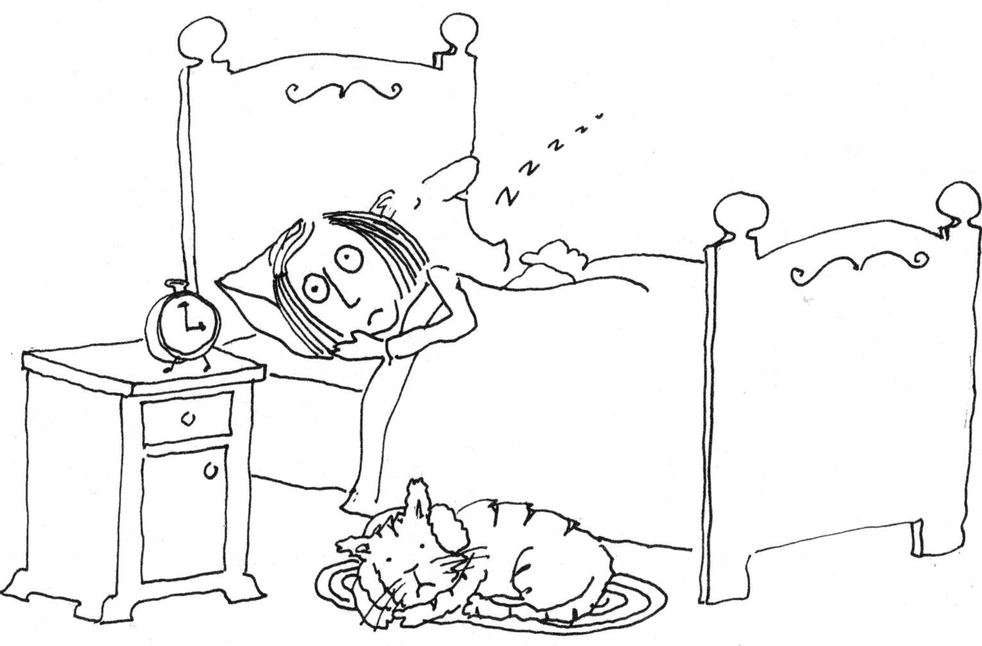

Does your husband snore so loudly
that he even keeps the cat awake?
Find the solution on page 402.

Saturated Fat

Truly Bad—Or Simply Misunderstood?

Saturated fats. They're the cause of all matters of disease, and maybe pestilence as well. At least that's what you may have been led to believe.

In truth, your body needs saturated fats. They help build neurons—the phone lines that allow your brain to communicate with every muscle in your body. "Without saturated fat, your brain couldn't tell your fingers to turn a page, nor could you remember what you read," says Michael A. Schmidt, Ph.D., visiting professor of applied biochemistry and clinical nutrition at Northwestern Health Sciences University in Bloomington, Minnesota, and author of Smart Fats.

The tricky part is getting the right amount. Eating too much saturated fat raises blood cholesterol levels, which cakes up arteries and may lead to heart disease and stroke. And since your body actually makes quite a bit of saturated fat, you don't need much more from your diet. In fact, experts recommend getting no more than one-third of your total dietary fat from saturated fats. The other two-thirds should come from monounsaturated and polyunsaturated fats, found primarily in unhyrogenated (liquid) vegetable oils.

Fortunately, there are five easy ways to fix your fat intake.

Have an olive, not a cow. To slice away 6 grams of saturated fat in one sitting, just substitute a tablespoon of mild-tasting olive oil (usually labeled "light") for a tablespoon of butter or other solid fat the next time you sauté foods or glaze baked goods.

Sizzle lean. The less white you see on a piece of red meat, the less saturated fat it contains. To keep this neuron builder at healthful levels (less than 4 grams per serving), choose lean cuts of beef—those with "loin" or "round" in their names like tenderloin or top round steak. Even better: Look for cuts marked "select." ››

MARGARINE OR BUTTER?

If a recipe calls for either butter or margarine, which should you use?

"Butter," says Mary Enig, Ph.D., a pioneer in trans-fatty acid research and director of Nutritional Sciences Division Enig Associates in Silver Spring, Maryland.

While it's true that butter contains lots of saturated fat, which may raise "bad" LDL cholesterol, it also raises "good" HDL cholesterol. But trans-fatty acids, also known as hydrogenated fats, not only raise LDL cholesterol, but research suggests that they also raise LP(a), the lipoprotein associated with an increased risk of heart disease, and lower HDL cholesterol. They may increase your risk for cancer as well.

What about trans-fatty-acid-free margarines? They contain many food additives. "You're still better off with butter, made entirely from natural ingredients," says Dr. Enig.

Natural or no, butter still contains 7 grams of saturated fat and 100 calories per tablespoon. So don't slather it on with a trowel.

These contain the least fat. "Choice" and "prime" cuts have more fat. In fact, 3 ounces of select top round contains just a tad more saturated fat than a 3-ounce skinless chicken leg. Avoid prime grade meats, like prime rib or prime chuck roast; they are the highest in fat.

Keep an eye on processed meats. Bacon, sausage, kielbasa, salami, pâté, and other processed meats are loaded with saturated fat. Instead, try smoked turkey, turkey pastrami, soy links, and other low-fat alternatives.

Stick with liquid oils. Since most foods contain a blend of saturated and unsaturated fats, you need to figure out which predominantly presides in your meal. Follow this rule of thumb: "In general, saturated fats are solid at room temperature," says Dr. Schmidt. "Unsaturated fats aren't." So a cup of beef fat, which contains lots of saturated fat, will harden if left out on your kitchen counter. On the other hand, a homemade vinaigrette, which contains unsaturated fats, will stay liquid. What's more, liquid oils such as canola and soybean oil are also high in omega-3 fatty acids. To read about their benefits, turn to page 317.

Save full-fat dairy products for special occasions. If you can't resist cream in your coffee, premium ice cream, ricotta cheese, brie, real Vermont Cheddar cheese, New England clam chowder, butter, cream cheese, cheese omelets, milkshakes, and other dairy delights, have just a little. These foods are not only high in saturated fat but they're also high in calories. ■

Sciatica

Stretch Away Crippling Pain

Mary Jo Marino was lifting her big bass fiddle into her car to go play jazz at a party. The instrument wasn't terribly heavy, but it was bulky—taller and wider than Marino's 5-foot 8-inch frame—and awkward to lift. She felt her back strain, but went on to the party anyway, where her back went into spasms.

Somehow Marino played her music and drove her stick-shift car home. "By then, I could barely make it into the elevator and into the apartment. I crawled in and asked my friend to unload the bass and park the car. I could hardly move. It was in total spasm and pain."

Marino should have known better. As one of only about 15 women out of 3,000 subway repair mechanics for New York City Transit, she was accustomed to heavy work. "I do everything—repair propulsion systems, power converters, doors, lights, and air-conditioning. We change air-conditioning motors that weigh 800 to 900 pounds." She knew how to lift and use equipment safely—on the job.

"It was a case of sloppy lifting," she admits about the bass-lifting incident.

Sciatica is the irritation of the sciatic nerve, or the lumbar nerve roots in the lower back. The discomfort can extend

Four Antidotes to Sciatica Pain

The following exercises can help you alleviate sciatica or prevent future episodes, says John E. Thomassy, D.C., a chiropractic neurologist in Virginia Beach, Virginia. Assuming your doctor gives you the green light, perform the exercises in the order given. Hold each position for 10 seconds, and repeat each exercise six times.

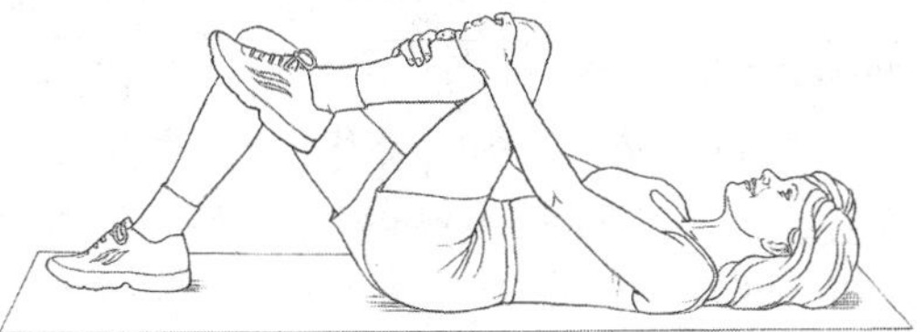

1. Lie on your back with both knees bent and feet flat on the floor. Press your lower back into the floor. Lift one knee and pull it up toward your chest. Repeat with the other knee.

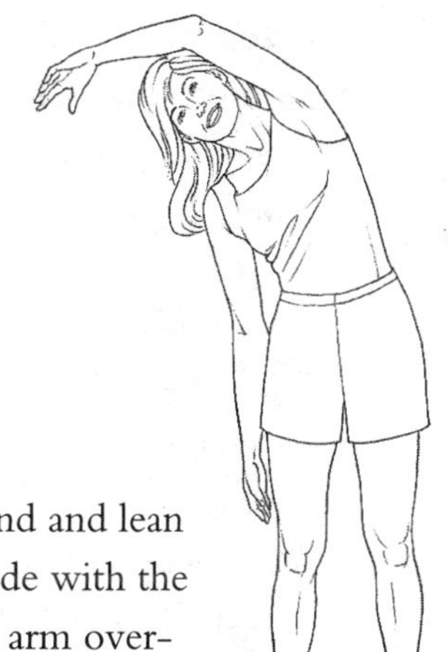

2. Stand and lean to one side with the opposite arm overhead, stretching the side of the raised arm.

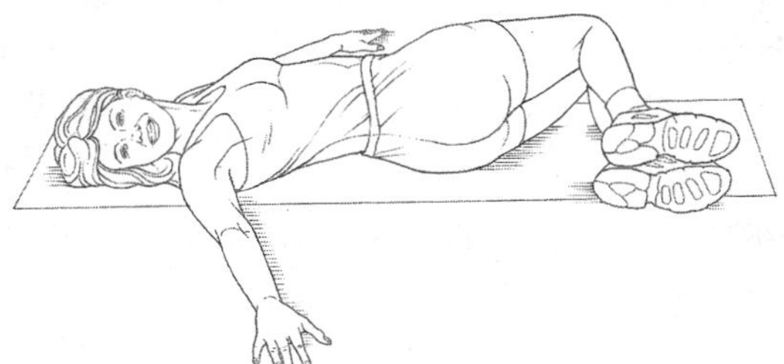

3. Lie on your back with your knees bent and feet together, arms out to your sides. Rotate your knees to one side and turn your head in the opposite direction.

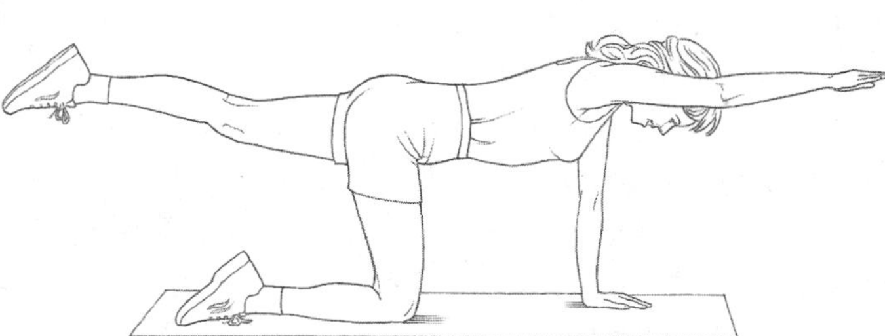

4. Get on your hands and knees. Keeping your back level, raise one arm and the opposite leg. Repeat with the other arm and leg.

from the lower back down to the foot. "It's a stabbing, knifelike pain. **The slightest movement can make it worse.** You may also feel pins and needles and numbness," says Marino's physician, Stuart Kahn, M.D., at Beth Israel Medical Center in New York City. In Marino's case, sciatica was caused by a herniated disk, which compressed and/or inflamed her ❯❯

nerves. But sciatica can also be caused by inflamed joints in the back that irritate the nerve root, or a spontaneous inflammation of the nerve.

Women who sit at a computer all day or drive trucks are as susceptible to sciatica as women who lift or carry things on the job, says Manish Suthar, M.D., of the Texas Back Institute in Plano.

If you have sciatic pain, your doctor will typically recommend rest, icing the back to prevent muscle spasms, over-the-counter anti-inflammatory medications such as aspirin, ibuprofen, or naproxen (unless you have stomach ulcers and bleeding disorders) and stretching and strengthening exercises. If the pain persists, corticosteroid injections may be required. Marino, for example, healed through a combination of rest, physical therapy, yoga, and exercises, which she continues to do faithfully. Surgery is a last resort.

If you have sciatica, ask your doctor which exercises would benefit you. Recommendations differ, depending on what's compressing your sciatic nerve and where, says Dr. Suthar. ■

Seat Belts

Buckle Up Your "Emergency Brake"

Professional race-car driver Shirley Muldowney makes a living driving one of the fastest machines on Earth. Her dragster can go over 300 miles per hour in less than 5 seconds, with the same gravitational force of a space shuttle leaving the launchpad. But whether Muldowney is piloting her road rocket on the track or driving her Cadillac STS around town, the four-time Top Fuel Winston world champion never forgets to buckle up.

"These days, with everyone jockeying for position on the highway, you need all the protection you can get," she says.

Seat-belt advocates like Carole Guzzetta wish every driver shared that attitude. As director of the National Safety Belt Coalition in Washington, D.C., Guzzetta finds it a challenge to convince the nation's drivers to always wear seat belts, even for a quick trip to the store. "No one likes to think that every time they get into a car there is a chance of a crash. But it's a possibility we can't afford to ignore," says Guzzetta.

Every state except New Hampshire mandates that front passengers wear seat belts. And with good reason—seat belts save 9,500 lives a year. So if you don't routinely buckle up, start now. And if you already buckle up, here's how to maximize your safety.

Wear the lap belt low on your hips over the pelvic bone—not riding across your tummy. Even a crash at a speed as low as 20 miles per hour could cause injury to vital organs like the spleen or stomach if the seat belt was not in its proper place, says Guzzetta.

Buckle up in taxis and airport shuttle vans. "All it takes is one person to click on her belt in an airport van. Each time I do, a chorus of clicks follow," says Guzzetta. And some taxicabs are equipped with recordings that ask passengers to buckle up as soon as they get into the cab. ■

Sensitive Teeth

A Cure for "Ice Cream Pain"

You know you have sensitive teeth if you bite into a Popsicle and your teeth immediately send a bolt of pain to the center of your brain.

The enamel shell that covers your teeth is the hardest substance in your body, providing a protective coating that shields the nerves in your teeth as you chew. Should this coating wear off, any hot or cold temperature can trigger pain, says Kimberly Harms, D.D.S, a dentist in Farmington, Minnesota, and consumer educator for the American Dental Association.

"The more you can do to preserve that enamel coating, the better," says Dr. Harms. "Otherwise, you start having problems."

Here's how to help keep your teeth hard and strong.

Use a soft toothbrush. Check the label.

Don't brush too hard. Bearing down on your teeth can wear away the enamel, particularly near the gum line, where it's not quite as thick.

Brush gently in a circular motion. The tips of the bristles should gently clean slightly below the gum line. The next time you go to the dentist, show the hygienist how you're brushing, to be sure that you're doing it right.

Floss daily to remove plaque. If allowed to accumulate, a sticky film of bacteria-laden dental plaque can prompt your gums to pull back a little. Since enamel covers your teeth only down to the gum line, the newly exposed tooth will be more sensitive.

Buy toothpaste for sensitive teeth. Widely available at supermarkets and pharmacies, these toothpastes contain substances that build up on the surface of your teeth, like an artificial coating of enamel. Be patient: You may need to use the paste for several weeks to notice improvement.

DON'T MAKE THIS MISTAKE

Chewing ice is extremely rough on your teeth. Not only can it wear away enamel but it can actually crack your teeth, exposing the sensitive dentin to the food, water, and air in your mouth. If you think you may have cracked a tooth, see your dentist right away.

Helpful Hints

Let your dentist know whenever your teeth hurt. If necessary, she may be able to seal them with a protective coating. And if you have just one tooth that's extremely sensitive, be sure to visit your dentist right away—it could be a damaged nerve problem, which calls for immediate treatment.

If you wake up mornings with clenched or tired facial muscles, you're grinding your teeth in your sleep and don't know it. Your dentist can fit you with a mouth guard to protect your teeth from further damage. ■

Sexy Hair

Styling Secrets for That Bedroom Look

You don't have to have thick, long hair—like women in the Victoria's Secret catalogs—to look sexy.

"The sexiest look is hair that looks unfinished," says Aidan Harty, a stylist in New York City who also moonlights as a stylist for off-Broadway theater productions. "It's low-maintenance hair that's loose and wild-looking. It says that the woman is not trying too hard and is just being herself."

Ironically, that sexy, unfinished look doesn't just happen. It takes a little effort. Whether your hair is long or short, thick or thin, here's how to achieve a relaxed and sexy look.

Start with a towel. After shampooing, tip your head over and towel-dry your hair well for at least a minute.

For long hair: Smooth in a light styling lotion or mist with volumizing spray. Then, holding your blow-dryer in one hand, grab your hair with the fingers of your other hand and gently pull and air-dry it at the roots. Continue for about 3 minutes, or until your hair is almost dry.

For short hair: Try for a spiky look. Run a styling gel through your hair after towel-drying, then finger-dry it by simply pulling up on it and holding it in place until it begins to dry.

For fine hair: Pin it up on top of your head. "That exposes the most beautiful part of a woman's body—her neck," says Harty. Leave a few loose fringes of hair out so it doesn't look too perfect.

To restore volume at the end of the day: Use a curling iron on the ends or hot rollers to add body.

For special occasions: Adorn your hair with a few delicate flowers, such as babies breath or rosebuds, in a semi-upsweep style.

Helfpul Hint

A blow-dryer can help revolumize your hair even when it's dry. "Women have the misconception they have to blow-dry their hair when it's wet," says Harty. "But hot forced air can pump up your hair even when it's dry, whatever you're trying to do." Wrap your hair around a round brush, put hair spray on it, and heat it up for 2 seconds. Then wait for 5 to 10 seconds and remove it. Focus on the top of your head—where the hairline begins to recede—and across your part. That will maximize volume—and the slightly messy look. ■

KNOW WHEN TO GIVE UP

If you're not getting the look you want, let it go. "Women often spend too much time on their hair when they are trying to get a certain look," says Harty. The more they keep fussing with it, the more frustrated they get. Meanwhile, their hair just gets weighed down. For the slightly unfinished look, Harty recommends spending no more than 10 minutes on short hair and 20 minutes on long hair.

Shift Work

Damage Control for Night Workers

For 27 years, Sherrill Dunning, R.N., has worked while the rest of us sleep.

"I've always liked working nights," says Dunning, an emergency room nurse in Watseka, Illinois. "It's easier to get your work done—you have more autonomy." Working nontraditional hours has also provided Dunning with a close band of coworkers, reduced her day care costs for her three daughters, and developed her appreciation for offbeat humor. "It's amazing what you find funny in the middle of the night," she says.

But shift work does have its drawbacks. Working the late shift or overnight disrupts the circadian rhythms that control when you eat, sleep, even ovulate, explains Martin Moore-Ede, M.D., Ph.D., founder and president of Circadian Technologies, a Cambridge, Massachusetts, company that trains workers how to adjust to nontraditional hours. Combined with rotating shifts and weekend work, stress due to circadian disruptions increases your risk of cardiovascular disease, insomnia, and digestive problems. It may also affect your reproductive cycles.

"Circadian rhythms trigger ovulation and other reproductive functions, which are driven by biological clocks," Dr. Moore-Ede says. "That's why flight attendants who cross time zones often have irregular periods. If you're having trouble conceiving, you may do better with a traditional shift."

Still, that's not always economically possible, Dr. Moore-Ede admits. In fact, about two-thirds of the women employed outside the home work something other than a 9-to-5, Monday-through-Friday workweek.

But you can minimize the health risks of shift work. Here's what experts recommend.

Prioritize sleep. Shift workers need sleep as much as day workers, but they have a much harder time getting it because of daytime distractions and the body's natural tendency to be awake in daylight. Make your bedroom as dark and quiet as possible: Buy light-blocking window treatments, turn off the phone, wear earplugs, and ask people not to call or ring the doorbell while you're sleeping.

Limit your caffeine intake. "People tend to drink lots of coffee when working nights to compensate for not having enough sleep—and caffeine is no substitute for sleep," Dunning observes. Plus, it interferes with your natural sleep cycle the next day after you get home.

If you must have caffeine, says Steve Mardon, editor of Circadian Technologies' *Working Nights* newsletter, limit yourself to 2 to 3 cups, with your last one coming no later than 4 to 5 hours before your shift ends so you won't be wired when you get home.

Eat lightly at night. "Your body's not really geared to be digesting food during the overnight hours, so you don't want to be having a cheeseburger at 4 A.M.," Mardon ❯❯

says. Instead, eat a light meal around 10:00 or 11:00 P.M. and supplement that with a healthy snack or two during the overnight hours. Good choices include complex carbohydrates such as whole grains, fish, lean poultry, fruits and vegetables, tofu, beans, low-fat dairy products, and complex carbohydrates such as pasta, rice, and potatoes.

Nap. If your workplace allows naps, numerous studies suggest that a 15- to 20-minute snooze will improve your alertness during the last half of your shift.

Energize with exercise. If you find yourself fading in the wee hours, get active. Take a walk through your building. Lift weights on your break. Climb a few flights of stairs. Some companies even provide exercise bikes for their workers.

Recover and readjust. After you end a stretch of night or evening shifts, give yourself a day to regroup and

Sinus Trouble

Relieve Sinusitis with Salt and Pepper

When they're working properly, the gutters on your roof help keep your home from becoming awash in rainwater. But when they become plugged with leaves, brackish water can overflow and cause a heap of trouble.

Your sinuses have a lot in common with your gutters.

Normally, these air-filled pockets behind your face and forehead constantly secrete mucus, which microscopic hairs in the sinuses push through tiny openings into the back of your nose. This sticky fluid humidifies the air you breathe and traps particles as it drains harmlessly down your throat.

But when the tiny openings to the sinuses swell shut—often because of a cold virus or allergies—the fluid can get trapped, says Richard Orlandi, M.D., assistant professor of otolaryngology at the University of Michigan in Ann Arbor and associate director of the Michigan Sinus Center in Livonia. As bacteria thrive in the bottled-up material, the sinuses can grow inflamed and infected. That's called sinusitis.

The main warning sign is greenish yellow mucus from your nose or throat, along with fever and pressure in your face or ears. If you have sinusitis, your doctor will probably prescribe antibiotics. If medication doesn't clear up the problem, you may need surgery.

It can take weeks or even months to completely clear a stubborn case of sinusitis. Here's how to feel better in the meantime.

Bottoms up. Above all, drink plenty of water—at least eight glasses a day—during sinusitis. Staying hydrated helps keep the mucus moist and flowing, says Charles P. Kimmelman, M.D., professor of otolaryngology at Weill Medical College of Cornell Uniget some extra sleep. A day or two before you start working nights again, stay up late and sleep late so your body begins to adjust to your nighttime schedule again.

Helpful Hint

Make time for your family; your nontraditional hours can be stressful for them, too. Among couples with children and a shift-working parent, the likelihood of divorce or separation is between three and six times higher than those with day-working parents, according to sociologist Harriet B. Presser, Ph.D., distinguished university professor and director of the Center on Population, Gender, and Social Inequality at the University of Maryland in College Park. Planning special family days or hanging a bulletin board where children can post art projects or schoolwork can help keep you connected. ■

versity in New York City.

Steam clean your sinuses. Another way to help moisten and loosen built-up material in your sinuses is to inhale steam through your nose. Just lean over a sink filled with hot water with a towel draped over your head and the sink to hold in the steam, and inhale deeply. Keep your face about 18 inches away from the water to avoid burns. Or, just use your stopped-up sinuses as a good excuse to linger in a hot, steamy shower.

Squirt them with saltwater. Washing your nasal passages with saltwater may loosen buildup and allow those tiny hairs in the sinuses to push the mucus along more efficiently, Dr. Kimmelman says.

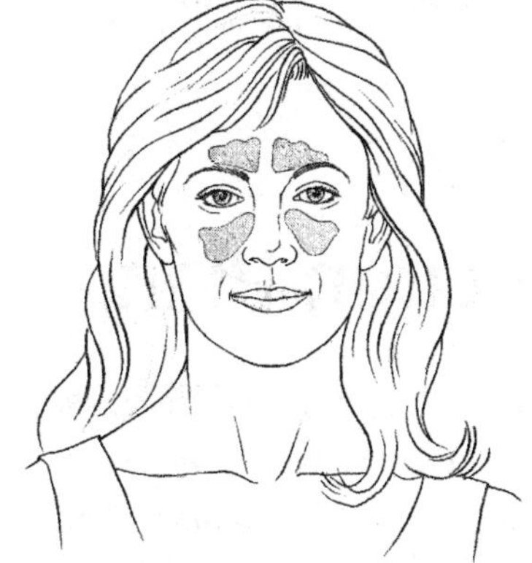

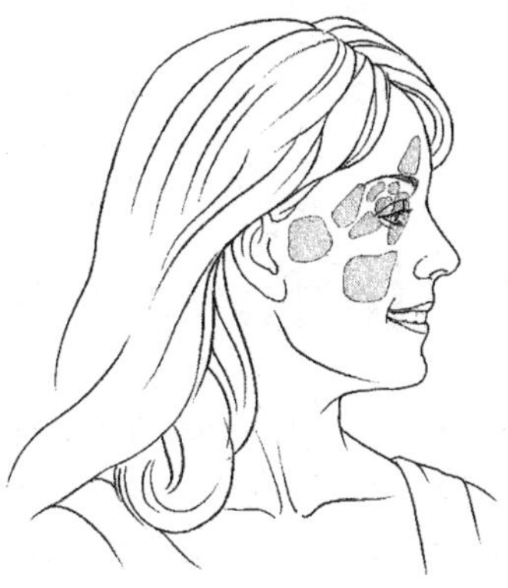

Sinusitis isn't limited to the hollow cavities underneath your cheekbones. Sinuses are also located above your eyes and nose, behind your forehead, and between your eye sockets (as shown), making it easy to see why sinus trouble can be such a pain.

You can use a spray mister or a squirt bottle to get the fluid into your nose; both are available at drugstores. You can also make your own by stirring a tablespoon of kosher salt into 8 ounces of water, then squirting it gently into your nostrils with a bulb syringe, also available at pharmacies. The liquid drains back out the nostril or into the throat, where it can be expelled through the mouth. ››

If the saline irritates your nasal passages, stop using it, Dr. Orlandi advises.

Pepper your problem. If you enjoy hot and spicy foods, now would be a great time to eat some. The capsaicin in hot peppers may open up your nasal passages and help ease your sinus congestion.

DON'T MAKE THESE MISTAKES

An over-the-counter decongestant in pill form or nasal spray is a tried-and-true way to quickly bring down swelling and open up your sinuses, Dr. Orlandi says. Be sure not to use a spray form for more than 3 days in a row, as your body may become dependent on it and need more and more to keep your passages open.

If your doctor prescribes antibiotics, be sure to finish all the pills even if your symptoms improve. If you don't, you might leave some stubborn bacteria behind that cause a chronic problem.

Helpful Hint

Take extra care to avoid colds, since they often lead to sinusitis. To protect yourself, wash your hands frequently, Dr. Orlandi says. And if you're allergy-prone, take steps to avoid whatever provokes your allergies. ■

Skin Cancer Prevention

A Lifetime Protection Plan

Sara Wise started lifeguarding at age 15. From childhood, she loved being in the sun and water. Her fair skin burned easily, but she paid little attention to protecting it. "I wanted a tan," Wise says. "That was more important than anything."

The high point of Wise's career was a summer lifeguarding in Orlando, Florida, at Walt Disney World, spending 40 hours a week in the sun for 3 months. She was 20 years old.

Then, at age 21, Wise noticed an ugly little bump under her left eye. She wanted it removed, so she went to her doctor. It was cancerous: basal cell carcinoma. Her doctor told her that this kind of cancer begins underneath the skin, not on the surface. Because it was so close to her eye, it could have blinded her.

Fortunately, the kind of skin cancer Wise had is the most treatable type, and she caught it in time. Now, Wise protects her skin with as much fervor as she used to worship the sun. She wears hats, sunscreens, and long-sleeved shirts and sees her dermatologist every 6 months.

DON'T MAKE THIS MISTAKE

Artificial tanners won't protect your skin from sun damage. You still need a lotion with an SPF of 15 or higher when you go outdoors.

How does Wise react now to seeing sunbathers seeking tans? "It makes me cringe," she says. "I've been through it. It can happen to anyone. I want women to understand that being pale can be beautiful."

You don't have to be a lifeguard to run the risk of skin cancer. Anyone who spends a

FAKE TANS THAT LOOK REAL

Want a healthy-looking tan without damaging your skin? Consider an artifical tanning gel. When used correctly, self-tanners look remarkably convincing, says Leslie S. Baumann, M.D., director of cosmetic dermatology at the University of Miami. They're especially convenient for women who want to go without stockings in summer but hate the way their legs look pasty white without a tan.

All self-tanners use the same active ingredient—dihydroxyacetone (DHA)—although the amount varies from product to product. Lotions are easier to apply than sprays. Here's how to get the best results.

• For the most natural-looking tan, don't be tempted to buy the darkest tanner you find. If your skin is very pale, use a lighter formula. If you have dark or olive complexion, select a medium or dark shade. Or start with a light shade and work up gradually.

• Remove your rings or other jewelry. Then take a shower or bath using an exfoliating scrub, giving special attention to your arms, legs, elbows, and knees. Finally, shave your legs. Your goal is to get rid of all the dead skin and hair that can cause an uneven application, explains Dr. Baumann.

• Apply the self-tanner to any area that you would normally tan—your arms, legs, top of feet and hands, neck, and face. Don't apply it to your underarms, though, because it will look unnatural. And go easy on your elbows and knees to keep them from getting too dark.

• Blend lightly on your face. Feather the tanner into your hairline and eyebrows.

• To eliminate tan palms, wash your hands thoroughly with an exfoliating scrub after applying to arms and legs.

• If you want tan hands, go back and apply the tanner to the tops of your hands with a cotton ball or a finger. Blend the edges of your hands and fingers.

• Apply a moisturizer after the tanner has dried—usually within a few minutes but up to ½ hour—to avoid uneven patches of color. Allow the lotion to dry thoroughly before you get dressed.

Helpful Hint: For even better results, use an alpha-hydroxy body lotion for 1 week prior to applying the self-tanning product. These lotions will eliminate dead skin so that the self-tanner will go on more smoothly, says Dr. Baumann.

lot of time in the sun is at risk.

"The definition of skin cancer prevention is sun avoidance," says Joseph Bark, M.D., a dermatologist in Lexington, Kentucky, and author of *Your Skin: An Owner's Guide.* "If sun doesn't hit your skin, you won't get skin cancer."

Not everyone who spends time in the sun gets cancer. Dr. Bark recommends sunscreens and hats as well as shirts or other cover-ups. "You can step into your sunscreen," says Bark. "Put it on and button it up."

"Protection should start at an early age," says Evelyn Placek, M.D., a dermatol- ››

ogist in Scarsdale, New York. So apply sunscreen liberally to your children every time they play outside. "Be careful not to skip any areas," she adds. You can find sunscreen with sparkles—children like wearing it, and you can see if you've covered their skin completely.

To protect yourself and your children from skin cancer:

• Avoid outdoor activities or use sunscreen when the sun is strongest, between 10:00 A.M. and 3:00 P.M. Or use the "shadow rule:" If your shadow is shorter than you are tall, the sun's rays are more likely to cause sunburn.

• Use a broad-spectrum sunscreen that blocks both ultraviolet A (UVA) rays and ultraviolet B (UVB) rays daily, year-round. (You can read more about sunscreens on page 421.)

• Apply sunscreen 30 to 45 minutes before sun exposure because it needs time to be absorbed by the skin.

• If you see changes in your skin—a new spot, a little notch, darker pigmentation, or

Smoking

A Painless Way to Quit—For Good

Your kids bring home treatises on the dangers of smoking, poke them under your pack of cigarettes, and cough loudly every time you light up. The last straw was the edict that you couldn't smoke at work anymore. You feel like a pariah huddled in the doorway as coworkers who used to join you for a smoke jog by on their lunch breaks.

Okay, it's time. You'll quit.

It ain't easy. Withdrawal symptoms such as cigarette craving, restlessness, increased appetite, depressed mood, anxiety, difficulty concentrating, irritability, frustration, anger, and difficulty sleeping often send quitters back to the pack.

If you've tried to quit a dozen times already, without permanent success, you might want to consider bupropion, a prescription antidepressant approved as a smoking cessation aid and sold under the brand name Zyban.

One study found that almost twice as many smokers who used bupropion were able to abstain from tobacco as those who used either the nicotine patch or a placebo. (A nicotine patch delivers enough nicotine through the skin to reduce withdrawal symptoms and help wean you off inhaled smoke that damages your heart and lungs.)

"Bupropion tends to decrease the severity of withdrawal symptoms," says Myra Muramoto, M.D., assistant professor of family and community medicine and medical director of the Arizona Program for Nicotine and Tobacco Research at the University of Arizona in Tucson and one of the researchers for this study. Bupropion affects the mood-regulating chemicals in the brain.

Bupropion may be of special benefit to women who are trying to quit. "Women are less likely to be able to quit smoking than men, says Dr. Muramoto. Yet women smokers, as well as men, did better on bupropion, so this drug may help to level the playing field. An additional a change in a lesion, wart, or mole—consult a dermatologist, says Dr. Bark.

Even if you don't see changes, get a skin screening from a dermatologist once a year. "A yearly screening is likely to pick up early skin cancer at its most treatable, entirely curable, stages," says Dr. Placek. ■

TANNING COFFINS?

Never use a sunlamp or tanning booth, and ignore tanning salons that claim to use "safe" tanning rays. There's no such thing. "We call tanning booths and beds the skin's 'doomsday machines,' " says Dr. Bark. "If you had a group of scientists figuring out ways to intentionally destroy human skin, they'd come up with a tanning parlor. You're nuking your skin, microwaving it, cooking it until it sizzles." If the risk of skin cancer isn't danger enough, Dr. Bark has seen women with herpes simplex sores on their buttocks and backs and fungus infections like ringworm on their legs from lying on unhygienic tanning beds.

DON'T MAKE THIS MISTAKE

If you're using a nicotine patch with or without bupropion, don't smoke—it can cause a heart attack on the spot. "Nicotine can constrict the blood vessels feeding the heart muscle, and may cause irregular heartbeats, so too much nicotine can lead to a heart attack," explains Paul Roberts, R.Ph., pharmacist at Kaiser Permanente in Santa Rosa, California, who teaches smoking cessation. Signs of too much nicotine include blurred vision, nausea, drooling, vomiting, and headaches. "If you wear a patch, and you smoke, and you get these symptoms, call 911, remove the patch—and of course, put the cigarette out," says Roberts.

If you get these symptoms and you're not smoking, the patch may be too strong for you. Remove it and call your health care provider. "Never cut the patch to decrease dosage," says Roberts. "The nicotine can leak out the cut end, which can be very dangerous. You can fold part of the patch back if you like. The strength of the patch is dependent on the surface contact with the skin."

benefit is that it prevents the weight gain usually associated with quitting smoking.

While bupropion does have some potential side effects—most notably, insomnia and headaches—these generally go away soon after you go off the drug (drug treatment is usually about 9 weeks).

Here are some additional tips from Dr. Muramoto.

Join a support group or enroll in a class. "The more help you get, the more likely you are to succeed," says Dr. Muramoto. Look for a smoking cessation class at your local hospital, or check with your HMO, the American Lung Association, or the American Cancer Society.

Tell yourself, "I am going to quit smoking," not "I'm going to *try* to quit." Motivation and confidence are strong predictors of success.

Get some kind of exercise. "Women who work out are conscious of their health and tend not to smoke," says Dr. Muramoto. ■

Snacking

Surprise! Between-Meal Treats Are Good for You

Kids aren't the only ones who snack. In yet another example of science confirming what we know to be true, a survey of 1,800 adults and children found that 98 percent of us snack. Whether we're hitting a vending machine, a convenience store, hotel minibar, gas-and-go food mart, or our own kitchen cupboards, three out of four adults (women included) snack at least once a day. Half us snack two to four times a day.

The most popular feeding times: late afternoon, when we like our snacks salty, and late evening, when we love to scarf scoopfuls of ice cream in front of the TV, says Audrey Cross, Ph.D., associate clinical professor at Columbia University's Institute of Human Nutrition in New York City. She has studied snacking as intensely as other scholars might study particle physics.

If you add up all the potato chips, popcorn, and party mix we pop into our mouths each year, it amounts to nearly 22 pounds per person.

Even Dr. Cross is surprised by Americans' increasing willingness to snack around the clock and in places where vittles once were verboten.

Like the classroom.

"When I was a student, you ate at mealtime," Dr. Cross says. "You didn't fumble with a soft drink and sandwich while trying to listen to the teacher."

Now that snacking is tolerated almost everywhere, including some churches and libraries, it's more important than ever to snack intelligently. In fact, snacking can be a valuable resource—a way to protect your health.

So what makes a healthy gnosh?

Raw vegetables and low-fat dairy products, says Barbara Whedon, R.D., a nutrition counselor at Thomas Jefferson University Hospital in Philadelphia. "American women typically don't eat enough of either," she says.

Phytochemicals in veggies are potent antioxidants, and the calcium in dairy products wards off osteoporosis. Some researchers have suggested that eating numerous well-balanced snacks throughout the day instead of three

DON'T MAKE THIS MISTAKE

Beware of mega-calorie snacks masquerading as health food. An inviting juice-bar smoothie can contain more than 400 calories. An innocent-looking muffin can contain 450 calories. And don't fall for chips that contain herbs like St. John's wort (used for depression), kava (a calming herb), or gingko biloba (a memory enhancer). To get a therapeutic dose of St. John's wort from one such product, you'd have to consume 1,400 calories' worth of chips.

squares can keep dieters on track and improve their blood cholesterol profiles.

"There's evidence that it works in rats, but rats are nibblers," says Judith S. Stern, Sc.D., professor of nutrition and internal medicine at the University of California at Davis. "Rats eat 11 or more meals a day."

If you're part of the human rat race, here are ways to work healthy snacks into your diet.

It all starts at the supermarket. "The real discipline occurs at the grocery store," Dr. Cross says. Here's an aisle-by-aisle guide to smart snacking.

Produce aisle: Think crunchy. Load up on apples, dried fruit, baby carrots, and fresh peppers.

Snack aisle: Skip crackers flavored with cheese and shaped like fish or dinosaurs. Instead, stock up on RyKrisp and other whole grain, high-fiber snacks. Buy fat-free sourdough pretzels, rice cakes, popcorn, and baked chips instead of full-fat chips.

Cereal aisle: Buy individual-size boxes of whole grain, nutritionally fortified cereals, like shredded wheat squares and low-fat granola and cereal bars. Choose oatmeal-raisin bars over chocolate chip—otherwise, you're really buying a candy bar.

Dairy aisle: Buy individually wrapped slices of fat-free cheese, soy cheese, and individual cartons of low-fat and fat-free yogurt.

At home, store munchies in designated snack areas. Keep cold cereal, dried fruit, nuts, pretzels, and low-fat crackers on a cupboard shelf. Place raw veggies, yogurt, and cheese in a plastic container in the fridge at eye level. Put fresh fruit in a bowl on the kitchen table. "Fruit is more flavorful at room temperature than cold," Dr. Cross says.

At work, add protein to your pleasure. Eat fruit with low-fat yogurt, fat-free cheese, or reduced-fat cottage cheese. If you don't have an office refrigerator, eat dried fruit with nuts. A little protein makes a snack more satisfying.

Keep your hands busy. If you're regularly blowing your diet by snacking in front of the TV, switch off the set. A good book or an engaging hobby can help keep your hands out of the chips bag. ■

YOUR BEST BET FROM THE HOTEL-ROOM MINIBAR

If you're famished by 4 o'clock in the afternoon and have no alternative but an office vending machine, go for the nuts. The same goes if your only choices are what's available in the hotel room minibar.

"Nuts are a healthier choice than cookies, chips, or candy," says Dr. Whedon. Nuts are high in phosphorus, potassium, the B vitamin folate, and vitamin E. English walnuts are also high in omega-3 fatty acids.

Snoring

Don't Ignore These Signals

So, you think you don't snore? Think again. Ever awaken with headaches? Morning fatigue? In women, these symptoms can be signs of sleep apnea, interruptions in sleep when you actually stop breathing several times a night.

"Snoring is a key sign of sleep apnea in men and women alike, but women are less likely to know they snore," says Joan Shaver, R.N., Ph.D., professor and dean of the College of Nursing at the University of Illinois at Chicago and one of the first researchers to study sleep problems in women. "If a man snores, his wife will complain and prompt him to find a solution. But if a woman snores, often the guy won't notice, because he's too busy snoring himself."

Snoring—and sleep apnea—are more than annoyances, says David J. Halvorson, M.D., clinical associate professor of surgery in the division of otolaryngology at the University of Alabama at Birmingham. Snoring can damage the nerves in your throat, leaving those muscles lax and you at risk for apnea. This disorder affects the quality of your sleep, making you restless during the night and tired during the day. And the stress of repeatedly stopping—and restarting—breathing may increase your

Soda

Make It a Treat, Not a Habit

Imagine an empty 56-gallon barrel in the middle of your kitchen. Now picture it filled to the brim with soda. If you're the average woman, that's how much soda you drink in just 1 year. If you chose regular sodas, you slurped down more than 50 pounds of sugar in the process. One can of soda alone yields 9.3 teaspoons of sugar—the equivalent of a candy bar—but no useful nutrients whatsoever. No vitamins, no minerals. No fiber. Just 150 empty calories.

If you had drunk that much orange juice instead, it would have given you more than three times as much vitamin C as you need each day, along with a bundle of other nutrients.

And if you drained a barrel of fat-free milk, you would've consumed more than two-thirds of the calcium you needed for the year.

Dietitians urge women to drink 8 to 10 glasses of fluid a day. No more than two glasses a day should be soda, says Molly Gee, R.D., manager of the Institute for Preventive Medicine at the Methodist Health Care System in Houston and a board member of the American Dietetic Association. Better yet, save soda for an occasional treat. Here's what to drink instead.

A frosty mug of milk. About 22 million American women have the bone-weakening condition risk of stroke, high blood pressure, or an enlarged heart.

As serious as apnea can be, it often goes unseen—or unheard—in women. One study estimates that 93 percent of women with apnea have not been diagnosed. "Even if women know they snore, they won't tell their doctors because it's not considered ladylike," Dr. Shaver says. And the longer it goes undetected, the worse it can be, because apnea gets worse with age. If you suspect you may have apnea, talk with your doctor.

If your problem is simply snoring, some of the same tips that experts recommend for men will work for you.

Sleep on your side. Sew a tennis ball into a pocket on the back of your night gown or pajamas; you're less likely to snore when you're not sleeping on your back.

Lose weight. Like men, women who are heavier have a greater risk of apnea.

Try an antisnoring device. Retainer-style mouthpieces that pull your jaw forward can be fitted by a dentist who specializes in this treatment. If you wake up tired, with headaches, and know that you snore heavily, ask your doctor to refer you to an accredited sleep center. They can assess and most often will prescribe a ventilator with a mask known as CPAP (continuous positive airway pressure) to keep ››

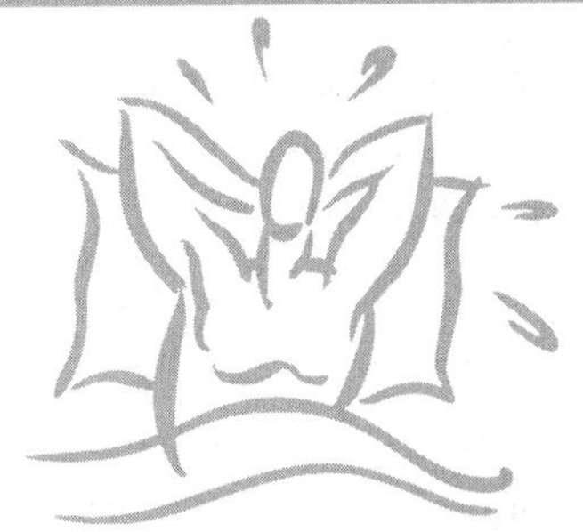

DON'T MAKE THIS MISTAKE

Switching to diet sodas will save on calories, but you won't necessarily lose weight. Researchers at the Centre for Human Nutrition in Sheffield, England, found that women who drink beverages loaded with artificial sweeteners such as aspartame may actually eat more food.

osteoporosis or are at extra risk for it. Swap a 12-ounce mug of fat-free milk for every can of soda you drink, and you'll add 453.6 milligrams of calcium to your diet.

Fruit or vegetable juice. While most juices contain a fair amount of calories—about 144 for a cup of cranberry or 127 for grape juice—you get a decent nutritional return for the investment. Cranberry juice contains substances proven to fight urinary tract infections. Grape juice contains flavonoids, which protect against heart disease . Tomato juice is a lightweight—supplying 41 calories per cup—but it contains lycopenes, which protect against cancer.

Reach for the bubbly. If you miss the satisfying zing of a carbonated drink, pour yourself a glass of sparkling water and add a twist of lime or lemon juice, Gee suggests. Avoid sweetened, flavored seltzer, though—it's just clear soda.

Helpful Hint

Drown your cereal in milk at breakfast and drink a glass of orange juice along with it. The vitamin C in the juice will help your body absorb the calcium from the milk better, Gee says. ■

your airways open and your sleep snore-free.

Congested? Try the strip. If you're snoring because of nasal congestion, try the Breathe Right strips found in most drugstores. They may keep your nasal passages open and stop your snoring, Dr. Shaver says. But they won't help women with true apnea because the disorder stems from problems in the throat and breath control, not the nose.

If all else fails, talk to your doctor. Surgery might be an option. ■

HOW BRITISH WOMEN KEEP THEIR HUSBANDS FROM SNORING

Imagine trying to sleep in the middle of rush hour in London. That's essentially what Julie Switzer did for more than 30 years. At 92 decibels, her husband Melvyn's snoring was equivalent to heavy traffic or thunder—so loud that he made it into *The Guinness Book of World Records.*

People sent the Switzers remedies from around the world, but nothing seemed to work—until they tried homeopathic drops containing wild yam (*Dioscorea villosa*) and common ginger (*Zingiber officiale*). Melvyn stopped snoring—at last.

The remedy that the Switzers used—called Y-Snore Anti-Snoring Nose Drops—is just one of various strategies that can help put an end to snoring, says Toni Bark, M.D., a homeopathic physician in suburban Chicago. Luckily, it's available at pharmacies in the United States.

Sodium

Not the Villain You Think It Is

Why all the fuss about sodium? The average woman has about 18 teaspoons of sodium in her body—about 90,000 milligrams. What's another couple of thousand milligrams from food?

"Sodium doesn't deserve its bad reputation," says John G. Gums, Pharm.D., professor of pharmacy and medicine at the University of Florida School of Medicine in Gainesville, who has studied sodium for about 15 years. "Like cholesterol—which is also misunderstood—we need a certain amount of sodium to function. It's not all bad."

Sodium maintains fluid levels in your body, attracting water to cells and other body tissues. Sodium balances other electrically charged essential minerals, like potassium (collectively called electrolytes). And sodium helps prevent muscle cramps. Adequate amounts of sodium allow muscles to contract easily. **A shortage of sodium can lead to nagging leg cramps.**

The Daily Value for sodium—the amount that experts recommend for good health—is 2,400 milligrams—

DON'T MAKE THIS MISTAKE

Sea salt is considered more "natural," but it has just as much sodium as table salt—2,000 milligrams of sodium per teaspoon. So it won't help reduce your sodium intake.

about as much as you get in ½ teaspoon of table salt, or sodium chloride, or about four servings of some processed foods (like canned soup).

For years, many experts considered sodium a major cause of high blood pressure. They noticed that in nations where men and women eat a lot of sodium, blood pressure seemed to be higher. Researchers now recognize, however, that high blood pressure (also called hypertension) is triggered by factors such as obesity, lack of regular exercise, consuming too much alcohol, and not getting enough potassium, calcium, and magnesium (minerals that help control blood pressure).

Doctors still recommend salt restriction for women who are salt sensitive. (Not everyone is.) Sodium intake affects their blood pressure levels. Cutting sodium intake in half will lead to a drop of 5 points (or more) in blood pressure in about half the women with high blood pressure, says Norman Kaplan, M.D., professor of internal medicine and chief of the hypertension division at the University of Texas Southwestern Medical Center in Dallas.

If you don't have high blood pressure, sodium is no big deal. But if you've been advised to cut back on sodium, Dr. Gums recommends three simple strategies.

- Taste your food before reaching for the saltshaker, and wean yourself off table salt.
- Switch to a salt-free substitute.
- Liven up your meals with savory herbs and spices such as basil, cilantro, oregano, garlic powder, dill weed, sage, and rosemary instead of routinely relying on salt for everything.

Helpful Hints

Sodium shows up in surprising places. So if you're trying to limit your sodium consumption to 2,400 milligrams or less, read labels carefully.

- A cup of corn flakes, for example, contains 298 milligrams of sodium—more than in an ounce of salted peanuts.
- Canned corn and green beans have more about 170 more milligrams of sodium per serving than frozen vegetables cooked without added salt.
- Rice mixes, banana cream pie, and instant cooked cereals are loaded with sodium. ■

Sore Feet

Great-Looking Shoes That Don't Hurt

When was the last time your husband came home from a party, kicked off his shoes in relief, and whined, "Ooh, my aching feet . . ."?

Probably never. Men, who wear roomier and more comfortable shoes than women, have only one-ninth as many foot problems. Men also have far less foot surgery.

Men's feet are no different than women's feet. Their footwear is another story. Eighty-eight percent of women wear shoes that are either too short or too narrow (or both).

Part of the problem is that women's shoes look like they were designed by someone who never saw a human foot: they taper at the front, where your foot is the widest.

"If you continue to put your foot in an ill-fitting shoe, ultimately, your foot starts to look like that shoe," says Cherise Dyal, M.D., orthopedic surgeon and chief of foot and ankle services at Montefiore Medical Center in New York City. "If your shoe is pointy, your big toe gets pushed toward your little toe, your little toe gets pushed toward your big toe, and there's no room for the other toes." Ill-fitting shoes cause or worsen problems such as hammertoe, bunions, corns, calluses, mallet toes, claw toes, neuromas, and ingrown toenails. High heels aggravate the problem, thrusting your foot—and the force of your body weight—forward onto your forefoot.

Over the years, more and more working women have made it a habit to wear low-heeled shoes at work. (One survey found that the higher the educational level, the lower the heel women wear—at least in fashion shoes.)

But let's be realistic. You're not going to wear your power suit or party dress with sneakers. Stephen Conti, M.D., assistant professor at the University of Pittsburgh School of Medicine and an orthopedic surgeon specializing in foot and ankle care, offers these tips for finding shoes that look great without killing your feet.

Length. When you stand in the shoe, there should be one thumb's width from the end of your longest toe to the end of the shoe.

Width. "Measure your foot by standing barefoot on a piece of paper and tracing your foot while you're standing," suggests Dr. Dyal. "Measure the widest part. Make yourself a card at that width. Take it to the shoe store." The widest part of the shoe should be as wide as the widest part of your foot.

Height. Choose a heel that's no higher than 1½ inches and as chunky as possible.

Flex. Take the shoe off and bend it in half. It should flex where your foot flexes so that the widest part of your foot is at the widest part of the shoe.

Toe box. Choose shoes with a roomy, rounded, toe box. Avoid pointy shoes that smash your toes together.

Heel fit. If a shoe that fits your forefoot is too wide at the heel, look for a combination-last shoe—the forefoot and

DON'T MAKE THIS MISTAKE

"Don't be a slave to size," says Dr. Dyal. Feet get longer and wider over the years, so a size that fit you in your twenties probably won't fit you 10 years later.

heel are different sizes. "The size will be given as two letters, like C/A—one wider, for the forefoot and one narrower, for the heel" says Dr. Conti.

Helpful Hints

Just because a particular shoe fits in one size, that doesn't mean that same size will fit the same among different manufacturers or even among different styles of the same manufacturer. **"So if you've found a shoe that fits, buy it in several colors,"** says Thomas M. Novella, D.P.M., associate professor of orthopedics at the New York College of Podiatric Medicine in New York City.

Also, wear high heels only for special occasions and short periods of time.

"Treat high-heeled shoes like a dessert," says Dr. Dyal. ■

Sore Throat

Easy-to-Swallow Solutions

Five nights a week, about 1.5 million people tune in to hear Delilah, a national nighttime radio host who listens to callers' troubles. But at least a few times a year, she has trouble of her own.

"When I get a sore throat, normally I just go on the air and apologize for sounding like a frog," she says.

Delilah's sore throat may be something of an occupational hazard caused by using her voice more than most people. But for the rest of us, throat pain is typically caused by viruses, such as colds or influenza, says Kevin Sherin, M.D., clinical associate professor of family medicine at the University of Illinois at Chicago.

For her pain, Delilah uses an over-the-counter throat spray. "It tastes hideous—I hate it. But it numbs my throat enough so I can talk. It's a staple among radio announcers. I go through a bottle a year," she says.

Such popular commercial remedies work just as well for the rest of us, too, says Dr. Sherin. So do medicated throat lozenges, especially those that contain zinc (which boosts immunity) and vitamin C (which fights viruses and acts as a natural antihistamine. But experts say you can also save yourself some money and use these effective home remedies the next time it hurts to swallow.

Sprinkle ¼ teaspoon of cayenne in a cup of hot tea. Cayenne subdues a body chemical known as substance P, which carries pain signals to the brain, and will lessen the discomfort you feel when you swallow.

Gargle with ½ teaspoon of salt in 4 ounces of warm water four times a day. The salt will help kill the bacteria that can infect your throat.

Drink at least 8 cups of water and other fluids a day. "If you're well-hydrated, the secretions of mucus that build up in your throat will become more thin and watery, and you'll feel better," says Dr. Sherin.

Try chicken soup. Chicken soup contains the amino ››

acid cysteine, which is similar to the chemical medications that are used in hospitals to promote drainage of the mucous membranes, says Dr. Sherin. In other words, it'll ease throat pain.

Turn on a humidifier to add moisture to the air. In cold weather, when the air inside your home is dry, you'll be more prone to sore throats. Running a humidifier, however, can keep the air moister, hydrating tissues in your throat and keeping them from causing pain. Just remember to clean the humidifier daily to prevent the spread of additional airborne bacteria.

Helpful Hint

Your grandmother's remedy of plain hot tea with lemon is still one of the best ways to ease a sore throat. The hot water relieves some of the inflammation and washes away nasal drainage that irritates the throat. And the lemon wedge, while too slight to provide much vitamin C, adds flavor. ■

Soy

How to Work More Soy into Your Diet without Eating Tofu

Call it a Soy Renaissance. Touted as the politically correct alternative to meat in the 1970s, soy is now being extolled for its extraordinary potential to relieve hot flashes and other menopausal symptoms and reduce cholesterol. It also may fight breast cancer, protect against colon cancer and endometrial cancer, and prevent stroke—among other life-extending benefits.

"There almost isn't a disease that soy can't help in some way," says John Glaspy, M.D., of UCLA's Jonsson Cancer Center in Los Angeles, who is studying soy's protective effect against breast cancer.

The "magic" ingredients responsible for soy's healing prowess? Isoflavones—specifically genistein and daidzein—estrogen-like compounds abundant in soybeans. Soy is "the" life extension food. Doctors and scientists add soy to their diets and advise women to do the same.

One of the richest sources of isoflavones (30 milligrams per ½ cup) is tofu—spongelike blocks of soybean curd sold in supermarkets. But if you're like many women, you know your family will never, ever eat it. (And you're not too fond of it yourself.) It's soft, mushy, and bland. No problem: **Here's a list of 15 other tasty ways to work soy into your diet without eating tofu,** starting with those with the highest isoflavone content per serving. (Isoflavone content varies from product to product.) Many are found in supermarkets; others, in health food stores.

- Soy cereal: 60 milligrams isoflavones per ¼ cup (sold under the brand name Nutlettes, it has a mild and slightly nutty flavor, like Grape-Nuts)

• Soy shakes: 52 to 57 milligrams isoflavones (smooth, creamy drinks from milk and fat-free ice cream)

• Soy protein bars: 49 milligrams isoflavones per bar (available in chocolate mint, peanut butter, and mocha)

• Canned soy beans: 38 to 41 milligrams isoflavones per ½ cup (chestnutty and creamy; works well in soups and chili)

• Tempeh: 36 milligrams isoflavones per ½ cup (sold in cakes; works well sliced, marinated, and fried)

• Soy milk: 30 milligrams isoflavones per cup (a slightly beany liquid best used in shakes, puddings, and hot cocoa; vanilla soy milk is tasty poured over cereal)

• Roasted soy nuts: 30 milligrams isoflavones per 3 tablespoons (look like tiny peanuts—delicious as a snack)

• Soy pudding: 30 milligrams isoflavones per ½ cup (chocolate almond is heavenly)

• Soy cheese: 9 milligrams isoflavones per ounce (used in cooking as a nondairy stand-in for the real thing)

• Soy burgers: 8 milligrams isoflavones per patty (an easy-to-digest substitute for beef that tastes a little like bean dip with vegetables)

• Soy flour: 8 milligrams isoflavones per tablespoon (replace up to a quarter of the flour in recipes for muffins and baked goods, and you'll never taste the difference)

• Soy hot dogs: 7 milligrams isoflavones per frank (resemble chicken burgers and work well with relish and other fixings)

• Soy ice cream: 5 milligrams isoflavones per ½ cup (comes in chocolate supreme, vanilla almond bark, and better pecan and tastes like premium ice cream)

• Soy iced milk: 3 milligrams isoflavones per ½ cup (sweet, ice-milk consistency, with a bit of an aftertaste)

• Miso: 2 milligrams isoflavones per 1 tablespoon (tastes a little like teriyaki)

Experts recommend you get 30 to 50 milligrams of isoflavones a day—a cinch with so much variety.

DON'T MAKE THIS MISTAKE

Not every soy product automatically supplies isoflavones. Avoid "soy protein concentrate"—most of the isoflavones may have been processed out. Instead, look for "isolated soy protein," "soy protein isolate," or "textured soy protein" on the label. (If you're unsure, write or call the manufacturer.) And don't count on soy sauce or soybean oil—they contain no isoflavones. Roasted soy butter has only 1 isoflavone per serving.

Helpful Hints

Plain soy milk is Band-Aid brown and beany tasting. Look for chocolate, vanilla, or other flavors. Or stir in some cocoa powder, coffee, almond extract, or whatever strikes your fancy. For example: Heat 1 cup soy milk in the microwave for 1 minute, add a little instant coffee or hot chocolate mix, and you have a healthy latte or hot cocoa.

If you don't like one soy cheese, try a different brand. Tastes and textures vary. ■

Spider Veins

Strengthen Broken Capillaries with Herbs and Blueberries

Like their insect namesake, spider veins are scary, but they pose no real threat. These tiny, red-purple veins that form a spider or star shape are simply capillaries that have become dilated or visible near the surface of the skin, says Luis Navarro, M.D., clinical instructor at Mount Sinai School of Medicine in New York City and founder and director of the Vein Treatment Center. They often just appear out of the blue on the outer thigh, inner knee, ankle or, less commonly, around the cheeks and nose. Though largely due to heredity, they can also appear as a result of hormonal changes such as pregnancy, menopause, oral contraceptives, or hormone replacement therapy.

A doctor who specialized in treating vein problems can virtually erase spider veins with sclerotherapy, a chemical injection treatment that causes the veins to close up and virtually disappear. Lasers are also used to treat unsightly veins, though they are more effective on the veins of the face than veins in the legs.

If you don't want to spend the money on a costly medical procedure, here are a few home remedies that may help alleviate the problem.

Butcher's broom. Best taken as a tincture or extract, this herb won't eliminate spider veins, but it may prevent new ones from forming by helping preserve the elasticity of the vein wall, says Mindy Green, director of education at the Herbal Research Foundation in Boulder, Colorado. She suggests taking 16 to 33 milligrams of standardized extract or tincture three times a day.

Ginkgo biloba. High in bioflavonoids, which strengthen your blood vessels and help make capillaries less fragile, this herb is effective for spider veins, says Green. Since dosage varies depending on strength, follow the label directions.

You'll also find bioflavonoids in dark-colored fruits like blueberries and cherries and in the white membranes of citrus fruit.

Do not use ginkgo with the following types of drugs: blood thinners, aspirin or other nonsteroidal anti-inflammatories, and antidepressants that are MAO inhibitors. Ginkgo in high doses (more than 240 milligrams of concentrated extract) can cause dermatitis, diarrhea, and vomiting.

Compression stockings or support hose. Gentle, graduated compression makes it difficult for blood to pool in any weak leg veins, so those veins are less likely to become stretched and stressed.

Exercise. Moving your legs encourages blood to keep moving, so get up from your desk every 45 minutes or so, and exercise three times a week for at least 30 minutes, says Dr. Navarro.

Helpful Hint

Keep both feet on the floor when sitting. Crossing your legs puts increased pressure on the veins and may increase your chances of developing vein problems in your legs. Propping your feet up on a footstool while working at a desk can also help keep blood flowing. ■

Split Ends

Why Using a Conditioner Is Futile

When the ends of your hair begin to look like hundreds of miniature tuning forks—each strand split in two—chances are it has been damaged by exposure to the sun, the cold, dry temperatures, hair coloring, chemical relaxers or permanent waves.

If you have split ends, your first inclination may be to pile on the conditioner. But that's a waste of time.

"All the conditioner in the world won't get rid of split ends, says Amy Everett, stylist at the Joseph Michael Salon in Chicago. "The best—and only—solution is to get your hair trimmed."

"Hair is a lot like a shrub," says hairstylist David Ramon, co-owner of David Gavin Salons in New York City. "If you don't keep cutting it, it splits, and the essential proteins and acids leach out. Cutting it regularly seals the hair shaft, and the hair grows thicker."

The moral of the story: Get your hair trimmed ½ to 1 inch every 6 weeks, whether it looks like it needs it or not, says Ramon.

If your hair tends to split easily, try these end-saving strategies.

Don't roughly towel-dry your hair after swimming or shampooing. Friction can cause ends to split. Instead, wrap a towel around your head and leave it there for a few minutes to absorb the moisture.

Wait till your hair is mostly dry before you brush or curl it. Hair is most susceptible to damage when it's wet.

Undo your ponytail. If you usually wear your hair tied back or in a ponytail, leave it down a few hours a day to take strain off your hair. And never sleep with any type of hair accessories, like clips or rollers.

Try an egg shampoo. Rub an egg yolk into your hair, let it coagulate, then rinse it out and shampoo. "Protein in the yolk helps your hair, which is also a protein," says Ramon.

Helpful Hint

Taking 1,000 micrograms of biotin (a B vitamin) three times a day for at least 4 to 5 months can promote healthy hair growth, says Diana Bihova, M.D, a dermatologist in New York City and author of *Beauty from the Inside Out*. ■

Sports Drinks

Who Really Needs Them?

Supermarket aisles are packed with sports drinks targeted to athletes. Originally formulated for major league football players, sports drinks are designed to replenish fluids and electrolytes (sodium and potassium) lost in sweat and provide energy for working muscles. The main ingredients are water, sugar, potassium, and sodium.

In fact, a typical 20-ounce bottle of Gatorade contains more sodium than a 1-ounce serving of potato chips. That's okay if you're working up a sweat for an hour or more, like cycling for the afternoon or running a 4-hour marathon. But if your Tour de France is more like a tour de neighborhood, a glass of water will more than meet your hydration needs, says Scott Montain, Ph.D., dehydration expert and research physiologist in the nutrition and biochemistry division at the U.S. Army Research Institute of Environmental Medicine in Natick, Massachusetts. And simply eating three regular meals a day provides all the sodium you'll need, says Dr. Montain.

For sustained, sweat-inducing exercise, sports drinks' real advantage over water is energy-packed carbohydrates. "Carbohydrates won't help you perform better, but they will help you perform longer," explains Dr. Montain.

The sugars in sports drinks—fructose, sucrose, and

Sprains

Twisted Ankle—Or Fracture? Don't Guess

Any sudden change in movement can twist your ankle: You trip wearing high heels. Miss the bottom step going downstairs. Land on a divot in the lawn playing volleyball. Or trip over the dog bringing groceries into the house. Without warning, your foot turns inward, and the ligaments on the outside of the ankle stretch or tear.

Twist your ankle badly enough, and it can break. Problem is, it's hard to tell the difference.

"If you have pain over a bone, difficulty walking, or swelling of the ankle, have it evaluated," says Cherise Dyal, M.D., orthopedic surgeon and chief of foot and ankle services at Montefiore Medical Center in New York City. And fractures often are accompanied by an audible "snap."

Diagnosis is tricky. **Bruising and pain alone are not reliable clues.** Both a sprain and a fracture turn black and blue from bleeding (either from torn ligaments and tendons or broken bones) and swelling. Both hurt when the part is moved.

Not all sprains are alike, complicating diagnosis, says Ellen Sobel, D.P.M., Ph.D., associate professor of orthopedic science at the New York School of Podiatric medicine in New York City. With a grade 1 sprain, you have a little pain, then the ankle returns to

MAKE YOUR OWN SPORTS DRINK

To make your own carbo-loading sports drink, minus the salt, start with a powdered drink mix, like Tropical Punch Kool-Aid. Add the recommended amount of water, but use only half the drink mix.

This will give you a thirst quencher with about a 6 to 8 percent sugar concentration—just like standard sports drinks. Anything sweeter will slow water absorption and prolong dehydration.

Drink ½ to 1 cup of your homemade power drink every 15 minutes whenever you exercise vigorously for an hour or more.

glucose—provide 125 calories per 20-ounce bottle—nearly half as much as the same size bottle of soda.

Helpful Hints

Avoid carbonated sports drinks—they are highly acidic and may upset your stomach or leave you bloated when consumed during strenuous exercise. Also, whether you're drinking a commercial sports drink or a homemade version, try it on a short ride or run or two before using it on a hard workout or race, because your tastes change when you are exercising, says Dr. Montain. You may like grape Gatorade with your lunch, but the flavor may be too sweet and overpowering during a run. ■

normal after a week or two. With a moderate sprain—grade 2—you have difficulty bearing weight. With a severe sprain—grade 3—the ligament is completely torn. Grade 3 sprains sometimes require surgery.

"You know when you have this—you can't get up and walk," says Dr. Sobel. **So forget the old saying that if you can't walk on it, it's broken.**

"Without taking an x-ray, it's not always easy to tell a break from a sprain, even for doctors," says Thomas M. Novella, D.P.M., associate professor of orthopedics at the New York College of Podiatric Medicine in New York City.

So if you twist your ankle and it's swollen and painful, go to the doctor. Only an x-ray can assess the real damage. ››

GO AHEAD—BUY YOURSELF NEW SHOES

Wearing old shoes isn't simply a fashion faux pas. It's dangerous—a major cause of ankle sprains, says Dr. Novella, who has treated thousands of dancers and athletes for foot problems.

His advice: If your shoes show signs of wear, replace them.

"Shoes tend to wear out in three places: at the front of the upper (the top of the shoe that's stitched to the sole), in the heel counter (the part of the upper surrounding the heel), or the outer heel," explains Dr. Novella. "When that happens, the bottom of the shoe tilts, and when you land, you twist your ankle."

Helpful Hint

If you've sprained your ankle, apply R.I.C.E., described on page 379. And don't be too quick to resume the activity that caused it, or you can reinjure yourself, advises Dr. Dyal. "You're jogging and you sprain your ankle. You go back to jogging while it's still painful, you hit a little pebble, and down you go," she says.

If it looks as if you have a fracture, "don't put weight on it and don't move it," says Dr. Novella. "If you must move to get assistance or to get out of imminent danger, the joint will need to be splinted in the position it took when the break occurred." Go to an emergency room immediately. ■

Stained Teeth

Smudge-Proof Your Smile

In nature, things that start out white and unblemished often don't stay that way for long.

Muddy footprints stain a fresh snowdrift. Inky letters mar a new sheet of paper. And a bright smile tends to gradually lose its sparkle.

It's normal for our teeth to take on a yellowish or greyish tone as we eat, drink, and grow older, says Sandra Rich, Ph.D, a dental hygienist and associate professor of periodontology at the University of Southern California in Los Angeles.

An off-white tint doesn't necessarily mean that your teeth aren't clean and healthy. And a few simple strategies will help you protect them from any future stains.

Kick the butts. Of all the things that you can put into your mouth that will discolor your teeth, cigarettes (and cigars) are the worst, Dr. Rich says. Smoking leaves a yellowish smear on the surface of your teeth that, over time, can be taken up by the enamel and become ingrained. So there's another incentive in an already lengthy list of reasons to avoid smoking.

By not smoking, you'll also cut your dental-care costs. Dr. Rich says that smokers need professional cleanings more frequently—three or four times a year—to remove tobacco stains.

Switch to herbal or green tea. Black tea and coffee do a nasty job of staining your teeth, Dr. Rich says. To cut down on discoloration, she advises tea- and coffee-drinking women to drink light-colored teas, such as green or chamomile or herbal tea mixtures such as orange-mango, instead.

Substitute white wine for red. If you drink wine, stick with a lighter type, such as a chardonnay or sauvignon blanc, says Dr. Rich.

Steer clear of vivid foods. Anything that leaves a color on your tongue can stain your teeth. If you want to keep your pearly whites pearly, avoid cola, frozen fruit bars, fruit juices, and brightly colored candies. Swishing water in your mouth after eating foods that stain or after drinking coffee, tea, cola, or red wine

DON'T MAKE THIS MISTAKE

You can purchase do-it-yourself bleaching kits at many drugstores to gradually lighten your teeth at home. But these can damage your teeth and gums. You'll get better—and faster—results from whitening gels available from your dentist. Depending on the tint of your teeth, you may start to see results in about a week.

can help minimize staining.

Brush and floss daily. Plaque, a sticky film that accumulates on the teeth, can soak up stains and transfer them to the teeth. Also gently brush your tongue, the roof of your mouth and the inside of your cheeks, Dr. Rich says.

Visit your dentist twice a year. Professional cleaning knocks off any plaque that you can't brush away yourself.

Helpful Hint

Bright berry-colored lipstick or other vivid shades may make your teeth look lighter by contrast. Yellow tints, such as coral, are the worst for contrasting stained teeth, says Dr. Rich. ■

Stiff Neck

The Right Way to Uncrick a Crink

After spending 8 hours hunched over an operating table, "I feel like I have a toothache in my neck," says Cheryl Riley, a physician's assistant in cardiothoracic surgery at Thomas Jefferson University Hospital in Philadelphia. "The pain radiates down my back as though someone were driving spikes into me."

When she leaves work and goes home, Riley soothes her neck and back with hot baths. She also does yoga and other exercises four or five times a week and tries to relax when she's off duty. Sleeping on a contoured neck pillow also helps enormously, she says.

Riley's approach makes sense, says Alison Lee, M.D., medical director at Barefoot Doctors Acupuncture and Natural Medicine Resource Center in Ann Arbor, Michigan. Anything you can do to relax helps—when you feel tense, the muscles around your neck go into spasm. Heat—including a hot bath—increases circulation to the ››

AVOID NECK ROLLS

Do not try to "uncrick" your neck by rolling your head in a circle, says Brian Casazza, M.D., of Charlottesville Orthopaedics Spine and Sports Medicine in Virginia. "That only makes it hurt more, and you could do more harm than good."

Instead, stand against a wall, tuck in your chin, keep your shoulders down and back, and press your lower back against the wall. Your feet should be shoulder-width apart, approximately 1 foot from the wall. Your shoulders, back, and buttocks should be touching the wall. Hold for 20 to 30 seconds and repeat three times.

Doing this will help place the spine in a neutral position, says Dr. Casazza.

area and loosens tight muscles. Mild, gentle exercises—like yoga—also increase circulation and relieve pain. And using a neck pillow helps support your neck as you sleep while keeping it in line with your spine.

If your neck pain persists longer than 1 to 2 days—or if it's caused by whiplash or other trauma—see your physician. Otherwise, try some heat. "My first suggestion if you wake up with a stiff neck after sleeping in a strange position or sleeping under a cold draft is to apply heat," says Patrick Waters, D.C., a chiropractor at the Waters Chiropractic Clinic in Dallas. Heat will relax the muscles of your neck and allow you to move more freely and feel less pain. Simply put a hot-water bottle wrapped in a thin towel on your neck. Heat shouldn't be applied to the skin longer than 20 minutes. Ten minutes is probably sufficient. ■

Stress

Dear Diary: I Feel So Much Better Now

You know it's going to be a bad day when your doctor calls in sick, your hairdresser is having a bad hair day, and your waitress takes her lunch break at the stroke of noon.

Feel stressed? You're not alone. Worldwide, women say they feel more stressed than men, according to a Roper Starch survey. The results don't surprise Simone Ravicz, Ph.D., a psychologist in Pacific Palisades, California, and author of High on Stress: A Woman's Guide to Optimizing the Stress in Her Life. *"We have so many demanding roles, and we're taught to be deeply involved in all of them, whether it's work, family, or both," the 37-year-old says. "We're caretakers, mothers, career women. When these roles conflict, it creates stress." But women worry about more than their own lives; they also fret over situations such as a friend's divorce or a family member's illness, Dr. Ravicz says. "These network-related events are very stressful for women, and they're also much more frequent than the events men report as stressful, such as financial trouble."*

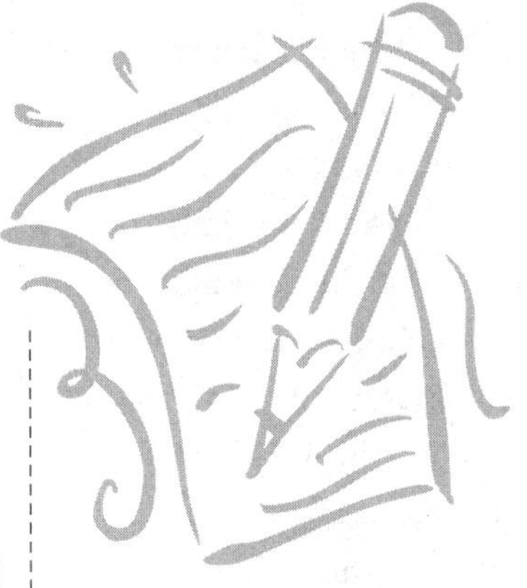

Regardless of the source of your stress, keeping a journal—even sporadically—can help you cope, emotionally and physically. "Writing forces a structure that thinking usually doesn't," says James W. Pennebaker, Ph.D., professor in the department of psychology at the University of Texas at Austin and author of *Opening Up: The Healing Power of Expressing Emotion.* "What

STIFF NECK? TRY A GINGER COMPRESS

To relieve a stiff neck caused by tired, sore muscles, Ian A. Cyrus, a registered acupuncturist at the Center for Integrative Medicine at Thomas Jefferson University Hospital in Philadelphia, recommends a ginger compress. Ginger has warming properties and will increase bloodflow to the area, increasing your circulation and loosening up those tight muscles.

Take a root of fresh ginger (available at supermarkets). Chop the root coarsely and blend 1 tablespoon well with 1 cup of water. In a large cooking pot, bring the mixture to a boil. Remove from the heat and let the mixture cool to a comfortable temperature. Then soak a clean hand towel in the warm ginger water. Ring it out and apply it to the stiff area.

writing does is bring it all together and give a situation a broader perspective." Healthwise, studies have shown that writing about stressful events can boost your immune system, reduce doctor visits, and lessen the symptoms of chronic diseases such as asthma or rheumatoid arthritis.

Yet women sometimes shy away from journaling. "They say, 'Oh, it will just dredge up bad feelings,'" Dr. Pennebaker says. "But the feelings are already there."

If you want to use pen and paper to manage the stress and emotions in your life, here's what journaling experts suggest.

Take 20. You don't need to write for hours to benefit from journaling; just 20 minutes once a week for 3 weeks improved the moods, grade point averages, and overall health of college freshmen in one study.

Don't self-censor. Journaling offers a wonderful opportunity to be emotionally honest. "You don't have to worry about hurting someone else's feelings, and you're not risking the nature of your relationship with another person. In some ways, writing is a little bit safer than confiding in people," Dr. Pennebaker says.

Write regularly. This is especially important for women writing about traumatic experiences. While your initial entry may leave your emotions topsy-turvy, those feelings will pass. "The more you write, the less impact an event has," Dr. Pennebaker says. "It won't have the same potency it did on the first day you wrote about it."

Keep a daily record. Sometimes negative thinking makes events more stressful than they need to be, Dr. Ravicz says. In a small notebook, jot down stressful events, followed by your feelings and the underlying fears causing those emotions. Then write down a more rational response to the situation and your resulting feelings. You'll learn to replace your stress-inducing reactions with more positive, rational thinking. ››

Write letters. If you have a troubled relationship with a friend or family member, write her a hypothetical letter but keep it to yourself. It may help you decide whether you want to reconnect or let go.

Get creative. Love the idea of journaling but hate putting pen to paper? Make a collage or talk into a tape recorder instead. You'll still be expressing your emotions—you just won't be worrying about those pesky punctuation marks.

Helpful Hint

If you're a pessimist, you need to do more than vent in your journal to reap writing's health benefits. After you write about a problem, spend 5 minutes jotting down coping strategies.

"Pessimists need structure to get away from the negative style they have," says Greg Nicholls, Ph.D., director of the Counseling and Personal Development Center at St. Joseph's University in Philadelphia. ■

Stretching

Bare-Minimum Stretches for Busy Women

Without stretching, fitness guru Karen Voight could not handle her daily life. The star of 11 videos, Voight's typical week includes a run-walk program (walking uphill and running on the flats) 4 or 5 days, teaching a couple of 2-hour aerobic classes (high- plus low-impact), cycling indoors, lifting weights, and doing yoga most days. She also may be rehearsing or taping one of her exercise videos, launching a health club, doing fitness demonstrations, or appearing on TV.

Voight credits stretching for keeping her safe and sane through her demanding schedule. "Stretching can help you release stress and tension in your neck, shoulders, and back, and it can improve your posture," says Voight. Thanks to stretching, she says she can exercise more intensely, without strain. She's convinced that if she didn't stretch, she would have injuries, aches, and pains, limited range of motion, and poor posture.

But stretching any old way won't give you these benefits, says Alice Lockridge, a Renton, Washington–based exercise physiologist who trains women's sports groups, fitness instructors, and electrical-company line workers. She offers these bare-minimum stretches that target the areas where women are typically tight.

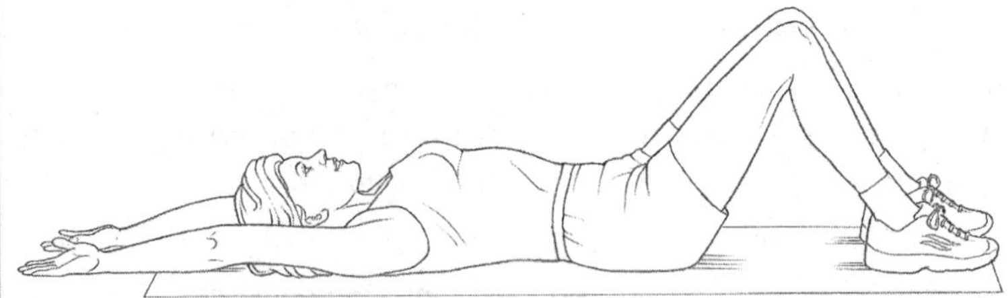

Shoulder (*above*): Lie on the floor on your back with your arms straight overhead, trying to touch the floor with your wrists. Keep your elbows straight, arms close to your head. Avoid arching your back.

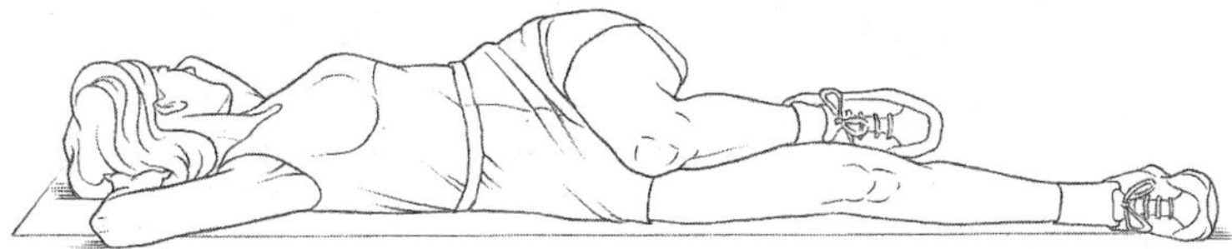

Full back (*above*): Lie on the floor with both legs straight and fingers interlaced behind your head. Bend one knee and cross your leg over your body. Try to keep your shoulders on the floor. Turn your head away from your bent knee. Relax. Repeat on the other side.

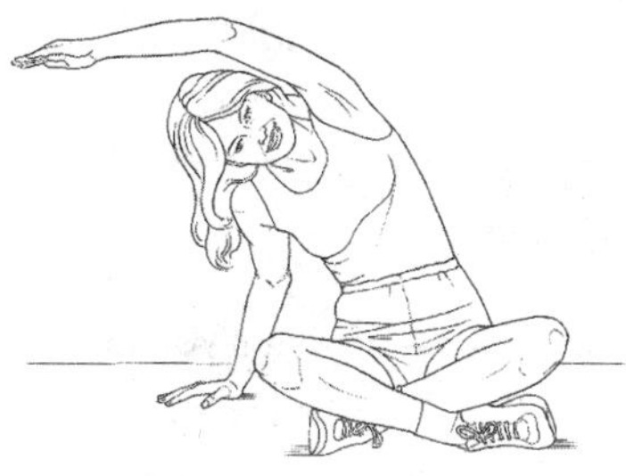

Sides (*above*): Sit on the floor cross-legged. Lift one arm overhead, leaning over to the side, arm up and over at a diagonal, so that if you were holding keys in your hand and you dropped your keys, they wouldn't land on your head. Reach until one buttock lifts off the floor.

Lower back (*right*): Sit on the floor, legs either out in front or crossed, hands on the floor. Round your back and bend forward.

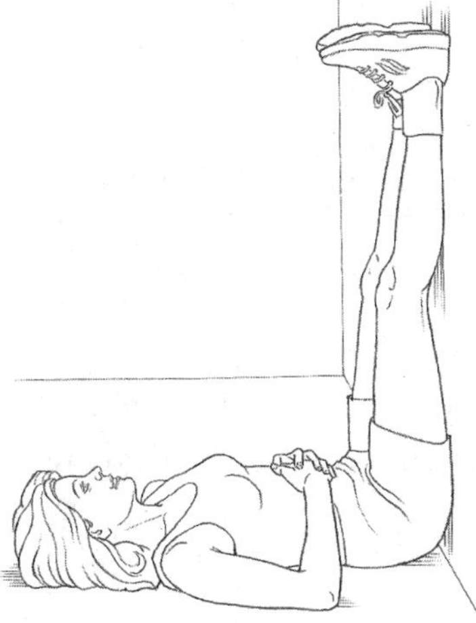

Back of thigh (*above*): Lie on your back on the floor with your tailbone against a wall, legs up on the wall, bent as much as necessary for comfort. Straighten your legs until you reach your limit.

Upper calf (*right*): Stand with your toes facing close to a wall and lean against it with your forearms so that your hands are at eye level. Bend the front knee as you step back with the other foot, keeping the back leg straight and the heel pressed down. (Position your back leg so that your toes point forward, not out to the side.) Relax and repeat on other leg. ››

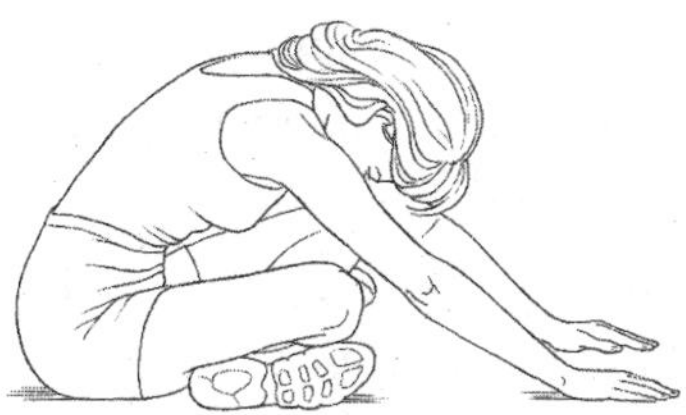

A SAFER WAY TO STRETCH

Stretch only to the point where you begin to feel the stretch, no farther, and hold for 10 to 30 seconds. You won't gain flexibility from stretching faster or farther—that only makes the muscle contract. If you want to increase your flexibility, you must hold stretches for at least a minute.

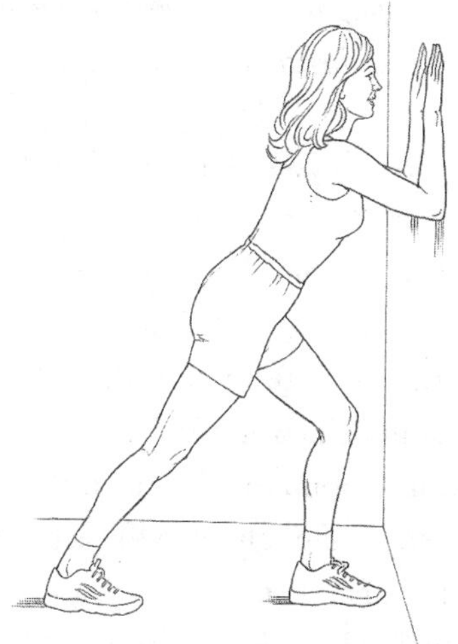

Lower calf (*right*): Use the same position as the stretch for the upper calf, but bring the back foot closer so that you can bend the back knee slightly.

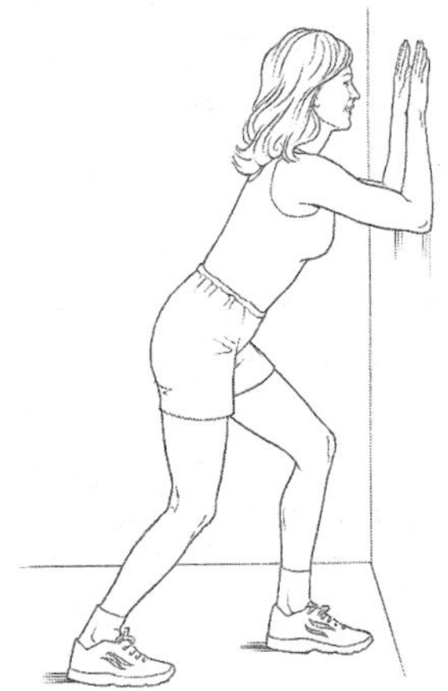

Helpful Hints

Stretch every day, even if you don't exercise daily, says Lockridge. To improve flexibility, stretch when your body is warm after exercise, play, or strenuous effort. To relieve physical or emotional tension or sore muscles, stretch any time and as often as you like—but go easy.

"When a muscle isn't warm, be gentle and move only within your range of motion, until you feel only a slight sensation of stretching," says Lockridge.

Many women stretch muscles that don't need it, such as the trapezius (upper back), and ignore muscles that are shortened (tight), such as the hamstrings (back of the thigh).

No matter how busy you are, says Lockridge, you, too, should stretch. ■

Sunburn

60-Minute Relief

Looking—and feeling—like last night's lobster?

If you have a bad sunburn, it'll be a few days before the red completely fades. But you can relieve the pain and swelling with ibuprofen (or even a couple of aspirin), says Leslie S. Baumann, M.D., director of cosmetic dermatology at the University of Miami.

When your skin is scorched by the sun, the blood vessels beneath your skin begin to leak fluid, leaving your skin tender and inflamed, says Dr. Baumann. The pain and swelling will respond to the same treatment you might give the ache and inflammation of, say, a sprained ankle. Nonsteroidal anti-inflammatory drugs (NSAIDs) such as ibuprofen (Advil or Motrin) or plain old aspirin work to quickly reduce the flow of this fluid.

As soon as you realize that you've had too much sun, take two 200-milligram tablets of ibuprofen or two 325-milligram tablets of aspirin, and then every 6 hours after that for 48 hours. You should feel better within the first hour, says Dr. Baumann. ■

DON'T MAKE THIS MISTAKE

Don't assume that if you tan easily you will be less prone to the damaging effects of the sun. UVA (ultraviolet A) rays penetrate deeply into unprotected skin, regardless of whether your complexion is fair or naturally dark. Chronic exposure to UVB (ultraviolet B) rays can cause skin cancer even in women with dark complexions, warns Dr. Buchness.

Sun Protection

Year-Round Damage Control

Your skin can burn after just 25 minutes of unprotected exposure to the sun. That's in New York City. In Orlando, Florida, or Vail, Colorado, you could burn even faster because the sun's rays are stronger the closer you get to the equator and the higher you climb in elevation.

With daily exposure, unprotected skin can undergo enough damage to contribute to wrinkles, freckle-like age spots, jowls, and precancerous changes. After years of exposure, you can look older than your years.

So go ahead and store your sandals, beach towels, and swimsuit when summer ends. But don't pack away your bottle of sunscreen. You may need sun protection in winter as well as in summer.

"Don't let the cold winter temperatures fool you," says Mary Ruth Buchness, M.D., chief of dermatology at St. Vincent's Hospital and Medical Center in New York City and president of the Women's Medical Association of New York City. "You should wear sunscreen every day, no matter the altitude or temperature."

You probably already know that you should avoid the sun during peak times, between 11:00 A.M. and 3:00 P.M., when the sun is at its brightest, during daylight savings time. And you probably already know that you should buy sunscreen with an SPF between 15 and 30. Sunscreens with SPF 15 protect against 94 percent of the sun's harmful rays, and those with SPF 30 protect against 97 percent.

Here's what else Dr. Buchness suggests for year-round sun protection.

• Look for sunscreens containing zinc oxide, titanium dioxide, or avobenzone. These block both ultraviolet B (UVB) rays—responsible for burning and tanning—and ultraviolet A (UVA) rays—the rest of the spectrum. They suit women with all types of skin, even the most sensitive.

While dermatologists don't yet know what the long-term effects of UVA rays are, Dr. Buchness advises that it's always best to use a sunblock that blocks both UVA and UVB rays.

• Apply sunscreen 30 minutes before you head outside and reapply every 2 hours or after you get wet from swimming or sweating.

• During the day, wear UV-protective sunglasses, especially when driving, since ultraviolet rays penetrate car windows.

• To protect your head, neck, and face from direct sunlight when you're outdoors, wear a hat with a brim no less than 4 inches wide.

Helpful Hint

Products with SPFs higher than 30 cost more, and they don't provide any more significant protection unless you're taking photosensitizing drugs such as some antibiotics. ■

Surgery

Speed Recovery with Mental Imagery

When Catherine Conant discovered she needed a hysterectomy, she panicked. "When I was 7 years old, I had an emergency appendectomy," she explains. "My parents didn't want to scare me, so they didn't tell me what was happening. As I was wheeled into the operating room, I was terrified." The experience left her so traumatized that she didn't speak for 2 months.

Yet, when she had her hysterectomy, Conant did fine. She needed only half the amount of pain medication her doctor expected, and she left the hospital a day early. One week later, she went out to lunch with friends. Two weeks later, she walked a mile. One month later, she felt happy and healthy.

Conant attributes her speedy recovery to a surgery preparation program developed by Peggy Huddleston, a psychotherapist and researcher at the New England Baptist Hospital in Boston and author of Prepare for Surgery, Heal Faster.

When women (and men, for that matter) learn that they need to have an operation, they get scared, anxious, fearful. It's a natural reaction, says Huddleston, but one that can backfire. "Being anxious and on edge can suppress your immune system," she explains, making surgery harder on your body and your recovery more difficult.

By the same token, being relaxed can ease your operation and your recuperation. "Before going into the operating room, the women who use this technique are much more calm. They often have a sense of serenity," says Dixie Mills, M.D., a breast surgeon at Women to Women, a clinic in Yarmouth, Maine, whose patients have used Huddleston's techniques. "They also report less pain, use less pain medication, and go home sooner. The nurses in the recovery room think they're not taking enough pain medication and try to get them to take more."

If you're anxiously facing the prospect of surgery, here's what Huddleston recommends to calm your nerves and expedite your recovery.

Learn to relax. Try a relaxation tape to teach your body and mind how to release tension. It will not only help you cope with the stress of upcoming surgery but it will also boost your immune system. To select the right tape, see page 373.

Visualize your healing. Instead of fixating on "going under the knife," imagine the hoped-for outcome. If you're having knee replacement surgery, for example, picture yourself dashing up the stairs. What does it feel like to live and move without pain? What does your new and improved body look like? "Take your worries and fears and turn them into positive healing imagery," Huddleston says.

Ask for support. Huddleston tells the women she counsels to ask their friends and families to surround them

SUPPLEMENTS THAT HEAL (AND SOME THAT HAMPER)

Surgery taxes your body's defenses just when you need them the most.

"Even relatively minor surgery depletes your immune system," says Judith J. Petry, M.D., a former plastic surgeon and current medical director of the Vermont Healing Tools Project in Brattleboro. Yet you need to be in top form to fight infection and heal your tissues.

Here's what Dr. Petry recommends to provide your body with the nutrients it needs to hasten your healing. Be sure to review all of these with your surgeon.

Vitamin C. After surgery, your body may be low on this antioxidant, but you need vitamin C to help your wounds mend and bolster your immune system. Take 1,000 milligrams daily for the week before and after your surgery. (Excess vitamin C may cause abdominal cramps and diarrhea in some people. If that happens, reduce your intake.)

Vitamin A. To prevent surgery from exhausting your immune system, take 10,000 to 25,000 IU of vitamin A daily the week before and after your operation, Dr. Petry says. (Don't do this if you're pregnant or have liver trouble, and check with your doctor before taking more than 10,000 IU of vitamin A.)

Zinc. "You can't heal a wound without it," Dr. Petry says. Take 15 to 30 milligrams daily the week before and after your surgery. (Talk to your doctor before taking more than 20 milligrams.)

Bromelain. This pineapple-plant extract prevents and eases bruising. To benefit from its anti-inflammatory and bruise-fading abilities, take bromelain on an empty stomach, with your first dose of 500 milligrams a few hours before your operation. (Get your surgeon's okay first.) Then take 500 milligrams twice daily for a week, or until your black-and-blue marks disappear.

On the other hand, if you're taking vitamin E, garlic, fish oil, selenium, hawthorn berry, or ginkgo supplements, stop a week before your surgery. They decrease the ability of your blood to clot, which is essential for healing. "You really want to be able to clot during and right after surgery," Dr. Petry says. Wait until your wound has healed before resuming these supplements.

in loving thoughts in the half-hour before their surgeries. Before her breast biopsy, Lorraine Vitagliano of Lynnfield, Massachusetts, suddenly felt so relaxed and peaceful, she thought the nurse had given her a shot of Valium. Then she looked at the clock and realized it was exactly 27 minutes before her operation—exactly when those she loved were thinking of her.

Helpful Hint

A classic study in the 1960s found that patients who spoke with their anesthesiologists for 5 minutes before surgery were calmer than patients who took sedatives. "This is the person to whom you're entrusting your consciousness," Huddleston says. "You need to feel a human connection with her." Even a brief conversation helps. ■

Swimmer's Ear

Infection Fighters from a Pro

Jane Katz, Ed.D., loves the water. The world-class competitive swimmer and professor of health and physical education at the City University of New York swims every day. Yet in more than 40 years of her swimming career, she has never had swimmer's ear, an infection of the outer ear caused, in part, by frequent exposure to water.

Katz is the exception, not the rule. Repeated exposure to water can break down the protective layering of the earwax, which coats the skin inside the ear. "Washing away this lubricating barrier causes dryness and flaking, shredding the protective tissue of the ear canal," explains Jim Miller, M.D., chair of the United States Masters Swimming Sports Medicine Committee. Then, when water gets into the ear, the bacteria or fungi that sometimes come with it can invade the broken skin, irritating the ear canal and causing painful swelling.

Women who swim frequently are particularly prone to swimmer's ear—their ears never quite dry out, so bacteria flourish. As with her swimming success, Katz owes her track record for infection-free ears to more than luck. She has figured out how to keep her ears dry and infection-free. Dr. Katz and Dr. Miller offer these tips for women who swim regularly for fun or exercise.

Pull the wool over your ears. Take a small amount of lamb's wool (found in the foot-care section of your local pharmacy), coat it with a little petroleum jelly, and stick it in your ears. "It takes a little practice to find just the right amount and comfort level," says Dr. Katz.

Lamb's wool acts like a sponge, absorbing the water but keeping it away from the ear. "If you press it, the water comes out and the piece of lamb's wool is dry again," Dr. Katz says. "It's like a repellent, a rain slicker for the ear." Cotton won't work.

Dry on low. The sooner you dry out your ears after a swim, the better your chance of eliminating the moisture that could promote bacterial growth. Right after swimming, use a blow-dryer on a lukewarm setting. Most women shower and dry their hair after swimming anyway, so this is a preventive step that you can easily add to your routine. "Just lower the heat and direct the air toward each ear," Dr. Katz says. Just don't hold it too close.

Mix your own eardrops. Take equal parts rubbing alcohol and white vinegar, mix them in an eardropper bottle, and you've got your own homemade solution for combating swimmer's ear.

"The alcohol serves as a drying agent to draw the water out, while the vinegar creates an acid environment, which helps retard the growth of bacteria," explains Dr. Miller. Use a few drops in each ear right after a swim. ■

DON'T MAKE THIS MISTAKE

If eardrops or other remedies don't help after a week or so, or if eardrops burn when you put them in your ears, see your doctor. If swimmer's ear gets out of control, it can cause severe swelling in the ear canal. You may need antibiotics to clear the infection and prevent hearing loss.

T-U-V

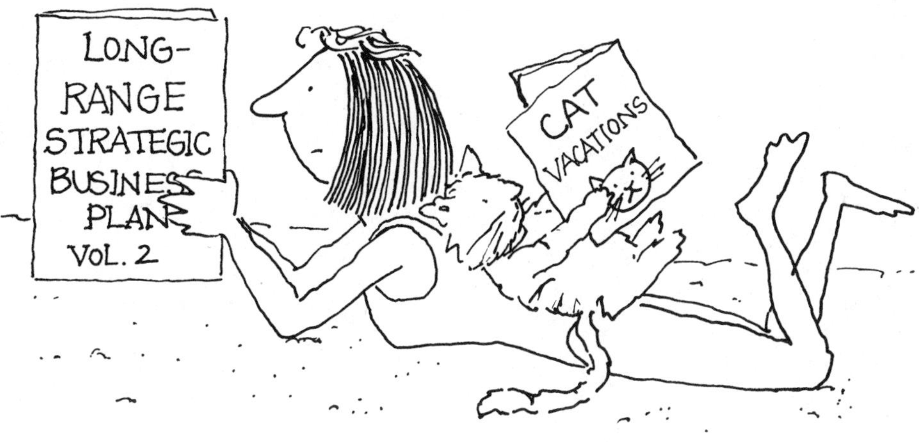

On vacation? Take a cue from your cat—
leave work behind.
See page 438 for details.

Tampons

Minimize the Risk While You Maximize Comfort

The average woman will use 6,700 tampons in her lifetime. More convenient than sanitary pads for collecting menstrual fluid, tampons are popular and safe, as long as you use them wisely.

Tampons got a bad rap in 1980, when they were linked to high incidences of toxic shock syndrome (TSS), associated with the bacterium Staphylococcus aureus, *which sometimes produces toxins. Symptoms of TSS include high fever, chills, vomiting, diarrhea, muscle pains, low blood pressure, dizziness, a sunburnlike rash, and, a week or two later, flaking and peeling skin, especially on the palms and soles.*

Experts estimate that in 1980, when TSS peaked, 38 women died of TSS and 800 others became very sick. Tampons don't cause the bacterial infection that may lead to TSS, but they do increase the risk, and the higher the absorbency of the tampon, the higher the risk.

"The infection rate peaked in 1979 and 1980 because of the introduction of the new Rely tampon, extremely absorbent, made of special material," explains Rana Hajjeh, M.D., medical epidemiologist for the division of bacterial and mycotic diseases at the Centers for Disease Control and Prevention. Rely tampons were taken off the market, and TSS cases decreased. Now, even super-absorbent tampons are only about half as absorbent they used to be, and therefore much safer. Since 1995, no women have died of TSS related to tampon use during menstruation.

Women who use tampons still need to take precautions to keep the risk low, says Dr. Hajjeh. Here are her tampon safety tips.

• Choose the lowest-absorbency tampon that meets your needs.

• Change tampons frequently. Try not to wear them for more than 8 hours.

• Don't go overboard by changing tampons too frequently (like every hour).

• Alternate tampons with pads.

• Wear tampons only when you're menstruating. Using tampons to control discharge or spotting at other times can dry out the vagina and cause irritation and tearing, ››

IGNORE INTERNET SCARES

Don't believe or pass along these Internet scares about tampons.

Cybermyth #1: Tampon manufacturers add asbestos to promote excessive bleeding (and therefore sell more tampons).

Fact: Tampons do not contain asbestos and never have.

Cybermyth #2: Tampons contain dioxin, which may cause cancer and damage to the reproductive system.

Fact: Dioxin—a toxic by-product of bleaching wood pulp with chlorine—is *not* a by-product of the specific bleaching processes used in the United States. Tampon use does not increase your risk of cancer.

DON'T MAKE THIS MISTAKE

If you have had TSS, it's better not to use tampons again, because 10 percent of women with TSS get a recurrence, says Dr. Hajjeh.

which can lead to infection.

• If you develop fever, a sunburnlike rash, dizziness, or nausea even 2 to 3 days after you stop using tampons, seek medical attention. "Early treatment is very successful," says Dr. Hajjeh.

Helpful Hints

If you have a teenage daughter, instruct her about the possible risks. Tampon companies have done a good job of alerting and educating people in the package inserts, says Dr. Hajjeh, but teenagers may not read it. ■

Temporomandibular Disorder

Press Away Jaw Pain with Acupressure

One day, a woman diagnosed with temporomandibular pain walked into the office of pain specialist Albert Forgione, Ph.D. In the course of their conversation, he put his hand on her forearm to console her. The woman screamed in pain. Assuming it was her arm that hurt, Dr. Forgione gently massaged the woman's arm to ease what he thought was a muscle spasm.

This time, the woman burst into tears of joy—somehow the pain in her face was gone. An acupressure treatment for temporomandibular disorder (TMD) was born.

Acupressure is a gentle treatment of massaging pressure points along meridians—energy channels often stimulated by needles in the related practice of acupuncture. As with acupuncture, the points stimulated during acupressure are often far away from what hurts.

TMD affects the jaw and muscles you use to chew food. This joint can be easily overstrained or injured, especially in women who clench their jaws or grind their teeth, causing pain in the neck, face, or shoulders. TMD pain is often accompanied by clicking or grating sounds in the jaw, says Dr. Forgione, director of research at the Gelb Craniomandibular Oral Facial Pain Center at Tufts Dental School in Boston.

Massaging the painful jaw muscles directly won't ease your pain. As Dr. Forgione discovered, what you need to press instead are special referral points in the arm that release and relax the aching jaw muscles.

If you have TMD pain, Dr. Forgione suggests pressing two points on your arms, depending on where your jaw hurts.

Cheek pain? Try this. To ease pain between your left cheek bone and the lower border of your jaw, find acupressure point M. Lay your left forearm on a table with your palm flat down. Put the fingers of your right hand on your left forearm, with your right index finger in the fold of your elbow and the rest of your fingers laying right next to each other (*below*). Then, wiggle your left middle finger. If you feel a ligament moving at the edge of your right ring finger tip, you're touching point M.

Press moderately hard on this point with your ring finger for 15 seconds. (The point will hurt if you have pain in your cheek.) You may have to do this three times in a row, pausing slightly in between. You'll experience a warm, tingling feeling in your facial muscles when they release. Find the same spot on your other arm and repeat three times.

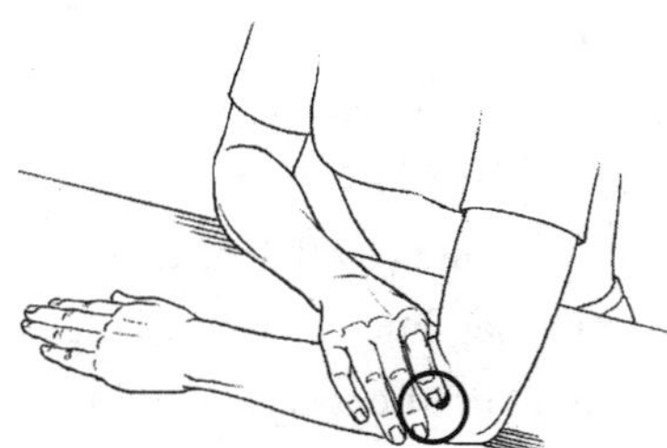

AVOID APPLYING ACUPRESSURE ON AN EMPTY STOMACH

If you haven't eaten for 3 to 4 hours, your body will be so tense that acupressure won't work very well, Dr. Forgione says. Eating something steadies your blood sugar, which can be low when you are in pain, so it helps your body relax. Be sure to eat, or at least drink an energizing beverage such as orange juice, before you press one of these referral points.

Temple pain? Press here. This point releases the temporalis muscles, which close your front teeth and spread like a fan on the sides of your head above your ears. To find point T, bend your left elbow 90 degrees. Curl the fingers of your right hand around your left bicep, with the end of your pinkie finger resting in the fold of your left elbow (*below*). Your right index finger will be touching point T. If it hurts when you press it, you have the point.

As with cheek pain, press hard on this point with your index finger for 15 seconds, three times, if necessary. Repeat on the opposite arm. You should feel a slow release of gentle warmth into the temporalis muscles, says Dr. Forgione.

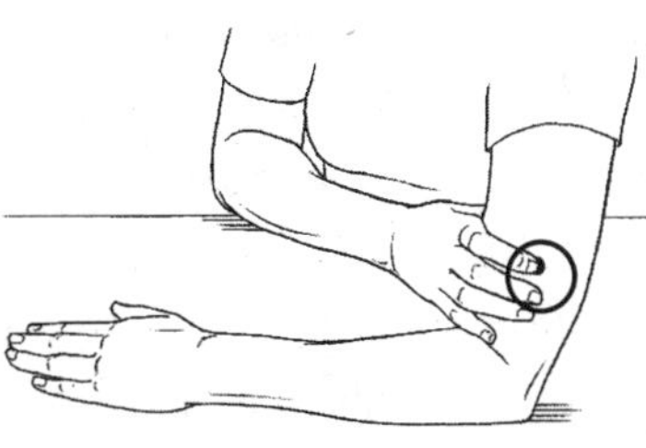

Helpful Hint

If these points are too painful to touch, rub them with ice first, says Dr. Forgione. Hold an ice cube on your skin for 30 seconds, then remove for 30 seconds. Repeat this four times.

If it still hurts to touch the point with your finger, relax the area using a vibrating massager, available at drugstores, Dr. Forgione says. They look like old-fashioned shower heads. Hold the massager on the point for 2 minutes four times a day. ■

Thinning Hair

Restorative Tips for Medically Induced Hair Loss

Some brave souls, like Irish singer Sinead O'Connor, have shaved all their hair off in the name of style. But most women would go to great lengths to keep their hair—or make it look as if they have—especially if it has begun to spontaneously shed, or gradually thin with age.

"Women definitely disguise hair loss better than men," says Marty Sawaya, M.D.,Ph.D., a dermatologist in Ocala, Florida, who specializes in hair loss. Yet the quest can be a tough one, given the number of factors that can cause temporary and long-term hair loss, including hereditary hormonal imbalances, oral contraceptives and other medications, chemotherapy, and even stress.

So what can you do, besides shop for a wig? It depends.

If you've just given birth or gone through a divorce, a move, or some other major stress:

Relax. All of these stress factors can cause your roots to close down and rest for 3 months. But after that, your hair should return to normal without help.

If your hair is coming out in patches, but you haven't experienced any life stresses:

Think about other changes. Have you started taking a new medication or changed your nutrition habits? Antithyroid drugs, anticonvulsants, diuretics, and even ibuprofen can trigger hair loss in some people. Chemotherapy causes temporary hair loss in many women. (It will grow back within 1 to 3 months after your last treatment.)

If you have no idea why you're losing your hair, promptly consult a dermatologist who deals with hair problems. "It's better to arrest the process as soon as possible instead of waiting for years, because it becomes more difficult to treat over time," says Dr. Sawaya.

Meanwhile, take these steps to conserve what you have.

• Don't perm, straighten, or color your hair until it's back to normal. Chemical treatments can inflame and irritate your scalp.

• Give your hair a break from tight braids and rollers, which can break the hair.

• Apply minoxidil, an over-the-counter hair-restoring treatment, to your scalp twice a day. It has been proven effective, especially for the 25 to 30 percent of women who lose their hair due to hereditary factors.

• Have patience. "Nothing restores hair loss in 6 weeks. It usually takes 6 months for the process to turn around," says Dr. Sawaya.

Helpful Hints

If you use birth control pills, ask your doctor to prescribe only those that contain the ingredients desogestrel or norgestimate, and avoid those that contain norgestrel or norethindrone, which promote hair loss, says Dr. Sawaya.

If you have no intention (or possibility) of becoming pregnant, ask your doctor if you would benefit from Propecia, a prescription drug that restores hair in men but is marketed only to men because it can cause birth defects. Some doctors prescribe it to women who are not trying to become pregnant. ■

Toe Pain and Discoloration

Help for Technicolor Toes

Blue. Black. Purple. Yellow. Nice colors for a swimsuit, but not your toes. Throw in pain, and you'll be seeing red.

Here's what causes female toenail problems, with advice on what to do from Thomas M. Novella, D.P.M., associate professor of orthopedics at the New York College of Podiatric Medicine in New York City, and Cheryl Burgess, M.D., of the Center for Dermatology and Dermatologic Surgery in Washington, D.C.

Nail Fungus

An infected toenail thickens and turns whitish, yellow, or sometimes blackish from tip to base. The color varies with the type of fungus, which originates in the soil and thrives in cozy, moist, dark environments like the toebox of your shoe.

Over-the-counter products won't get rid of nail fungus. They don't penetrate the nail. See your doctor for an oral antifungal prescription drug. To prevent future problems, use a hair dryer on a cool setting to dry your toenails before puting on your shoes and socks, especially after bathing or before spending all day in a warm, damp environment.

Also, were leather or canvas shoes, not vinyl.

Black or Jammed Toe

If you run in ill-fitting shoes, you may end up with bruising or dark red hemorrhaging that looks like splinters stuck up the nail. If you wear hiking boots, ski boots, or other athletic footwear that's too loose or too tight, your toes will hit the front of the toebox again and again, leaving the toe and possibly the nail black. "The toe hits and it jams," says Dr. Burgess.

If your toe is bruised or black, you don't have to do anything. The hemorrhage will grow out with the nail. If it doesn't, seek medical attention promptly. And do get better-fitting shoes or boots so that it won't happen again.

DON'T MAKE THESE MISTAKES

Don't use the same nail clipper on a healthy toenail or fingernail if you've just trimmed an infected nail, says Dr. Novella. And don't share nail clippers. You may spread the fungal infection.

Helpful Hints

"If the nail is loose, you or a professional can carefully trim the loose bit off so that it doesn't tear the part that is still connected to the bed," suggests Dr. Novella.

As a rule, keep your toenails clipped back or filed down so that your toe acts as a cushion and your nail doesn't hit the shoe directly, suggests Dr. Burgess. Cut your toenails straight across, then file the corners to eliminate sharp edges and keep nails from cutting into your toes. ■

Trans Fatty Acids

Hydrogenated Fats Don't Fool Your Arteries

Before you toss that bottle of salad dressing or loaf of bread in your shopping cart, scrutinize the ingredients label. A fair amount of processed foods—notably margarine, pastries, mayonnaise, salad dressings, white bread, and even some breakfast cereals, contain trans fatty acids.

Trans fatty acids start out as liquid polyunsaturated vegetable fats, like soybean oil. Hydrogen atoms are added, turning the oil from liquid to semisolid. The firmer the fat, the more hydrogenation, the more trans fatty acids. Vegetable shortening is always partially hydrogenated, for example.

Trans fatty acids act like saturated fat in your body, raising total blood cholesterol. But trans fatty acids not only raise "bad" LDL cholesterol but research suggests that they also raise LP(a), the lipoprotein associated with an increased risk of heart disease, as well as lower "good" HDL cholesterol. Some studies suggest that they may even increase your risk of cancer.

Avoiding trans fatty acids comes down to two simple strategies.

Read labels. Until manufacturers are required to report the amount of trans fatty acids on the label, you'll need to do a little simple math, says Mary Enig, Ph.D., a pioneer in trans fatty acid re-

Traveler's Diarrhea

Don't Take Antibiotics as "Vacation Insurance"

Maria Coria, an intrepid traveler based in New York City, describes traveler's diarrhea to a T:

"You feel like your whole body is melting," she says. "You find it difficult to keep your eyes open. You want to be either sitting on a toilet or a foot away from it. You're cramping. You wish you could sleep, but you can't, because you're constantly running to the bathroom. You feel like you have no control."

Coria markets medical products internationally, so she has to travel a lot. She had been to Mexico four times before and had gotten sick once. When she was pregnant, she had to make a return trip to Mexico for a week. She didn't want to take any chances, so she took preventive measures and stayed healthy.

Traveler's diarrhea is caused by bacteria that you can get from contaminated food and water. This is very common in countries with poverty and poor sanitation. "The key is prevention," says Keith Armitage, M.D., infectious diseases physician at Travelers Health Care Center in Cleveland.

Here are Dr. Armitage's rules for avoiding traveler's diarrhea. (Even if you've heard them before, pay attention—it only takes one slipup to send your bowels into an uproar.)

search and director of the Nutritional Sciences Division of Enig Associates in Silver Spring, Maryland. When a label lists the grams of saturated, polyunsaturated, and monounsaturated fatty acids, just add the numbers and subtract from the total fat grams on the label. The difference is the amount of trans fatty acids that are in the product.

Eat as little processed food as possible. French fries contain trans fatty acids, for example. But oven-baked potatoes don't. Neither do unprocessed whole grains, beans, and fresh vegetables and fruits. When a product is processed and contains partially hydrogenated oil, it will contain trans fatty acids, says Dr. Enig. ■

FRIENDLIER FRIES

French fries are a major source of trans fatty acids, indicted for contributing to heart disease and cancer. So make your own. Preheat the oven to 475°F. Coat a baking sheet with nonstick spray. In a large bowl, combine 1 tablespoon olive oil, ½ tablespoon of your favorite dried seasoning, and ¼ teaspoon black pepper. Cut three large baking potatoes lengthwise into ½" wedges, add to the bowl, and toss. Arrange in a single layer on the baking sheet and bake, turning occasionally, for 20 to 30 minutes, or until the potatoes are lightly browned and tender.

Do not drink water unless it's bottled (with the seal intact) or boiled for 5 minutes. Coffee, tea (hot, not iced), and soft drinks (straight from the sealed bottle or can) are safe, provided you wipe the top of the can or bottle rim first. Ice is not safe.

Be careful about accidentally drinking water. Brush your teeth with bottled water. Don't swallow any water in the shower. Do not drink from glasses, which may have been washed inadequately.

Do not eat raw fruits or vegetables unless you ❯❯

A STRATEGY THAT CAN BACKFIRE

It's okay to ask your doctor for a prescription for antibiotics and carry them with you as an insurance policy in case you get sick. Do not take the antibiotics as prevention, however. Taking antibiotics when you don't need them can suppress your body's natural flora.

If you get sick, take the antibiotic for 3 to 5 days. "See a doctor if you have persistent bloody diarrhea or persistent fever after 2 to 3 days," says Dr. Armitage.

Most antibiotics are photosensitizing, so don't lie out on the beach and work on your tan if you're taking them.

You can also carry Imodium, an over-the-counter antidiarrheal, with you. But use it only if you have diarrhea and are taking antibiotics for it. It's not a preventive. If you take it without antibiotics, it can make your condition worse, especially if you have fever or bloody diarrhea.

peel them yourself. Cooked fruits and vegetables that are still hot are usually safe. The highest risk is probably raw food from a street vendor.

Take the pink stuff as a prevention. Bismuth subsalicylate (such as Pepto-Bismol) "coats the intestines, and the bacteria can't adhere," explains Dr. Armitage. To be effective, you have to take it every 4 to 6 hours.

Follow the guidelines until you're safely home. "Food and water on an airplane that originates in the country of risk may be unsafe," warns Dr. Armitage. "Don't throw caution to the wind when you board the plane home. That's a famous pitfall."

Most types of traveler's diarrhea will make you sick right away. Giardia, for example, waits a while before kicking in and can last for weeks if not treated. "If you were fine on your trip but start to get diarrhea and cramping after you've been home for a few days, go to your doctor," says Dr. Armitage. ■

Ulcers

Get Rid of That Stomach Pain for Good

Researchers once believed that demanding bosses, jealous coworkers, and other forms of job stress were responsible for ulcers. But it's now known that 90 percent of ulcers are caused by a smaller life form: the spiral-shaped bacterium Helicobacter pylori (H. pylori). *The other 10 percent are caused by overuse of nonsteroidal anti-inflammatory drugs (NSAIDs) such as aspirin and ibuprofen.*

Unlike most bacteria, H. pylori *actually thrive in the stomach's acidic environment. When these nasty little bugs burrow too deeply into the stomach's protective mucus layer, they expose the delicate underlying tissue to the corrosive effects of stomach acid and pepsin, a digestive enzyme.*

The resulting ulcer can lead to such life-threatening complications as bleeding, perforation, and obstruction.

If you have the most common ulcer symptom—chronic pain between your breastbone and belly button—quitting your job won't relieve it. The only way to cure an ulcer is to kill *H. pylori*, says Melissa Palmer, M.D., a gastroenterologist in Plainview, New York. You'll need a powerful antibiotic such as clarithromycin or metronidazole with a prescription acid blocker such as Prilosec or Prevacid. If you're like 90 percent of those treated with this combination, a week or two of medication will leave you ulcer-free for life.

If your ulcer was caused by NSAIDs, the cure is even simpler. Stop taking the offending drug and start taking a prescription acid blocker to speed healing. "Over-the-counter antacids aren't as good, but even they may do the trick," Dr. Palmer says.

Here are some steps you can take to ensure that you get the

DON'T MAKE THIS MISTAKE

Even if your ulcer has apparently vanished after a few days of antibiotic treatment, don't stop taking your medicine. Unless you empty the prescription bottle, *H. pylori*—and your ulcer—could come roaring back.

best possible treatment and outcome.

Insist on the deluxe diagnostic test. Although blood and breath tests can detect the presence of *H. pylori*, the most accurate test is an upper endoscopy. During this procedure, a doctor runs a fiber-optic tube down your throat, takes a gander at your stomach, and snags a snippet of tissue for analysis.

Bag the coffee. All coffee (decaf included) increases stomach acid production, which promotes the proliferation of *H. pylori*, so avoid it during treatment. The same goes for any food or substance that causes stomach pain. Some prime offenders: cola, citrus, alcoholic beverages, tobacco, and dairy products.

Give your gut some natural assistance. To relieve ulcer symptoms, drink 2 or 3 cups a day of fresh cabbage juice, recommends Patrick Donovan, N.D., a naturopathic physician in Seattle. Cabbage juice contains considerable amounts of two ulcer-fighting compounds, glutamine and s-methyl-methionine, which studies have shown improve ulcer symptoms. Or chew some licorice, he suggests. Deglycyrrhizinated licorice (DGL) is a natural product available in health food stores or wherever herbal preparations are sold. (Don't confuse it with licorice root, which you should avoid if you have diabetes, high blood pressure, liver or kidney disorders, or low potassium levels.) Before or after meals, slowly chew two tablets of DGL extract or swallow ½ teaspoon of the powder form. This herb contains several anti-ulcer compounds that protect the lining of the stomach and small intestine.

Help yourself to lactobacillus. To minimize side effects from antibiotic treatment, Dr. Donovan recommends taking ½ teaspoon of powdered lactobacillus twice a day during treatment and for two weeks thereafter. He recommends that women use Monistat or some other anti-yeast cream daily during treatment to help prevent an overgrowth of *Candida* or other yeast during treatment for *H. pylori*.

Helpful Hint

Provided you're not lactose intolerant, you might be able to prevent an ulcer by eating more yogurt. In some people, fermented milk products such as yogurt appear to protect the stomach lining from *H. pylori*. ■

Urinary Incontinence

Regain Control of Your Bladder and Your Life

If you've experienced embarrassing leaks, you're not alone. Millions of women have the same problem. Hormonal and physical changes during childbirth, menopause, and aging can cause urinary incontinence. But you don't have to live with leaks.

"Urinary incontinence is very common, but it's not normal, and women need to seek treatment," says Patricia S. Goode, M.D., medical director of the continence program at the University of Alabama at Birmingham.

Perhaps you leak only when you exercise, laugh, sneeze, or cough, a condition known as stress incontinence. If you feel immediate, uncontrollable urges to urinate and often can't make it to the bathroom in time, you may have urge incontinence. Or, you could be experiencing a combination of the two.

Experts recommend these self-care strategies.

If you smoke, quit. Between the smoker's cough and nicotine's ability to trigger bladder spasms, a woman who smokes puts herself at risk for stress and urge incontinence, says Christine LaSala, M.D., a urogynecologist at University of Connecticut Health Center/Hartford Hospital.

Cut out caffeine (if you have urge incontinence). Like nicotine, "caffeine is a horrendous bladder irritant," Dr. LaSala says. If you get withdrawal headaches when you try to give up caffeine, Dr. Goode recommends gradually reducing your caffeine intake by 25 percent weekly.

Avoid artificial sweeteners. Like caffeine, they irritate the bladder and contribute to urge incontinence, experts say.

Lose weight. Carrying extra pounds, especially if you're apple-shaped and tend to gain weight in your midsection, puts pressure on your pelvic organs and makes stress incontinence more likely.

Keep a bladder diary. Recording when, why, and what you ate or drank before you urinated will help you and your doctor determine physical or dietary reasons for accidents and make lifestyle adjustments. Maybe you're waiting too long between bathroom breaks. Perhaps you leak only during aerobics or after drinking wine. One study found that women who kept a bladder diary and met regularly with a nurse practitioner about their incontinence reduced their accidents by 39 percent, without medication or behavioral treatment.

Schedule bathroom breaks. To train your bladder when to empty, try to keep increasing the intervals between bathroom visits, says Dr. LaSala. Steadily lengthen that

DON'T MAKE THIS MISTAKE

Don't let urinary incontinence rule your life, keeping you from exercising, traveling, or socializing. And don't wait until your doctor asks you about it. If you have a problem, speak up.

STOP A LEAK BEFORE IT HAPPENS

If you feel the urge to urinate, Susan Scanlon, M.D., director of an incontinence clinic at Women's HealthFirst in Buffalo Grove, Illinois, suggests you try "quick flicks": Do four fast squeezes of your pelvic muscles, relax, and then do four more fast squeezes. "This tactic helps women relax spasms in the bladder and get to the bathroom before they leak," she says.

time by a few minutes every few days until you can last about 4 hours. If you keep up this regimen during the day, you'll probably find that you'll make fewer nocturnal bathroom visits, also.

Do Kegels. Described on page 248, Kegel exercises strengthen the pelvic floor muscles essential to bladder control.

If these approaches fail to work as well as you'd like, talk to your doctor. She may recommend other treatments, such as incontinence devices, biofeedback, medications, vaginal estrogen creams, collagen injections, or—if necessary—surgery. ■

Urinary Tract Infections

Ironclad Ways to Stop the Burn

Unfortunately, you know the feeling. A constant urge to go to the bathroom—and when you do, excruciating, burning pain. You have a urinary tract infection (UTI), and you just want the agony to end. Now.

"So many women are just crippled by UTIs," says Martha Roach, M.D., a urologist specially trained in female urology in Atlanta.

To some extent, women get UTIs simply because of their anatomy. "In women, the rectum, vagina, and urethra are within centimeters of each other, making it easy for infection-causing bacteria such as E. coli *to enter the vagina, travel up the urethra, and get into the bladder," explains Christine LaSala, M.D., a urogynecologist at University of Connecticut Health Center/Hartford Hospital. Women should consult a doctor whenever they suspect they have a UTI. Treatment usually consists of a 1-day or 3-day dose of antibiotics. To ease the pain and protect yourself from future infections, follow this expert advice.*

Sip cranberry juice at the first twinge of pain. Cranberries contain unique substances, called condensed tannins, that make it more difficult for bacteria to adhere to the lining of your urinary tract.

Drink more water, not less. You may be tempted to drink less because urinating afterward is so painful. But if you drink a gallon of water within 24 hours of discovering UTI symptoms, you might be able to flush the bacteria out of your system, Dr. Roach says.

Urinate every 2 hours. Emptying your bladder will decrease the number of bacteria in your bladder as they multiply.

Wash your underwear in color-safe all-purpose bleach. Dr. Roach tells the women she counsels to wash their underwear with a laundry bleach such as Clorox to kill any ››

UTI-causing bacteria that may be coming in contact with their bodies. Then double-rinse them, to get rid of any final traces of bleach, which can be irritating.

Wear underwear with a cotton crotch. A breathable fabric, cotton doesn't trap moisture, which can foster bacterial growth, explains Patricia Stockert, R.N., associate professor at St. Francis Medical Center's College of Nursing in Peoria, Illinois.

Don't sit around in wet bathing suits or sweaty workout gear. They, too, promote bacteria.

Practice good hygiene. After going to the bathroom, wipe yourself from front to back, recommends Stockert. Before having sex, wash yourself with a washcloth and warm soapy water, and rinse thoroughly, says Dr. LaSala. Otherwise, a penis can transfer a woman's own bacteria into her body during intercourse, causing a UTI.

Urinate within 2 hours after sex. It can dislodge UTI-causing bacteria that may have

Vacations

A Busy Woman's Guide to the Perfect Getaway

As travel agents, Maija Ositis of San Francisco and Vickie Eddington of San Antonio, Texas, plan excursions for others. They skillfully map out itineraries, book flights, hotel and car rental reservations, and provide inside tips on the destined city. And when it comes time to plan their own vacations, they put all of their professional skills to good use.

Not every woman is lucky enough to make a living planning the perfect getaway. In fact, it's downright difficult for some women to truly leave responsibilities of job and family for a week or even a weekend. Besides a suitcase of clothes, they often pack beepers, cellular phones, and laptop computers to stay connected with the office.

"It's easy to get trapped into feeling that nobody can do it as well as we do, or that feeling of guilt of leaving others behind to do the work," says J. Crit Harley, M.D., a behavioral medicine physician and former emergency room physician in Hendersonville, North Carolina. "But we all need vacations to shut off the dreaded stress response and improve our immune systems."

For seekers of true leave-all-obligations-behind vacations, Ositis and Eddington, along with the well-traveled Dr. Harley, offer these inside pointers on how they spend their days off.

Really leave the office behind. For a guilt-free vacation, Dr. Harley recommends setting up your office e-mail with a message indicating your departure and return dates, special instructions, and the name of who is in charge while you're gone. Also, write a memo to whoever is in charge, describing who needs to know what, do what, and by when. "It is always easiest to leave work when you provide adequate instructions for your coworkers," says Dr. Harley.

entered your body during intercourse. If you have recurrent UTIs that seem to be linked to sexual activity, your doctor may prescribe a preventive antibiotic for you to take each time you have intercourse.

Helpful Hints

If you have a childhood history of UTIs, tell your doctor. It may help her determine any underlying causes that could be making you susceptible to UTIs.

If you're in your forties, you may want to ask your doctor about estrogen cream. It helps your body maintain a normal vaginal environment and helps the urethra to produce mucus; both of these protect against bacterial infections such as UTIs.

If you get symptoms of UTIs frequently, your doctor may need to check you for interstitial cystitis, a chronic condition that mimics the symptoms of UTIs but calls for very different therapy. ■

Take relaxation gear only. Put some of the time you usually devote to your job into preparing for your vacation. The obvious step is to make up a list of things you need to take, such as a camera and sunscreen. Don't leave any room in your luggage for your laptop and beeper.

Adjust your attitude. Before and during the vacation, make it a goal to enjoy your time away from work. If you're task-oriented, regard the vacation as the break you need to be able to function more efficiently when you return to work, says Dr. Harley.

Build in transitional time. When Eddington plans to take a Caribbean cruise, she often takes a day off before the trip and a day off after the trip. "The day before, I do my running around, like getting my nails done, my hair styled, and my things packed. When I return, I take a day off to rest so that I can go back to work feeling truly refreshed," says Eddington.

Don't overbook your time. "Being on a tight schedule and rushing around to see everything under the sun is not a real vacation," Ositis says.

Make time for yourself. Whether they travel solo, with a friend, or in a group, both Ositis and Eddington book free time for themselves. "I enjoy waking up without an alarm clock, sitting on the deck, and just letting my mind rest for a while," says Ositis.

Eddington is a self-described sun, sand, and water person who loves a morning jog on the beach, reading a few chapters of a novel, and reveling in the simple pleasures of an ocean breeze. ■

DON'T MAKE THIS MISTAKE

Avoid traveling in groups of three or more whenever possible. Ositis says that trying to satisfy the vacation desires of so many different people creates too many conflicts over what to see and do. If it can't be avoided, at least make sure that you all agree to have one day where each of you goes off by herself to do her own thing.

Vaginal Dryness

The Best Lubricants

When a woman reaches menopause, her vagina may become dry enough to cause discomfort, especially during sex.

That's because estrogen levels are at an all-time low. Without enough of this female hormone, vaginal tissues tend to become weak, thin, and easily traumatized. Intercourse may hurt, even if you've allowed enough time for your vagina to become moist during foreplay.

You may be tempted to reach for the petroleum jelly. Not a good idea. Petroleum jelly can break down condoms. Plus, it isn't water-soluble, so it remains in the vagina, where it can harbor yeast and other infection-producing microbes.

The better options? Prescription creams or over-the-counter products. Here are the pros and cons of each.

Estrogen creams. These prescription creams are applied directly into the vagina. They relieve dryness by keeping vaginal tissue moist, healthy, and strong, says Brian Walsh, M.D., director of the menopause clinic at Brigham and Women's Hospital in Boston. Because the hormone stays mostly in the vagina, it doesn't raise blood levels of estrogen, making this an attractive option if you experience breakthrough bleeding or other undesirable side effects from estrogen in pill form.

Vaginal ring. About the size of a diaphragm, the ring is inserted into the vagina by either you

Vaginal Infections

To Blast Bacteria, Try This Herb-Vitamin Combo

If you develop an itchy discharge or other symptoms of a vaginal infection, you should:

a.) Assume that it's yeast and buy an antifungal cream.

b.) Call your gynecologist.

c.) Wait to see if it goes away by itself.

The correct answer is b, call your gynecologist. Buy an antifungal cream only if you've had a yeast infection before, and you know the symptoms *(see page 483)**. Otherwise, get a proper diagnosis.* Candida albicans*—the fungus that causes yeast—aren't the only bugs in town. And waiting to see if the infection goes away on its own will only make matters worse.*

If you have a vaginal infection, most likely your doctor will check you for bacterial vaginosis or trichomonas—two very stubborn bacterial infections that won't go away unless treated properly, says Beverly Yates, N.D., a naturopathic physician at Natural Health Care Group in Seattle.

Bacterial vaginosis causes a yellowish, fishy-smelling discharge. Trichomonas is characterized by itching, burning, and a frothy green or yellowish, foul-smelling discharge. A prescription for or your doctor and kept there for up to 3 months, where it releases a steady, low dose of estrogen, says Dr. Walsh. Studies show that it works well to relieve both vaginal dryness and urinary tract complaints. Some women prefer the ring over the creams because it's less messy.

Vaginal moisturizers. Available over the counter, feminine moisturizers such as Replens hydrate the vagina and relieve irritation for 2 to 3 days. They're available in suppositories or single-use applicators for convenience. And they're estrogen-free, pH balanced, nonirritating, and safe to use with condoms. (Check product labeling.)

The moisturizers won't strengthen or build up weakened vaginal walls. Only estrogen can do that, says Dr. Walsh.

Lubricants. Vaginal lubricants such as Astroglide and K-Y Jelly are designed to relieve friction during sex by coating your vaginal walls. Unlike the moisturizers, they tend to evaporate and often need to be reapplied during intercourse.

Helpful Hint

If you smoke, quit. Women who smoke complain of vaginal dryness and painful intercourse a lot more than nonsmokers do. The reason? Smoking restricts bloodflow necessary for a clitoral erection, engorgement of the vaginal walls and labia, and lubrication. So much for those sexy cigarette ads. ■

antibiotics is probably in order.

"These infections are stubborn," says Dr. Yates. "Sometimes, it takes more than one round of medications to get the job done. While you'll need specific prescription medicines to fight the infection at hand, building up your immunity can increase your chances of a full recovery with one course of treatment."

There are some natural remedies you can use to complement the treatment prescribed by your doctor. Here is what Dr. Yates recommends.

Goldenseal and astragalus. These herbs work in tandem. Goldenseal activates macrophages, specialized white blood cells that fight and destroy invading bacteria, says Dr. Yates. (Don't use it if you have high blood pressure.)

An immune system tonic, or strengthener, astragalus calls white blood cells into action and also produces antibodies and interferon—another immune system agent—to ward off intruders. For bacterial infections, Dr. Yates prescribes two capsules of each—350- to 400-milligram capsules of goldenseal and 250- to 300-millligram capsules of ››

DON'T MAKE THIS MISTAKE

If your doctor prescribes medication for a vaginal infection, never stop taking it before finishing the full course of treatment, even if your symptoms subside. Your vaginal infection will come back with a vengeance, because the most resistant bugs are always the last to die.

astragalus—three times a day, taken with food, for 2 weeks.

Mission-critical vitamins and minerals. Buy some zinc, vitamin C, vitamin E, and beta-carotene. They're renowned infection fighters that work hard to rev up your immune system.

Zinc generates new white blood cells to kill bacteria. Vitamin C boosts interferon levels. Vitamin E and beta-carotene—both powerful antioxidants—gobble up cell-damaging free radicals. Beta-carotene, in particular, protects the thymus gland, the main headquarters where a certain type of white blood cell matures and learns to recognize foreign bacteria.

If you have a vaginal infection, Dr. Yates suggests taking 10 to 20 milligrams of zinc a day with food; 1,000 milligrams of vitamin C; 400 IU of vitamin E; and 25,000 IU of beta-carotene. ■

Varicose Veins

Herbs That May Save You from Surgery

Clothing styles come and go, but varicose veins—those blue, swollen, protruding veins that appear mainly on the lower legs and feet—seem to affect women generation after generation. Blame heredity (although pregnancy, the use of oral contraceptives or hormone replacement therapy, lack of exercise, jobs that require constant standing, and obesity also play important roles).

What exactly makes a vein go varicose?

"The veins lose their elasticity," says Luis Navarro, M.D., founder and director of the Vein Treatment Center and clinical instructor at Mount Sinai School of Medicine in New York City. "Valves in the veins sometimes become weak, so that blood cannot be effectively pumped back toward the heart. Instead, it pools in the lower leg, stretching the vein and causing it to swell and bulge."

Your doctor can treat varicose veins using several methods, says Dr. Navarro.

Large veins can be removed surgically. Smaller veins qualify for sclerotherapy, wherein a chemical is injected into the vein, causing it to close up. Laser treatments work better on tiny varicose veins of the face than the leg.

If you're not ready for surgery, here are some treatments you can try at home that may reduce symptoms or halt progression.

Horse chestnut. Available in tincture form at health food stores, this herb can really improve stressed veins by helping strengthen and repair blood vessels that have lost their elasticity, says Mindy Green, director of education at the Herbal Research Foundation in Boulder, Colorado. Studies have shown that taking 250 to 312.5 milligrams of the standardized extract twice daily is effective in relieving symptoms. Taking 600 milligrams of horse chestnut whenever your legs will be in a stressful situation, such as walking all day in the heat or sitting through a long flight, will help prevent swelling. Don't try homemade concoctions of horse chestnut. It's toxic at high doses. So use only the manufactured form, where strength is carefully controlled. Horse chestnut may interfere with the action of other drugs, especially blood thinners such as warfarin (Coumadin). It may also irritate the gastrointestinal tract. Do not use horse chestnut during pregnancy or while nursing.

Butcher's broom. This herb contains natural steroid-like compounds that decrease inflammation and constrict blood vessels. It helps shrink varicose veins by strengthening and constricting the walls of the vein, according to Green. She suggests taking 16 to 33 milligrams of standardized extract or tincture three times a day.

Garlic, cayenne, and ginger. These aid in improving circulation, so if you have varicose veins, include them in your diet as often as possible, suggests Green.

Helpful Hint: Foods rich in flavonoids are believed to increase the tone of the veins, especially the walls. You'll find flavonoids in red wine and in fruits and vegetables that are brightly colored.

What Else You Can Do

Try water therapy. In the shower, or using compresses, alternate between applications of comfortably hot and cold water on your legs, suggests Green. Gradually switch temperatures at 1- to 3-minute intervals and repeat three times. The changing temperature will expand and contract the blood vessels and get pooled blood moving.

Make sure you get plenty of fiber in your diet. Drink plenty of water, too. Together, they're your best strategies for staying regular. Chronic constipation can lead to varicose veins, since "pushing" during a bowel movement puts extra pressure on the valves in your legs.

TAKE A CUE FROM FLIGHT ATTENDANTS

Being crammed into a tiny airline seat, barely able to move, causes the blood in your legs to pool, resulting in swelling and puffiness, especially if you have varicose veins.

Next time you take to the skies, don a pair of support hose first. One study at Johns Hopkins University in Baltimore and UCLA School of Medicine showed that flight attendants who wore support hose or graduated compression hose experienced far less swelling, fatigue, and aching in their legs.

Redouble your efforts to exercise. Thirty minutes of activity three times a week will help strengthen the muscles of your legs and increase venous circulation. ■

Vegan Diets

Busy Women Can Go All Vegetarian

A growing body of evidence suggests that the fewer animal foods we eat, the better. A study done at Georgetown University in Washington, D.C., for example, found that men and women with non-insulin-dependent diabetes who ate a low-fat diet consisting exclusively of vegetables, grains, and other plant foods (no meat, eggs, or dairy) reduced their blood sugar significantly, despite reduced or discontinued use of their medication. And they lost an average of 16 pounds each. They fared better than those on a very low fat diet that contained meat and dairy food.

Other research suggests that, chosen wisely, low-fat, all-vegetarian diets yield other benefits, including protection against high blood pressure, heart disease, and cancer, among other health problems.

Coined in 1944, the word vegan *(vee-gun) means a philosophy of compassionate living that includes a totally plant-based diet. Like other vegetarians, vegans eat no meat, but they also abstain from products that come from or may have harmed an animal—from milk to gelatin—as a way to show compassion toward all living beings. So true veganism is a lifestyle, not just a diet. Vegans avoid leather shoes, fur coats, snakeskin handbags, and the like.*

If you're interested in trying a vegan diet—or your teenage son or daughter suddenly announces that he or she is swearing off all animal products—it doesn't have to turn your life upside down, says Joanne Stepaniak, author of The Vegan Sourcebook *and* The Uncheese Cookbook.

While it may be difficult to avoid every last iota of animal product in your life, you can avoid the major animal foods and by-products, says Stepaniak. Here are some ways to follow a vegan diet.

Stick with your old favorites. Fill your kitchen with pastas, tomato sauces, canned and dry beans, grains, fresh fruits and vegetables, breads, peanut butter, nuts, and seeds.

Seek out meat substitutes. "For most foods that people are familiar with, there are now vegan options, and they're incredible," Stepaniak says. Many supermarkets sell at least some form of vegetable-based meat alternatives, which can resemble ground beef, burgers, sausage, bacon, or cold cuts. Products like "veggie ground round" look, feel, and taste so much like the real thing, you can use them in tacos, spaghetti sauce, curries, and other dishes, and you'll never know the difference.

Try nondairy milks and cheese substitutes. You can also replace cow's milk in your glass, cereal bowl, and recipes with milk made from soybeans, rice, nuts, or grains. Some stores carry vegan substitutes for cheese, cream cheese, and Parmesan, as well as yogurt and sour cream, says Stepaniak.

Help yourself to Toffuti. If you love ice cream and want to go vegan, try Tofutti, a totally soy-based ice cream sold in most supermarkets. It looks and tastes like the real thing, yet it contains no animal products at all.

Try tofu, tempeh, or seitan. Use firm tofu—blocks of white cheese made from soy milk curds—in stir-fries and soups, and silken tofu, which is creamier, in shakes, puddings and other soft foods. If you buy water-packed tofu that's refrigerated at the store, be sure to change the water daily after you open the package, and it will stay fresh for 5 to 7 days. Tempeh is made from fermented soybeans, while seitan is a chewy food made of wheat gluten, and both can take the place of meat in recipes.

Check for these at your supermarket or natural-foods store.

Read labels for traces of animal products. Watch out for ingredients like calcium stearate, casein, lactose, lactic acid, oleic acid, stearic acid, suet, tallow, and whey. These animal substances are hidden in a wide variety of processed foods.

Helpful Hints

Generally speaking, vegan alternatives to meats, dairy foods, and condiments will keep as long in the refrigerator or freezer as their animal-based counterparts. Some nondairy milks come in "drink boxes"—like aseptic packages, which you can keep unrefrigerated for several months. Once you open them, though, they must be refrigerated. ■

Vegetable Oils

The Best Way to Lubricate Your Food

If you squeezed a turnip hard enough, you could squeeze out a tiny speck of oil. In fact, most of the plants we eat contain at least a trace of oil, and some yield enough of it to bottle and sell at the supermarket.

You won't find turnip oil on the shelves. But you will find oil from olives, peanuts, corn, soybeans, safflower, sunflowers, sesame seeds, walnuts, grapeseed, flaxseed, and even coconuts. Most are some combination of three different types of oil—monounsaturated, polyunsaturated, and saturated (so named because of their chemical makeup). Olive oil, for example, has a lot of monounsaturated fat (77 percent) and comparatively little saturated fat (14 percent). Coconut oil, by contrast, has very little monounsaturated fat (6 percent) and quite a bit of saturated fat (92 percent, even more than lard).

The proportions of each oil make a big difference in how healthy they are for you and how you can cook with them. Oils that are high in saturated fats, like coconut and palm, are the hardest on your body—they tend to raise blood levels of cholesterol, increasing your risk of heart disease. They're found mostly in processed foods and have little reason to be in your kitchen, says Jane Rubey, R.D., a California dietitian who educates through her Nutritiously Gourmet Web site.

On the other hand, oils that are high in *un*saturated fats ››

SURFING THE SLIPPERY SMORGASBORD OF OILS

Oils supply a fair amount of calories. But chosen smartly, vegetable oils can add valuable nutrients, like omega-3 fatty acids, to your diet. And they make other healthy foods—like tomatoes, greens, stir-fried vegetables, and whole wheat pasta—taste better. Here's what various oils have to offer. You should keep your daily intake of oil at or below 1 teaspoon of oil. Omega-3 fatty acids make up a portion of the polyunsaturated fats in an oil, so the percentage of omega-3's represents a percentage of the polyunsaturated fat rather than a percentage of the total fat.

OILS	% MONOUNSATURATES	% POLYUNSATURATES	% SATURATES	% OMEGA-3 FATTY ACIDS
Top Choices				
Hazelnut	82	10	8	0
Olive	77	9	14	0.63
Canola	62	31	7	9.73
Peanut	48	34	18	0
Sesame	42	43	15	0.3
Walnut	24	66	10	10.92
Flaxseed	21	68	11	55.8
Use Occasionally*				
Corn	25	62	13	0.73
Soybean	24	61	15	7.1
Grapeseed	17	73	10	0.1
Avoid				
Coconut	6	2	92	0

SOURCE: USDA Nutrient Database

*Safflower and sunflower oils should also be used only occasionally, but actual values vary from manufacturer to manufacturer. Check labels for nutrition information.

can improve the cholesterol in your blood. Monounsaturated fat lowers the "bad" LDL cholesterol in your blood that forms plaques on your artery walls. To some degree, polyunsaturated fats lower cholesterol, too, but they also lower the "good" HDL cholesterol that can slow the growth of plaques. So even among vegetable oils low in saturated fat, some are better for you than others. Sunflower seed oil and nut oils, for example, are good sources of vitamin E, an antioxidant that protects the heart.

As a bonus, some vegetable oils—notably canola and walnut oil—are high in omega-3 fatty acids, which seem to protect against a host of diseases, including cancer, heart disease, depression, asthma, even Alzheimer's disease. In contrast, soybean, safflower, grapeseed, and corn oils contain omega-6 fatty acids, which hinder the work of omega-3's when consumed in excess.

All things considered, your best bet is avoid coconut oil, use corn, safflower, grapeseed, and soybean oils sparingly, and focus on oils high in monounsaturates, omega-3's, and vitamin E. Here's how.

Olive and canola oil. If you're going to use just two oils, stick with these, Rubey says. Both are high in monounsaturated fat. As a bonus, canola oil is also a source of omega-3 fatty acids, which may also help cut your risk of heart attacks by making your blood less sticky and likely to form clots in your bloodstream.

How you use them is a matter of taste. Extra-virgin olive oil is more expensive, strong-tasting, and sensitive to heat, so use it just as a flavoring instead of in cooking. On the other hand, canola oil and the virgin and light olive oils have a blander taste and are suitable for stir-frying and cooking.

Peanut oil. This oil is about half monounsaturated and one-third polyunsaturated. It has a high smoking point and holds up well in high-temperature cooking, like stir-frying.

Nut and seed oils. You can give sauces and salad dressings a rich zing of flavor with a bit of sesame, walnut, or hazelnut oils, which vary from oil to oil in their balance of poly- and monounsaturates. Since these oils have a strong flavor and don't hold up well in high temperatures, drizzle small amounts of them over a salad or other cold dishes.

Flaxseed oil. Though rich in omega-3's, flaxseed oil is difficult to use because it goes rancid very quickly. Rubey recommends purchasing flaxseeds in small quantities, grinding them in a coffee grinder, and baking them in muffins or other foods that will conceal their gritty texture.

DON'T MAKE THESE MISTAKES

While some oils are better for you than others, all oils contain 120 calories per tablespoon. So if you're watching your total fat and calorie intake, don't go hog wild.

And don't be fooled by the term "hydrogenated vegetable oil" on food labels. Hydrogenation solidifies any vegetable oil, converting it into the equivalent of lard.

Helpful Hint

When oils get warm stored in your pantry, they can lose some of their nutrients, including vitamin E and omega-3's, and turn rancid. Buy your oils in small bottles and keep them in your refrigerator. Some, like olive oil, will solidify when they're cool. You can pour them into a widemouth jar and just spoon out what you need, Rubey suggests. It will liquefy again as it warms. ■

Vegetables

How to Sneak "Three-a-Day" into Your Diet

Most women eat plenty of vegetables. More often than not, though, we're eating french fries, potato chips, and iceberg lettuce, which supply far fewer vitamins, minerals, and other health-building nutrients than dark green and deep yellow vegetables like broccoli and squash.

It makes some nutritionists gnash their teeth.

"There are so many vegetables to choose from," says Megan McCrory, Ph.D., a research associate at Tufts University's Energy Metabolism Laboratory in Medford, Massachusetts. From artichokes to yams, vegetables yield a multitude of benefits: Vegetables are a key source of essential vitamins and minerals, such as beta-carotene and other carotenoids, vitamin C, and potassium. Cruciferous vegetables such as broccoli contain phytochemicals. Among those are a number of protective plant substances that enhance your body's ability to eliminate the cancer-causing chemicals you encounter daily.

Eating your vegetables may even help you lose weight. One study found that people who eat a greater assortment of vegetables tend to be leaner.

No wonder nutrition experts recommend we eat at least three vegetable servings a day.

Yet for a lot of women, that's easier said than done.

"Some don't like the taste of vegetables," explains Susan Lutz, R.D., Ph.D., who has researched ways to successfully encourage people to eat more fruits and vegetables. "If you buy fresh produce, it can spoil before you have a chance to eat it. For others, it never even crosses their minds to try to eat more veggies."

The key to eating more vegetables is to think beyond dinner, and work vegetables into your diet at every meal—and in between, suggests Dr. Lutz. Here's what she suggests.

Breakfast

Vege-size your omelette. Put diced tomatoes and peppers, cut broccoli, or other veggies in your morning omelette.

Anytime

Opt for vegetable juice. In one study, women who drank carrot, tomato, or vegetable juice had higher blood levels of certain protective carotenoids (such as alpha-carotene and lutein) than women who ate equivalent amounts of raw or cooked vegetables. The researchers suggest that these vitamins may be more easily absorbed in juice than in either raw or cooked vegetables.

Lunch

Start with a salad. If you must choose fast food, hold the fries and get a salad instead.

Pile extra tomatoes and lettuce on your sandwich. And make it romaine. Dark leafy greens have seven times as much beta-carotene as iceberg lettuce.

Snacks

Make extras for Mom. If you're trying to get your kids to eat more vegetables, remember that you should try, too. "When you pack small bags of cut carrots and other bite-size vegetables for school lunches or snacks, pack a bag for yourself too," says Dr. Lutz. Then if you get the munchies between meals, snack on veggies first instead of chips or cookies.

Dinner

Pile steamed veggies on your pizza. Ask for extra mushrooms and peppers instead of sausage and pepperoni. Even better, try broccoli florets, chopped spinach, and roasted peppers. Or have a salad with your piece of pizza.

Don't reserve sweet potatoes for Thanksgiving. Bake, boil, mash, or oven-fry these instead of white potatoes.

Stir vegetables into sauces and soups. Try adding grated carrots to spaghetti sauce or lasagna. "You won't even know they're there," says Dr. Lutz. Mix chopped cauliflower or broccoli into your favorite soups. Stir a few tablespoons of plain canned pumpkin into soups as a thickener.

Sprinkle broccoli sprouts on salads. Half a cup of these sprouts have 20 times the cancer-fighting power of broccoli, says Jed Fahey, faculty research associate in the Brassica Chemoprotection Laboratory at Johns Hopkins University School of Medicine in Baltimore.

Helpful Hints

Research shows that if you have more of a variety of foods available, you'll eat more than if you have limited options. The same applies to vegetables. If you keep a variety of veggies around the house, you'll eat more of them because you won't get tired of the same taste. What's more, it's believed that the disease-fighting nutrients found in various vegetables work synergistically: You're better off eating a lot of different vegetables than sticking to a few standards week in and week out.

So visit farmers' markets, says Dr. Lutz. "Vegetables are so fresh and displayed so lavishly at farmers' markets that it makes you want to eat more of them." And try one new vegetable a week. You'll discover new favorites and possibly boost the phytochemical power of all the fruits and vegetables you eat. ■

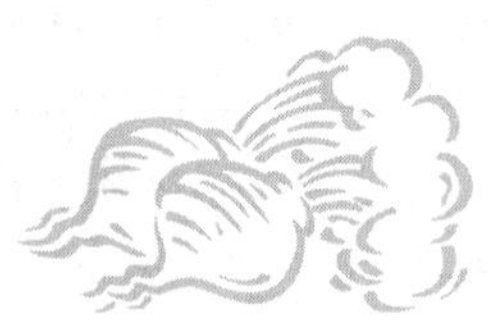

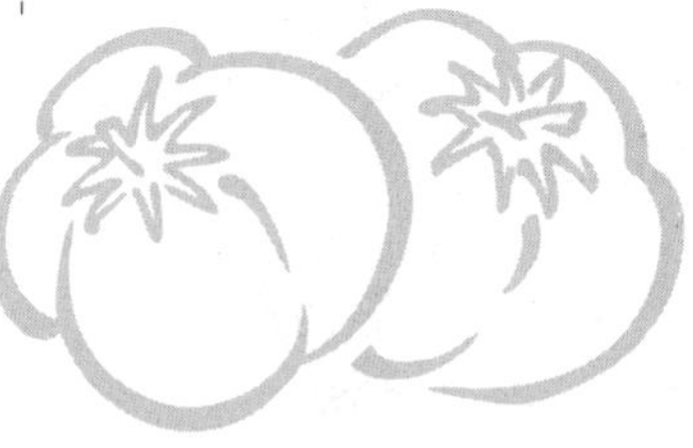

Vegetarian Diet

10 Meatless Meals Your Family Will Love

Mealtime just wasn't the same for Vesanto Melina after she became a vegetarian in the late 1970s. Once she turned away from pork chops, burgers, and holiday turkey, she found that her diet offered nothing but sheer . . . variety.

As she shared meals with vegetarian friends, she discovered Indonesian and Mediterranean dishes. She learned to love lentils and packed her pantry with new products.

A registered dietitian in Vancouver, Melina emphasizes that becoming vegetarian doesn't mean living on grains and salads. She has written two cookbooks to prove it: Becoming Vegetarian *with Brenda Davis and Victoria Harrison and* Cooking Vegetarian *with chef Joseph Forest.*

Women decide to cut down on meat—or eliminate it altogether—for various reasons. Some want to cut down on animal fats, which are associated with an increased risk of heart disease and cancer. Others object to consuming meat for moral, philosophical, or religious regions. Some are worried about antibiotics and hormones used to raise commercial meats. Some eat meat themselves but are trying to accommodate a teenage son or daughter who suddenly announces they're going vegetarian.

If you decide to part ways with meat for whatever reason, try these easy-to-make meatless versions of standard fare.

1. Serve veggie burgers on whole grain Kaiser rolls, topped with lettuce and tomato, accompanied with potato salad. Many supermarkets carry a wide variety of heat-and-eat meatless burgers made from mushrooms, vegetables, beans, soy, wheat, or a combination of ingredients.

2. Spear cherry tomatoes, mushrooms, and red and green peppers into a veggie kabob and cook it on the grill. For protein, you can also stick on cubes of firm tofu or tempeh (a fermented soy product) that have been marinated in teriyaki sauce. Serve with rice.

3. Stir-fry sliced onion, carrots, broccoli, and chickpeas in a skillet in a bit of vegetable oil and season with soy sauce, ginger, and honey. Serve over brown rice or noodles.

4. Cook a pot of spicy, tasty chili. Use pinto or kidney beans, canned tomatos, chili powder, and cumin—your usual recipe—but instead of meat, toss in soy crumbles, which look like browned ground beef. Serve with crusty whole grain bread and a salad.

5. You can make tacos with soy crumbles instead of meat. Heat the crumbles in a skillet with taco seasoning, then scoop them into tortillas or hard taco shells with shredded dairy

DON'T MAKE THIS MISTAKE

Opting for cheese instead of meat is one way to get protein and calcium. But don't go overboard, or you'll inadvertently load up on fat and calories, cancelling out some of the benefits of going meatless. Save full-fat cheese for special occasions, and use reduced-fat versions on a daily basis.

cheese or soy cheese, cubed avocado, diced tomatoes, bits of lettuce, and sprouts.

6. Build a Mediterranean-style meal around hummus, a dip made of ground chickpeas and sesame seed paste that many supermarkets carry premade. Serve the hummus with wedges of pita bread, accompanied with minestrone or vegetable soup.

7. Roll up a soft tortilla filled with black bean stew, rice, salsa, and cilantro.

8. Load tomato sauce with vegetables like onions, garlic, carrots, mushrooms, sweet green peppers, and zucchini, along with cooked red lentils for protein and basil and oregano for flavor. Serve over pasta.

9. Prepare an easy one-pot soup. Start by heating some scallions and fresh ginger, garlic, curry powder, and cumin seeds in a little oil in a saucepan. Add ½ cup red lentils, 2 cups vegetable stock, and a can of stewed tomatoes and simmer for 40 to 45 minutes, or until the lentils are tender. Stir in some thyme (fresh or dried), and a spoonful of white vinegar. Simmer for 10 minutes longer. Serve with whole wheat bread.

10. Mix together black beans, corn, cilantro, chopped tomatoes, onion, and some ground cumin. Use it as a topping for a baked potato. If you'd like, add a little grated low-fat Cheddar cheese and microwave it until the cheese melts. ■

Visualization

Create Your Own Healing Image

Laurie Nadel, Ph.D., used to be a TV news writer in New York City. At age 38, she was struck by debilitating chronic fatigue. She had memory loss, constant sore throats, fever, and brief spells of unconsciousness. She couldn't drive for a year and could barely take a shower. "My immune system had broken down. There was nothing doctors could do," says Dr. Nadel. No longer able to work, she went on disability pay.

A board certified doctor of clinical hypnotherapy, Dr. Nadel asked her unconscious mind for an image of why she was sick. "I saw this picture like a cartoon—my cells were walking around with picket signs, saying, 'We're on strike!'" She realized that her body was overloaded with stress and fatigue. Aided by meditation, visualization, and nutrition, she released enough stress to heal.

A few years later, she developed severe adult-onset asthma. Again, she used visualization to help heal her body. "Sometimes the asthma comes back, but it isn't crippling," says Dr. Nadel.

Now a psychotherapist specializing in mind/body therapies for stress-related conditions, Dr. Nadel helps others learn visualization and other techniques that helped her heal.

Visualization may help trigger healing in some types of diseases, says integrative medicine specialist Andrew Weil, M.D., director of ›› the program in integrative medicine and clinical professor of internal medicine at the University of Arizona College of Medicine in Tucson. "Visualization and guided imagery work with the connection between the visual brain and the involuntary nervous system," he says. "When this portion of the brain is not occupied with input from the eyes, it seems to be able to influence physical and emotional states."

Healing visualizations help relax you and reduce the stress and emotional turmoil that make symptoms worse, says Dr. Nadel. The immune system can function better, rebalance, and produce healthy new cells where needed. Visualization can also be helpful for unblocking feelings of helplessness. "Sometimes, when you're very sick and can't do anything physically, shifting to your inner world helps you feel unstuck," says Dr. Nadel.

Here are Dr. Nadel's steps for creating your own healing visualization.

1. Get in a calm, relaxed state. To do that, remember a time when you felt calm and relaxed and imagine you are there again.

Vitamin C

Your All-Day Pollution Shield

Back in grade school, we all learned that scientists discovered our need for vitamin C by accident, when British sailors deprived of fresh fruits and vegetables developed scurvy. Today, we need more vitamin C than ever. Vitamin C naturally battles toxins, fortifying us against cigarette smoke, exhaust fumes, smog, and other pollutants that—except for the occasional volcanic eruption—didn't exist back in the Stone Age.

"Smokers need more vitamin C than nonsmokers because what they are inhaling is essentially highly polluted air," says Robert A. Jacob, Ph.D., a research chemist for the USDA Western Human Nutrition Research Center.

Even if you don't live in a smog capitol like Los Angeles or spend hours in bumper-to-bumper traffic, you need vitamin C. This water-soluble antioxidant helps detoxify your system by activating glutathione, a sulfurlike antioxidant, inside the body. Antioxidants eliminate cell-damaging molecules known as free radicals.

"Vitamin C not only neutralizes free radicals by itself but it also works with glutathione to eliminate other potential toxins you might take in through food or drugs," adds Dr. Jacob. Vitamin C

DON'T MAKE THIS MISTAKE

Regularly taking doses in excess of 1,000 milligrams of vitamin C can cause diarrhea, nausea, abdominal cramps, and even kidney stones in people who are prone to them. If vitamin C seems to cause you trouble, take less.

2. Imagine that you're looking at a TV monitor at an image of the sick or injured part of your body. See what it looks like. (It doesn't have to be anatomically correct).

3. Say, "I want to talk to the part of me that knows how to heal. Show me an image of what needs to happen for my body to be healthy and what it will look like when it's healthy."

4. Make that healthy image the size of a postage stamp, superimposed on the unhealthy image.

5. Imagine that you have a remote control that shifts the two images so that the healthy postage-stamp image gets large, bright, and colorful, and the unhealthy image shrinks, becoming smaller and darker, until the healthy image replaces the unhealthy image.

Helpful Hints

You can enhance the effects of your visualization by drawing a picture of what is going on in your body before and after the visualization, suggests Dr. Nadel. ■

EASY WAYS TO LOAD UP ON VITAMIN C

The Daily Value for vitamin C is 60 milligrams. (You need 100 milligrams if you smoke.) You can easily meet those amounts and combat pollutants with these vitamin C–packed foods.

Papaya (1 medium, fresh)	187 mg
Yellow bell pepper (1 cup chopped, raw)	170 mg
Red bell pepper (½ cup chopped, raw)	141 mg
Peaches (½ cup sliced, frozen)	117 mg
Cantaloupe (½, fresh)	116 mg
Hot green chile pepper (1 raw)	109 mg
Orange juice (¾ cup, fresh)	93 mg
Orange (1 medium)	69 mg
Cranberry juice cocktail (¾ cup, bottled)	67 mg
Grapefruit juice (¾ cup, fresh)	62 mg
Broccoli (½ cup, cooked)	58 mg
Strawberries (½ cup sliced, fresh)	47 mg

also helps your immune system protect you against infectious and chronic illnesses.

Pound for pound, women need less vitamin C than men. That's because vitamin C is used by muscle, not fat, and since women typically have less muscle mass, we need less vitamin C to derive the same benefits. However, Dr. Jacob recommends that women and men both get at least 60 milligrams of vitamin C a day. Smokers should get 100 milligrams a day.

Helpful Hint

Your body can absorb only so much vitamin C at a time. So if you take supplements, try to spread out the amount of vitamin C you take throughout the day. ■

Vitamin D

The "Other" Bone-Friendly Hormone

Way back in 1922, at the University of Wisconsin in Madison, professor Elmer McCollum discovered vitamin D in cod liver oil, earning himself the title "Father of Vitamin D." More than 70 years later, vitamin D is still a hot research topic on the Madison campus, where three generations of scientists have studied the nutrient.

Leading the latest wave of researchers is Hector DeLuca, Ph.D., chair of the biochemistry department, who has studied vitamin D since 1951. More than four decades later, he remains intrigued by this vitamin and its benefits in the body.

Technically, vitamin D is a hormone, not a vitamin, says Dr. DeLuca. And while estrogen gets all the attention for protecting your bones, your body relies on vitamin D to fully absorb calcium, keep bones strong, and prevent osteoporosis. Vitamin D targets the intestines, the kidneys, and bones, which all respond by making calcium available for bone growth.

"In a sense, vitamin D acts like a chauffeur, driving calcium to where it is needed in the body," says Dr. DeLuca. "I believe all life originated in the sea where calcium was abundant. Today, we live on land, where calcium is not so abundant. I think vitamin D has evolved to help us with this calcium shortage."

DON'T MAKE THIS MISTAKE

Avoid taking more than the recommended amount of vitamin D. Taking large amounts—2,000 IU or more of vitamin D a day over several months—can cause high blood levels of calcium, kidney damage, and calcium deposits in the heart and lungs, and which can be fatal. And if you take combination calcium/vitamin D supplements, make sure you keep your daily calcium intake under 2,500 milligrams.

Even if you drink milk, eat yogurt or other calcium-fortified foods, and take calcium supplements, you need to make sure you're getting enough vitamin D—400 IU a day—especially in winter, says Dr. DeLuca. Your body uses sunlight to produce vitamin D. So spending as little as 10 minutes a day in the summer sun is enough to soak up a whole day's worth of D. Using sunscreen will interfere with the production of vitamin D, and sunblock will completely prevent it. Yet you don't want to forgo protection during peak hours. The best solution is to drink in those rays after 3:00 P.M. when the sun isn't so damaging, and wear sunblock the rest of the time.

If you live in northern areas of the country, squeezing out even 200 IU of vitamin D from the sun can be difficult, however. "If it's cold and snowy for weeks, and you don't get out, your vitamin D may be totally depleted by April," says Dr. DeLuca. Sunlight pouring through a window won't do because glass filters out the rays that you need most for vitamin D. To winterize your bones, he suggests that you:

Help yourself to salmon and mackerel. They're rich in vitamin D. You should also drink 2 cups of vitamin D–fortified milk a day.

Take a supplement that supplies calcium and vitamin D. If you're not sure you're getting enough vitamin D, Dr. DeLuca recommends taking a supplement once a day that provides 400 IU of vitamin D along with the recommended intake of 1,000 to 1,200 milligrams of calcium you need. ■

Vitamin E

Natural Supplements Are Twice as Good

A generation ago, vitamin C topped the Hit Parade of vitamins, says Maret Traber, Ph.D., associate professor in the department of nutrition and food management at Oregon State University in Corvallis. These days, vitamin E gets all the attention.

Dr. Traber ought to know: She is the principal investigator for the Linus Pauling Institute, and she rates vitamin E an "E for Excellent" when it comes to helping prevent heart disease and cancer. It can also clear the lungs of air pollutants—if you get enough, that is.

As premier member of a class of nutrients known as antioxidants, vitamin E protects your body against the harmful effects of oxidation by taking a spare electron from the harmful free radical molecules inside cells. In your lungs, vitamin E protects you against nitrogen dioxide, ozone, and other pollutants that can oxidize cells in your lungs, so you can breathe more easily.

The Daily Value for vitamin E is 30 IU, but medical experts who've studied the benefits of E recommend 100 to 200 IU a day—more than you can realistically expect to get from even the richest dietary sources. You'd have to eat 6 cups of peanuts or 39 cups of boiled spinach to get 100 IU.

DON'T MAKE THIS MISTAKE

Large doses of vitamin E may increase the risk of bleeding problems and lead to strokes. Before taking vitamin E supplements, check with your doctor, especially if you have high blood pressure, if you smoke, if you have had a stroke, or if you take blood thinners (anticoagulants) or regular doses of aspirin for a heart condition.

"Even in the healthiest of diets, we don't get enough vitamin E," says Dr. Traber. "So supplements are important."

Which vitamin E supplements are better: natural or synthetic? Several studies support the use of vitamin E in its natural form, d-alpha-tocopherol, over its synthetic ›› form, dl-alpha-tocopherol. For one thing, it's twice as active—you'd need 400 IU of synthetic vitamin E to equal 200 IU of natural vitamin E. **Your body also retains natural vitamin E three times as long as the synthetic,** which means that it can build up to and maintain higher levels of protection.

Natural vitamin E supplements start with the letter "d" such as "d-alpha-tocopherol." Synthetic vitamin E products start with the letters "dl."

Helpful Hint

Foods contain not one but eight types of vitamin E molecules—alpha-, beta-, gamma-, and delta-tocopherols, and alpha-, beta-, gamma-, and delta-tocotrienols. So even if you partially rely on supplements, experts say you should aim to include good sources of vitamin E in your diet: soybean, corn, and canola oils; avocados, peanut butter, wheat germ, and sunflower seeds. ■

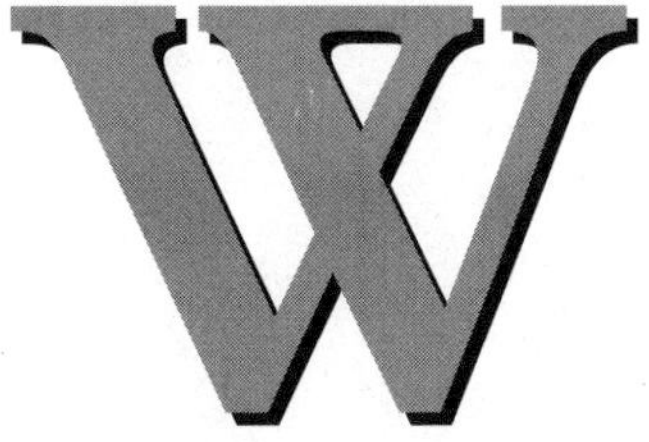

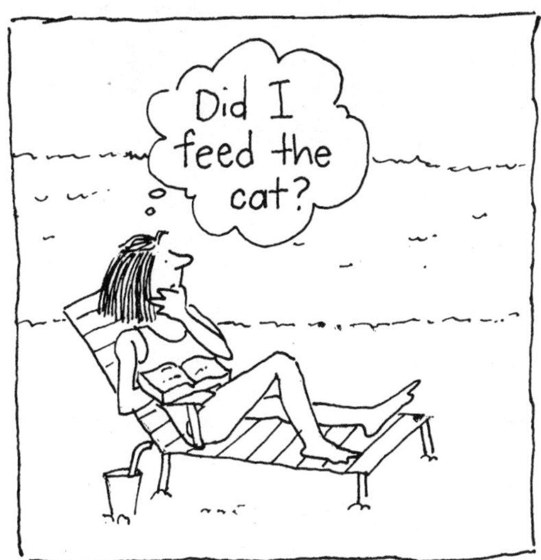

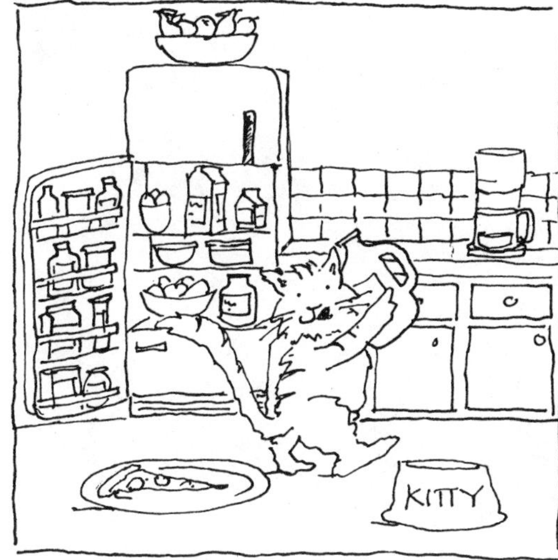

Worrying about things that are beyond your control?
For a 10-second cure, see page 477.

Walking

Get the Most Power Out of Your Daily Stroll

Looking for an easy, inexpensive, and low-risk fitness investment with the highest health returns? How about a super-efficient workout that burns a fair amount of calories instead of your precious time?

"Just put one foot in front of the other at a brisk pace," says Elaine Ward, managing director of the North American Race Walking Foundation and walking coach of the Southern Cal Walkers in Pasadena, California. Fitness walking is convenient, cheap, easy, and safe for just about everyone at any age. And walking for just 30 minutes a day, every day, delivers tremendous health and body benefits. Not only does it shave off pounds and cut your risk for cardiovascular disease, diabetes, cancer, and arthritis, it relieves stress, tones muscles, elevates mood, and boosts energy. (If you're fairly overweight and are accustomed to little or no exercise, it might be a good idea to get your doctor's okay before you get started.)

To get the most mileage out of your daily 30-minute walk (that is, to burn more calories per minute and give your whole body a better workout), follow these tips:

Shift out of the stroll mode and into high gear. Walk like a woman on a mission—or like you're on the verge of being late for an appointment (we all know what that feels like). That is, walk fast enough to break a sweat (or at least get a little clammy) and step up your heart rate, but not so fast that you can't carry on a conversation. If you're equipped with a pedometer and wristwatch, time yourself. If you're walking briskly, you might be able to log a mile in 15 minutes or less.

Do some fancy footwork. With each step you take, come down on your heel and push off with your toe. You'll tone and strengthen your shin and calf muscles and slim down your legs. This technique also will enable you to pick up the pace and burn more calories.

Head for the hills. "Walking hills at a safe pace will increase the intensity of your workout, just like walking faster on level ground," explains Ward. It revs up your body's fat-burning potential. Plus, it will strengthen and tone your hips, butt, quadriceps (muscles in front of your thighs), hamstrings (muscles in back of your thighs), and calf muscles, and boost your endurance.

Engage in speed play. Walk for 15 minutes at a brisk pace to warm up, then kick up your speed for 1 minute. Slow to your brisk pace for 2 minutes, then speed up for another minute. Repeat until you've completed 30 minutes.

Pump your arms. Moving your upper and lower body simultaneously makes for a high-intensity, vigorous aerobic activity.

Keep your shoulders down and relaxed. Bend your elbows at an 85-degree angle, close to your body. Your fists should be loosely closed. Know you have the right angle when you feel your thumb brush your waistband with each forward and backward stroke. ■

Warts

A Scientific Approach to Toady-Looking Bumps

Among the more bizarre folk remedies for warts is one that recommends rubbing the wart with a tadpole tail, then standing on a tree stump at night and letting the light of a half-moon fall on the wart so it will disappear. And of course, there's the opposing notion: That you can get warts from touching a frog.

"Neither is true, of course," says Seth Matarasso, M.D., a dermatologist in San Francisco. A wart is spread by a virus and, just like the virus that causes the common cold, it can't be cured by moonlight, tadpoles, or other superstitious notions. "But you can treat it symptomatically" and reduce your risk of contracting one, says Dr. Matarasso.

"First, recognize a wart for what it is, because the longer you leave a wart untreated, the bigger it will grow," he says. A wart tends to be a dry and craggy or highly irregular growth. Here's what to do.

• Soak the area where the wart appears in tepid water, then take a pumice stone or an emery board and file it down. "That will help create a hostile environment, encouraging the wart virus to regress," says Dr. Matarasso.

• Apply Compound W or a similar over-the-counter wart treatment, which will cause the wart to blister, scab, and fall off. Simply wash the skin where the wart appears, then dry it. Apply the applicator to the wart and let dry.

Repeat daily or twice a day until the wart disappears, but for no more than 12 weeks. Warts that are unresponsive to over-the-counter products may not actually be warts. If there is no response within a few weeks, see your dermatologist.

• If the wart persists, or you want a faster-acting treatment, consult a dermatologist. Most will perform an in-office procedure, called cryosurgery, in which they freeze the wart with liquid nitrogen, causing it to turn white, blister, scab, and fall away. The treatment is likely to sting for a moment, but it is effective.

To reduce the risk of contracting a wart:

• Wash your hands frequently, especially in public places. "This will reduce your exposure time to the virus in case you got it from someone else," says Dr. Matarasso.

• Use a moisturizer. This will help eliminate the tiny lacerations that come with dry skin and can serve as a port-of-entry for the virus.

• Keep your cool. "Warts like warm, moist areas," says Dr. Matarasso. After exercising, take off your shoes and socks so that your feet can dry. Or use a foot powder in your sneakers. ■

DON'T MAKE THIS MISTAKE

Because warts are unsightly, you may be tempted to be overzealous in your use of over-the-counter wart treatments. These products contain acid, which can seriously damage your skin if overused. Thoroughly wash off any wart compound after use, and rub the dead tissue away before reapplying.

Water

Simple Ways to Get Eight Glasses a Day

In a world where change has become the status quo, there's one piece of health advice that has remained constant: Drink eight 8-ounce glasses of water every day.

"Water is necessary for every single function in your body," says Barbara Dixon, R.D., nutrition educator in Baton Rouge, Louisiana. It boosts your energy. It prevents headaches, constipation, urinary tract infections, and kidney stones. It regulates body temperature, sharpens your concentration, and can help you lose weight. By drinking eight 8-ounce glasses of ice water a day, your body will burn an extra 123 calories while it warms it up to a cozy 98.6°F.

"Water is responsible for healthy hair and a glowing complexion," Dixon adds. "So the next time you water your favorite plant, take time out to drink some water yourself, because you're just as fragile as your plant."

Still haven't poured yourself a glass? Admittedly, drinking eight glasses a day can feel like a formidable task. So here are some simple, creative—and tasty—ways to ensure your daily water quota.

Start every workday with a liter of water on your desk—or, if you work at home, place the bottle in clear view on the kitchen counter. Be sure to drink every drop by 5:00 P.M. A liter contains 33.8 fluid ounces—that's just over four glasses.

Drink from a colorful water goblet. Each time the goblet catches your eye, drink up.

Include one or two 8-ounce glasses of iced or hot herbal tea, decaffeinated coffee, or milk in your daily water quota.

Carry an 8-ounce cup of water to all meetings. Make sure it's empty when the meeting adjourns.

DON'T MAKE THIS MISTAKE

Don't buy pre-sweetened bottled waters. What you'll end up with is a high-sugar, high-calorie drink.

Enjoy a light, low-sodium broth or non-cream-based soup for lunch or a mid-afternoon snack. Check your supermarket or health food store for many varieties of healthy soup in a cup. Just add boiling water to the cup and eat up.

If you have a morning commute, tote along an 8-ounce or 16-ounce bottle of water instead of that coffee travel mug. Drink it all before you reach your destination.

For a healthy alternative to soft drinks, mix 4 ounces of sparkling water with 4 ounces of 100 percent tropical fruit juice. Or, for an even lower calorie drink, squeeze a wedge of lemon, lime, or orange into a tall glass of sparkling water.

Drink one glass of water for every alcoholic beverage you sip. Every time you order a cocktail (or glass of wine or beer), order a glass of water » with a twist of lemon or lime. And when you motion for a refill, make it water, not alcohol.

Don't leave home without a 16-ounce bottle of water in your handbag or tote. Take a sip every chance you get.

Snack on fruit—especially the high-water varieties. Watermelon is the most obvious choice. But all melons, as well as grapes, pineapples, apples, oranges, and grapefruits are 85 to 95 percent water. So eat up and enjoy!

Drink a glass of water first thing in the morning and last thing before you go to bed.

Take a drink of water for at least 10 seconds every time you pass by a water fountain.

Spruce up your fluid intake with sugar-free bottled waters that contain fruit essences.

As you can see, getting your fill of the water you need each day isn't that difficult. Drinking a little water here and a little water there will eventually add up to 64 ounces before you even realize it. ■

Water Retention

A Natural Diuretic from Your Pantry

Feeling puffy a day or so before your period? Could be you're retaining water. During the last phase of your menstrual cycle, fluid that normally flows through the body in blood vessels sometimes gets trapped in the tiny spaces between cells, causing swelling—often most noticeable in the hands, feet, and ankles. This may also be the cause of breast tenderness. (Heart and circulatory problems, among other medical conditions, can also cause fluid retention, but that's beyond the scope of self-care.)

For simple, temporary water retention, Sharol Tilgner, N.D., a naturopathic physician and president of Wise Women Herbals in Creswell, Oregon, suggests sipping parsley seed tea. "Parsley is a diuretic, which means that it will help flush out the excess fluid in your system," says Dr. Tilgner.

To make the tea, steep ½ to 1 teaspoon of parsley seeds in a covered cup of boiling water for 20 minutes, let cool to a palatable temperature, and drink three times a day.

If the problem persists, consult your doctor. And don't use parsley seed tea if you have kidney disease or if you're pregnant—it may stimulate uterine contractions. ■

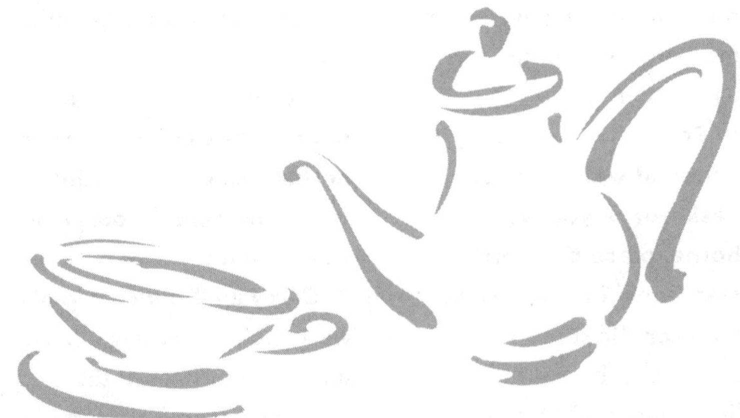

Weight Loss

Weird (but Safe) Diet Strategies

Here's a weight loss strategy you won't hear from your doctor: The next time you're ready to make a meal out of a carton of Häagen-Dazs, strip naked in front of a full-length mirror. Then study your thighs, hips, butt, and stomach while savoring every bite.

Unless you're built like Cindy Crawford, chances are that decadent treat will lose its appeal—fast.

Welcome to the world of unusual—and sometimes bizarre—weight loss strategies.

"Eating three sensible meals a day and avoiding crash diets are tried-and-true ways to lose weight," says Jan McBarron, M.D., a weight-control specialist and director of Georgia Bariatrics in Columbus, Georgia. "But to beat boredom and stay motivated, you sometimes need exciting, new ways to keep the weight off."

What follows is a smorgasbord of clever, zany, amusing, or downright weird weight-loss strategies from real women, offered with Dr. McBarron's blessing.

Wacky Ways to "Weigh" Yourself

- Stack magazines in the corner of your room, equivalent to the number of pounds you want to lose. For every pound you drop, remove one pound of magazines. As the weight disappears, so will the magazines.
- String paper clips together, each one representing a pound you want to lose. For every pound you shed, remove one paper clip. Begin a new chain of paper clips for the pounds you've lost. As you see the pounds-to-lose chain get shorter and the pounds-lost chain get longer, you'll stay motivated to slim down.
- Buy yourself a charm bracelet. For every 10 pounds you lose, buy a pretty charm as a reward.
- Put $1 in a piggy bank for every mile you walk, run, or cycle each day. At the end of 1 month, buy yourself some earrings or other clothing accessories.
- Buy a box of color-coated stars and a calendar. Stick a star on the calendar for each day you exercise. If you dropped the amount of weight you wanted to lose by week's end, give yourself a gold star.
- Wear a watch with a second hand when you eat dinner. Halfway through the meal, put your knife and fork down, place your hands on your lap, and don't touch another morsel for 60 seconds. Work up to doing this three to five times in one sitting. You may delay your meal by as long as 5 minutes, which will give your brain enough time to tell your stomach that it's full. And you won't overeat.
- Put on some pants and cinch a belt snugly around your waist before you sit down for dinner. When your waistband starts to dig into your stomach, stop eating. **››**

No-Sweat Motivators

• Hang a pair of your large-size jeans on or next to your refrigerator door. Whenever your willpower slips, let the jeans remind you of the size you no longer want to wear. Needless to say, another piece of cake won't look so tempting.

• Hang a pair of your dream-size shorts in front of your treadmill, stationary bike, or other exercise equipment. Whenever you work out, picture yourself wearing those sexy shorts when you achieve your goals.

• Plop a scale on the floor right in front of the goodie cupboard. Fattening treats won't look as scrumptious after you've stepped on the scale and crunched the numbers.

Burn Fat While You Cook

• While standing at the stove preparing dinner or waiting for something in the microwave, do half-knee bends to strengthen and tone your quadriceps and buttocks muscles. Do two or three sets of 10 repetitions as often as possible. "The more the better," says Dr. McBarron. Be sure to keep your feet shoulder-width apart, and make sure your knees don't extend over your feet.

• Spend 15 fast or 30 leisurely minutes on your treadmill or stationary bike while dinner is in the oven. You'll burn a fast 150 calories and keep your metabolism revved up while you eat your meal.

Work Out While You Clean House

• Do alternating lunges as you push your vacuum cleaner from room to room. Lunges will tighten and tone your quadriceps and buttocks muscles. For proper form, keep your knees in line with your heels.

• Even if you don't have two wicked stepsisters, scrub some floors for 20 minutes. You'll burn about 150 to 377 calories.

Goof Off, Lose Weight

• Do seated calf raises—the "bouncy horse"—with your child. A small child can work your calves to the max. Do two sets of 10 repetitions as often as possible throughout the week.

• Do telephone aerobics. Pace back and forth while gabbing on the phone with your girlfriend. Before you know it, 30 to 60 minutes will fly by, along with quite a few calories.

Fool Your Food

• Talk to your food. Ask that chunk of cheesecake or bag of potato chips, "Do I really want you badly enough to wear you on my hips, butt, and thighs?" Nine times out of 10, the answer will be *heck* no.

• Make a snack food your side dish. If you really crave potato chips, corn chips, popcorn, or a bite-size chocolate bar, eat it with part of your main meal, not as a meal in itself. More than likely, you'll eat a smaller portion of the main meal and will be less likely to binge on the snack later.

Make a Deal

• For every pound you lose in a week, ask your husband or

significant other to give you a massage, do your chores, or take you out for a night on the town. If you don't lose the weight, do the same for him.

• Buy yourself an outfit one size too small. Try it on once a week until it fits. The goal is to get into it in 4 weeks. Realistically, that's the shortest amount of time it takes to lose a dress size, says Dr. McBarron.

Sweat as You Samba

• Head to the music store and buy some dance music from a decade you loved. Pop in those CDs or cassette tapes and dance yourself silly for 30 minutes or more five times a week. You'll burn 200 to 300 calories or more a session as you relive the good ol' days.

• Take up ballroom dancing. Twirling around and shuffling your feet while doing the swing, cha-cha, fox-trot, waltz, tango, samba, and mambo can burn 200 to 300 calories or more in 30 minutes.

Can't dance? Take lessons. Dance classes are shimmying their way in to studios across the country more than ever before. ■

Weight Machines

The Right Way to Train

Your first encounter with a weight machine can be perplexing. Where does the metal pin go? How much weight should I lift? Do I have to use all *the machines, or just the ones that work my trouble spots?*

Relying on guesswork—or muddling through on your own—isn't the best approach to weight training. You could hurt yourself. What's more, if you don't work out correctly, you also miss out on some of the slimming benefits.

"Over the long run, those perks include improved muscle tone, loss of unwanted weight, and a higher metabolism—the rate at which your body burns calories during and after the workout," says Wayne Westcott, Ph.D., a strength training consultant to the American Senior Fitness Association and the National Youth Sports Safety Foundation. Weight training pays off in other ways, too. It helps prevent osteoporosis, reverses the loss of strength that women experience after age 25, lowers the risk of adult-onset diabetes, prevents lower-back problems, and can help relieve arthritis pain, says Dr. Westcott.

As with most skills, there's a right and a wrong way to weight train. Ideally, you should ask a certified weight training instructor to teach you how to use the weight machines and perform the exercises properly. Fitness experts warn against the 10 most common mistakes women make when using weight machines and explain what to do instead.

1. Skipping the warmup and stretch. Warming up and stretching reduce the risk of injuries and enable you to ›› lift more effectively. Walk briskly on a treadmill, pedal on a stationary bike, or jump rope for 5 minutes. Then, before the workout, stretch the muscles you're going to strengthen.

2. Lifting too much weight. Heavy weights can stress muscles, joints, and tendons and cause injury, says Dr. Westcott. Start by lifting the lightest weight on the stack.

If you can perform more than 12 repetitions with little or no effort, increase the weight in 1- or 2-pound increments until you can lift 8 to 12 repetitions with some effort, says Victoria Johnson, a certified personal trainer and president of Victoria Johnson International, a fitness consulting group in Portland, Oregon.

3. Lifting weights that are too light. Training against too little resistance won't build any muscle or increase your metabolism or calorie burn. Try the lightest weight first. If you don't feel resistance in the muscle you're targeting, increase the weight by 1- or 2-pound increments until you do. You know you're lifting the proper amount of weight

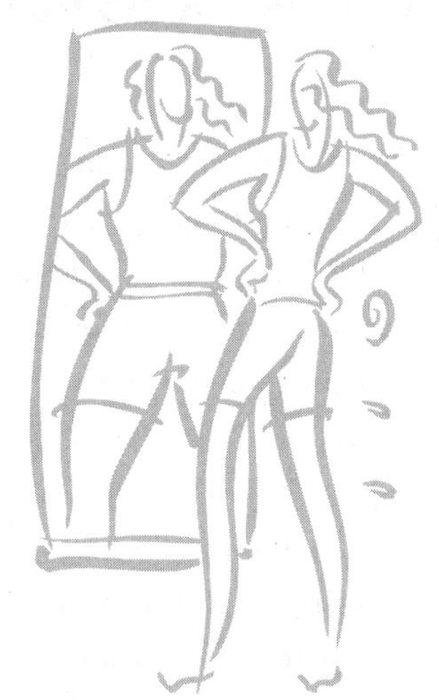

if your 10th repetition is tough to perform. If it's too easy, you need more weight.

4. Performing the exercises too fast. If you rush through the workout, you won't fully benefit from training, plus you run the risk of injuring your muscles and joints, completely sidelining your exercise regimen. Ask a trainer to coach you on how fast you should lift and how to coordinate your breathing with your repetitions, depending on your body type, joint flexibility, strength, arm and leg length, and height. Then work at the pace recommended for you.

5. Not completing the full range of motion. This usually happens when you're trying to lift too much weight—you don't follow through with the entire move. But if you cut the move short, your muscles will be stronger in one area and weaker in others. Switch to a lighter weight so you can complete a full range of motion.

6. Focusing on some muscles but neglecting others. This can cause muscle imbalances that can lead to injury. So strengthen opposing muscle groups. If you strengthen your abdominals, work your lower back; if you work your quadriceps (on the front of the thighs), don't forget your hamstrings (on the back of your thighs). Your workout should be aimed at strengthening and conditioning your whole body.

7. Drinking after your workout, but not before. Muscles that are well-hydrated can be trained more effectively. Drink at least one 8-ounce glass of water before, during, and immediately following the workout to sustain your energy, help build muscle strength, and keep cool.

8. Overdressing. Maybe you that think the more you sweat, the more calories you'll burn. (You won't.) Or maybe you work out in a heavy sweatsuit because you're self-conscious about your shape or size. Either way, you won't get as good a workout if you're overheated and uncomfortable, says Dr. Westcott. Instead, wear a sports bra plus a T-shirt and shorts or tights to keep cool while you train.

9. Working out on an empty stomach. Strength training takes effort, and effort takes fuel. You should eat a substantial but light snack about 20 to 30 minutes before the workout. A bagel, apple, yogurt, or banana are good choices.

10. Listening to music on headsets. Music can distract you from counting your repetitions, paying attention to form, and listening to your body. It hinders the overall quality of your workout. Instead, concentrate on your workout and do your best to focus on your exercise task at hand. ■

Weight Training

An At-Home Whole-Body Workout

Weight training can tone your muscles, strengthen your bones, and help you lose unwanted pounds. But it doesn't have to be a big production. You can work your whole body with a simple pair of lightweight dumbbells. They're inexpensive, portable, convenient, a cinch to store, and easy to use.

You can burn about 250 to 300 calories an hour while using dumbbells—just as many as you burn using a weight machine. And the more muscle you build, the more calories you burn—day and night.

"Adding just 2 to 3 pounds of muscle forces your body to burn at least an extra 70 to 105 calories a day over and above the calories you burn by doing the exercises," says Wayne Westcott, Ph.D., a strength training consultant to the American Senior Fitness Association and the National Youth Sports Safety Foundation.

All you need for this whole-body workout is a pair of 2- to 5-pound dumbbells and a weight bench. Then do the exercises on pages 468 to 471 in the order given. Start with two sets of 8 to 12 repetitions, two to three times a week. Once you can complete more than 12 reps easily, increase the weight in 1- to 2-pound increments.

Helpful Hint

Your muscles are 75 percent water. So make sure you drink at least one 8-ounce glass of water before, during, and immediately following your weight-training workout. Otherwise, you'll tire easily and won't build as much muscle, says Dr. Westcott.

If you develop pain in your joints, stop doing the exercise right away and check with your physician if the pain persists. Also, be sure to maintain proper posture while doing the exercises. Exhale when you lift the dumbbells and inhale when you lower them. Keep the dumbbells moving, and don't hold them in a forced position for more than a second or two. ››

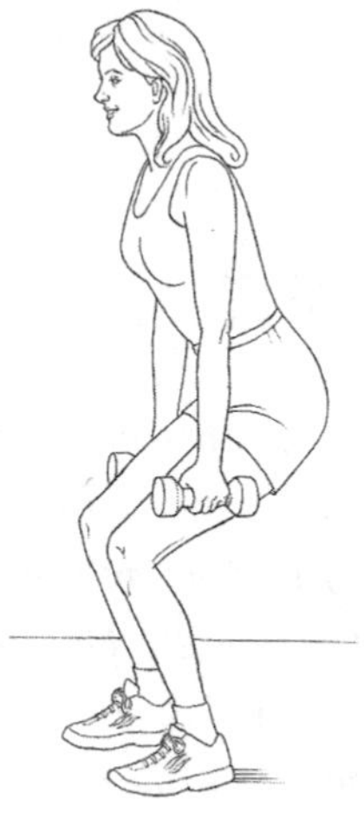

Dumbbell squat (strengthens your buttocks, hamstrings, and quadriceps muscles): Hold the dumbbells with your arms hanging at your sides, feet pointing forward and slightly wider than hip-width apart. Looking straight ahead and keeping your torso erect, bend your knees until your thighs are almost parallel to the floor, as if you were about to sit in a chair. Slowly rise back up to the starting position, pushing through your heels. Don't bend forward at the waist or round your back. Don't let your knees move out in front of your toes.

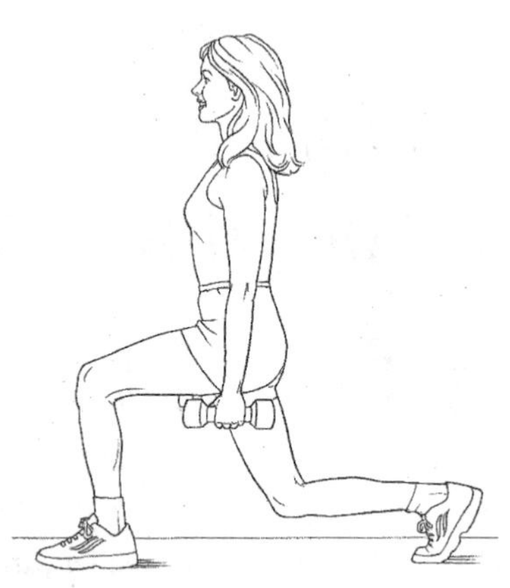

Forward lunge (also strengthens your buttocks, hamstrings, and quadriceps muscles): Stand holding your dumbbells with your arms hanging at your sides, feet hip-width apart. Look straight ahead and step forward with your left foot so that your knee is bent directly over your heel and your right leg is outstretched behind you. With your weight distributed evenly on both feet, bend your right knee until it almost touches the floor. Push off of your left foot and return to the starting position. Do one set, switch legs, and repeat. Remember to keep your torso erect throughout the lunge.

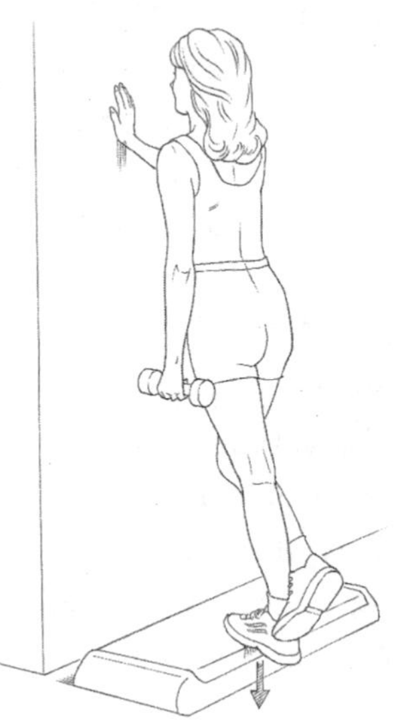

Single-leg calf raise (sculpts your calf muscles): On the edge of a 4- to 6-inch step, balance on the ball of your left foot, holding a dumbbell in your left hand; rest your right hand on a wall or other fixed object. Wrap your right foot around your left heel. Don't lock your knee. Slowly lower your left heel as far as you can without it touching the floor. Then, rise up as high as you can on your toes. Do one set, switch legs, and repeat. Don't let your ankle roll out as you rise up.

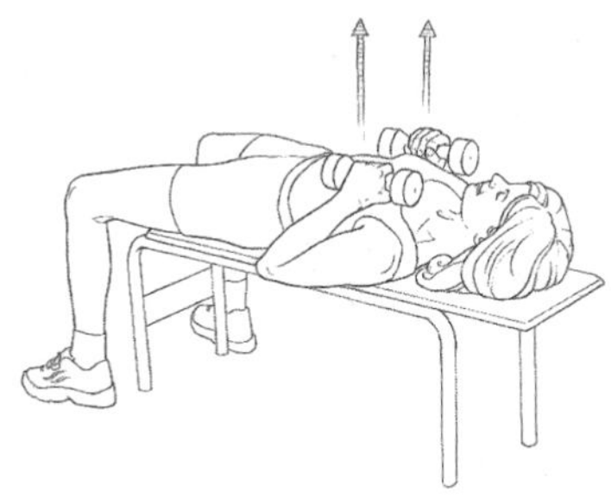

Dumbbell bench press (works the chest, triceps, and front shoulder muscles): Lie faceup on a bench with your abdominal muscles taut, knees bent, and feet flat on the floor. Hold your dumbbells with an overhand grip and extend your arms directly over your chest. Don't lock your elbows. Slowly lower the dumbbells until they are even with your chest, keeping your elbows in. Press back up to the starting position and repeat. To put extra emphasis on your upper chest, adjust your bench to a 45-degree incline. To strengthen your lower chest and give your breasts a lift, do the exercise while lying at a downward slant. Concentrate on contracting your chest muscles at the very top of the movement.

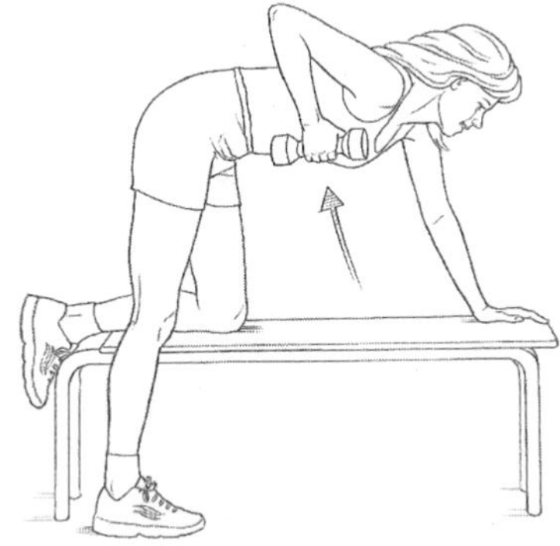

One-arm bent row (strengthens your upper and middle back, rear shoulder, and biceps muscles): Place your left knee on a bench so that your lower leg is supported. Bend at the hips until your chest is parallel with the bench. Support yourself with your left arm (elbow unlocked), and contract your abdominal muscles. Hold a dumbbell in your right hand with your palm facing you and your arm extended directly under your shoulder. Bend your right arm, leading with your elbow to lift the dumbbell to waist level. Slowly lower, do one set, switch arms, then repeat. When you lift, keep your arm and the dumbbell close to your body.

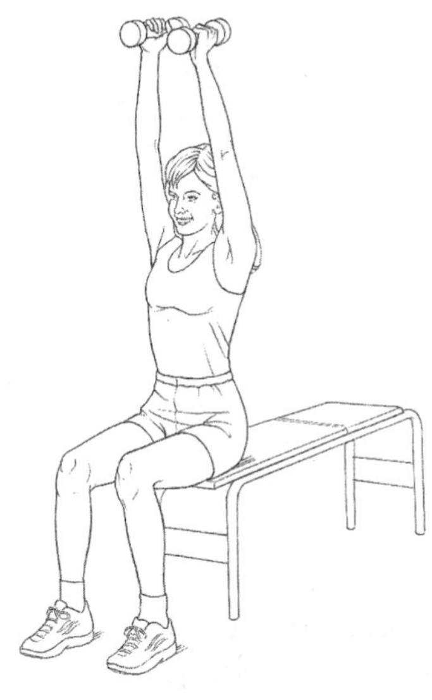

Shoulder press (works your middle- and front-shoulder and upper-back muscles): Sit on a bench with your feet flat on the floor. Hold the dumbbells at shoulder level, palms facing your body, elbows bent and pointing down. Squeeze your shoulder blades together, then press the weights up until your arms are straight but not locked and the weights are slightly in front of you. Lower them slowly to the starting position and repeat. ››

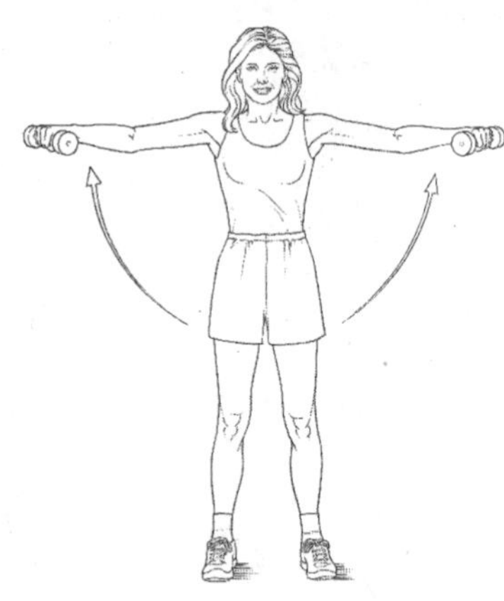

Lateral raise (works your middle- and front-shoulder muscles): Stand holding your dumbbells with your arms hanging at your sides, feet pointing forward and slightly wider than hip-width apart. With your palms facing your body, raise both dumbbells straight out from your sides until they're at shoulder level. Pause, then lower. Keep your elbows moderately bent.

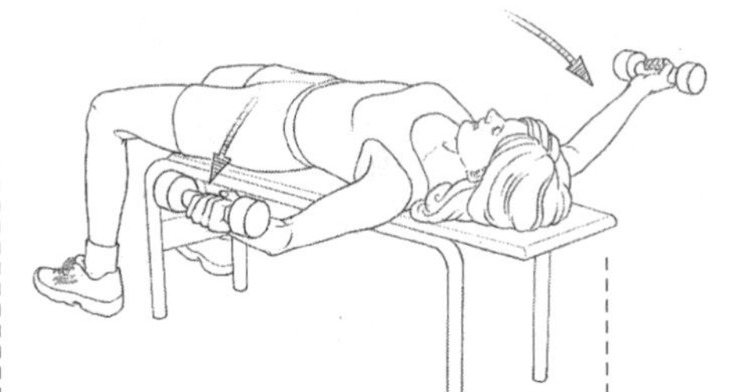

Chest fly (works chest and front-shoulder muscles): Lie on a bench with your legs more than shoulder-width apart and feet firmly on the floor. Hold two dumbbells above your chest, palms facing each other. Your dumbbells should be nearly touching each other above your chest. Your back should be straight and firm against the bench, with elbows unlocked. This is your starting position.

Slowly lower your dumbbells out and away from each other in a semicircle motion (as if you were hugging a tree). Keep your wrists straight. Lower until the dumbbells are just above chest level. Your elbows should be slightly bent, and your back should remain in contact with the bench. Slowly raise the dumbbells, again in a semicircle, to the starting position.

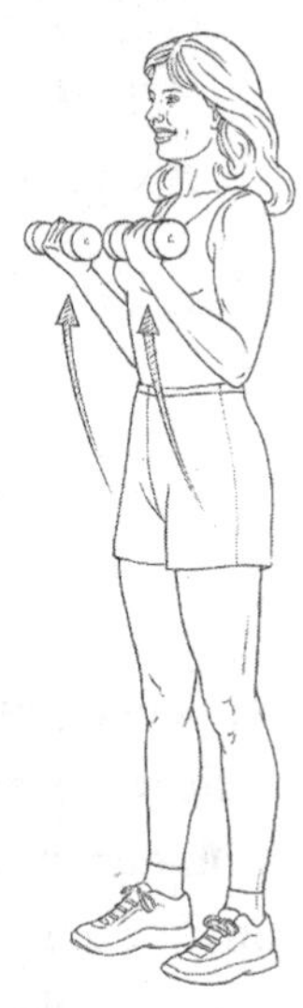

Biceps curl (strengthens your biceps muscle): Stand with your feet hip-width apart. Hold your dumbbells, palms facing your body. Let your arms hang at your sides. Bend your elbows and lift the weights to chest level, rotating your hands until your palms face your chest, keeping your elbows in place at your side. Slowly lower to the starting position, rotating your hands back to their original position. Repeat.

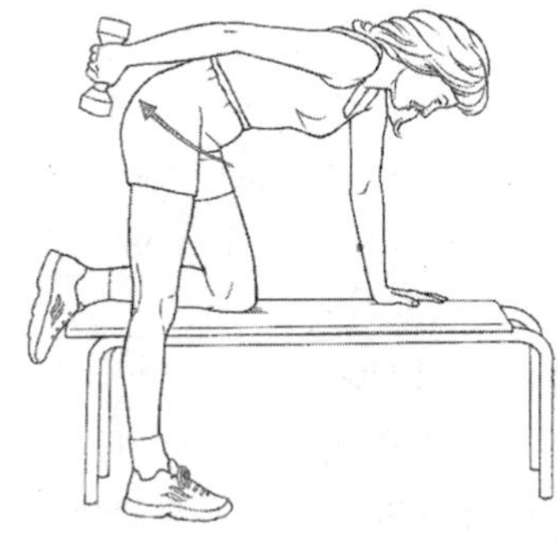

Triceps kickback (firms your triceps muscles): Place your left knee on a bench so that your lower leg is supported. Keeping your abdominals contracted, bend at the hips until your chest is parallel to the bench. Support yourself with your left arm (elbow unlocked). Hold a dumbbell in your right hand with your palm facing you. Bend your right arm and bring it up to rest lightly against the side of your waist. Keep your lower arm perpendicular to the floor. Straighten your lower arm behind you, keeping your shoulder, upper arm, and elbow in place. Return to the starting position. Do one set, switch arms, then repeat. ■

Wine

The Perfect Match

Wine lovers often select bottles based on taste, varietal, vintage, and sometimes, price. But the next time you buy wine, think "redder is better" and make a side trip down the candy aisle.

Wine and chocolate just may be the perfect combination for your heart.

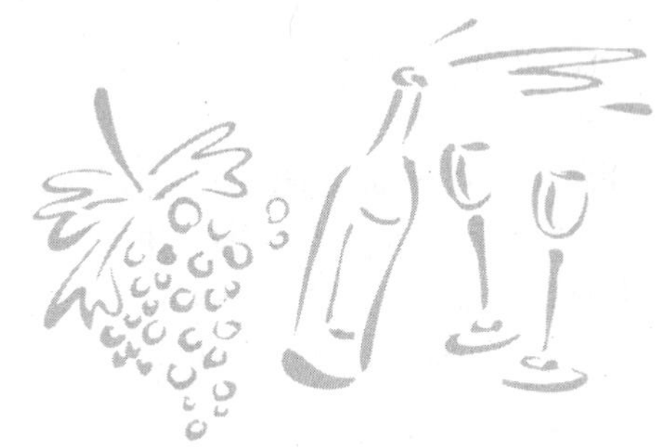

Research has found that both red wine and dark chocolate contain a type of antioxidant called phenolics, which have the ability to neutralize free radicals, unstable oxygen molecules that create harmful cholesterol. Over time, this damaged cholesterol clogs arteries, leading to blood clots and heart disease.

"While chocolate often gets a bum rap as a sinful food, our research suggests that a small piece of dark chocolate isn't going to hurt you. In fact, the antioxidants in it may help you," says Andrew J. Waterhouse, Ph.D., wine chemist and assistant professor in the department of viticulture and enology (wine making) at the University of California, Davis. "When combined with a glass of dark red wine, it may help you even more."

As a cofounder of the Scharffen Berger Chocolate Maker and a family practice physician in San Francisco, Robert Steinberg, M.D. is personally interested in the benefits of this interesting mix. He agrees that combining the advantageous ingredients in chocolate with those offered in red wine will result in a healthy dose of antioxidants.

All wines contain antioxidants, but dark red wines, ››

Winter Itch

The Best (and Worst) Time to Shower

Europeans think that Americans bathe to the point of obsession. We bathe to relieve stress, to soothe sore muscles, and to wash off the grime of exercise or the residue of a workday sweating out deadlines. And in our quest for cleanliness, skin can become a casualty. Women who take a couple of hot showers a day may notice that their skin is noticeably drier in winter, leaving them with a distinct crawly sensation known as winter itch.

"Bathing strips away the natural moisture in our skin," says Lieutenant Colonel Scott Norton, M.D., a dermatologist stationed with the U.S. Army at Fort Huachuca, Arizona, known for its desert dry air. "People don't realize that bath-water can actually dry out their skin."

In the winter, cold, dry outdoor air (or indoor heating systems) steal even more moisture from skin. Hot or cold, dry air makes the water in your skin cells evaporate. And as you age, your oil glands shrink, making you more susceptible to dry skin.

You don't have to give up bathing until April to soothe winter itch. Simply change the way you shower.

especially cabernet sauvignons, petite sirahs, and merlots, seem to offer higher levels. In laboratory tests, red wines can prevent anywhere from 46 to 100 percent of LDL cholesterol from oxidizing, far exceeding what white wines can do.

That's because red wines remain in contact with skins and seeds during the wine-making process longer than white wines. The skins and seeds contain the healthy phenolics.

For an interesting blend, Dr. Steinberg suggests this daily regimen:

- One 5-ounce glass of red wine
- One ounce of dark chocolate (about two-thirds of a standard size candy bar)
- One vitamin E capsule containing 400 IU

Dr. Steinberg adds, "the darker the chocolate, the better."

Helpful Hint

If you're not fond of red wine, drink purple grape juice. ■

DON'T MAKE THIS MISTAKE

More is *not* better!

Moderation is key, especially when it comes to drinking, says Dr. Waterhouse. Too much wine and chocolate will only cancel the health-rendering effects and can, in fact, create health problems, including cirrhosis, pancreatitis, obesity, and digestive problems.

Take only one 5-minute shower a day. The longer and more frequently you bathe, the more opportunities your skin has to lose moisture.

Turn down the heat. Hot water removes oil, so there's less to lubricate your skin. Lukewarm water will get you just as clean without drying out your skin as much.

Use a moisturizing or nonsoap cleanser. Many dermatologists recommend Dove, Purpose, or Cetaphil. Avoid unmoisturized, pure soaps or perfumed soaps—dermatologists say they're too harsh and drying.

Lather only where needed. Your face, hands, underarms, groin, and feet probably need a thorough washing. Your arms and legs can often get by without being soaped every time you shower.

Pat yourself dry. Rubbing will only irritate your skin. So go easy.

Moisturize within 1 minute. If applied while your skin is still damp, moisturizing lotion will seal in water that your skin absorbed during the shower. ■

DON'T MAKE THIS MISTAKE

Avoid luxuriating in a long, hot bath, says Dr. Norton. The more water to which you expose your skin, the drier it can get.

Winter Weight Gain

Stay Slim for Spring

The weather update has just announced the 10th consecutive day of below-freezing temperatures. You can't remember the last time you weren't wearing a turtleneck and long johns. And when you look outside, all you see is white. The absolute last thing you feel like doing? Exercising.

"For men and women alike, activity levels drop precipitously in the winter," says Pamela M. Peeke, Ph.D., a metabolism researcher at the National Institutes of Health and author of Fight Fat After Forty. *"It's hard to walk on slippery sidewalks. It's uncomfortable—you have to put on 85 layers to go outside. Maybe Norwegians are accustomed to that, but not Manhattanites." So you stay inside—and too close to temptation. "If you're home, you're going to be around the kitchen more. Ask anyone who has started working at home. You nosh more," she explains. Add the usual holiday indulgences, and you can expect to gain anywhere from 5 to 10 pounds in the winter.*

Here's what she and others suggest to halt your hibernating and keep that winter weight off.

Lift weights. "Winter is a golden opportunity to work out with weights because you're stuck indoors," Dr. Peeke says. By lifting weights two or three times weekly, you'll increase your lean body mass and enjoy a host of benefits. "You'll feel warmer and stronger, you'll cruise through your aerobic exercise, it'll boost your metabolism, and by spring, your clothes will fit better," she adds. See page 467 for a weight-training routine that any woman can do.

Rent exercise videos. "If it's miserable outside, do a video instead," says Marilyn Bach, Ph.D., a fitness consultant in St. Paul, Minnesota, ›› where snowstorms can strike as late as April, and author of *ShapeWalking*. Check your local video store for tapes of low-impact aerobics, yoga, cardio kickboxing or another exercise routine you've been wanting to try.

Pay yourself to stay active. Every time you do something active, put a dollar in a piggy bank. Buy yourself a new workout outfit or exercise video with your earnings.

Slurp some soup. When you feel chilly, you may feel tempted to munch. "When you eat, you get warmer because your body has to convert that food into fuel," Dr. Peeke explains. But it only takes an extra 500 calories a day to pack on a pound a week. Instead, have some soup. It's the perfect answer to the wintertime warmth dilemma, says Dr. Peeke. "It's warm, it fills you up, and it feels good. Just don't eat half a loaf of bread with it."

Reorganize. Take advantage of a snowy day by conquering the clutter in your attic, closets, or basement. "All of that hoisting, pulling, and pushing adds up in terms of calorie burning and shouldn't be negated," Dr. Peeke adds.

Meet friends at the mall. If you enjoy walking but fear icy sidewalks, try your local indoor shopping mall. Joining a mall-walking club can give you the social incentive and group accountability you may need to keep up your wintertime exercising.

Buy a treadmill. "You can achieve your aerobic goals in the warmth of your home without having to go outside," says Dr. Peeke.

Helpful Hint

Even if you don't have seasonal affective disorder (a condition where you feel depressed and lethargic because of winter's shorter days and less natural light), you can increase your energy level and lift your mood by exercising in a brightly lit room or gym. ■

Women's Health Centers

Comparison Shopping Pays Off

Today, you can find ads in newspapers and local magazines across the country for women's health centers. How does a women's health center differ from a traditional doctor's office? Is it something you should consider?

"Health care institutions are courting women because women use health care more than men and are the main health care shoppers for their families," explains Nancy Milliken, M.D., codirector of the Women's Health Center at the University of California in San Francisco.

"The beauty of these centers is that they look at women's health throughout her life span," says Donna Shelley, M.D., medical director of Women's Health Management Solutions at Mt. Sinai Medical Center. Some centers offer ultrasounds (for pregnant women), mammograms (for breast cancer diagnosis and screening) and bone density testing (for osteoporosis) all on the same site. "There's a continuity of care that is missing in health care in general," says Dr. Shelley. "And things don't fall through the cracks. There's better collaboration and communication between your doctors."

Not all women's health centers are alike. To find one that meets your needs, shop around. Here's what to look for.

Comprehensive care. Many centers focus narrowly on breast care or reproductive health. Look for a center with a staff of psychiatrists or clinical psychologists, nurses, internists, gynecologists, and a social worker, says Carol Weisman, M.D., professor of health management and policy at the University of Michigan and author *Women's Health Care*. If you have a chronic condition or other special need, make sure there's a specialist on staff or affiliated with the center who can take care of you.

Physicians committed to caring for women. This is a little trickier to determine. "There is no card-carrying credential in women's health," says Dr. Milliken. Ask if the doctors at the center have extra training in areas like women's mental health or if they have taken electives on diseases like osteoporosis that are common to women.

Patient education programs. To take the best care of yourself, you need information. So look for a center that provides written materials or offers seminars on health topics.

An attitude that patients are partners. "You should find a sensitivity about your need to be talked to and ›› listened to," says Dr. Shelley. This is more important than ever, since doctors are often pressed for time.

A link to a good hospital. Look for a center that's affiliated with a well-regarded hospital, since that is where you would be admitted if you required hospital care. Teaching hospitals offer some advantages. "Anything that is cutting edge is going on at a university," says Cynthia Silber, M.D., a gynecologist with the Jefferson Center for Women's Medical Specialties in Philadelphia.

Other services important to you. Some centers offer alternative medicine, and some even provide child care while you have your appointment.

Helpful Hint

As you shop, trust your instincts. You'll know when it feels right. As Dr. Milliken says, "Women are very savvy consumers. They know whether they're getting window dressing or the real thing." ■

Worry

Fret-Free, Finally

"How can I ever face her again after what I said?"

"What if I bomb in my presentation tomorrow?"

"Did I remember to pack everything?"

"Will my dinner guests like each other? What if I burn the roast or run out of wine?"

Psychologists call those kinds of guilt-laden thoughts "endless mental replays," and anxious what-if's "perseveration." But regardless of what you call it, obsessive thinking can drive you crazy.

"Most often, the average woman calls it worry—a continuous thought that keeps interrupting your mode of thought and that you find it hard to get away from," says Tina Tessina, Ph.D., a psychologist in Long Beach, California, and author of The 10 Smartest Decisions a Woman Can Make before 40. *"If it's continuous and not focused on any one thing, we tend to call it anxiety."*

Doing something functional and practical is better than worrying, which is not only useless but also harmful. "Worry drains and wastes your energy and makes you less likely to make good decisions," says Dr. Tessina. "If you take that same energy you're using running around in mental circles, and you do something productive with it, it'll serve you better." Here's Dr. Tessina's advice for when, how, and why women typically worry.

Late-night worry: "Get out of the habit of using your brain as a memo pad," says Dr. Tessina. "The best sleep aid I know is a pencil and paper by your bed to write down whatever is bugging you." If you're worried about forgetting something, write it down. If you're anxious about something you have to do, organize it with a written plan or checklist.

"What if" worry: Fretting about what might happen? Figure out what you would do in case the hypothetical disaster occurs, suggests Dr. Tessina.

Endless replay worry: If you regret something you said or something that happened, then figure out how you could

A 10-SECOND CURE FOR WORRY

Dr. Tessina offers this three-step remedy for overcoming an obsessive thought.

1. Write it down.
2. Ask yourself, "Is there anything I can do about this right now?"
3. If your answer is yes, do it. If your answer is no—that is, if you're worried about something that's beyond your control—distract yourself by shifting your focus to something else.

handle that situation better next time. "Practice it over and over until you feel confident that you know what you're doing," says Tessina.

Obsessive thinking is common, more so in women than men. But if it's interfering with your ability to function, get help, advises Dr. Tessina. If obsessive thinking keeps you from leaving the house or working productively, or if you're not sleeping well (or sleeping all the time), or it's disrupting your relationships, then consult a licensed therapist. **"As emotional problems go, obsessive thinking is simple to fix,"** she says. ■

Wrinkles

The Real Deal on Anti-Aging Creams

Alpha hydroxy acids. Beta hydroxy acids. Vitamin C. Collagen. Wrinkle creams feature a cornucopia of ingredients that promise to smooth your skin and erase years from your face.

"It's such a competitive market," says Grace Pak, M.D., a cosmetic dermatologist in New York City. "Someone comes up with something new every day."

Over time, age and exposure to sunlight break down collagen (the protein that gives your skin structure) and elastin (the protein that keeps your skin pliable). So does smoking. When collagen and elastin break down, a wrinkle forms. At the same time, surface cell turnover slows, giving your skin a dull appearance. Wrinkle creams attempt to repair either kind of damage in various ways.

Here, in order of potential effectiveness, is a primer on popular wrinkle cream ingredients.

Tretinoin. The active ingredient in Renova and Retin-A (prescription-only creams) tretinoin is proven to rejuvenate the skin structure with continued use. Tretinoin helps your skin produce new collagen, form new blood vessels, and shed layers of dead skin. It can be irritating, though, causing peeling, flaking, sun sensitivity, and redness.

Retinol. Retinol is a retinoid (a vitamin-A derivative) used as an ingredient in some over-the-counter wrinkle creams. "We don't know yet if the effects are comparable, but it's worth a try for a woman whose skin can't tolerate tretinoin," Dr. Pak says.

Alpha hydroxy acids (AHAs). "Basically exfoliating agents, alpha hydroxy acids help to 'unglue' the layer of dead skin cells that tends to accumulate and give skin a lackluster appearance," Dr. Pak explains. With continued use, they, like tretinoin, also stimulate the development of ›› new collagen, which is what makes your skin look and feel "plumper."

Glycolic acid is the most common AHA.

Beta hydroxy acids (BHAs). Also known as salicylic acid, BHAs have been used in acne treatment for years. They also help wrinkling by sloughing off the layers of dead skin, which in turn stimulates healthy cell turnover. However, they may not have the same tightening effect as AHAs, Dr. Pak says.

Vitamin C. Vitamin C is an antioxidant, theoretically protecting your skin against sun damage done by ultraviolet rays and unstable molecules known as free radicals they introduce. Problem is, vitamin C breaks down when exposed to light, making it tough to package vitamin C in a bottle and effectively deliver it topically to your skin. It's best used in conjunction with retinoids, AHAs, or BHAs, and sun protection, which have proven anti-aging results, says Dr. Pak.

Vitamin E. As an antioxidant, vitamin E should have the same effect on skin as vitamin C, but there's no proof that vitamin E does anything more for your wrinkles than serve as a moisturizer, says Dr. Pak. If your skin is dry and crinkly, any lotion will temporarily reduce the appearance of your fine lines and wrinkles.

Coenzyme Q_{10}. This coenzyme also acts as an antioxidant, neutralizing free radicals that lead to skin damage. While no published studies exist on the effectiveness of wrinkle creams supplemented with coenzyme Q_{10}, "there's good reason to believe that coenzyme Q_{10} might be helpful," says Valerian Kagan, Ph.D., a biochemist at the University of Pittsburgh.

Furfuryladenine. Use of this plant-growth hormone results in skin that looks and feels better with some improvement in fine lines, but without irritation says Kathy Fields, M.D., clinical instructor of dermatology at the University of California in San Francisco. However, there has been no independent research verifying how it compares with tretinoin.

Melibiose. This sugar molecule can temporarily help skin appear firmer, but no one knows if melibiose can make a long-term difference, Dr. Pak says.

Collagen and elastin. Derived from animal sources or produced synthetically, collagen and elastin molecules are too big to penetrate the skin. They only work if injected—an office procedure.

Helpful Hints

If you use these anti-aging creams, wear an SPF 15 sunscreen daily and 30 SPF for extended sun exposure. Retinoids, AHAs, and BHAs all make your skin more sensitive to sun. And, if you smoke, quit. "None of this is worth doing if you continue exposing yourself to the things that generated the skin-damaging free radicals in the first place," Dr. Pak says. ■

X-Y-Z

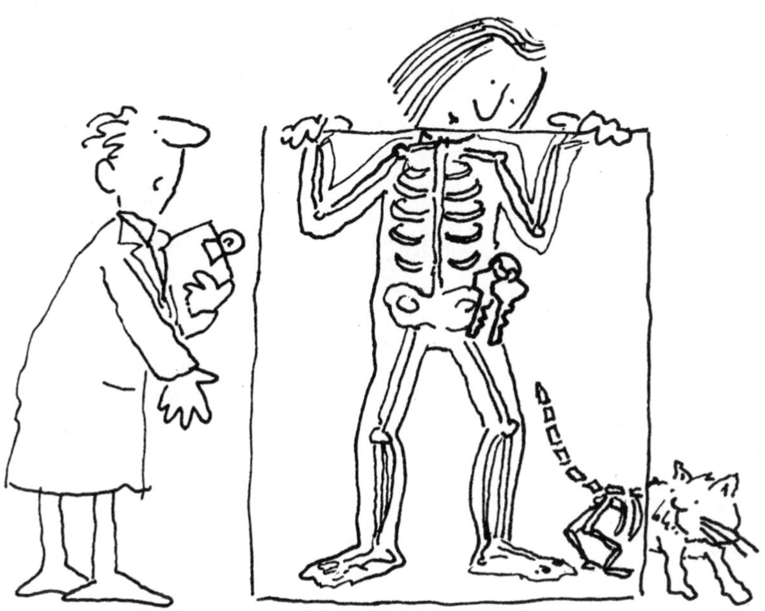

An x-ray can help you find your car keys.
But is it safe?
The answer is on page 482.

Xanax

Do You Really Need It?

Car payments. Sick pets. Deadlines at work. Parent-teacher meetings. Forgotten birthdays. These are just a few of the endless ingredients that can add up to anxiety.

A little anxiety can be a good thing, though, when it motivates you to meet your deadlines, pay your bills on time, and remember those birthday cards.

But when too much anxiety weighs you down and interferes with your ability to live your life—or when you experience panic attacks, which are sudden bouts of unreasonable fear—many women seek help. When they do, their doctors may prescribe alprazolam (Xanax), a mild sedative used for anxiety, insomnia, and panic disorders. Or women ask for it outright.

"Xanax isn't a drug to be taken lightly," says Scott Woods, M.D., associate professor in the department of psychiatry at Yale University School of Medicine and director of its treatment research program. It's a hypnotic, which means that it can cause drowsiness and impaired coordination. And, like other drugs in this category—collectively known as benzodiazepines—your body could develop a dependence on it, leading to difficulty when you want to stop taking it.

Here's how you can help ensure that you're using the medication properly.

Make sure you really need it. Be sure your doctor prescribes the drug for a specific condition, such as anxiety or panic disorder, not just an occasional case of nerves, says John Marshall, M.D., professor of psychiatry at the University of Wisconsin Medical School in Madison and director of its anxiety disorders clinic.

Otherwise, another drug may be safer and more effective. "With the advent of newer antidepressants like Prozac, Zoloft, and Paxil, drugs like Xanax, which can be addictive, are being used less and less," says Leah Dickstein, M.D., director of attitudinal and behavioral medicine at the University of Louisville School of Medicine in Kentucky.

Follow dosage instructions to the letter. Your doctor should also tell you how often to take it, instead of a vague recommendation of "when you feel a little nervous," says Dr. Marshall.

Be regular. This is a short-acting drug, so you need to take it at regular intervals to keep a steady level in your body. Don't concentrate your doses at bedtime to help you sleep, or you may become anxious the next day as the effects of the drug fade.

If you're still anxious, speak up. Most women find that they need less and less Xanax as time goes on, says Dr. Marshall. If you feel like you need more of the medication, discuss it with your physician, Dr. Woods says. ››

DON'T MAKE THIS MISTAKE

Never take more Xanax than you're prescribed, and don't borrow pills from someone else.

Back away from it slowly. If you stop taking any benzodiazepine, including Xanax, abruptly, your body may protest. You may start feeling your original symptoms again, including shakiness and nervousness and, rarely, seizures. So don't stop taking the drug on your own, even if you feel better. Discuss with your doctor the best way to gradually taper off the amount you use.

Helpful Hint

Be sure to tell your doctor if you've had problems with any other drugs or alcohol. Anyone who has had earlier substance-abuse problems is more likely to misuse Xanax. ■

X-Rays

Don't Let Fear Cloud Proper Diagnosis

Sooner or later, every woman encounters some kind of diagnostic x-ray: An annual mammogram. Baseline dental x-rays. A broken ankle.

Are you at risk for overexposure?

Not likely, say experts.

"Despite horror stories of radiation causing cancer and mutations, the adverse effects are all associated with high doses of radiation, not the low doses used in diagnostic radiology, explains Wayne Hedrick, Ph.D., a medical physicist specializing in radiation safety at Aultman Hospital in Canton, Ohio.

There's a huge difference between the amount of radiation you get with diagnostic x-rays and therapeutic x-rays. Diagnostic x-rays show an image that helps the doctor diagnose a disease or a bone problem. The radiation dose is very low. Diagnostic x-rays have no observable effect on people x-rayed, says Dr. Hedrick.

Therapeutic x-rays, on the other hand, are radiation treatments to combat a disease. The amount of radiation may be thousands of times greater than diagnostic x-rays. The aim may be to kill cancer cells in a solid tumor, for example.

Scientists look at what happens with high radiation levels and extrapolate what might happen in lower doses. To be safe, they recommend limiting your exposure.

"We're assuming they *may* be at some risk, extrapolating from populations that have received high doses," says Dr. Hedrick. "For example, let's say we give several people 100 aspirin each, and we see adverse effects. So we say that maybe aspirin can cause problems. But people don't have problems taking two aspirin."

Keep in mind that diagnostic imagery gives your doctor information that she needs to figure out what's wrong with you and treat it properly.

"Our imaging technology

has improved greatly over the past 20 years," says Dr. Hedrick. "It saves lives." Case in point: A mammogram uses low-dose radiation and is carefully regulated and strictly monitored. Compared with groups of women not screened with mammography, there are far fewer deaths from breast cancer in groups of women who have periodic mammograms.

So if an x-ray is called for, don't fight it. But don't try to convince your health care provider that you must have an x-ray if you don't really need it.

There's no way of keeping track of your lifetime exposure to x-rays and setting any kind of limit. Dr. Hedrick suggests asking your health professional these questions when diagnostic x-rays are advised.

- What are we trying to find out or rule out?
- What other exams can possibly provide this information?
- Is this the best exam to determine the suspected diagnosis?

By all means, let the technologist know if you're pregnant or might be pregnant before being exposed to x-rays. (They'll ask.) That way, they can take steps to protect the fetus, such as shielding with a lead apron, limiting the number of films, and restricting the x-ray beam.

Ultrasound, used to monitor the fetus, is considered safe. It's not even radiation, but sound waves, and no harmful effects have ever been documented.

FYI: Despite rumors to the contrary, an ultrasound is not a substitute for a mammogram. ■

Yeast Infections

Itching Like Mad? Ditch the Sweets

What do a candy bar, a jelly doughnut, and a glass of milk have in common? All three can contribute to recurrent yeast infections.

If you get one yeast infection after another, you know the symptoms all too well. A white cottage cheese–like discharge and intense itching and burning. The cause? A decrease in the "good" bacteria that keep the vagina healthy and an increase in the "bad" bacteria, or Candida albicans—*the fungus that causes the infection.*

DON'T MAKE THIS MISTAKE

Vaginal antifungal creams and suppositories containing miconazole break down latex condoms. If you use an antifungal remedy with a condom, the condom may burst.

Trying to avoid sweets might keep you from getting so many.

Candy bars are loaded ››

with sugar, which yeast thrive on. Milk contains the sugar lactose. "So if your vagina is already low on the good bacteria, and you eat a lot of sweets, it will become more acidic, which is the perfect environment for the yeast to grow and flourish," says Pamela Sky-Jeanne, N.D., a naturopathic physician at Choose to Be Healthy, a clinic in Gresham, Oregon.

What's more, too much sugar may weaken your immune system, so your body can't fight off a yeast invasion, says Jennifer Brett, N.D., a naturopathic physician and chair of botanical medicine at the University of Bridgeport College of Naturopathic Medicine in Connecticut.

Other sugary fare that may contribute to yeast infections include dried fruit, pastries, cake, and glazed doughnuts filled with custards or jellies.

If you're prone to yeast infections, you should consult your doctor for treatment. But some naturopathic physicians also recommend that you avoid or at least eat less sugary fare. Other foods that may also contribute to the problem include:

Milk, cheese, and other dairy foods. Dairy products tend to make mucus thicker, which keeps your body from getting rid of yeast naturally. The high-fat content of milk and cheese lowers immunity. And some naturopaths believe that eating cheese that was fermented during processing can contribute to a yeast population explosion.

Peanuts, melons, and mushrooms. These foods contain molds and yeast, which can set off an infection, says Dr. Brett.

Alcoholic beverages. Alcohol offers a double whammy. It automatically turns to sugar in your body, and it raises estrogen levels, which creates a breeding ground for yeast, says Dr. Brett.

Helpful Hint

Yogurt is an exception to the no-dairy rule. But it has to be the right kind. Eating one cup a day of plain, unsweetened yogurt that contains live cultures of *acidophilus* will keep yeast away. These live cultures will help restore your vagina's natural pH level (acid-base balance) and healthy bacteria. Look for wording stating that it contains live *acidophilus* cultures.

For external itching, apply a yogurt compress. Place ½ cup plain yogurt on a clean cloth or towel and place it on the outside of your vagina for 15 minutes. Rinse off the yogurt with warm water, then use a blow-dryer on the warm setting to make sure that you're totally dry. Don't hold it too close. ■

BUY YOUR GUY SOME POLYURETHANE CONDOMS

Allergies to latex condoms may be associated with increased susceptibility to yeast infections, says Margaret Polaneczky, M.D., assistant professor of obstetrics and gynecology and medical director of women's health at New York Hospital/Cornell Medical Center in New York City. So, if you use condoms for protection and get frequent yeast infections, consider switching to a nonlatex brand.

Yogurt

Seven Amazing Benefits from One On-the-Run Food

If you're like a lot of women, you've probably been eating yogurt for so long that you forgot why you started. Sure, yogurt is loaded with bone-strengthening calcium—a typical 8-ounce cup contains about one-third of your daily requirement. And you've read that the friendly bacteria found in yogurt—Lactobacillus bulgaricus, Streptococcus thermophilus, Lactobacillus bifidus, and Lactobacillus acidophilus—are good for your digestion. But yogurt helps women stay healthy in seven amazing ways.

1. It lowers cholesterol. If you're battling to get your cholesterol out of the danger zone, start by looking in the dairy case. No one knows why, but studies show that "1 to 2 cups of yogurt a day tend to reduce the total amount of cholesterol in the blood—increasing HDLs while lowering LDLs," says Khem M. Shahani, Ph.D., professor of food science and technology at the University of Nebraska in Lincoln. And improved cholesterol levels over time reduce your risk of heart disease.

2. It boosts your Bs. Another way yogurt may help prevent heart disease: By increasing levels of folate and vitamin B_{12}. "When yogurt cultures grow, they produce lots of vitamins, especially folic acid and vitamin B_{12}," says Dr. Shahani. How much? It varies from person to person, but every bit counts. After all, few women consume enough of these vital vitamins that lower the risk for heart disease and ensure proper brain development in fetuses.

3. It strengthens your immune system. Yogurt works behind the scenes to prevent cancer, says Dr. Shahani. It feeds your white blood cells to keep them working at their best.

4. It unleashes extra calcium. Although 8-ounce servings of yogurt and milk contain about the same amount of calcium, your body retains more of this bone-strengthening mineral when you eat yogurt. That's because calcium (and iron) are tangled up in other milk components—sort of like fish in a net. Yogurt cultures apparently release them, making them easier for your body to absorb. And, over time, that may mean a reduced risk for not only osteoporosis but also atherosclerosis, heart disease, and arthritis, says Dr. Shahani. ››

TRAVELING? STEER CLEAR OF YOGURT SHAKES

To reduce your odds of coming down with traveler's diarrhea on your next vacation, steer clear of blended yogurt and fruit drinks. A study conducted in Nepal looked at factors that may affect travelers to developing countries. Researchers found that yogurt smoothies were a major contributor to traveler's diarrhea and recommended that international travelers avoid these to help prevent diarrhea. Eating fresh fruit and plain yogurt separately didn't pose a problem.

5. It battles bad bacteria. Your upper intestine is home to 100 to 500 trillion bacteria—both good and bad. Antibiotics kill many of the good guys along with the bad. To replenish the good guys and keep the bad guys in check, include a cup of yogurt in your daily diet while on antibiotics.

6. It's colon-friendly. Eager to add some calcium to your diet, but all too aware that milk makes your intestines do the macarena? Switch to yogurt with live *acidophilus* cultures. It's kinder to your colon—especially if you're lactose intolerant—for two reasons: While the yogurt sits in your cup, its "good" bacteria are busy producing lactase—taming the intestine-twisting effects of the milk sugar lactose before you eat it. Plus, yogurt cultures continue to produce this lactose-neutralizer long after they've gone down the hatch—helping you metabolize more of that evil lactose in your gut.

7. It soothes your belly. Spent the last day or so sprinting to the bathroom with diarrhea? Once again, the "good" bacteria in yogurt ride to the rescue—curing and even preventing diarrhea. Many experts believe it helps by producing natural antibiotics that inhibit the growth of bad bacteria that cause stomach distress. A cup a day should get the job done.

Herbed Yogurt Cheese Dip

2 cups fat-free plain yogurt
2 ounces reduced-fat cream cheese
1½ tablespoons finely chopped fresh chives
1 tablespoon finely chopped fresh basil
¼ teaspoon coarsely ground black pepper

Line a sieve with 2 layers of cheesecloth and set over a large bowl. Spoon the yogurt into the sieve. Cover and refrigerate for at least 12 hours, or until the yogurt is the consistency of cream cheese. You should have about 1 cup of yogurt cheese and 1 cup of drained liquid. Discard the liquid.

Place the yogurt cheese, cream cheese, chives, basil, and pepper in a food processor. Process until well-blended. Spoon into a small bowl. Cover and refrigerate for at least 1 hour to allow the flavors to blend.

Makes 1 cup

Note: Use yogurt that does not contain gums as thickeners; they will prevent it from draining.

Helpful Hints

Look for "live active cultures" on the label, and check the expiration date on yogurt you buy. The fresher the yogurt, the more active the cultures.

For building bone or boosting immunity, flavored yogurt is as good as plain, unsweetened yogurt, as long as it contains live and active cultures. If you're watching your dress size, be aware that flavored, sweetened yogurt has nearly twice the calories of plain yogurt. Best bet: Blend ½ cup of fresh or frozen fruit, like blueberries, with a cup of plain yogurt.

Using yogurt in recipes is fine, but be aware that heating yogurt destroys many of its therapeutic qualities and doesn't provide the same benefits as eating it chilled. ■

Yo-Yo Dieting

Stop Rebound Weight Gain—Forever

For years, you've been losing—and regaining—the same 20 to 30 pounds. It's always the same story: You go on a diet, you shed a few pounds, and then the scale creeps back up. No matter what you eat or do, you just can't keep the weight off. You try diet after diet—commercial programs, diet pills, special food plans—in search of one that will work for you.

For you, even the sensible approach—eating less and exercising more—seems to fail. Eventually, you gain everything back—and then some.

"If you want to gain weight, go on a calorie-restricted diet," says Gloria Kensinger, R.D., a registered dietitian in Wheaton, Illinois, who has worked extensively with women struggling with weight control. For many, and perhaps you, keeping the pounds off requires more than simply eating less and exercising more; it involves dealing with the other issues—psychological, emotional, stress-related—behind the overeating.

"For women who weight-cycle, food represents more than an energy source," says Sue Popkess-Vawter, R.N., Ph.D., professor of nursing at the University of Kansas School of Nursing in Kansas City. It's a stress reliever, a tie to happier times, and it represents love, acceptance, and celebration when we feel good. Food is a comfort and a good friend when we feel bad, she adds. "If you have a bad day at work, you turn to food. But comfort food is like alcohol; it temporarily makes you feel better, but it leaves you with a hangover. You need to learn to handle the ups and downs of life without turning to food."

Without those coping skills, diets just put you on an emotional and physical roller coaster. So before you go on another diet, follow these suggestions from experts who have helped women just like you overcome emotional eating.

Make time for you. Anne M. Fletcher, R.D., author of *Thin for Life*, tells a story that illustrates how important it can be for women to make sure their needs are met. It's about a missionary's daughter who had learned to take care of everybody but herself. "It left a hole inside of me, and I filled it up with food," she told Fletcher. Once she learned that it was okay to take time for herself, she lost more than 40 pounds—permanently.

Reconnect with your hunger signals. Kensinger says that many of the women she counsels no longer remember what it feels like to be hungry, because they're eating so frequently. If you don't know when you should eat, you may eat more than you need, even after you're full.

Identify problem situations. When do you overeat? At family dinners? When you're home alone? After a stressful day at work? If you you're craving food when you're not physically hungry, ask yourself what's going on before heading to the fridge. Perhaps you're angry or lonely. Instead of using ›› food to numb those feelings, allow yourself to experience your emotions. Write down your feelings in a personal journal. Learn to fight fair instead of "stuffing" your anger and hurt. Learning to separate eating from feelings is the first important step in stopping the yo-yo diet cycle.

Replace food-oriented socializing with more active events. It's easy to overindulge when you're having dinner with friends, especially for weight-cyclers. Ask your friends to go for a walk with you instead.

Discover new ways to deal with stress. Instead of reaching for food, call a friend. Techniques such as yoga, meditation, or progressive muscle relaxation also might be helpful.

Helpful Hint

If you overeat in response to anger, depression, anxiety, or stress and need help learning new ways to manage emotion-driven eating, consider counseling. Talking with a therapist or a registered dietitian may help make the kind of lasting, fundamental changes that guarantee permanent weight control. ■

Zinc

The Last Word in Preventing Colds

Scientists continue to search for a cure for the common cold. But until they find it, the closest thing to a cure may be zinc. In fact, some experts believe that this essential mineral may fight the sniffles, scratchy throat, and other symptoms better than the much-heralded cold-fighter vitamin C.

"Zinc helps your body in so many ways," says Judith Turnlund, R.D., Ph.D., a research nutrition scientist for the USDA Human Nutrition Center. Zinc works with more than 300 enzymes in the body to help in normal growth, sharpen night vision, and hasten wound healing.

Meanwhile, science is learning more every day about zinc's cold-fighting prowess. In a Cleveland Clinic study, men and women with colds who sucked on zinc gluconate lozenges every 2 hours cleared up their symptoms 4 days sooner than the group who didn't use the lozenges. To keep a cold at bay, you may need to take a zinc lozenge every 2 to 4 hours, starting as soon as you feel the symptoms of a cold coming on and continuing until the symptoms subside. Let it dissolve completely in your mouth for maximum benefit.

The Daily Value for zinc in adults is 15 milligrams per day. While you can get your daily zinc needs with supplements, it's best to get zinc directly from food, which contains a balance of other nutrients. Red meat is a solid source of this vital nutrient. Four ounces of lean, broiled ground beef provides 7.1 milligrams; a 4-ounce broiled sirloin contains 7 milligrams of zinc. For those who shun red meat, Dr. Turnlund suggests including these zinc-rich foods in your daily diet:

- 4 ounces of Steamed oysters (205.8 mg.)
- ½ cup of Toasted wheat germ (15.5 mg.)
- ⅓ cup of Oil-roasted unsalted peanuts (3 mg.)
- ⅓ cup of Unsalted roasted cashew nuts (2.1 mg.)
- ⅓ cup of Dry-roasted salted almonds (2.3 mg.)
- 3 ounces of Steamed Dungeness crab (4.6 mg.)
- 4 ounces of Roasted dark turkey meat (5 mg.)
- 1 cup of Low-fat yogurt (2 mg.)
- 1 ounces of Pumpkin Seeds (2.1 mg.)
- 3 ounces of Steamed clams (2.3 mg.)
- 3 ounces of Steamed Alaskan King crab (6.5 mg.)

Helpful Hints

It's best to take a zinc supplement with food to avoid stomach upset. ■

DON'T MAKE THIS MISTAKE

As important as zinc is for your body, don't think that more is better. Long-term doses (for more than 2 weeks at a time) of 50 milligrams or more a day of supplemental zinc can lower your immunity and interfere with your body's absorption of two other essential minerals—copper and iron.

Index

Underscored page references indicate boxed text. **Boldface** references indicate illustrations.

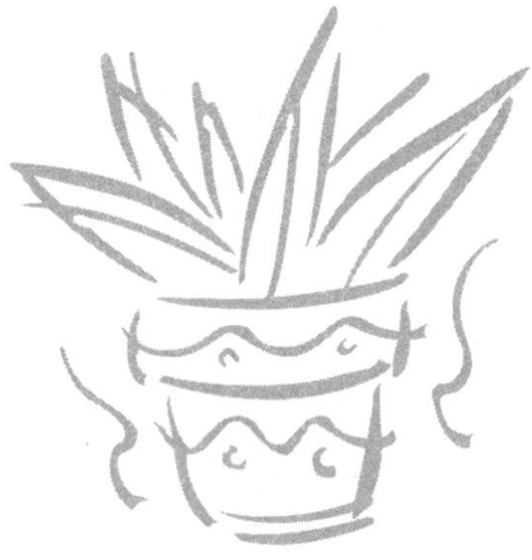

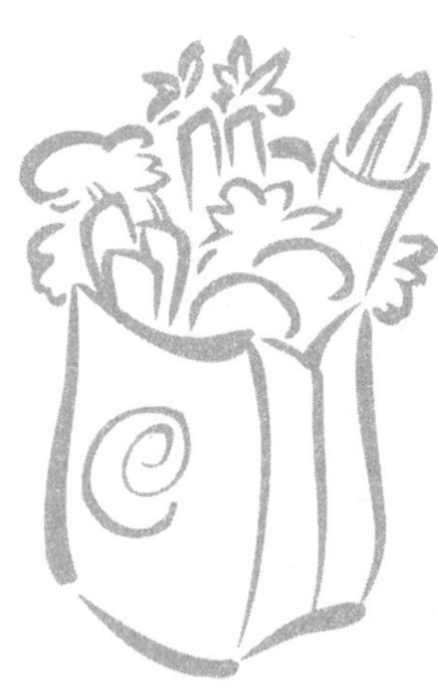

B

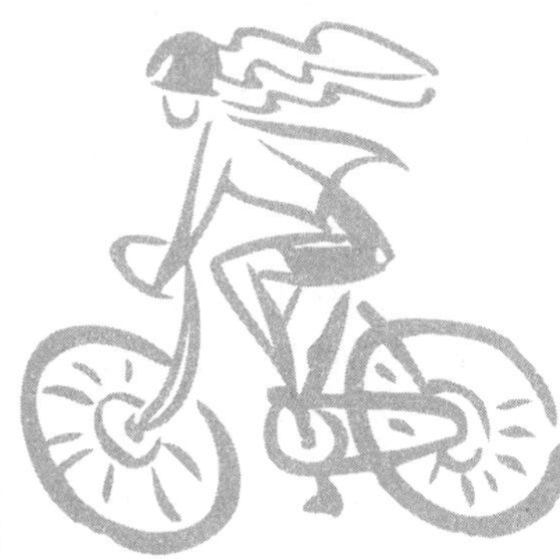

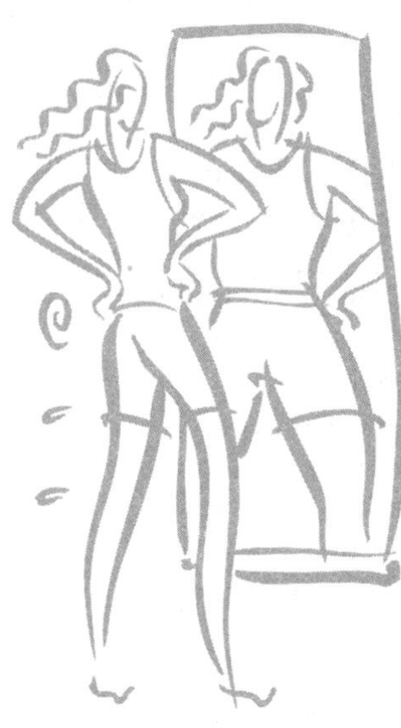

C

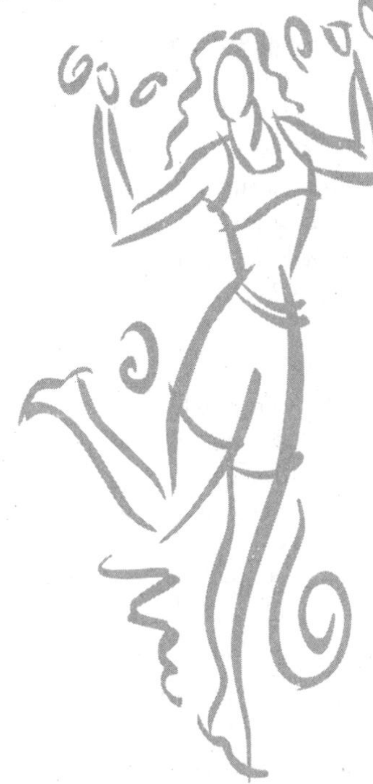

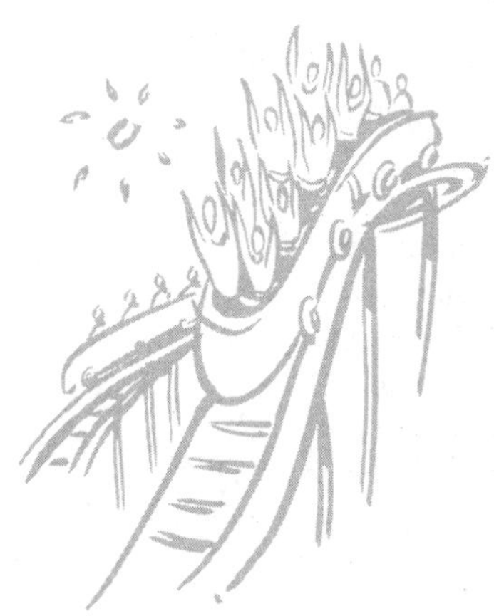

D

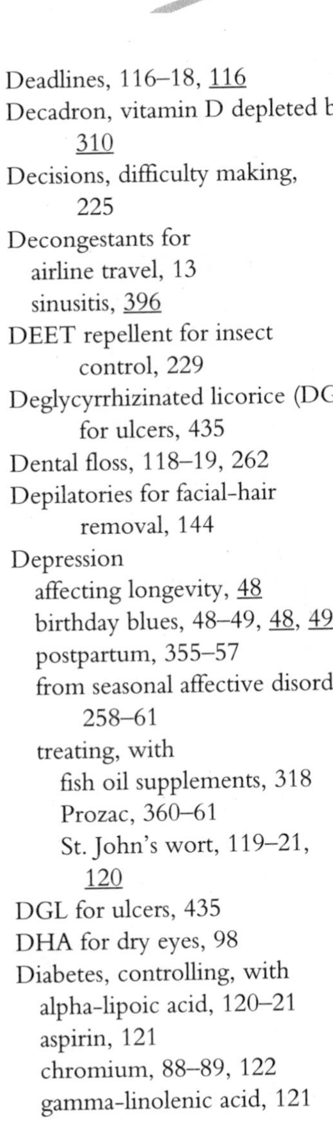

E

F

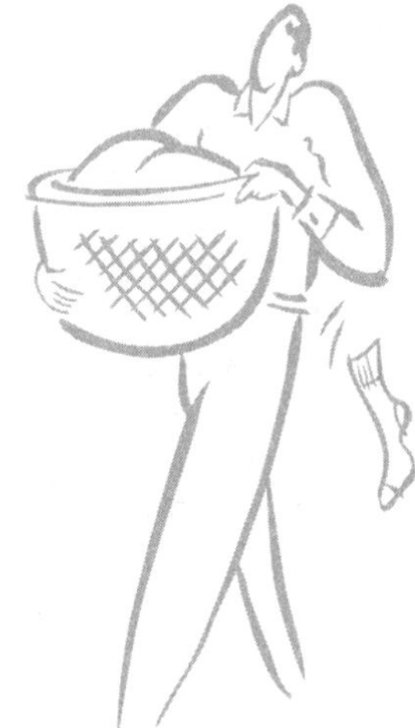

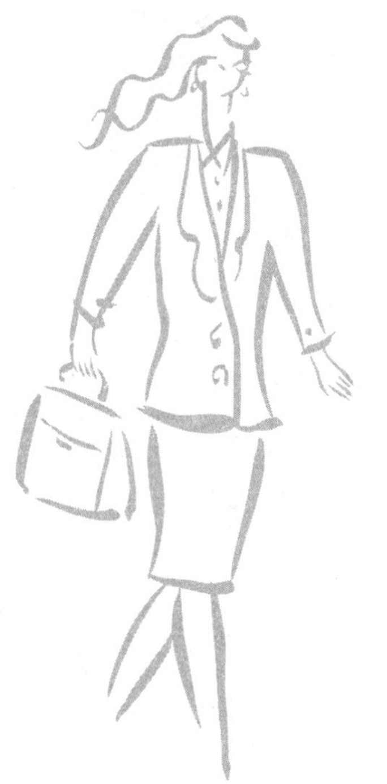

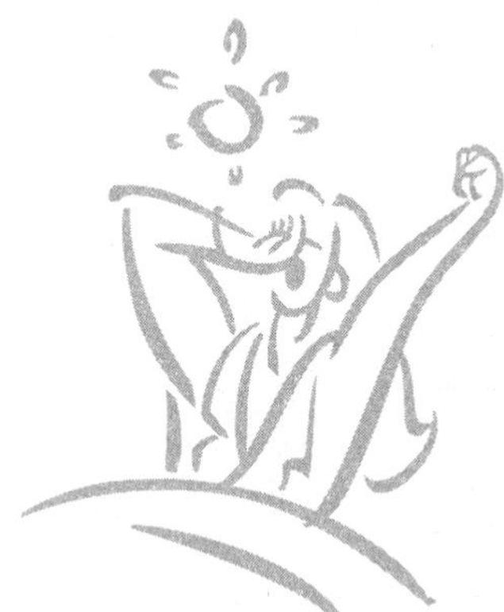

H

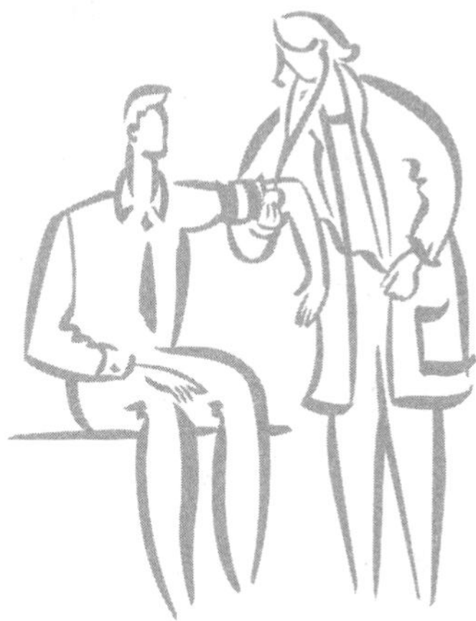

I

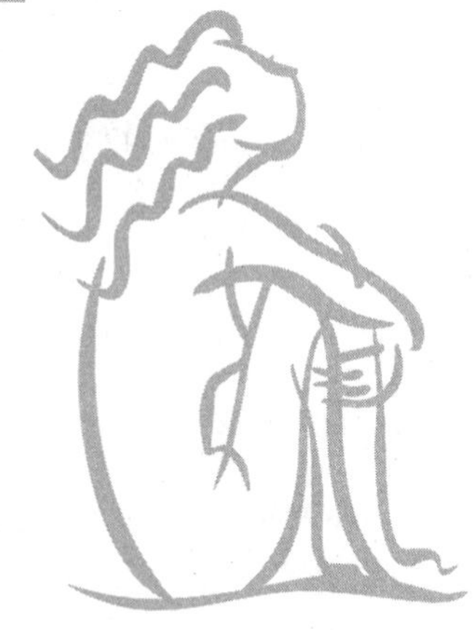

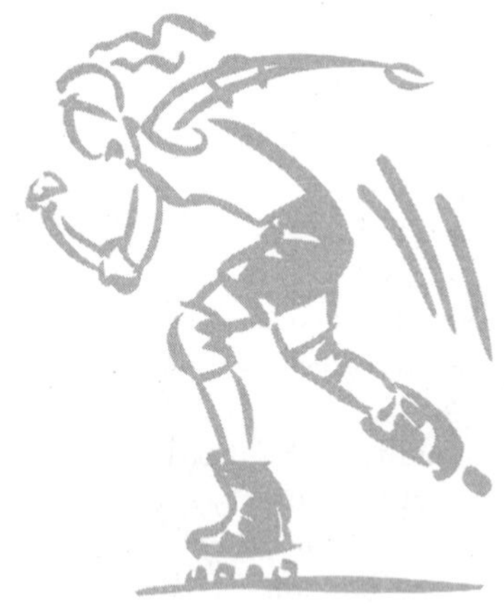

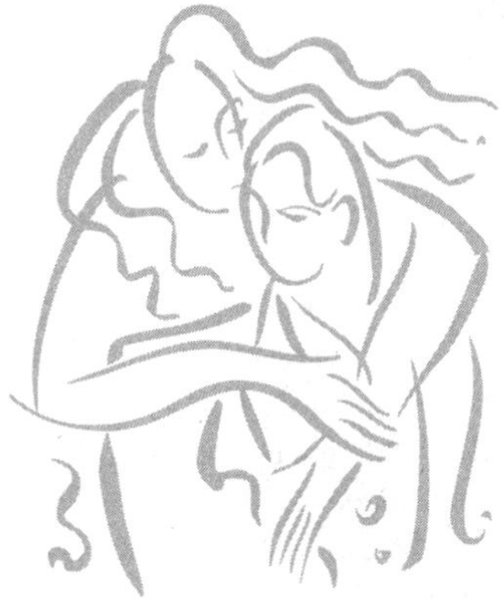

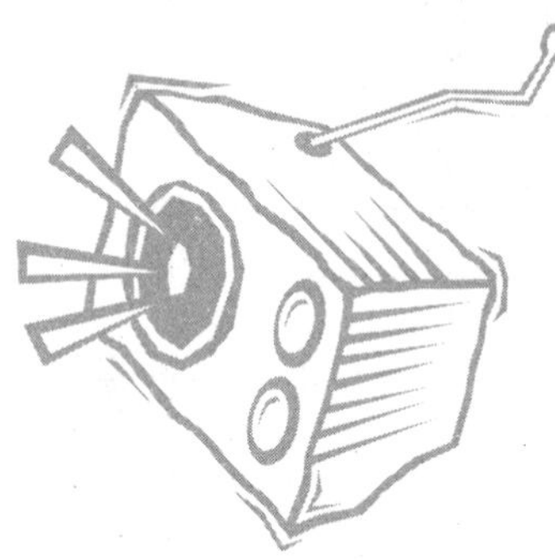

N

O

P

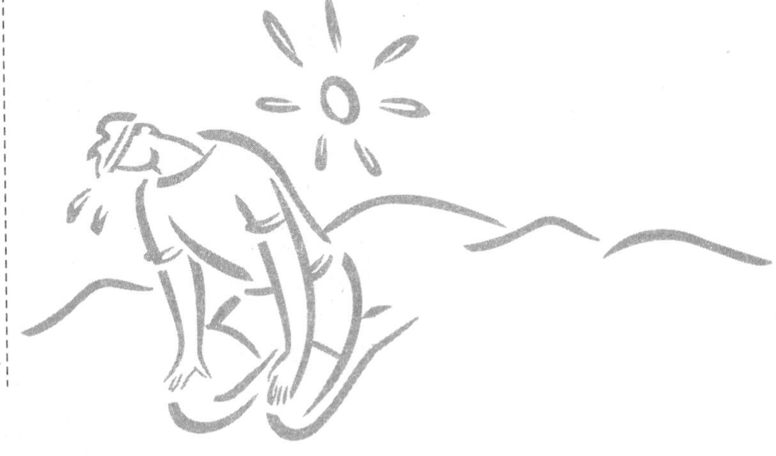

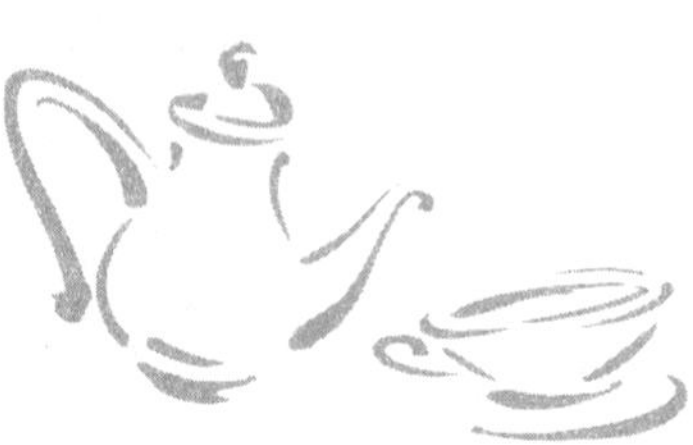

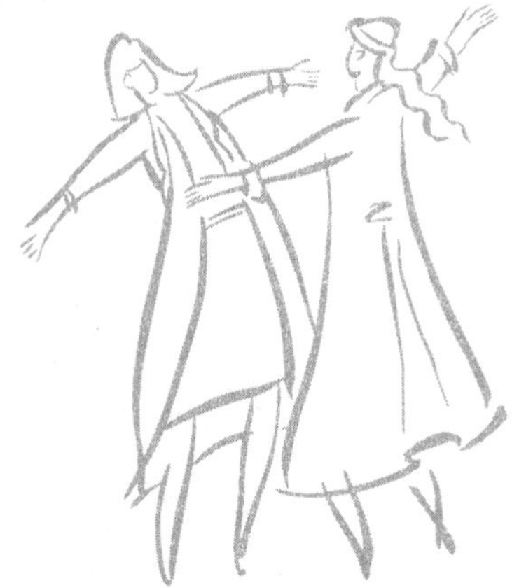

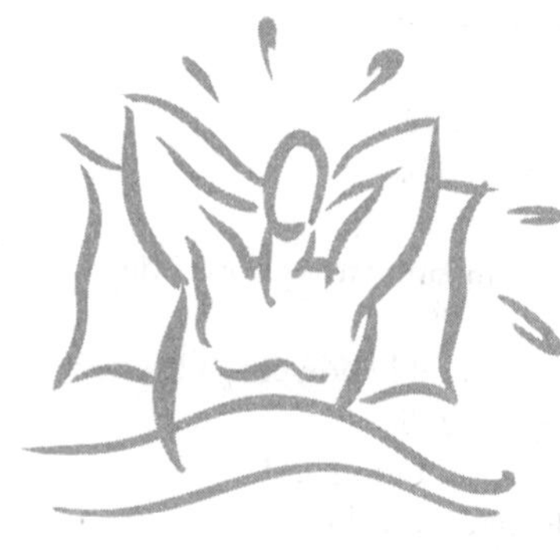

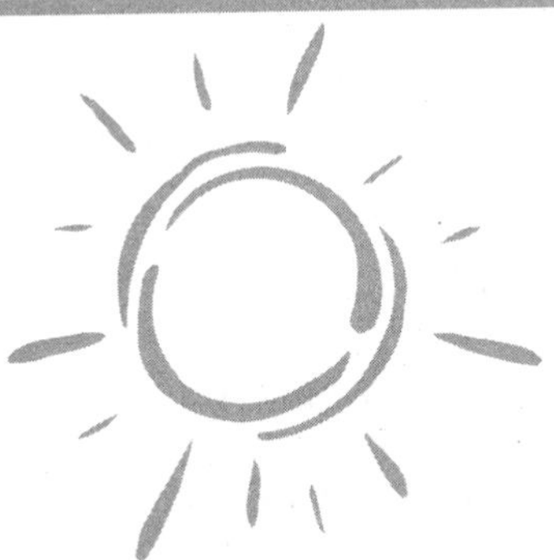

U

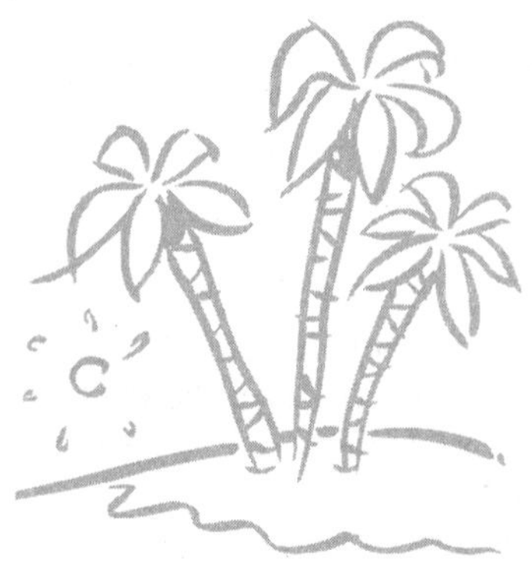

V

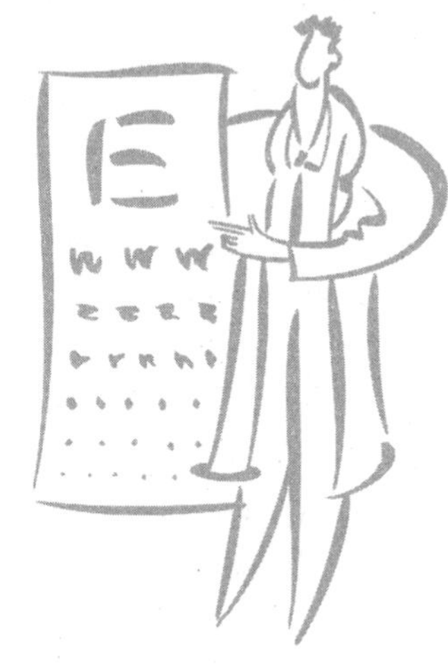

W

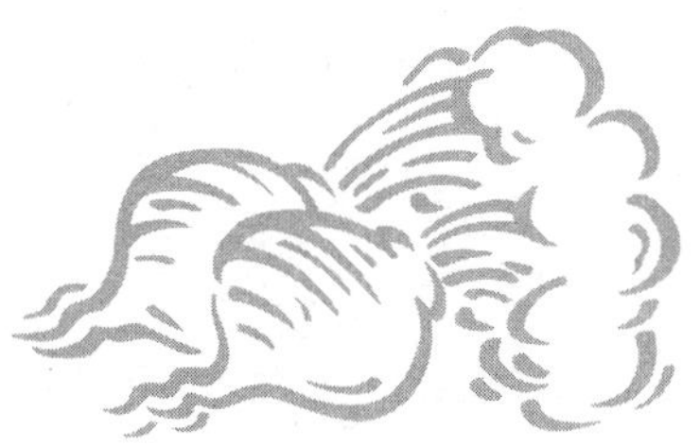